NEUROLOGICAL COMPLICATIONS OF THERAPY:
Selected Topics

Edited By:

Allen Silverstein, M.D.

Associate Clinical Professor of Neurology
Mt. Sinai School of Medicine
New York, N.Y.

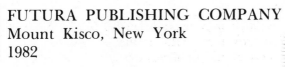

FUTURA PUBLISHING COMPANY
Mount Kisco, New York
1982

Dedication

To Pamela, Suzanne,
Russell, and Robin,
who helped.

© Copyright 1982
Futura Publishing Company, Inc.

Published by:
Futura Publishing Company, Inc.
295 Main Street, P.O. Box 330
Mount Kisco, New York 10549

LC #: 81-71801
ISBN #: 0-87993-171-X

Contributors

Paul S. Berger, M.D.
Assistant Clinical Professor of Radiation Therapy, Albert Einstein College of Medicine; Director of Radiotherapy, Bridgeport Hospital, Bridgeport, Conn.

Roger C. Duvoisin, M.D.
Professor and Chairman, Department of Neurology, University of Medicine and Dentistry, Rutgers Medical School, Piscataway, N.J.

Gordon J. Gilbert, M.D.
Clinical Associate Professor of Neurology, Clinical Professor of Physiology, Department of Medicine, University of South Florida, College of Medicine, Tampa, Florida.

Norman Godin, M.D.
Gastroenterology Fellow, Mt. Sinai School of Medicine, New York, N.Y.

Christopher G. Goetz, M.D.
Assistant Professor, Department of Neurological Sciences, Rush Presbyterian-St. Luke's Medical Center, Chicago, Ill.

Gerald T. Golden, M.D., F.A.C.S.
Assistant Clinical Professor of Surgery, The University of Virginia Medical Center, Charlottesville, Va.; Chief of Surgery, City Hospital, Martinsburg, W. Va., Consultant in Surgery, U.S. Veteran's Administration Hospital, Martinsburg, W.Va.

Sandra J. A. Golden, R.N.
Director of Clinical Research, The Shenandoah Surgical Group, Martinsburg, W. Va.

Peter A. Gross, M.D.
Professor of Medicine, UMDNJ — N.J. Medical School, Newark, NJ.; Director, Department of Medicine, Hackensack Medical Center, Hackensack, N.J.

Sidney A. Hollin, M.D.
Clinical Professor of Neurosurgery, Mt. Sinai School of Medicine, and Attending Neurosurgeon, Mt. Sinai Medical Center

Julius H. Jacobson, II, M.D.
Clinical Professor of Surgery, Mt. Sinai School of Medicine, and Director, Vascular Surgical Service, Mt. Sinai Medical Center

Harold L. Klawans, M.D.
Associate Chairman, Department of Neurological Sciences, Rush Presbyterian-St. Luke's Medical Center, Chicago, Ill.

Amos D. Korczyn, M.D., M.Sc.
Associate Professor and Chairman, Department of Neurology, Tel Aviv Medical Center, and Department of Physiology and Pharmacology, Sackler School of Medicine, Tel Aviv University, Ramat-Aviv, Israel.

Jack H. M. Kwaan, M.D.
Associate Clinical Professor in Surgery, University of California, Irvine, Ca.; Chief, Vascular Surgery Section, Veterans Hospital, Long Beach, Ca.

Mitchell E. Levine, M.D.
Resident in Neurosurgery, Mt. Sinai Medical Center, New York, N.Y.

Julio Messer, M.D.
Gastroenterology Fellow, Mt. Sinai School of Medicine, New York, N.Y.

Anthony B. Minnefor, M.D.
Clinical Associate Professor of Preventive Medicine and Community Health, UMDNJ — N.J. Medical School, Newark, N.J.; Associate Chairman, Department of Pediatrics; Chief, Section of Infectious Diseases, St. Joseph's Hospital and Medical Center, Paterson, N.J.

Michael F. Parry, M.D., F.A.C.P.
Assistant Clinical Professor of Medicine, Columbia University College of Physicians and Surgeons, New York, N.Y.; Director of Infectious Diseases and Microbiology, Stamford Hospital, Stamford, Conn.

David H. Rosenbaum, M.D.
Assistant Professor of Neurology, Mt. Sinai School of Medicine, New York, N.Y.

I. Richard Rosenberg, M.D.
Assistant Clinical Professor of Medicine in Gastroenterology, Mt. Sinai School of Medicine, New York, N.Y.

Allan E. Rubenstein, M.D.
Assistant Professor of Neurology, Mt. Sinai School of Medicine, New York, N.Y.

Allen Silverstein, M.D.
Associate Clinical Professor of Neurology, Mt. Sinai School of Medicine, New York, N.Y.

Kyösti A. Sotaniemi, M.D.
Assistant Chief, Department of Neurology, University of Oulu, Oulu, Finland.

Michael H. Sukoff, M.D.
Chief of Neurological Surgery, Western Medical Center, Santa Ana, Ca.

William E. Wallis, M.D., F.R.A.C.P.
Visiting Neurologist, Auckland Hospital, Auckland, New Zealand.

E. Jane Woolley, M.D.
Anesthesiologist, Verdugo Hills Hospital, Glendale, Ca.

Dean F. Young, M.D.
Associate Attending Neurologist, Memorial Sloan-Kettering Cancer Center, New York, N.Y., Associate Professor of Clinical Neurology, Cornell University Medical College, New York.

Foreword

During the past quarter century biochemical research has provided the clinician with a considerable number of new diagnostic and therapeutic tools. Diseases previously not definable in their early stages or to their full extent can now be readily detected and many not felt remediable can be treated. However, as is often the case with new and potent weapons in medicine, risk factors exist. Indeed we must be as knowledgeable of the untoward effects of these new approaches as of the benefits to be derived.

Systemic physiological changes, whether produced by disease or alterations in the environment either within the body or outside of it, use the nervous system to express themselves. That many of these are reflected by signs and symptoms of neurological dysfunction is not unexpected. Symptoms may be as specific as focal loss of motor or sensory function or as diffuse as disordered mentation, mood, or level of consciousness. Though they may be indicative of primary involvement of the nervous system, it is not infrequent that they signal dysfunction in other organs. Hence, in the preparation of this volume Dr. Silverstein has wisely drawn not only on the expertise of neurologists but those from the varying branches of medicine that are involved in the use of these therapeutic modalities. The choice of topics is extensive and no doubt reflects Dr. Silverstein's own wide neurological experience. It also highlights the interactive role which clinical neurologists are involved in with other branches of medicine. The comprehensive scope of this text should have wide appeal and prove useful for all practicing physicians.

MELVIN D. YAHR, M.D.
Professor and Chairman
Department of Neurology
Mt. Sinai School of Medicine
New York, N.Y.

Preface

Among the several oaths taken by most of us when we accepted the Doctorate of Medicine or its equivalent, was the promise to "do no harm." Yet this ancient Hippocratic oath is violated several times a day by current practitioners of medicine and surgery. As medical science develops and medical knowledge increases and technology improves, ever increasingly newer forms of medical and surgical therapies have appeared. These newer therapies, as well as older, more established ones, are sometimes followed by complications. Fortunately, most of these side effects are mild, transient, and usually, readily reversible. Because the benefits to be gained by these therapies by far exceeds the possible adverse effects, these medical and surgical forms of treatment have continued.

Not infrequently, these complications of therapy have involved the nervous system, both central and peripheral, and the muscular system as well. The recognition, prevention if possible, and treatment of these neurological side effects of therapy is the concern not only of the neurologist who may be called in consultation, but also of the physician who initially employed the particular treatment. In an attempt to collect the varying neurological complications of some forms of therapy in one publication, and to assist the physician in his or her awareness and management of these problems, this book has been compiled.

At the suggestion and urging of the publisher, the editor invited several distinguished physicians in varying specialties to contribute chapters to this book. Most of these authors had already published on some aspect of the neurological complications of therapy in the medical literature; others are prominent clinicians and researchers in their respective fields of interest. The editor is indebted to all the authors who agreed to take part in this venture and did so. I would especially like to thank them for submitting their manuscripts to me within the time allowed — or at least, very close to the deadline.

The authors were given considerable freedom in the development of their individual chapters. Thus, there is considerable overlap in this book. As examples, the neurological side effects of adreno-cortical-steroids are discussed in the chapters related to Cardiovascular Medication (Chapter II), Cancer Chemotherapy, (Chapter III), and Gastrointestinal Drug Therapy (Chapter XI), and the neuropathies induced by improper positioning are described in the sections dealing with Anesthesia (Chapter VII) and General Surgery (Chapter VIII).

It is sincerely hoped that the material presented in this book will be of assistance to clinicians who have patients who develop neurological complications from therapy. It is also hoped that the information presented in this book will *not* be used by those who seek to take advantage of the current climate of the medical-legal milieu concerning malpractice claims, at least in the United States. I certainly hope this is so; but somehow, today (July 1981), I have my doubts.

ALLEN SILVERSTEIN, M.D.
New York, N.Y.

Table of Contents

Chapter I

Antibiotic Neurotoxicity

Michael F. Parry, M.D.

Introduction

Adverse reactions to drugs account for 5% of all hospital admissions and up to 25% of hospitalized patients experience a drug reaction during their hospitalization. Antimicrobial agents occupy a prominent position in the lists of such drugs and account for between 20% and 30% of all adverse reactions.

Drug toxicity may occur in a variety of ways: (1) Irritative local effects at the site of administration are regularly seen; (2) Superinfection is common; (3) Direct toxic effects on one or more organ systems occur frequently; (4) Hypersensitivity reactions account for fever, rash, and some other manifestations of toxicity; (5) Finally, inhibition of cellular metabolic activity and interference with elimination, distribution, or metabolism of other drugs account for a large proportion of adverse reactions. The last two are important mechanisms for antibiotic toxicity and cause the majority of those reactions referable to the nervous system.

The manifestations of antibiotic neurotoxicity can be conveniently categorized (Table I). The rest of this review is organized by antibiotic rather than adverse reaction. Minor side effects occurring in association with antibiotic administration such as nausea, headache, and unpleasant taste may be neurologically mediated but are not discussed in this chapter as significant manifestations of neurotoxicity.

Aminoglycoside Antibiotics

Neuromuscular Toxicity

Aminoglycoside antibiotics interfere with peripheral neuromuscular function by direct neuromuscular blockade or by producing electro-

1

Table I

Neurotoxicity of Antibiotics

Benign intracranial hypertension
Ampicillin
Nalidixic Acid
Sulfonamides
Tetracycline

Encephalopathy/myelopathy
Aminoglycosides (IT)
Amphotericin (IT)
Cycloserine
Ethionamide
Metronidazole

Meningitis/meningoencephalitis
Aminoglycosides (IT)
Amphotericin (IT)
INH
Miconazole (IT)
Penicillin
Sulfonamides

Neuromuscular dysfunction
Aminoglycosides
Capreomycin
Clindamycin
Lincomycin
Polymyxin
Tetracycline
Viomycin

Optic neuropathy
Chloramphenicol
Ethambutol
INH

Ototoxicity
Aminoglycosides
Chloramphenicol
Erythromycin
Minocycline
Polymyxin
Vancomycin

Peripheral neuropathy
Chloramphenicol
Ethambutol
INH
Metronidazole
Nitrofurantoin
Sulfonamides

Seizures
Cephalosporins
Cycloserine
INH
Metronidazole
Nalidixic Acid
Penicillins

IT = intrathecal

lyte disturbances which manifest themselves as neuromuscular dysfunction.

Gentamicin administration may produce hypokalemic alkalosis, hypomagnesemia, and hypocalcemia due to accelerated renal losses of divalent and monovalent cations.[1] This effect is unrelated to nephrotoxicity and is associated with high dose regimens. Many, but not all such patients, have other reasons for electrolyte derangements including diuretic administration and cancer chemotherapy.

Clinical presentations vary according to the predominant cation deficit. Hypokalemia is manifest by muscular weakness and hypocalcemia by tetany and paresthesias. In most cases there is depletion of all three ions with predominating clinical signs of hypocalcemia. The effects of hypocalcemia are exacerbated by concomitant hypokalemia and alkalosis, shifting ionized to unionized calcium. Cation replacement will reverse the clinical abnormalities although magnesium replacement may also be necessary for restoration of normal serum calcium concentrations.

The activity of aminoglycoside antibiotics on the neuromuscular junction is well described. All aminoglycosides have been implicated although neomycin association seems most common, perhaps due to its most frequent use in surgery and the additive effects of aminoglycoside neuromuscular blockade and anesthesia. Experimental data vary, but gentamicin, neomycin and streptomycin seem to produce more neuromuscular blockade than kanamycin, amikacin, or tobramycin.[2] The role of anesthesia is discussed in Chapter VII of this book.

Several hundred cases of neuromuscular blockade have been recorded.[3] Although usually reported in association with anesthesia and/or concomitant non-depolarizing neuromuscular blocking drug administration, clinical neuromuscular blockade is now seen in other situations. Potentiation of neuromuscular dysfunction in botulism, myasthenia gravis, and Guillain Barré syndrome have all been noted. The most pronounced effects are on respiratory function, leading to hypoxia, increased respirator dependence, increased risk of aspiration pneumonia, and respiratory arrest. Depression of the gag reflex, decrease in spontaneous movement, and generalized weakness are also described. Patients with non-neuromuscular disease, such as chronic obstructive pulmonary disease, may also be at risk for manifesting neuromuscular blockade due to aminoglycoside antibiotics.

Although high antibiotic blood levels may be expected to produce more blockade (especially with intraperitoneal instillation and absorption during surgery) such blockade may be clinically apparent with normal doses in the presence of normal renal function and normal blood levels. Clinical deterioration occurs rapidly after administration of the aminoglycoside but is reversible within 12 to 24 hours of stopping the drug. In one study, seven of eleven patients with infant botulism needed intubation within 48 hours of initiating aminoglycoside therapy.[4]

Aminoglycoside antibiotics competitively inhibit the action of acetylcholine at the neuromuscular junction.[5] They produce a nondepolarizing, flaccid paralysis in in vitro muscle preparations or in experimental animals. Such effects are enhanced by anesthesia, other neuromuscular blocking agents (especially d-tubocurarine and pancuronium bromide), and magnesium ions. The aminoglycoside activity can be effectively antagonized by calcium ions, but only slightly by neostigmine. Electromyographic studies reveal patterns similar to those produced by magnesium or curare.

The exact mechanism of action of aminoglycoside antibiotics remains to be clarified. Although spontaneous prejunctional activity is not diminished under usual conditions, there is marked depression of acetylcholine release after stimulation. This appears due to aminoglycoside competition with calcium ions resulting in decreased acetylcholine release which is antagonizable by excess calcium ions (usually above physiologic range). In addition to the prejunctional effect, aminoglycoside antibiotics decrease the postjunctional end plate sensitivity to acetylcholine. The combined pre- and postjunctional effect explains the activity of aminoglycoside antibiotics in a variety of clinical situations where neuromuscular dysfunction is observed.

Management of neuromuscular blockade consists primarily of an awareness and avoidance of such drugs for the treatment of infections in patients with neuromuscular disease, especially if these individuals are not receiving ventilatory support. If neuromuscular blockade occurs, reversal is usually prompt on discontinuing the offending aminoglycoside. Calcium ions may reverse the blockade experimentally, but usually at levels greater than those achievable in men ($>$ 8 meq/L). Neither calcium nor neostigmine has proven predictably effective in humans.

Ototoxicity — Experimental

Aminoglycoside eighth cranial nerve toxicity may occur in two forms: labyrinthine or vestibular toxicity, and cochlear or auditory toxicity. These are lumped together under the term "ototoxicity."

Animal models of aminoglycoside ototoxicity have shown a great deal of relevance to human toxicity. However, methods of testing vary from study to study and usually employ massive doses of drugs to produce rapid physiologic and pathological effects in the experimental animal. In contrast, human toxicity occurs with much lower doses over time and may be delayed by days or weeks. This makes direct applicability of animal data less certain. Indeed, there is some evidence to suggest that massive doses of aminoglycoside antibiotics given intravenously to animals may produce eighth nerve toxicity secondary to systemic hypotension due to a direct cardiac depressant effect of the high drug levels achieved.[6]

In the experimental animal, aminoglycoside antibiotics cause destruction of neural end organ hair cells in the labyrinth (Crista ampulare) and cochlea (organ of Corti) by an unknown mechanism. At a sub-cellular level, two major effects of the aminoglycosides have been proposed to account for their neurotoxicity.[7] Firstly, aminoglycoside antibiotics interfere with ATPase activity in the stria vascularis, altering electrolyte transport between the endolymph (potassium 140 meq/L; sodium 10 meq/L) and perilymph (potassium 6 meq/L; sodium 140 meq/L). The sodium/potassium gradient sustains electrical activity and its impairment (e.g., by aminoglycoside antibiotics) disrupts neural conduction, and may be partly responsible for toxicity. In addition, aminoglycosides interact with phosphoinositides, binding to these lipid components of the cell membrane and displacing calcium ions. This interaction disrupts membrane integrity and may produce hair cell damage. Decreased oxygen consumption and inhibition of protein synthesis have also been measured and may be separate consequences of aminoglycoside activity or due to the above effects. However, these abnormalities are of uncertain relationship to the hair cell damage that is seen both pathologically and functionally.

Pathologically, in the cochlea of animals, aminoglycoside antibiotics cause preferential destruction of hair cells in the basal turn, corresponding to high frequency sound reception. Within each turn, outer hair cells are more susceptible to damage than inner hair cells. With increasing dose and time of exposure, hair cell damage progresses from basal to apical turns corresponding to loss of high frequency reception (15-20,000 cycles/sec) progressing to low frequency reception (< 500 cycles/sec). These changes are seen with systemic (IM or IV) administration or topical administration of aminoglycoside to the inner ear.

Microscopically, degeneration of hair cells begins with nuclear and mitochondrial clumping, progresses to merging of the sensory hairs and bulging of the cell surface membrane, and ends with disintegration of the cell.[8] Similar changes occur with chronic, "low" dose, parenteral administration (100 mg/kg of gentamicin per day) as with acute, "high" dose, topical administration (10 mcg in 0.2 ml) to the middle ear, although nuclear changes are more prominent with the latter. Both vestibular and cochlear hair cells are affected in a similar fashion.

The pathologic changes of aminoglycoside ototoxicity correlate well with functional changes as assessed by a variety of behavioral tests in the experimental animal.[9] Objective evidence can be obtained by demonstrating changes in cochlear nerve action potentials in response to auditory stimuli. These also correlate well with pathologic findings.

The occurrence of aminoglycoside ototoxicity is best explained by the peculiar pharmacokinetics of aminoglycoside antibiotics in the inner ear. Not only are high concentrations of aminoglycoside reached in the perilymph fluid of the inner ear, but these levels are maintained for a considerable period of time.[10,11] After administration of a dose of aminoglycoside antibiotic, levels in the perilymph rise slowly, peaking 4 to 6 hours after the dose (Fig. 1). Peak concentrations in the perilymph are higher than simultaneous serum concentrations, and decay with a long half-life of 8 to 12 hours (for gentamicin, tobramycin, and amikacin). Concentrations are linearly related to dose and peak serum level, are bilaterally equal, are increased in the presence of otitis media, and are unchanged by diuresis. Conflicting data exist as to whether perilymph concentrations of aminoglycoside accumulate with long-term treatment in the absence of renal failure. However, perilymph concentrations certainly increase with rising serum concentrations during long-term treatment if renal disease supervenes. Finally, there is a direct relationship between perilymph (and endolymph) concentration of aminoglycoside and ototoxicity as measured pathologically and functionally. The highest perilymph concentrations are achieved with local aminoglycoside application to the middle ear and these are associated with the most profound ototoxicity.

There is little data regarding reversibility of toxicity in animal experiments. In most cases, toxicity seems irreversible, but high doses are used to produce rapid pathological and functional changes. Furthermore, much of the objective data accumulated by these studies cannot be obtained without death of the animal. Further insight into the reversibility of toxicity, therefore, remains to be achieved.

Comparative ototoxic studies in animals, using large parenteral doses of aminoglycoside, demonstrate that gentamicin, streptomycin, and sisomicin cause predominant labyrinthine damage, whereas kanamycin, amikacin, and neomycin produce predominant cochlear damage. Tobramycin produces similar effects on both the labyrinth and cochlea. Although gentamicin produces more ototoxicity on a weight for weight basis in the experimental animal than either kanamycin, streptomycin, or amikacin, proportionately lower doses of gentamicin are used clinically. The ototoxicity of tobramycin in the guinea pig is less than that of gentamicin, and may in part be related to lower perilymph concentrations. An investigational aminoglycoside, netilmicin, produces even less ototoxicity and minimal change in cochlear action potential despite massive doses (150 mg/kg).

Concomitant administration of an aminoglycoside antibiotic and a loop diuretic (ethacrynic acid or furosemide) produces profound ototoxicity in the experimental animal. Furosemide or ethacrynic acid when given alone produce transient decreases in cochlear potential, but when

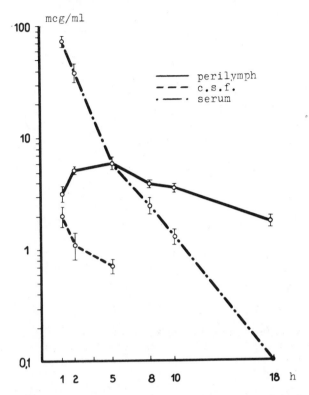

Figure 1. Concentrations of tobramycin in perilymph, C.S.F. and serum after subcutaneous injection of 50 mg/kg in guinea pigs. From Federspil P, Schatzle W, Tiesler E: *J. Infect Dis* **134**:S200-S204, 1976, with permission.

given together with kanamycin, produce permanent deafness (Fig. 2).[12] A similar interaction occurs between streptomycin and ethacrynic acid and vestibular function. The exact mechanism of interaction between the diuretic and aminoglycoside antibiotic is unknown.

Ototoxicity — Clinical

Clinical ototoxicity in humans has been extensively documented. However, the frequency with which it occurs depends upon the populations studied, the definition of ototoxicity (number of decibels, unilateral or bilateral, conversational loss only, etc.), the technique and sensitivity of measurement, and the vigor for which ototoxicity is sought. The variability amongst these factors has resulted in widely disparate estimates of toxicity. A literature review shows the quoted risks of genta-

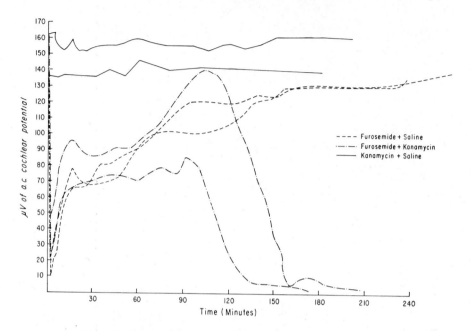

Figure 2. Effect of furosemide (100 mg/kg) and kanamycin (400 mg/kg) on the a.c. cochlear potential that is generated in response to a 1000 Hz continuous tone. From Brummett RE, Traynor J, Brown R: *Acta Otolaryngol* **80**:86-92, 1975, with permission.

micin ototoxicity, for example, to range from 0 to 30%. The truth lies somewhere in between. The Boston Collaborative Drug Surveillance Group showed that aminoglycoside antibiotics were the most frequent cause of drug-induced deafness in the hospital setting, accounting for 13 cases per thousand patients exposed, or 1.3%, exceeding the rates for aspirin (1.1%), ethacrynic acid (0.7%) and quinidine (0.3%).[13]

Early reports of ototoxicity suggests a higher incidence than that reported recently. In 1967, reliable estimates of gentamicin toxicity were 9% of patients exposed. This was revised in 1971 to 2.8%, and in 1974 to ≤ 1%.[14] This decrease can be accounted for mainly by an improved understanding of aminoglycoside pharmacokinetics and the risk factors for toxicity.

Aminoglycosides differ in their potential for causing either auditory or vestibular toxicity in man. Streptomycin and gentamicin produce predominantly vestibular toxicity,[15] whereas amikacin,[16] kanamycin, and neomycin produce predominantly auditory toxicity. Tobramycin[17] produces roughly equal auditory and vestibular toxicity. These human data are very similar to the experimental results obtained from animal studies (q. v.).

Auditory toxicity is readily detectable audiometrically, but conversational hearing loss rarely occurs. Abnormal audiograms, defined as bilateral decreases of $\geqslant 15$ decibels, occur in approximately 20% of kanamycin treated patients but in only 5% of tobramycin treated patients (Table II). Conversational hearing losses occur in 1 to 2% of kanamycin treated patients, but in less than 0.5% of tobramycin treated patients. Audiometric studies show initial loss of high frequency reception which progresses to loss of lower, or conversational, frequencies if the drug is continued. Prompt detection of early high frequency loss will usually prevent loss of lower frequency reception. Dead hair cells are not replaced, so that added importance is stressed on early detection via audiograms. Apparently, the initial early decrease in high frequency reception does not always mean hair cell death, since 40 to 60% of patients will reverse their hearing loss after terminating the drug. An occasional patient will progress but fortunately this is rare. Delayed (> 1 week) onset deafness is also rare but has been described in aminoglycoside treated patients who return to a noisy environment after treatment, and is a peculiar feature of dihydrostreptomycin therapy. This drug is no longer available because of the high incidence of its auditory toxicity.

The vast majority (> 80%) of audiogram abnormalities occurring during treatment are bilateral. Evaluation of the audiogram requires a pretreatment study since the patient population being treated has a high incidence of pretreatment audiogram abnormalities, in some series up to 75%.[18] Although the initial manifestation of toxicity may be tinnitus, in only one-third of patients does tinnitus precede or coincide with decrements in audiometric function. Neither the watch test nor whispered voice have been useful in detecting early losses of high frequency reception.

Vestibular toxicity may occur as the only manifestation of eighth nerve toxicity or may accompany auditory toxicity. In gentamicin-treated patients, for example,[16] auditory toxicity accompanied vestibular toxicity as often as it occurred alone (16% each). Most studies have evaluated vestibular toxicity clinically (subjective vertigo or dizziness) rather than by actual measurement. Electronystagmograms and caloric studies are 3-4 times more sensitive than subjective complaints or gross physical abnormalities in the same way that audiograms are more sensitive indicators of auditory toxicity than complaints of conversational hearing loss (by a factor of 10 or more). Subclinical hair cell damage occurs in both situations.

Clinical vestibular toxicity occurs most commonly with strepto-mycin and gentamicin (Table II). It may present as an acute Meiniere's syndrome, or more insidiously as vertigo or unsteadiness. Onset usually occurs during therapy but it occasionally (5-15% of cases) appears up to 10-14 days after stopping the drug, and in these cases, usually with genta-micin.[14] Only 50% of patients with vestibular toxicity due to gentamicin reverse, but 75-90% of cases attributed to tobramycin or netilmicin are said to be reversible. This perhaps accords with animal studies showing more profound hair cell loss in the stria vascularis with gentamicin than tobramycin, amikacin, or netilmicin. However, even those cases that do persist are usually well compensated for in 6-12 months by visual and proprioceptive adjustments in life style.

Risk factors for ototoxicity are debated in the literature. However, there is general agreement that the most important three risk factors are total dose received, duration of therapy, and aminoglycoside blood con-centrations. Although pre-existing renal disease is also related to increased toxicity, it may only be indirectly related by causing increased blood concentrations and not as an independent risk factor.[14]

Both high peak blood levels and high trough blood levels are asso-ciated with increased risk of ototoxicity. Definitions of peak and trough vary from study to study, and therefore, interpretation of specific numbers varys. Peak levels, anywhere from 0 to 30 minutes after comple-tion of an intravenous infusion or 1 hour after an intramuscular injec-tion, represent the highest blood levels achieved after equilibration; and trough levels, defined anywhere from 5-30 minutes prior to the next dose, represent the lowest blood levels. In early gentamicin studies,[15] 53% of ototoxic cases had peak blood levels $\geq$ 8 mcg/ml and 37% were $\geq$ 16 mcg/ml, compared to 22% and 6% of the non-ototoxic group. Trough blood levels $\geq$ 2 mcg/ml, or in other studies $\geq$ 3 mcg/ml, are associated with increased risk. Both high peak and high trough blood levels increase the area under the curve, perhaps the most significant, but rarely available, measurement. Blood levels for risk with tobramycin have not been as well defined but appear similar to those published for gentamicin and are usually accepted as peak levels $>$ 10 mcg/ml and trough levels $>$ 2 mcg/ml. Such blood levels are rarely exceeded by recommended doses of gentamicin or tobramycin (3-5 mg/kg/day) in patients with normal renal function. However, routine measurement of aminoglycoside blood levels should be standard procedure, both to achieve therapeutic levels and avoid toxicity. This is particularly impor-tant in the elderly because aminoglycoside antibiotics are excreted solely by glomerular filtration and pre-existing abnormalities in GFR (not necessarily reflected in the serum creatinine concentration) may result in rapid elevations in aminoglycoside blood concentrations (and peri-lymph concentrations), superimposed nephrotoxicity, and ototoxicity.

Amikacin blood levels associated with increase risks of ototoxicity are peak levels > 32 mcg/ml and trough levels > 10 mcg/ml. Individualized dosing with frequent blood level monitoring, permitting effective but non-toxic concentrations, can minimize toxicity to < 0.1% of patients receiving gentamicin.

Non-parenteral administration of aminoglycoside antibiotics can occasionally produce ototoxicity. Systemic absorption of neomycin has been shown after administration topically to burn wounds, orally for the treatment of hepatic encephalopathy, and as a colonic or wound irrigant. Deafness due to neomycin under these circumstances is almost always associated with either very prolonged (frequently months) administration of the drug or concomitant renal insufficiency.[20] Paromomycin may produce toxicity in a similar fashion.

Age, especially over 60 years, is an important risk factor for toxicity. In part this is due to declining creatinine clearance with age. It is estimated that creatinine clearance falls by one ml per minute from normal (100 ml per minute) for each year over 20 years of age. This may not be reflected in serum creatinine concentrations due to decreasing muscle mass with age. Age less than 10 is negatively correlated with toxicity. Aside from renal function, this may also be due to the fact that the volume of distribution is increased in children, resulting in markedly lower blood levels after similar mg/kg doses. Indeed, children less than five years of age require about twice as much gentamicin as children over 10 years old or adults to achieve similar blood concentrations.[21] Clinical studies of newborns show no significant differences in ototoxicity between aminoglycoside treated and control patients,[22] although gentamicin, kanamycin, and neomycin have all been reported to cause isolated cases of deafness in the newborn. Neonatal sepsis and meningitis, for which these antibiotics are used, however, has a clearly greater impact on whatever neurological sequelae occur than does the use of an aminoglycoside antibiotic.

Recent or concurrent administration of other aminoglycoside antibiotics is an independent risk factor for ototoxicity. The role of concomitant loop diuretics is unclear, but impressive anecdotal reports suggest that large doses of such drugs, especially ethacrynic acid, given to a patient with renal insufficiency while receiving an aminoglycoside antibiotic, is likely to produce irreversible ototoxicity. Animal studies support this (q. v.). Whether the presence of renal insufficiency alters the blood/perilymph/endolymph gradient or just raises the blood concentration of antibiotic is not clear from published studies.

Finally, it is not clear that any of the following are independent risk factors for aminoglycoside ototoxicity: Daily dose in mg/kg, sex of the patient, prior history of noise exposure, abnormal pretreatment audiogram, or patient's size (weight).

Table II
Incidence of Toxicity (Percent)*

Drug	Abnormal Audiogram	Clinical Auditory	Clinical Vestibular
Streptomycin	2-10	< 0.2	2-10
Kanamycin	20-25	1-2	< 1
Gentamicin	8-10	0.5-1	2-4
Tobramycin	4-6	< 0.5	< 1
Amikacin	10-20	0.5-1	< 1
Netilmicin	4-6	< 0.5	< 1

*Most reasonable estimate based on literature review.

Miscellaneous Neurotoxocity

Circumoral paresthesias have been described in association with streptomycin, kanamycin, and amikacin administration. These are usually transient, associated with peak blood concentrations, and not reported with other aminoglycoside antibiotics. Their etiology is unknown and the occurrence does not seem related to other forms of neurotoxicity.

Intraventricular or intrathecal administration of aminoglycoside antibiotics seems to be remarkably free of toxicity. Ototoxicity has not been reported and would therefore seem to depend more upon serum than CSF levels, especially since ventricular CSF levels can exceed 40 mcg/ml after intraventricular administration, and cisternal levels can exceed 10 mcg/ml after intralumbar administration, well in excess of the < 1 mcg/ml levels achieved after parenteral administration. However, assessment of toxicity has been difficult because patients receiving aminoglycosides directly into the cerebrospinal fluid are profoundly ill and have high neurological morbidity and mortality from their central nervous system infections.

Intrathecal administration of both kanamycin and gentamicin has been shown to cause polyradiculitis. This appears due to direct irritation by the injected drug, or its diluent. Reported cases used preparations intended for intravenous use, which contain preservatives. Preservative free material is currently available for intrathecal injection. Whether it produces less radiculitis is unknown since the number of reported cases is so few. Preservatives in these preparations include phenol, paraben derivatives, EDTA, sodium bisulphite, and benzyl alcohol.

Intraventricular aminoglycoside antibiotic must be administered either through an indwelling reservoir or by repeated punctures (usually in neonates). Neonatal meningitis treated with intravenous and intraventricular aminoglycoside has a worse prognosis than when treated with intravenous aminoglycoside alone.[23] This may be due to the trauma of needle injury or to a direct local toxic effect of the aminoglycoside. Experimental studies have shown axonal degeneration, myelin swelling, and glial cell necrosis after intracisternal administration of gentamicin. Similar lesions were noted in the brain stem of a patient treated with intrathecal gentamicin[24] and were reproduced in a rabbit model given high doses of intracisternal gentamicin. The implication of these findings for other patients receiving either intraventricular or intrathecal aminoglycoside is not yet clear.

Antifungal Agents

Amphotericin

Amphotericin B is the most effective systemic antifungal agent currently available. It is a polyene antibiotic, a complex cyclic fatty acid which binds to sterols in the cell membrane of fungal and mammalian cells. Its affinity for the major sterol of fungal cells, ergosterol, is much greater than its affinity for mammalian cholesterol, accounting for its differential toxicity. Treated, susceptible cells develop pores and leaky cell membranes with resultant loss of potassium and other intracellular constituents.

The binding of amphotericin B to cholesterol in mammalian cell membranes accounts for its toxicity. Although nephrotoxicity and hematologic toxicity are predictable and most important, neurotoxicity occasionally occurs. Peripheral neuropathy has been reported after intravenous administration on one occasion but neurotoxicity is more commonly seen after intrathecal or intraventricular administration. These routes are necessary for the successful treatment of many fungal infections of the central nervous system. Chemical meningitis after intraventricular administration has been reported. Intrathecal administration has led to severe myelopathy with paresthesias, weakness, nerve palsies, and paraplegia.[25] Although arachnoiditis may occur, myelopathy is more likely due to direct damage to the spinal cord or its vascular supply. Short of administration by other routes there are no known ways to lessen the risk of such neurotoxicity. Neurologic deficits may remain after stopping the drug.

Miconazole

Miconazole is an imidazole derivative with broad spectrum antifungal activity. Its recent introduction provided hope of avoiding the toxicity of amphotericin B, although its proper place in the antifungal armamentarium is yet to be established.

Intravenous miconazole frequently produces hyponatremia due to inappropriate ADH secretion. Concomitant depression of CNS function may occur if the electrolyte disturbances are not recognized and corrected. Independent of electrolyte derangements, light headedness, euphoria, anxiety, hyperesthesia, blurred vision, weakness, and toxic psychoses have been observed. Arachnoiditis and chemical meningitis may occur after intrathecal or intraventricular administration but myelopathy has not been described.[26]

Antituberculosis Drugs

Cycloserine

Cycloserine is a structural analog of D-alanine, and as such, competetively inhibits the incorporation of D-alanine into the bacterial cell wall. Although active against several species of mycobacteria and some other microorganisms, its severe neurotoxicity has limited its use to the treatment of drug-resistant tuberculosis.

Administration of 1 gram of cycloserine per day produces neurotoxicity in 10% of patients.[27,28] Acute psychiatric disturbances such as confusion, depression, hallucinations, and manifestations of abnormal behavior frequently occur, especially in those individuals with underlying mental instability. In addition, tremor, myoclonic jerks, and major motor seizures may develop. Dysarthria, vertigo, and peripheral neuritis have also been described. All symptoms of neurotoxicity are dose related and are rapidly reversible on stopping the drug. Reducing the daily dose to < 500 mg decreases the incidence of neurotoxicity to < 5%. Underlying seizure disorders increase the risk of convulsive neurotoxicity.

The etiology of cycloserine neurotoxicity is not known. A direct effect of the drug on the central nervous system is most likely. Reduced CSF levels of calcium and magnesium have been found and may also be related to its toxicity. Beneficial effects of large doses or pyridoxine have been reported both therapeutically and prophylactically but experience is limited.

Ethambutol

Introduced in 1961, ethambutol has achieved widespread use for the treatment of tuberculosis where its main value lies in the rarity of adverse reactions. Its only major toxic effect is optic neuritis, the frequency of which has been minimized in recent years by appropriate selection of dosage.

At currently recommended doses of ≤ 15 mg/kg/day the incidence of optic neuritis is considerably less than 0.1%. Indeed, toxicity has never been convincingly documented at this dose. At 25 mg/kg/day the incidence is perhaps 2-3%. Optic neuritis is predominantly a feature of the levoisomer, therefore current preparations of ethambutol employ solely the dextroisomer.

The clinical manifestations of optic neuritis due to ethambutol are decreased visual acuity and decreased ability to perceive green color. Purely central scotomas may be present and rarely constriction of visual fields may occur. These changes are bilateral in almost all cases. As long as the drug is stopped at the earliest sign of toxicity the abnormalities are reversible, although recovery may take several months. Blindness is only reported at doses above 15 mg/kg/day with continuance of the drug in the face of worsening visual symptoms. Ophthalmoscopic exam is usually normal. Occasionally, edema, hyperemia, and blurred disc margins are noted and optic atrophy may be seen if permanent visual impairment remains.

Pathologically, demyelination of the optic chiasm and adjacent optic nerves has been described. In animal studies, similar predilection for the optic chiasm has been noted with vacuolization and dilatation of axons.[29] The reason for this peculiarly local effect and the mechanisms for toxicity are unknown. Neither retinal nor cortical abnormalities occur.

Peripheral neuritis has also been described as a rare complication of ethambutol therapy. It may occur alone or together with optic neuritis and appears dose related. It is reversible when ethambutol is withdrawn but its histopathology and etiology are unknown.

Ethionamide

Ethionamide is a derivative of isonicotinic acid and is useful in the treatment of drug–resistant tuberculosis or infection due to atypical mycobacteria. Neurotoxicity is rare but peculiar mental disturbances and encephalopathies do occur.[27,28] Depression, anxiety, psychosis, dizziness, visual disturbances, peripheral neuritis, and convulsions are all reported. Encephalopathy is characterized by tremor, loss of recent memory, confusion, and apathy. Recovery may be slow after withdrawing the drug but pyridoxine has been reported to speed recovery. Little further information regarding the basis for its toxicity exists since its use at present is quite limited.

Isoniazid

Isoniazid (INH), introduced in 1952, remains a mainstay for the treatment of tuberculosis. Although gastrointestinal intolerance is common, major toxicity is rare. Hepatitis (1-2 per hundred exposed) and neurotoxicity (1 per 400 exposed) are the major adverse reactions.

Isoniazid mediates its neurotoxicity through interaction with pyridoxine (Vitamin B_6). Inhibition of the phosphorylation of pyridoxine and its derivatives to form the active coenzyme pyridoxal phosphate, and chelation of pyridoxal phosphate itself, are direct effects of INH. Chronic ingestion of low doses of INH preferentially inhibits phosphorylation and produces peripheral neuritis. In contrast, acute ingestion of high doses preferentially chelates pyridoxal phosphate and produces convulsions.[30]

Acute neurologic toxicity is manifest by tonic-clonic seizures which are usually generalized but may be focal. They are frequently preceded by hyperreflexia, confusion, ataxia, or slurred speech, and are usually intractable to standard anticonvulsant therapy. Acute toxicity occurs in newborns, and in adults as a manifestation of overdose ($>$ 6 grams in a single dose) or with high doses ($>$ 5 mg/kg/day) in the presence of renal failure, an underlying seizure disorder, malnutrition, or alcoholism. Although the seizures of acute INH toxicity do not respond readily to phenytoin or phenobarbitol administration, pyridoxine in large doses usually aborts seizure activity within 8 to 12 hours.

Pyridoxal phosphate is an important cofactor in the transamination and decarboxylation of amino acids. The acute convulsive toxicity of isoniazid is probably due to depletion of this coenzyme with inhibition of glutamate decarboxylase and diminished levels of γ-amino-butyric acid (GABA) within the central nervous system. Decreased levels of GABA result in diminished activity of inhibitory synapses and the appearance of seizure activity. There may also be important effects on other central decarboxylation and transamination reactions that require pyridoxal phosphate as a cofactor. Such seizure activity is due to functional derangements. No pathologic abnormalities have been described in association with acute INH toxicity in humans.

Peripheral neuropathy occurs in approximately 0.3% of patients receiving isoniazid. The degree of toxicity and the time of onset are dose dependent. It is rarely seen at less than 6 mg/kg/day unless alcoholism, or malnutrition, or both are present. However, it is estimated that 40% of patients at $>$ 15 mg/kg/day and 10% at 6-15 mg/kg/day will develop neuropathy. The time of onset may be as little as 1 month in the high dose group or as long as 12 months in the lowest dose group after therapy has started. Slow acetylators are at greatest risk of toxicity since blood and tissue levels are highest in this group. Slow acetylation is common (50%) in Europeans and Africans but rare in Asians. Although liver disease would be expected to increase INH levels by decreasing its metabolism, this is only important at bilirubin levels > 2.0 mg/dl. There is no information on the role of renal disease in the development of neuropathy due to isoniazid.

INH peripheral neuropathy may be motor, sensory, or optic. The lower extremities are mostly affected. Numbness, tingling, and burning sensations with or without weakness are the presenting complaints. Myalgias and ataxia may also occur. Pyridoxine administration leads to prompt (within 1-4 weeks) improvement in neuropathy and ultimate recovery is usually complete. Prophylactic pyridoxine may also prevent the occurrence of neuropathy and is recommended for all patients receiving over 5 mg/kg/day or who are malnourished.

Pathologically in man and animals, denervation atrophy of muscle and Wallerian degeneration of nerve fibers, both myelinated and unmyelinated, are present. Schwann cell abnormalities are also described.[30] Although peripheral neuropathy can be prevented by prophylactic administration of pyridoxine, the role of pyridoxine–dependent enzyme systems in maintaining the integrity of the peripheral nervous system is unknown.

An acute hypersensitivity meningoencephalitis has also been described due to isoniazid, similar to that observed with sulfonamides or penicillin derivatives. This may occur independently or as a manifestation of drug-induced systemic lupus erythematosis. The onset is usually acute, and consists of headache, fever, confusion, and a stiff neck accompanied by a CSF pleocytosis, elevated protein, but normal sugar. A prompt response is seen upon withdrawal of the isoniazid or administration of adrenocorticosteroids.

Isoniazid administration may decrease the clearance of phenytoin through inhibition of its metabolism, thereby producing toxicity and necessitating downward adjustment of the anticonvulsant dose, especially in slow acetylators. Because of the risk of seizure activity with isoniazid administration, it is not recommended that phenytoin be discontinued in patients receiving this drug for the underlying seizure disorder.

Other Antituberculosis Drugs

Rifampin, pyrazinamide, and para-aminosalicylic acid have not been described to cause neurotoxicity. Viomycin and capreomycin are infrequently used parenteral agents. They possess vestibular toxicity, auditory toxicity, and neuromuscular blocking activity similar to the aminoglycoside antibiotics.[27,28]

Chloramphenicol

Optic neuritis is the most common neurologic manifestation of chloramphenicol toxicity. It is only seen with chronic, continuous administration, usually oral, in doses generally in excess of 100 grams (2 gm/kg) over several weeks or months. Most cases occur in children or young adults with cystic fibrosis, perhaps because this group commonly receives long-term oral chloramphenicol, although nutritional factors have also been implicated.

Clinically, patients present with sudden onset of blurred vision and orbital pain. Physical examination reveals tender globes, sluggish pupillary reflexes, and funduscopic abnormalities of papillitis.[31] Optic disks are hyperemic and edematous with indistinct margins, vessels are tortuous and engorged, nerve fibers are thickened and readily visible, and retinal striations are prominent. Visual acuity is decreased bilaterally with impaired color perception, especially red-green (long wave length) discrimination. Central or secocentral scotomata are present. Visual evoked responses to photic stimulation are delayed in parallel to subjective complaints, indicative of decreased optic nerve conduction. These delays are more prominent with red light stimulation than with blue-white light stimulation, confirming the subjective impairment in red-green discrimination.

Pathologically there are changes in the optic nerve and retina. Ganglion cells in the macular and peri-macular regions are lost. Edema followed by gliosis and atrophy of the papillomacular bundle and the optic nerve may be present. Despite such abnormalities, patient's visual functions recover promptly upon withdrawal of the drug. The physical and laboratory abnormalities, however, may persist to some degree. Constriction of visual fields, mild decreases in acuity, disk pallor and decreased retinal vascularity are the usual residua.

The biochemical bases for chloramphenicol optic neuropathy are unknown. Theories implicate hypercapnea (in patients with cystic fibrosis), nutritional deficiencies, or hypersensitivity. There is little to support any of these theories, but the direct neurotoxic effect of chloramphenicol seems important since clinical improvement occurs only upon cessation of the drug.

Peripheral neuropathy has also been noted, usually along with optic neuritis. It is associated with high dose, long-term therapy (over months) and presents as numbness and dysesthesia of the distal extremities. Reflex changes are not usually present. Pathologically, nerve fiber loss and gliosis are seen. In a fashion similar to chloramphenicol optic neuropathy, the mechanisms of toxicity are unknown, but the disease is reversible in almost all cases.

Chloramphenicol ototoxicity has been reported after topical therapy to the middle ear. Only a few episodes have been reported after systemic therapy and it is probable that the underlying disease (meningitis) or concomitant chemotherapy was responsible for hearing loss in these cases. Animal models have not produced ototoxicity after systemic administration of chloramphenicol.[32]

After topical therapy to the middle ear in experimental animals, sensorineural hearing loss can be promptly detected. Decreased cochlear oxygen consumption, decreased endocochlear action potentials, and pathological damage to the hair cells of the organ of Corti can be demonstrated.[33] The toxicity is predominantly auditory and may be permanent. The mechanisms and patterns of hearing loss in humans have not been well studied due to its rarity, but they appear similar to those of aminoglycoside ototoxicity.[34]

Chloramphenicol elevates the blood and tissue levels of both phenytoin and phenobarbitol by inhibiting their conjugation in the liver. The clearances of phenytoin and phenobarbitol in individuals receiving 3-4 grams of chloramphenicol per day are decreased by 60% and 30% respectively, resulting in marked elevation in anticonvulsant blood levels.[35] The effect is rapid, occurring within hours of chloramphenicol administration, and requires immediate adjustment in anticonvulsant dose to avoid toxicity. Similarly, the effect is reversible, with clearances falling to normal within three days after stopping chloramphenicol.

Clindamycin and Lincomycin

Lincomycin and its 7-chloro derivative, clindamycin, are antibiotics frequently used for the treatment of infections due to aerobic gram-positive and anaerobic microorganisms. Most recent attention has focused on their propensity to cause pseudomembranous colitis but hypersensitivity reactions, hepatotoxicity, and neurotoxicity also occur.

Neurotoxicity due to these compounds is rare. However, neuromuscular paralysis has been described both in vitro and in vivo. Clinical observations suggest that this effect, usually manifest as prolonged paralysis after anesthesia, is 10-fold less common than that associated with aminoglycoside antibiotics.[36]

Clindamycin, the more commonly used derivative, produces direct muscle relaxation by inhibiting contractility. As such, it acts in an additive fashion with non-depolarizing blocking agents like d-tubocurarine and, in contrast to aminoglycoside antibiotics which act primarily on neuromuscular transmission, its activity is not reversed by calcium or neostigmine.[2,36] In addition, experimentally, it produces an initial twitch augmentation. The biochemical basis for this aurgmentation and the decrease in contractility is unknown. Lincomycin seems to produce both muscle relaxation and neuromuscular blockade. Evidence for the latter is its increased interaction with d-tubocurarine and its partial reversal by calcium ions.[2] Both drugs produce clinically relevant paralysis after anesthesia. This is most appropriately managed by prolonged respiratory support until the effects of one or both agents dissipate. Further work remains to define the biochemical bases and sites of action of both antibiotics in the production of neuromuscular paralysis.

Erythromycin

Erythromycin has little potential for neurotoxicity. Rare instances of ototoxicity have been described, but these have never been reported after oral administration of usual doses ($\leqslant$ 2 grams per day).

Topical administration of erythromycin to the middle ear produces profound ototoxicity in experimental animals. However, the ototopical administration of this drug in humans is rare and has not recently been reported as a cause of eighth nerve toxicity. High doses of intravenous or oral erythromycin may produce tinnitis and bilateral deafness, without vestibular toxicity, but to date this has always been reversible upon withdrawal of the drug.[37] Liver disease, with resultant elevation of erythromycin blood levels due to diminished hepatic metabolism, seems to increase the risk of ototoxicity.

Pharmacologic interaction of erythromycin and carbamezepine (Tegretol) has recently been described. Rapid elevation in blood concentrations with resultant carbamezepine toxicity (confusion, ataxia, nausea and vomiting, diplopia) occurs when given together with erythromycin or troleandomycin. It is suggested that close clinical observation and monitoring of anticonvulsant blood levels be performed in all patients given concurrent erythromycin.

Metronidazole

Metronidazole is an imidazole derivative active against a variety of protozoal and anaerobic pathogens. Its notariety as putative mutagen and carcinogen have overshadowed its value as a chemotherapeutic agent and its other, less prominent, toxicities.

Metronidazole, however, is generally well tolerated. Gastrointestinal upset is the only frequent adverse reaction. Dose related minor neurologic side effects such as dizziness, headache, and depression are uncommon and reversible.[38]

Convulsions have been reported in three patients receiving massive doses (6 gm/day) of metronidazole.[39] None of these patients had an underlying seizure disorder. Risk factors other than dose are unknown, but renal insufficiency does not lead to drug accumulation since metronidazole is metabolized in the liver and only 7% is excreted unchanged in the urine. Convulsions have been shown to occur in experimental animals given high doses of the drug. Reversible ataxia, encephalopathy, and peripheral neuropathy are also described after metronidazole administration. Sensory neuropathy occurs after long-term therapy, and although ultimately reversible, paresthesias may persist for months.

Central nervous system concentrations of metronidazole obviously contribute to its neurotoxicity. The drug is well absorbed from all sites of administration and reaches CSF and brain concentrations 30 to 50% of simultaneous blood concentrations. Animal studies show distribution of radio-labelled metronidazole to brain, spinal cord, and dorsal root ganglia. Purkinje cell lesions and peripheral axonal degeneration have been seen but other studies report no histopathology despite functional abnormalities. Further definition of the risks, manifestations, and pathophysiology of metronidazole neurotoxicity remains to be achieved.

Nalidixic Acid

Nalidixic acid is a urinary antiseptic active against a variety of gram-negative bacilli. Adverse gastrointestinal, dermatologic, and neurologic reactions are frequently associated with the administration of this compound (NegGram) and its close relative, oxolinic acid (Utibid).

The most common neurologic aberrations associated with nalidixic acid administration are visual and psychological.[40] Visual disturbances occur in 10-20% of patients receiving the drug and include blurring of vision, scintillating scotomas, halo vision, changes in color perception, and visual hallucinations. These symptoms are associated with high peak blood levels and are rapidly reversible (within hours) after withdrawing the drug. The mechanism of action is unknown but may be due to generalized central nervous system stimulation. Mental disturbances occur frequently and may be as mild as drowsiness or confusion or as severe as acute delirium and toxic psychosis. These disturbances also appear related to peak blood level and are reversible. Mental abnormalities are more common in patients with underlying mental instability and care should be taken when prescribing nalidixic acid to such patients. Since the drug is excreted primarily by renal mechanisms its administration in renal insufficiency is not advised.

Convulsions occur with nalidixic acid administration but have not been reported with oxolinic acid. They are generalized, major motor seizures and are frequently accompanied by hyperglycemia, although the relationship of seizures to blood sugar is not established. In the presence of an underlying seizure disorder, seizures occur in the absence of hyperglycemia. Convulsions are related to dose and blood level, are more likely to be seen with overdose, and disappear after withdrawing the drug.

Benign intracranial hypertension is also described with nalidixic acid. It is rare and usually seen in infants. Typical clinical manifestations of pseudotumor cerebri develop after a few days of therapy and include irritability, vomiting, headache, and papilledema. Sixth nerve palsies have been described. Signs and symptoms resolve quickly after stopping the drug, although papilledema may persist for months.

Nitrofurantoin

Nitrofurantoin is a hydantoin derivative commonly used in the management of urinary tract infections, both therapeutically and prophylactically. A multitude of toxicities have been ascribed to its use, although pulmonary toxicity, gastrointestinal dysfunction, allergic reactions, and hepatotoxicity are the most common.[41] It is estimated that 10% of patients receiving nitrofurantoin develop significant adverse reactions. Although uncommon, neurotoxicity due to nitrofurantoin is well described and represents approximately 2% of adverse reactions to the drug, or about 0.2% of all patients receiving the drug.

Polyneuropathy presents as a sudden onset, predominantly sensory neuropathy in the distal extremities, lower greater than upper. It ascends in a bilaterally symmetrical fashion with subjective complaints of pain, numbness, and tingling sensations. Vibratory and position sense are usually more affected than pain or thermal sensation. Motor neuropathy follows symmetrically on the sensory deficit, with findings of weakness, atrophy, and areflexia in severe cases. Peripheral neuropathy is usually the exclusive neurologic abnormality, although retrobulbar neuropathy and emotional lability have been described in rare cases.[42]

Patients developing neuropathy are usually elderly and female. These patients receive lower daily doses of drug (mean, 150 mg/day) for a longer period of time (50% over 1 month) than other types of nitrofurantoin toxicity.[41] Most cases (80%), however, develop symptoms after less than 45 days of therapy,[42] although the toxicity may not be recognized until after the drug is stopped. The role of renal insufficiency as a risk factor is not clear. Literature reports cite the incidence of renal insufficiency in patients developing polyneuropathy as 30%[41] to 85%.[42]

Laboratory abnormalities are not associated with nitrofurantoin polyneuropathy. This is not an allergic manifestation of toxicity and, in contrast to nitrofurantoin pulmonary toxicity, eosinophilia is not seen. The spinal fluid is normal in 75%. The remaining 25% have slight increases in protein and no pleocytosis.

Thirty-five percent of patients experience total recovery after withdrawal of nitrofurantoin and another 50% have partial recovery. Only 15% show no change.[42] Recovery takes several days to several months, typically occurring over 4-8 weeks. Prognosis is most directly related to severity of neuropathy at diagnosis, and perhaps blood levels of nitrofurantoin. It is not related to total dose, duration of therapy, age, or sex. Continuing the drug in the face of neuropathy leads to worsening of signs and symptoms and has led to death from widespread motor neuropathy, weakness, and respiratory failure.

Pathologically there is demyelination, axonal swelling, and Wallerian degeneration in peripheral nerves. Abnormalities in dorsal root ganglia, demyelination of both dorsal and ventral roots, and chromatolysis of anterior horn cells has also been reported. These changes occur in the absence of local inflammation. Electromyography confirms denervation in distal musculature. Even in the absence of clinical toxicity and after only two weeks of therapy in individuals with normal renal function there are detectable decreases in both sensory and motor nerve conduction velocity.

The etiology of nitrofurantoin polyneuropathy is unknown. Clearly a direct, toxic, usually subclinical, effect on neurologic function is detectable in almost all patients but the biochemical basis for this toxicity remains unknown.

Penicillins and Cephalosporins

The neurotoxic potential of penicillin and cephalosporin derivatives is well established. Neurotoxicity is directly related to cerebrospinal fluid concentrations of drug and was first reported in association with direct intrathecal administration of penicillin. Although this route of administration has generally been abandoned, high CSF levels may still be achieved with massive doses (usually > 20 million units) of penicillin administered intravenously.

Neurotoxicity has been described due to penicillin G, ampicillin, methicillin, oxacillin, cloxacillin, carbenicillin, cephalothin, cephaloridine, cephalexin, and cefazolin (Fig. 3). Penicillin G is the most eleptogenic on a weight basis and has been responsible for most reported cases.[43] The biochemical basis of toxicity is uncertain but they may exert their effects in part by inhibition of the sodium/potassium pump. Neurotoxic symptoms usually begin within 24-72 hours after starting penicillin and terminate within 24-48 hours after stopping the drug. Seizures

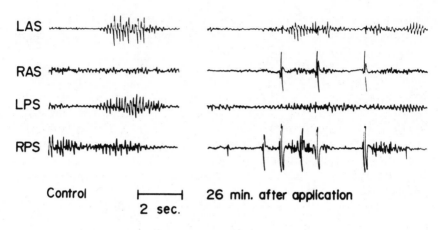

LAS

RAS

LPS

RPS

Control   ├────────┤   **26 min. after application**

2 sec.

Figure 3. Electrocorticogram of a cat before and 26 minutes after topical application of cephalothin. There is extensive high-voltage spike activity on the right side. From Garretson HD, Reid KH, Shields CB, et al: *J Neurosurg* **50**:792-797, 1979, with permission.

are refractory to usual anti-convulsant therapy, although intravenous paraldehyde has been useful on occasion.

Myoclonus is the most common clinical sign of toxicity and is seen in 70-75% of cases.[44] It varies from ocular twitching to continuous jerking of all muscles. Seizures, either focal or generalized, ensue in 60% and coma occurs in 40%. Hyperreflexia, hallucinations, and asterixis are also seen. Sudden death may occur in association with other neurologic manifestations, but is rare. Seizures are clearly of cortical origin, reflecting the effects of high concentrations of penicillin in the CSF. Myoclonus, however, may originate at subcortical or spinal cord levels.[45] It may be multifocal, asymetrical, and may occur in the absence of EEG abnormalities.

Renal insufficiency (BUN > 25) is the most important risk factor for penicillin neurotoxicity and is present in 77%,[46] to 84%[44] of cases. In fact, adults with normal renal function only develop myoclonus, not seizures. The most obvious explanation for the increased toxicity in azotemia is decreased penicillin clearance, resulting in high blood (> 300 units/ml in 70%) and CSF (> 25 units/ml in 75%) concentrations. The half-life of penicillin G increases from 20 minutes to 7 hours in renal failure, requiring major adjustments in dose to prevent such blood and tissue accumulation. Upper dosage limits can be calculated by the formula:[47]

$$\text{Dose (millions of units)} = 3.2 + \frac{\text{creatinine clearance}}{7}$$

Not only are high blood concentrations in uremia directly productive of high CSF concentrations, but the decreased capacity of uremic serum to bind acidic drugs results in increased free drug concentrations available for diffusion into the CSF. In addition, there is evidence of an impaired blood: CSF barrier in azotemia, perhaps further promoting increased CSF concentrations of penicillin and cephalosporin derivatives. Parenthetically, probenecid may increase CSF levels and promote toxicity by decreasing both renal secretion and active transport of penicillin out of the CSF via the choroid plexus.

Although age and underlying central nervous system disease are reported to increase the risk of penicillin neurotoxicity, there is little objective data to support this. Autopsy studies of patients suffering from penicillin neurotoxicity reveal normal or unremarkable central nervous system pathology in 73%.[44] Furthermore, in meningitis, seizures do not develop in the vast majority of patients despite increased permeability of the blood:brain barrier and decreased choroid plexus transport of penicillin out of the CSF.

Neurotoxicity has been seen frequently during cardiopulmonary bypass in patients receiving prophylactic penicillin. Experimental studies suggest increased permeability of the blood:CSF or blood:brain barrier due to microemboli or blood stasis. Similar explanation for penicillin neurotoxicity may apply to other vasculopathies such as endocarditis, systemic lupus, or gram-negative sepsis.

Continuous infusion of penicillin is more toxic than intermittent infusion. Forty percent of patients in one review received penicillin by this now fairly uncommon method.[44] Continuous infusion seems to produce higher CSF concentrations of antibiotic, perhaps by interfering with or saturating the active transport of penicillin from the CSF.

Procaine penicillin G can cause a constellation of bizarre neurologic symptoms which are directly related to high blood levels of free procaine.[48] Most cases are due to inadvertent intravenous administration where aqueous penicillin G was prescribed, or accidental intravenous injection during intramuscular administration. The manifestations of procaine toxicity occur within minutes of administration and are characterized by anxiety, dizziness, tinnitis, violent behavior, and generalized major motor seizures (Table III). Allergic manifestations (hives, bronchospasm, etc.) are not present and hypotension is not a feature of this syndrome.[49] The reaction rate in a venereal disease clinic population receiving intramuscular procaine penicillin is approximately 1%.

Diffuse muscle weakness due to hypokalemia is seen with administration of the sodium salts of penicillin and its derivatives. This may be profound, especially where high doses of the disodium derivatives carbenicillin and ticarcillin are used. Hypokalemia is due to the renal effects of secreted, non-reabsorbable anion resulting in accelerated losses of potassium. Potassium values < 2 meq/liter are reported and have led to respiratory failure due to intercostal muscle weakness.

Table III
Neurologic Manifestations of Procaine Toxicity in 21 Patients
Receiving Procaine Penicillin G

Manifestation	Number	Percentage
Dizziness	13	62
Weakness	5	24
Tinnitis	5	24
Violent behavior	4	19
Tremors	4	19
Seizures	3	14
Hallucinations	3	14
Headache	3	14
Dyspnea	3	14
Disorientation	2	10
Syncope	2	10

Polymyxins

Polymyxin B and colistin (polymyxin E) are polypeptide antibiotics used therapeutically in the 1960's for systemic gram-negative bacillary infections. Polymyxins bind to phospholipids in cell membranes resulting in toxicity to both bacterial and mammalian cells. Since the development of potent, less toxic, aminoglycoside antibiotics, polymyxin is now used primarily for topical therapy. However, their important neurotoxicity after parenteral administration deserves mention. There is negligible absorption after topical therapy to wounds or mucous membranes although neurotoxicity has been reported after this route of administration.[50]

Neurotoxicity occurs in 5-10% of patients receiving parenteral polymyxin. Paresthesias account for half of these reactions. They may be facial or peripheral, are benign, transient, and unrelated to other forms of neurotoxicity.

Neuromuscular blockade occurs in 2% of patients receiving polymyxin or colistin.[51] On a weight basis, these drugs are more potent than aminoglycoside antibiotics in producing experimental neuromuscular blockade and their effects are not reversed by either calcium or neostigmine.[2,5] Their mode of action appears related to their surface active properties on biologic membranes. Experimentally, the presynaptic release of acetylcholine is not diminished, but the sensitivity of the postsynaptic membrane to acetylcholine is decreased.

The usual manifestation of polymyxin neuromuscular blockade is apnea. Most reported cases are not associated with concomitant anesthesia or other neuromuscular blocking drugs in constrast to those associated with aminoglycoside administration.[50] The onset may occur within one day of starting therapy or after several days and may appear suddenly, without premonitory manifestations of neurotoxicity. It is more common in the elderly and occurs almost exclusively in patients with renal insufficiency. Minor manifestations of neuromuscular blockade may be seen without respiratory paralysis. These include generalized weakness, diplopia, and ptosis. Although there is a paucity of pharmacokinetic data in toxic patients, the risk of toxicity appears related to peak blood concentrations and total dose of polymyxin received.

Ototoxicity is not a commonly described adverse effect of polymyxin therapy. Decreased hearing does occur after topical therapy to the middle ear but is not described after parenteral therapy. Administration of polymyxin to animals produces deafness and its topical use in otitis should be cautioned, especially if perforation of the tympanic membrane is present. Reversible ataxia has also been reported. Such patients either have had renal insufficiency or received massive parenteral doses of polymyxin. Vertigo, nausea, and vomiting begin 1-4 days after starting therapy and nystagmus, decreased position sense, and staggering gait are the prominent physical findings. All signs and symptoms have disappeared upon withdrawal of the drug.[52]

Sulfonamides

To the sulfonamides are attributed a formidable list of untoward reactions. Most common (approximately 5% of patients exposed) are hypersensitivity reactions including rash, drug fever, serum sickness, and vasculitis. The latter two may include, as part of their systemic manifestations, neurologic abnormalities such as headache, altered mental status or aseptic meningitis.

Other neuropsychiatric disturbances may occur with sulfonamide administration that are not clearly part of a systemic hypersensitivity response. Such disturbances probably occur in less than 0.1% of patients receiving sulfonamides. Confusion, muscle weakness, vertigo, ataxia, tinnitus, tremor and convulsions are all reported. Rarely, an acute toxic psychosis may occur, especially in those individuals with a prior history of mental illness. Peripheral neuropathy has been reported in a handfull of cases. Both motor and sensory disturbances are described, together or independently, and are usually reversible.[53] The etiology of these neuropathies is not clear. Similar reactions may be seen with the fixed dose combination sulfamethoxazole-trimethoprim (Bactrim, Septra) due to its sulfonamide component. Neurotoxicity has not been attributed to trimethoprim.

Adverse reactions other than hypersensitivity phenomena are related to high doses of sulfonamide and blood levels over 50 mcg/ml. Eighty percent of reactors are slow acetylators and have a lower drug clearance and higher blood and tissue concentrations than fast acetylators. Adjusting the dose of sulfonamide in such patients may lead to disappearance of toxicity, including neuropathy, while the drug is continued at a lower dose if necessary.

Sulfonamides decrease the hepatic clearance of phenytoin resulting in elevated blood levels and possible toxicity. Blood levels of anticonvulsant drugs should be monitored closely in patients taking sulfonamides.

Tetracycline

Tetracycline derivatives cause pseudotumor cerebri in infants and young children, manifest by irritability, vomiting, and bulging fontanelles. Rarely, this syndrome is seen in older children and young adults where visual disturbances and headache predominate. Papilledema is described in approximately half the cases and sixth nerve palsies may appear. The syndrome results in no permanent neurologic deficit and remits within a few days after withdrawing the drug, although papilledema, if present, may persist for days to weeks. Pseudotumor cerebri has also been described in association with penicillin, ampicillin, and nalidixic acid administration (q. v.).

Minocycline is a semi-synthetic tetracycline with unique lipid solubility accounting for its large volume of distribution and the highest blood:brain ratio of any tetracycline derivative.[54] These characteristics probably account for its pronounced vestibular toxicity. Animal studies have shown no pathologic changes in the inner ear, however, so the exact mechanism of neurotoxicity is unknown.

The incidence of vestibular toxicity due to minocycline varies. Early reports, prior to 1974, suggested a lower incidence (average 7%, range 0-18%) than more recent data (average 70%, range 40-90%), perhaps in part due to vigilance in its detection or increased awareness of its occurrence leading to suggestive questioning of study participants. Placebo controlled studies[55] place the most reasonable estimate of vestibular toxicity at 50%: 30% of male recipients and 70% of female recipients.

Vestibular reactions are manifest by the second or third dose if a loading dose of 200 mg is given, or by the second or third day if no loading dose is given. This is consistent with achieving a threshhold blood level (the half-life of minocycline is 13.5 hours). The apparent greater susceptibility of females to vestibular toxicity is perhaps due to their smaller size and 25% higher blood levels on a fixed dose regimen (100 mg b. i. d.). The most common symptoms of toxicity include light headedness, vertigo, unsteady gait, nausea, and lack of concentrating ability. Some patients complain of weakness, headache, and loss of appetite. The electronystagmogram is of little help in detecting or standardizing toxicity because it correlates poorly with patient's subjective symptoms. Vestibular toxicity is more likely to occur in patients with prior vestibular disease, but is transient, and usually disappears within 48 hours of stopping the drug. However, patients with severe side effects may continue to have symptoms for three to five days.

Tetracyclines produce neuromuscular blockade experimentally[5] and in this context can potentiate the effects of d-tubocurarine. This blockade has been attributed to the interaction of tetracycline and calcium ions and its reversibility by calcium administration has been documented.[2] No decrease in acetylcholine release is seen and the site of action would appear to be postsynaptic. However, despite this experimental data, there is little evidence that tetracycline neuromuscular blockade is clinically important.

Vancomycin

Vancomycin, introduced in 1958, is a glycopeptide antibiotic active against almost all gram-positive bacteria. Although infrequently used after the introduction of β-lactamase-resistant penicillin derivatives in 1960, vancomycin has recently experienced a dramatic resurgence in use due to its activity against methicillin-resistant and tolerant staphylococci, enterococci, and *Clostridium difficile* (the cause of pseudomembranous colitis).

Vancomycin has a well established record of neurotoxicity. Ototoxicity, which is exclusively auditory, occurs frequently. Recent experience suggests that clinically decreased hearing is rare, perhaps less than 2% of treated cases, but abnormal audiograms characterized by decrease in high frequency sound reception occur in up to 20% of patients receiving the drug.[56] Hearing decrements may be transient, permanent but sub-clinical, or clinically significant, even progressing after the drug is stopped. Deafness occurs most frequently in the elderly and may or may not be preceded by tinnitus. The location of its toxic effect and the pathology of its toxicity are not well known.

Auditory toxicity occurs most frequently when vancomycin blood levels exceed 90 mcg/ml and is rarely seen at the serum levels less than 30 mcg/ml. After a usual dose of 500 mg intravenously in a patient with normal renal function, peak blood concentrations reach 15-20 mcg/ml. However, vancomycin is solely dependent upon glomerular filtration for excretion so that the half-life increases from 6 hours to 7 days in renal failure. Mild abnormalities of renal function, therefore, can lead to significant accumulation of the drug and increased risks of ototoxicity. Serial tests of renal function are indicated in all patients receiving the drug. Blood levels must be measured and serial audiograms performed in any patient with renal insufficiency, or the drug avoided under these circumstances. Daily maintenance doses to avoid peak blood levels above 20 mcg/ml can be estimated by the formula:

$$\text{Daily dose (mg)} = 150 + \text{creatinine clearance} \times 15$$

Toxicity occurs only after intravenous administration. Absorption after oral administration is negligible and serum levels after 2 gm/day orally for over two weeks remain less than 0.6 mcg/ml, even in anephric patients. In meningitis, CSF levels reach 10% of simultaneous serum levels but are less than 1% of serum levels in the absence of inflammation and seem to play little role in toxicity.

Transient paresthesias have been described after rapid intravenous administration of vancomycin. These are not associated with decreased hearing or other neurologic sequelae. Neuromuscular blockade has not been ascribed to vancomycin.

References

1. Bar RS, Wilson, HE, Mazzaferri EL: Hypomagnesemic hypocalcemia secondary to renal magnesium wasting — A possible consequence of high-dose gentamicin therapy. *Ann Intern Med* **82**: 650-658, 1975.
2. Singh YN, Harvey AL, Marshall IG: Antibiotic-induced paralysis of the mouse phrenic nerve-hemidiaphragm preparation, and reversibility by calcium and by neostigmine. *Anesthesiology* **48**:418-424, 1978.
3. Paradelis AG: Aminoglycoside antibiotics and neuromuscular blockade. *Antimicrob Chem* 5:737-738, 1979.
4. L'hommedieu C, Stough R, Brown L, et al: Potentiation of neuromuscular weakness in infant botulism by aminoglycosides. *J Pediatr* **95**:1065-1070, 1979.
5. Pittinger C, Adamson R: Antibiotic blockade of neuromuscular function. *Ann Rev Pharmacol* **12**:169-184, 1972.
6. Brummett RE, Brown RT: Tobramycin ototoxicity: A second look. *Arch Otolaryngol* **101**:540-543, 1975.
7. Bendush CL, Senior SL, Wooller HO: Evaluation of nephrotoxic and ototoxic effects of tobramycin in worldwide study. *Med J Aust Specl Supp* **2**:22-26, 1977.
8. Wersall J, Lundquist PG, Bjorkroth B: Ototoxicity of gentamicin. *J Infect Dis* **119**:410-416, 1969.
9. Hawkins JE, Johnsson LG, Aran JM: Comparative test of gentamicin ototoxicity. *J Infect Dis* **119**:417-426, 1969.

10. Federspil P, Schatzle W, Tiesler E: Pharmacokinetics and ototoxicity of gentamicin, tobramycin, and amikacin. *J Infect Dis* 134:S200-S204, 1976.
11. Christensen EF, Reiffenstein JC, Madissoo H: Comparative ototoxicity of amikacin and gentamicin in cats. *Antimicrob Agents Chemother* 12: 178-184, 1977.
12. Brummett RE, Traynor J. Brown R: Cochlear damage resulting from kanamycin and furosemide. *Acta Otolaryngol* 80:86-92, 1975.
13. Boston Collaborative Drug Surveillance Program: Drug-induced deafness. *JAMA* 224:515-516, 1973.
14. Hewitt WL: Gentamicin: toxicity in perspective. *Postgrad Med J* 50: Suppl 7:55-59, 1974.
15. Jackson GG, Arcieri G: Ototoxicity of gentamicin in man: A survey and controlled analysis of clinical experience in the United States. *J Infect Dis* 124:S130-S137, 1971.
16. Lane AZ, Wright GE, Blair DC: Ototoxicity and nephrotoxicity of amikacin. *Am J Med* 62:911-918, 1977.
17. Neu HC, Bendush CL: Ototoxicity of tobramycin: A clinical overview. *J Infect Dis* 134:S206-S218, 1976.
18. Fee WE, Vierra V, Lathrop GR: Clinical evaluation of aminoglycoside toxicity: tobramycin versus gentamicin, a preliminary report. *J Antimicrob Chemother* 4:Suppl A 31-36, 1978.
19. Smith CR, Lipsky JJ, Lietman PS: Relationship between aminoglycoside-induced nephrotoxicity and auditory toxicity. *Antimicrob Agents Chemother* 15:780-782, 1979.
20. Berk DP, Chalmers T: Deafness complicating antibiotic therapy of hepatic encephalopathy. *Ann Intern Med* 73:393-396, 1970.
21. Siber GR, Echeverria P, Smith AL, et al: Pharmacokinetics of gentamicin in children and adults. *J Infect Dis* 132:637-650, 1975.
22. Finitzo-Hieber T, McCracken GH, Roeser RJ, et al: Ototoxicity in neonates treated with gentamicin and kanamycin: Results of a four-year controlled follow-up study. *Pediatrics* 63:443-450, 1979.
23. McCracken GH, Mize SG, Threlkeld N: Intraventricular gentamicin therapy in gram-negative bacillary meningitis of infancy. *Lancet* 1: 787-791, 1980.
24. Watanabe I, Hodges GR, Dworzack DL, et al: Neurotoxicity of intrathecal gentamicin: A case report of experimental study. *Ann Neurol* 4:564-572, 1978.
25. Carnevale NT, Galgiani JN, Stevens DA, et al: Amphotericin B-induced myelopathy. *Arch Intern Med* 140:1189-1192, 1980.
26. Stevens DA: Miconazole in the treatment of systemic fungal infections. *Am Rev Respir Dis* 116:801-806, 1977.
27. Moulding T, Davidson PT: Tuberculosis II: Toxicity and intolerance to antituberculosis drugs. *Drug Therapy*, Feb 1974, pp 39-43.
28. Addington WW: The side effects and interactions of antituberculosis drugs. *Chest* 76S:782S-784S, 1979.
29. Lessell S: Histopathology of experimental ethambutol intoxication. *Investig Ophthalmol* 15:765-769, 1976.
30. Blakemore WF: Isoniazid. In: Spencer PS, Schaumburg HH, eds: *Experimental and Clinical Neurotoxicity* Baltimore, Williams and Wilkins, 1980, pp 478-489.

31. Godel V, Nemet P, Lazar M: Chloramphenicol optic neuropathy. *Arch Ophthalmol* **98**:1417-1421, 1980.
32. Beaugard ME, Asakuma S, Snow JB: Comparative ototoxicity of chloramphenicol and kanamycin with ethacrynic acid. *Arch Otolaryngol* **107**:104-109, 1981.
33. Proud GO, Mittelman H, Seiden GD: Ototoxicity of topically applied chloramphenicol. *Arch Otolaryngol* **87**:34-41, 1968.
34. Mittelman H: Ototoxicity of "ototopical" antibiotics: Past, present, and future. *Trans Am Acad Ophthalmol Otolaryngol* **76**:1432-1443, 1972.
35. Koup JR, Gibaldi M, McNamara P, et al: Interaction of chloramphenicol with phenytoin and phenobarbital. *Clin Pharmacol Ther* **24**: 572-575, 1978.
36. Wright JM, Collier B: Characterization of the neuromuscular block produced by clindamycin and lincomycin. *Can J Physiol Pharmacol* **54**:937-944, 1976.
37. Nicholas P: Erythromycin: Clinical review. *NY State J Med* **77**:2088-2246, 1977.
38. Roe FJ: Metronidazole: review of uses and toxicity. *J Antimicrob Chemother* **3**:205-212, 1977.
39. Frytak S, Moertel CG, Childs DS: Neurologic toxicity associated with high-dose metronidazole therapy. *Ann Intern Med* **88**:361-362, 1978.
40. Gleckman R, Alvarez S, Joubert DW, et al: Drug therapy reviews: Nalidixic acid. *Am J Hosp Pharm* **36**:1071-1076, 1979.
41. Holmberg L, Boman G, Bottiger LE, et al: Adverse reactions to nitrofurantoin. *Am J Med* **69**:733-738, 1980.
42. Toole JF, Parrish ML: Nitrofurantoin polyneuropathy. *Neurology* **23**: 554-559, 1973.
43. Garretson HD, Reid KH, Shields CB, et al: The effect of topical application of antibiotics on the cerebral cortex. *J Neurosurg* **50**:792-797, 1979.
44. Fossieck B, Parker RH: Neurotoxicity during intravenous infusion of penicillin. A review. *J Clin Pharmacol* **14**:504-512, 1974.
45. Sackellares JC, Smith DB: Myoclonus with electrocerebral silence in a patient receiving penicillin. *Arch Neurol* **36**:857-858, 1979.
46. Nicholls PJ: Neurotoxicity of penicillin. *J Antimicrob Chemother* **6**: 161-172, 1980.
47. Bryan CS, Stone WJ: "Comparably massive" penicillin G therapy in renal failure. *Ann Intern Med* **82**:189-195, 1975.
48. Green RL, Lewis JE, Kraus SJ, et al: Elevated plasma procaine concentrations after administration of procaine penicillin G. *N Engl J Med* **291**:223-226, 1974.
49. Galpin JE, Chow AW, Yoshikawa TT, et al: "Pseudoanaphylactic" reactions from inadvertent infusion of procaine penicillin G. *Ann Intern Med* **81**:358-359, 1974.
50. Lindesmith LA, Baines RD, Bigelow DB, et al: Reversible respiratory paralysis associated with polymyxin therapy. *Ann Intern Med* **68**: 318-327, 1968.
51. Koch-Wesser J, Sidel VW, Federman EB, et al: Adverse effects of sodium colistimethate. Manifestations and specific reaction rates during 317 courses of therapy. *Ann Intern Med* **72**:857-868, 1970.

52. Wolinsky E, Hines JD: Neurotoxic and nephrotoxic effects of colistin in patients with renal disease. *N Engl J Med* **266**:759-762, 1962.
53. Weinstein L, Madoff MA, Samet CM: The sulfonamides (concluded). *N Engl J Med* **263**:952-957, 1960.
54. Allen JC: Minocycline. *Ann Intern Med* **85**:482-487, 1976.
55. Fanning WL, Gump DW, Sofferman RA: Side effects of minocycline: A double-blind study. *Antimirob Agents Chemother* **11**:712-717, 1977.
56. Cook FV, Farrar WE: Vancomycin revisited. *Ann Intern Med* **88**: 813-818, 1978.

Chapter II

Neurological Complications of Cardiovascular Medication

Gordon J. Gilbert, M.D.

Introduction

Among all medications used to treat cardiovascular diseases, it is most unusual to find an isolated effect upon the cardiovascular system. Instead, these drugs characteristically have only a relative tissue specificity, and thus not infrequently manifest significant deleterious effects upon other body organs, including particularly both the central and peripheral nervous systems. That the nervous system becomes the target of these toxic side-effects is not surprising, since neural tissue exhibits delicate sensitivity to metabolic and toxic environmental pertubations. Moreover, these drugs frequently have potent hemodynamic effects capable of causing significant alterations in cerebral blood flow that result in diffuse or even focal cerebral ischemic manifestations. Resulting neurological symptoms are frequently prominent and devastating, and may include weakness, numbness, dizziness, confusion, delirium, agitation, muscular twitching and convulsive seizures, headaches and visual disturbances. The neurological manifestations of cardiovascular drug toxicity thus often present as important problems in therapy.

Diuretics

Of those drugs used to treat cardiovascular disorders, the diuretics are among the most commonly prescribed. Accordingly, the frequency of neurological complications due to diuretics is unusually high. Symptomatic hyponatremia is not uncommon in the patient treated with thiazide diuretics, furosemide or ethacrynic acid. Diuretically induced hyponatremia may be distinguished from other causes of hyponatremia by the associated hypokalemia and alkalosis. The presenting symptoms of the diffuse, metabolic encephalopathy are weakness and lassitude. As the severity of hyponatremia worsens, there is increasing lethargy, confusion, and finally coma.[1] Asterixis may be found in the presence of only mild to moderate degrees of hyponatremia and should be sought whenever hyponatremia is suspected; when the patient holds his arms in front of him with wrists hyperextended, flapping movements appear at the wrists, symmetrically or asymmetrically, constituting an instability of extensor posturing of the wrists. Asterixis may betray the presence of even a mild hyponatremia, while in more severe hyponatremia, there may be myoclonic jerkings of the extremities; more often, the patient will simply become increasingly lethargic and finally comatose.[1]

Hyponatremia may also present with quite focal paralytic neurological manifestations. In a personally observed case,[2] a 72-year-old woman was seen with confusion, weakness, visual hallucinations of ants crawling on the walls, and left-sided hemiplegia. A stroke with left hemiparesis two years earlier had been followed by considerable recovery, so that the patient could walk but was deficient in the fine use of her left hand. She had been on a low-salt diet for two years, and two weeks before admission daily hydrochlorothiazide (Esidrix) was started. Neurologic deterioration began at that time and progressed steadily to the time of the admission; the serum sodium was then 105 mEq/L, the potassium 2.3 mEq, and the chloride 51 mEq/L. Correction of this electrolyte imbalance resulted in dramatic improvement within 48 hours, and the left extremities regained their usefulness.

The diagnosis of focal paralytic manifestations of hyponatremia may be suspected at the bedside and before the serum electrolytes have been determined. An important clue to the underlying metabolic encephalopathy is the association with a marked organic confusional state disproportionate to that commonly found in simple hemiplegic stroke.[2] Such is also true of other metabolic encephalopathies and is not at all specific for hyponatremia. There may be further evidence of a more diffuse cortical hyperirritability, such as the visual hallucinations seen in the patient described above, or bilateral, small myoclonic jerks of the four extremities. This patient had no evidence of a new stroke, and in fact, her recovery was complete immediately upon correction of her hyponatremia.

A further case of an acute, reversible hemiparesis precipitated by two intravenous injections of furosemide (40 mg) was more recently described.[3] The serum sodium level fell to 116 mEq/L, and the patient became stuporous and then comatose, with a right hemiparesis and hemisensory deficit. Upon correction of her hyponatremic state, the neurological deficit resolved, and when her serum sodium reached 123 mEq/L after six hours of intravenous 5 percent saline, she became arousable and her neurological signs resolved completely. Faris and Poser were able to induce metabolic hemiparesis experimentally; hyponatremia was produced in dogs that had previously undergone ligation of the left middle cerebral artery and were allowed to make complete neurological recovery.[4] When such dogs were rendered hyponatremic, right hemiparesis reappeared and could be immediately and dramatically abolished by the intravenous infusion of sodium.

Fichman has demonstrated the mechanism of thiazide-induced hyponatremia to be an initial depletion of body potassium which triggers an inappropriate secretion of antidiuretic hormone, resulting in both dilutional hyponatremia and enhanced renal salt losses.[5] Because of this, the administration of potassium may be quite useful in reversing diuretic hyponatremia, and the restriction of fluid intake to 900 cc or less per 24 hours will also promote more rapid recovery. In addition, the judicious administration of hypertonic saline solution (e.g., 300 ml of 3 percent saline) is often useful.

In addition to their hyponatremic manifestations, diuretics may adversely influence cerebral function by producing an acute depletion of blood fluid volume, or a chronic hypotension. This volume depletion may result in orthostatic hypotension, such that the patient becomes light-headed upon standing up, and may experience presyncope or actual syncope. Characteristically, the orthostatic hypotension is at its worst immediately upon arising from a chair and while standing still rather than walking; a typical attack will occur in an individual who has been supine or sitting for 10 minutes or longer, then arises quickly, experiences light-headedness and syncope. The serum sodium may be perfectly normal in such hypotensive patients whose only other symptoms may be lethargy and mild weakness but may progress to a severe confusional state. The orthostatic hypotension is best treated initially with the use of elastic stockings and a tight belt, but if such measures do not suffice, then a reduction in diuretic dosage may be indicated.

A third major problem produced by the thiazide diuretics is hypokalemia, presenting neurologically as increasing and diffuse muscular weakness leading to paralysis. The weakness induced by hypokalemia has been shown to correlate with certain ultrastructural changes in muscle, including swollen, condensed, and disintegrated mitochondria and dilatation of the transverse tubules and sarcoplasmic reticulum with vacuole formation.[6]

Such weakness generally has a myopathic distribution, affecting proximal muscles of the limb girdles more severely than the distal muscles, with early weakness of the deltoid, the external rotators of the shoulders, and the hip flexors. When such hypokalemic weakness is severe, there may be prominent elevation of the serum creatine kinase, aldolase, and SGOT, as well as myoglobinemia and myoglobinuria, the results of rhabdomyolysis.[7] Characteristically, hypokalemic proximal weakness is painless, but when more severe and associated with rhabdomyolysis, may be painful and associated with muscle cramps.

Hypokalemia may also induce a further variety of syncope due to Stokes-Adams attacks.[8] When a patient on diuretic medication experiences syncope, one must particularly suspect orthostatic hypotension, but if such is not found, and if hypokalemia is present, then Stokes-Adams attacks may be responsible for the syncope, and a Holter monitor study may be of diagnostic value.

It is distinctly unusual for diuretic medication alone to cause symptomatic hypokalemia; accordingly, in the presence of a severe hypokalemia, the physician should seek out a second contributing cause such as chronic ingestion of licorice, corticosteroid medication, Cushing's disease, vomiting, diabetic ketoacidosis, or certain antibiotics, such as carbenicillin, gentamicin, nafcillin, and methicillin. All of these agents or disorders may themselves produce hypokalemia, which may then be only intensified by the concomitant use of a thiazide diuretic. Of course the specific diuretic is of much consequence, and if, for example, spironolactone is the diuretic used, there will be no tendency toward hypokalemia, but instead, hyperkalemia may occur and may itself cause weakness.

It has recently been suggested that diuretic hypokalemia may be a significant cause of mental depression.[9] Such would presumably relate to the cerebral effects of hypokalemia and might be considered when a patient on diuretics becomes seriously depressed.

Cardiac Glycosides

Neurotoxicity is, after G.I. symptoms, by far the most common manifestation of digitalis overdosage, and headache and fatigue are particularly frequent symptoms.[10] The central nervous system manifestations do not always precede evidence of cardiac toxicity and do not correlate well with serum glycoside levels, but it is important that they be recognized as glycoside-induced, so as to prevent severe toxicity.[11] Digitalis delirium has been provoked by varied glycosides, including Digoxin, Gitalin, and Digitoxin.[12] It was originally described in 1874 by Duroziez,[13] who also emphasized the occurrence of coma as a more severe manifestation.

The primary form of digitalis neurotoxicity, digitalis delirium, relates to the toxic influence of digitalis upon the cerebral cortex, an influence that has both depressive and irritative components. Included among the cortical depressive components are giddiness, drowsiness, fatigue, weakness, disorientation and confusion, progressing to coma. Irritative symptoms of restlessness, headache, nervousness, agitation, hallucinations, psychotic episodes and convulsions are frequently found in association with these depressive symptoms.[11] When multiple etiologies contribute to a confusional state, the significance of the contribution by the cardiac glycoside may be overlooked.

Digitalis delirium frequently is associated with visual changes, including blurred or hazy vision, a green or yellow flickering amblyopia, scotoma, photophobia, and red-green color-blindness. Notable features of the delirium include a more common occurrence in older age groups, a frequent association with aortic valve lesions, and the influence of the premorbid personality upon the type of psychosis provoked by digitalis intoxication.[12] Digitalis delirium may be the earliest and possibly the only sign of intoxication, and occurs in the absence of electrolyte imbalance, sedation, anoxia, and Cheyne-Stokes respirations. Its resolution, even when delirium is caused by a short-acting glycoside, may be remarkably slow, requiring up to two weeks after discontinuation of the glycoside.

Douglas et al described a remarkable case in which momentary blackouts that began at age 72 were found to be electroencephalographically associated with diffuse bursts of 3 Hz spike-and-wave activity.[14] This paroxysmal EEG abnormality was due to digitalis intoxication, and cleared when digitalis was discontinued. Thus, the finding of paroxysmal epileptiform activity in the EEG of a patient on a digitalis preparation should raise a question of digitalis intoxication. The topical and intravenous administration of ouabain has been effective in the experimental production of cortical epileptiform activity,[15] experimentally demonstrating the cortical irritative effect of cardiac glycosides. By inhibiting sodium-potassium-dependent adenosine triphosphatase, ouabain causes a decrease in membrane potential and thus enhances a tendency to self-sustained seizure activity.

There have been several reports of a more localized neurotoxicity involving the trigeminal nerve or nucleus. Trigeminal neuralgias and paresthesias may occur as a manifestation of digitalis neurotoxicity.[16] Digitalis-induced bradyarrhythmia may have caused an occurrence of transient global amnesia,[17] a condition of temporarily impaired memory-recording that is thought to have a medial temporal lobe ischemic or epileptic etiology.[18]

Coronary Vasodilators

Headache is the most common neurological manifestation of the nitrites and nitrates used to treat angina pectoris. It is common at effective dose levels but is less frequent when dosage increments are gradual.[19,20]

Caused by extracranial dilatation in the distribution of the external carotid arteries, it is a natural consequence of effective vasodilation. Patients subject to the vasodilatory headaches of migraine (constituting up to 20 percent of the population) are particularly susceptible. In fact, it is remarkable that headache is not a more frequent or constant problem in vasodilator treatment. Typically throbbing, it tends to disappear after several days to weeks of nitrate therapy,[21] and also responds to reduction in dose.

Nitrites and nitrates not infrequently produce some degree of orthostatic hypotension, but in some patients this may be severe. Light-headedness, syncope and stroke may occur, particularly when vasodilator therapy is used for an acute attack.[19] In patients reporting light-headedness when these drugs are taken, it is wise prophylaxis to recommend the supine position prior to use, and elevation of the legs may be of further aid. Elastic stockings may ameliorate the orthostatic fall in cerebral blood flow.

In a small proportion of patients in whom perhexiline maleate is used in the treatment of angina pectoris, a sensorimotor peripheral neuropathy develops. Those individuals developing peripheral neuropathy are probably slow metabolizers of the drug, and develop unusually high blood levels. The mechanism of this toxic neuropathy is one of Schwann cell damage resulting in segmental demyelination and slowing of nerve conduction velocities.[22] The initial symptoms of distal paresthesias are accompanied or followed by weakness, and appear first in the toes and later in the fingers. It is a slowly progressive neuropathy and may produce severe disability. Electrophysiologic studies reveal slowed nerve conduction velocities which become faster when the perhexiline maleate is discontinued. The dosage and duration of perhexiline maleate vary from case to case, but patients always recover when the drug is discontinued. Improvement begins within two weeks and continues for weeks or months. The recognition of the distal paresthesias and weakness that are the earliest manifestations of perhexiline maleate neuropathy must lead to prompt discontinuation of the drug. While the proportion of symptomatic cases is small, a subclinical neuropathy, chracterized by slowed nerve conduction velocities and electromyographic changes, may be quite common. It is advisable to obtain baseline nerve conduction velocity studies in patients selected for therapy with perhexiline maleate, and to order further nerve conduction velocity studies at yearly intervals in patients undergoing chronic treatment with this drug.

Antiarrhythmic Medications

Quinidine may cause an acute confusional state. Used primarily in the treatment of atrial fibrillation and certain other cardiac arrhythmias, quinidine is well recognized to be a dangerous as well as an effective drug. Occasionally, the introduction of even small doses may cause tinnitus, vertigo, visual disturbance, headache, and acute confusional state.

Quinidine is a toxic drug whose effect on the myocardium reflects a more generalized cellular toxicity. It affects many biological systems and has been referred to as "a general protoplasmic poison." Quinidine is toxic to many bacteria and other unicellular organisms, such as yeast, plasmodia, and spermatozoa. It depresses excitability, contractility and conduction velocity of the heart, increases the muscular weakness of patients with myasthenia gravis, [23,24] and may induce a syndrome resembling lupus erythematosus. Cinchonism, a combination of headache, visual and auditory disturbances, is generally seen in the early stages of quinidine usage and responds to reduction in dosage. Well-recognized manifestations of quinidine toxicity include nausea, vomiting, cramps, diarrhea, tinnitus, vertigo, and blurred vision. Not as well recognized is a group of symptoms referred to as "central nervous system symptoms," consisting of difficulty in speaking, confusion and excitement or somnolence, followed by unconsciousness alternating with delirium.[25] Coma and generalized convulsions may occur. Manifestations of pyramidal tract involvement, including Babinski signs, have been described.

In addition, quinidine has been demonstrated to be a cause of chronic and progressive dementia. In the initial case of this quinidine dementia syndrome,[26] a 72-year-old woman who had taken quinidine for 14 years after an acute myocardial infarction was hospitalized with severe memory loss and chronic confusion of several years duration, manifested by disorientation for time and place and greatly impaired memory, inability to perform household tasks, to cope with small sums of money, remember a short shopping list, find her way about indoors or along familiar streets, or recall recent events. The syndrome included impaired regard for the feelings of others, purposeless hyperactivity, and marked emotional lability, with a tendency to sexual misdemeanor. Only over the last several of the 14 years that she had consumed quinidine daily had the patient undergone progressive dementia. The relationship of her dementia to quinidine usage was distinct, and not only was her dementia inexorably progressive over this period of several years, but it improved remarkably within 24 hours of discontinuing quinidine, and progressively recovered over the ensuing six months. In fact, the patient regained her intelligence level approximating that of two years earlier. Her improvement was well documented by serial studies of orientation and intelligence. Electroencephalographic changes present during the period of quinidine dementia also cleared after discontinuation of quinidine.

Early adverse effects of quinidine are likely to be detected and corrected by reducing or eliminating its use. When, however, a confusional state develops in a patient who has taken quinidine for many years, it is not surprising that the possible relationship of quinidine to this evolving confusional state might be overlooked in the search for a more expected cause of progressive dementia. When thorough neurological evaluations fail to disclose a cause of progressive dementia, the discontinuation of a usual quinidine regimen should be considered. In essence, when after thorough neurological evaluation no cause of a progressive dementia has been established, it behooves the physician to attempt the discontinuation of any medication that has been used throughout the period of evolution of this dementia.

Further cases of quinidine dementia, including cases in physicians, are known to the author. Generally, such cases have had thorough neurologic evaluations, often including potentially hazardous studies such as arteriography, prior to recognition that the chronic use of quinidine itself caused the dementia.

Quinidine can also produce a myopathy,[27] manifested by proximal weakness and elevation of serum muscle enzymes, including CPK, aldolase, SGOT, and LDH. This myopathy may be caused by increased sarcoplasmic concentration of unbound calcium.

Finally, quinidine syncope should be suspected when a patient receiving quinidine suddenly loses consciousness or complains of light-headedness. Quinidine syncope may be due to a variety of factors, including vasodilatation, orthostatic hypotension, or arrhythmia.

Procainamide (Pronestyl) may also cause light-headedness and syncope due to hypotension. Of greater frequency and significance is a lupus erythematosus syndrome which appears in approximately 20 percent of patients taking Procainamide. Eighty to ninety percent of patients receiving this drug develop antinuclear antibodies after three to six months of procainamide therapy; these clear when the drug is discontinued, as does the lupus-like syndrome. Commonly encountered in this procainamide-lupus syndrome are confusion and disorientation, but no other neurologic problems are reported.[28]

Propranolol (Inderal) may cause hypotension with light-headedness and syncope. Its use in hypoglycemia is contraindicated, since it will suppress the sympathetically mediated rebound response, and may mask associated symptoms of sweating and tachycardia. Propranolol readily crosses the blood-brain barrier and has sedative and anticonvulsant effects upon laboratory animals. In some patients mood and affect are altered. Most neurologic side effects have occurred when propranolol was used, over long periods and in large doses in the treatment of hypertension.[29] Most common among the central nervous system effects are fatigue and lethargy. while less common are vivid dreams, insomnia, depression, hallucinations and peripheral neuropathy.[30] There is a rare report of acute confusional state complicating the induction of propranolol therapy. A newer beta adrenergic blocking agent, metoprolol, may, like propranolol, also induce depression and fatigue.

Phenytoin (Dilantin), a drug primarily used in the treatment of seizure disorders, has also been of use in the treatment of cardiac arrhythmias. Whenever phenytoin is used, it is of particular importance that the serum level be monitored. The major side effects of phenytoin are neurological, and correlate closely with blood levels above 20 μg/ml. Because the efficacy of hepatic detoxification of phenytoin may vary markedly from patient to patient, the final serum phenytoin level cannot be predicted readily on the basis of total daily dosage. After phenytoin therapy is initiated, up to 10 to 14 days will be required at a fixed dosage level in order to attain a steady blood level. As the serum phenytoin level rises above 20 μg/ml, nystagmus and ataxia are found, while at still higher blood levels, drowsiness, stupor, chorea and coma ensue. Further discussion of phenytoin neurotoxicity can be found in Chapter XIII in this book.

The major side effects of lidocaine also relate to its central nervous system effects.[31] At plasma levels above 5 μg/ml, drowsiness, dizziness, and agitation may occur. Somnolence and parasthesias often precede the more severe reactions including euphoria, disorientation, psychosis, coma and convulsive seizures. Somnolence and paresthesias may thus be important early warnings of the imminence of these more severe neurological side effects.[30]

Disopyramide (Norpace) may cause light-headedness and syncope due to an induced hypotension, and urinary retention through its anticholinergic effects. It may also produce a toxic psychosis which remits following discontinuation of the drug.[28,30]

Bretylium (Bretylol) may also cause hypotensive dizziness and syncope, and problems of cerebral ischemia may appear as a result of systemic hypotension. This drug, like many of the others described in this section, may also cause a toxic psychosis manifested by disorientation, confusion, and hallucinations.[28,30]

Verapamil, a papaverine derivative, may cause hypotensive light-headedness, dizziness, and syncope, as well as headache.[30,32]

An adverse effect of the antiarrhythmic agents as a class upon the disease myasthenia gravis has long been recognized.[23,24] Among the agents that can precipitate clinical myasthenia in a susceptible individual, or worsen pre-existing myasthenia gravis, are quinidine, procainamide,[33] trimethaphan, and several of the beta adrenergic blocking agents.[34] The effect is mediated through an interference with neuromuscular transmission. Quinidine can unmask or aggravate myasthenia gravis and can cause a delayed postoperative respiratory depression due to its interaction with muscle relaxants. Its L-isomer quinine, has well-known neuromuscular blocking effects, and at one time was used in a provocative test for the diagnosis of myasthenia gravis. Procainamide exerts a post-synaptic curare-like effect.[33] Among the beta adrenergic blockers, propranolol, oxyprenolol, and practolol[35] have all been reported to induce a myasthenia gravis syndrome or to unmask latent myasthenia gravis.[36] At concentrations comparable to those used therapeutically, propranolol produces a post-synaptic curare-like effect. Even phenytoin has been shown experimentally to interfere with neuromuscular transmission through a combined pre-synaptic and post-synaptic action,[37] and a myasthenic syndrome has occurred in some patients taking this drug, as has an exacerbation of myasthenia gravis.[38]

Anticoagulants

When a patient receiving anticoagulant therapy develops a sudden, subacute or slow neurological deterioration, the physician should suspect intracranial hemorrhage, acute or chronic subdural hematoma, spinal epidural hematoma, or hemorrhagic femoral neuropathy. In a group of over 600 patients receiving anticoagulant drugs at New York Hospital, 23 were found to have "CVA's".[39] Of these, nine proved to be cerebral hemorrhages, five subdural hematoma, and nine cerebral embolism. In the anticoagulated patient, relatively slight head trauma may lead to subdural hematoma,[40] particularly when the prothrombin time is excessive. Hypertension also acts to increase the incidence, severity, and mortality of intracranial bleeding in the anticoagulated patient, as does cerebral angiitis.[41,42-44]

The neurological complications of anticoagulation are often severe. While occurring more often in patients whose prothrombin time or partial thromboplastin time has been allowed to become excessively high, they may also be seen when these indices are in the therapeutic range. Headache in the anticoagulated patient should always suggest intracranial bleeding. Cerebral hemorrhage is always suspect in the anticoagulated patient presenting with a stroke-like syndrome, headache, or stiff neck.[40] Pure subarachnoid hemorrhage presenting with severe headache, stiff neck, and back pain will be diagnosed by careful lumbar puncture. The best method for diagnosis of cerebral hemorrhage is by computerized tomographic (CT) brain scan, which can reveal practically all parenchymal hemorrhages.

If a CT scanner is not readily available, other diagnostic studies short of arteriography may be useful in ruling out intracranial hematoma. Skull x-rays or an echoencephalogram may show a pineal shift away from the hematoma. The electroencephalogram may reveal localized flattening of amplitude over a subdural hematoma, and focal slow wave activity, sharp waves or spikes related to intracranial hemorrhage. The isotope brain scan may display a characteristic picture in subdural or intracerebral hemorrhage.

Subdural hematoma occurs with increased frequency in the anticoagulated patient and is usually apparent on CT brain scan. Characteristically, subdural hematoma produces obtundation, but there may also be focal neurological signs, papilledema, or pupillary asymmetries. Bilateral subdural hematoma can be a particularly difficult diagnostic problem, since, when subacute, the hematoma may on the CT scan appear isodense with the brain, and when bilateral may produce no shift of the ventricular structures. The "hypernormal" CT scan, in which the ventricles are unusually small, may suggest subacute, isodense, bilateral subdural hematoma, but carotid arteriograms may be necessary in order to establish that diagnosis. In contrast, the unilateral subdural hematoma, is almost always apparent on the CT scan and is thus readily diagnosed in the obtunded, anticoagulated patient.

More rarely, anticoagulation may promote the formation of a spinal epidural or subdural hematoma which will characteristically present with progressive cord compression, requiring prompt surgical decompression in order to prevent permanent paraplegia. The clinical picture is of severe back pain at the level of the lesion and leading to a rapid onset of paraparesis which progresses to paraplegia over a period of several hours or days. A myelogram should be ordered on an emergency basis when spinal epidural hematoma is suspected. CT scan of the appropriate spinal level may also prove diagnostic.

The treatment of intracranial subdural hematoma and of spinal epidural or subdural hematoma is surgical, but craniotomy or laminectomy should be postponed until blood coagulation mechanisms have been controlled. When anticoagulation must be stopped and reversed rapidly because of hemorrhage, there is no increased risk of rebound thromboembolism.[45]

In the anticoagulated patient, retroperitoneal hematoma not infrequently presents as a femoral neuropathy.[46] The femoral nerve passes through a discreet compartment beneath the inguinal ligament and may be compressed at this site. A similar syndrome occurs in hemophilia. In a personally observed case,[47] a 58-year-old man, anticoagulated with Coumadin, presented with a prothrombin time of 52 seconds and excruciating pain localized to the right inguinal region and radiating to the medial aspect of the lower leg anteriorly. This was associated with numbness of the anterior aspect of his right thigh and the anteromedial area of the right lower leg, marked weakness of the hip, and an inability to extend the right knee. The pain characteristically was relieved by maintaining his right hip in a position of complete flexion. The observed pattern of hypalgesia was in the distribution of the long saphenous branch of the femoral nerve. In cases of hemorrhagic femoral neuropathy, there is characteristically a flaccid paralysis of the quadriceps muscle and loss of the knee jerk. There may be exquisite sensitivity over the femoral nerve at the inguinal ligament, and palpation in this area may reproduce the pain pattern.[48] Hot packs to the inguinal area may provide dramatic pain relief, and the prognosis is favorable once the prothrombin time has been normalized.

Further discussion of the neurological complications of anticoagulants will be found in Chapter XIV.

Clofibrate

Clofibrate (Atromid-S), used in the treatment of hyperlipemia, may cause a reversible, dose-related myositis as an uncommon reaction that will necessitate the discontinuation of the drug.[49] Other symptoms more rarely produced by clofibrate are drowsiness, giddiness, and weakness. Clofibrate myositis characteristically begins with muscular pain and stiffness, weakness and malaise.[50,51] The myositis usually begins acutely within three days of starting therapy; the proximal muscles, and particularly those of the hips, thighs, and low back are found to be tender. The deep tendon reflexes may be hypoactive. In addition to stiffness and weakness, muscle pain in the arms and legs may become severe, leading to an inability to walk. The muscles are tender both to palpation and during passive limb movements. Consistent with the diagnosis of myositis, there may be elevation of the erythrocyte sedimentation rate, serum glutamic-oxalacetic transaminase, serum pyruvate transaminase and lactic dehydrogenase, while serum levels of creatine phosphokinase may exceed 12,000 units. In more severe cases, there is myoglobinemia and myoglobinuria. The electrocardiogram may show evidence of an associated cardiomyopathy, [52] and death has been reported. Once clofibrate has been discontinued, a good recovery of strength may take a month or more, but there is often prompt relief of the muscular pain and tenderness.

Onset of disability is more gradual in some cases and may take the form of a progressive myopathy, with proximal muscle wasting and weakness. In such cases, the deep tendon reflexes may be hyperactive, yet nerve conduction velocities slowed, indicating a peripheral motor neuropathy. This pattern appears to be more frequent when clofibrate is administered in the presence of uremia. Again, symptoms and signs tend to clear within two months after the clofibrate is withdrawn.

The efficacy of clofibrate may depend upon an increase in lipoprotein lipase activity, and the myopathy is probably due to the production of toxic plasma levels of 3-chlorophenoxyisobutylic acid.[53] Clofibrate myositis appears more often in patients having a low serum albumin (to which clofibrate is firmly bound), so that the percentage of unbound serum clofibrate is elevated. The myositis is also more common in patients with poor renal function,[54,55] since 95 percent of clofibrate is conjugated with glucuronic acid in the kidney and excreted in the urine. Thus, impaired renal function results in the elevated serum clofibrate levels which seem necessary to produce the reversible dose-related myositis. Chronic renal failure is an absolute contraindication to the use of clofibrate for the treatment of co-existing hyperlipidemia. Clofibrate myositis also occurs with increased frequency in the presence of hypothyroidism, and the drug should not be administered when untreated hypothyroidism is present.

Antihypertensive Medications

The neurological complications of antihypertensive medication must be considered to include those related directly to its effective antihypertensive action. Thus, hypotension, and particularly orthostatic hypotension, is a potential complication of almost all antihypertensive therapies.[56]Moreover, enthusiastic antihypertensive medication in the elderly may result in strokes. Under the heading "inappropriate antihypertensive therapy in the elderly," Jackson et al[57] reported six patients, aged 64 to 84, previously asymptomatic, all of whom became comatose within a week of beginning varied antihypertensive regimens. Each of these patients initially had symptoms of orthostatic hypotension, and one suffered a residual occipital infarction. Antihypertensive treatment should be initiated cautiously, particularly in the elderly, with gradual increments over periods of weeks or months based upon clinical response. The regular use of elastic stockings is often useful in reducing the severity of orthostatic hypotension.

The diuretics are discussed separately because of their multiple uses. Other aspects of orthostatic hypotension due to medication will be presented in Chapter XVI.

Diazoxide, administered in the treatment of hypertensive crisis, will occasionally cause headache, but may precipitate cerebral ischemia in up to one percent of patients, and cerebral infarction with hemiplegia has been reported.[58] An oral dosage form of diazoxide has been developed, and with the long-term administration of this agent, extrapyramidal symptoms of a parkinsonian type may develop.

Reserpine has a modest antihypertensive efficacy but may produce major neurological complications. The drug may worsen migrainous vasospastic attacks, while reducing the incidence of migraine headaches.[59] The chronic use of daily reserpine may induce a parkinsonian syndrome that is indistinguishable from idiopathic Parkinson's disease, but will usually clear completely within a month after discontinuing the reserpine. This drug-induced parkinsonism will respond to medications used in the treatment of Parkinson's disease, including levodopa and trihexyphenidyl. It is considered best, however, to discontinue reserpine when parkinsonism occurs in the course of its use. Epileptic seizures, including grand mal convulsions, have at times complicated the use of reserpine and are reason enough to discontinue reserpine. Psychic depression is a much more frequent side effect of chronic reserpine therapy and at times will become so severe as to lead to suicide. A history of depression is an absolute contraindication to the use of reserpine.

Methyldopa (Aldomet) also has many possible neurologic effects, including sedation, headache, orthostatic hypotension, depression, insomnia, nightmares, and hallucinations. Most of these can be considered effects upon the cerebral cortex and are adequate reason to discontinue methyldopa. Impaired concentrating ability, dyslexia, dyscalculia, and amnesia-like attacks may occur in the patient on methyldopa. Adler[60] described five professionals with symptoms of this type, all clearing within 96 hours of discontinuing methyldopa. Methyldopa dementia was reported by Kurtz[61] in a 36-year-old, intelligent nurse taking 750 mg daily. After 43 days of therapy, she developed forgetfulness and recent memory impairment, which began to recover within two days of discontinuing methyldopa and completely cleared within two weeks. A Parkinson-like syndrome may also complicate the use of methyldopa and is characterized by a predominance of rigidity and akinesia, frequently in the absence of tremor, making it more difficult to diagnose. Characteristically such patients present with "weakness" and falling. Subsidence of these symptoms may take several weeks following discontinuation of methyldopa.

Propranolol (Inderal) can reduce exercise tolerance, perhaps by causing a mild myopathy. Propranolol may also mask hypoglycemic symptoms in diabetics receiving insulin therapy. Among the central nervous system side effects of propranolol are insomnia, nightmares, hallucinations, fatigue, depression, paresthesia, ataxia, and dizziness.[62] It is frequently possible to relieve the insomnia and bad dreams by avoidance of a late evening dose of propranalol. Drowsiness and depression are relatively infrequent in comparison with such agents as reserpine, methyldopa, and clonidine.

Metoprolol (Lopressor), a newer beta-adrenergic antagonist released for clinical use in the United States in 1978, has caused tiredness and dizziness in about 10 percent of patients, and depression in five percent.[63] Early reports have also mentioned headache, insomnia, and nightmares. Like propranalol, metoprolol can mask some of the clinical signs of hypoglycemia.

Clonidine (Catapres) has been reported to cause mental confusion. A 72-year-old man receiving clonidine, 0.3 mg daily, developed dementia characterized by memory loss, confusion, aggressiveness, incontinence, and unsteady gait, which cleared completely within a week of discontinuing clonidine.[64] A 33-year-old man receiving clonidine, 0.2 mg daily experienced lethargy, agitation, disorientation, confusion, and impaired short-term memory . These symptoms began to clear within 24 hours of discontinuing clonidine and had completely subsided within 72 hours.[65] The use of clonidine in children has been reported to cause a syndrome of lethargy, bradycardia, confusion, and epileptic seizures.

The sudden discontinuation of clonidine may result within 12 to 48 hours in a severe withdrawal reaction manifested by restlessness, insomnia, irritability, tremors, and headaches. Similar symptoms may ensue following the paroxysmal release of its catecholamine content by a pheochromocytoma. Because of this withdrawal syndrome, largely neurologic in nature, clonidine should never be discontinued abruptly, but should be gradually tapered. Patients receiving clonidine should be warned never to discontinue the drug abruptly. Deaths due to hypertensive encephalopathy have been reported after abrupt withdrawal of the drug. Generally, anxiety and nervousness are prominent warnings in such patients and headache is often present. Laboratory studies reveal urinary and blood catecholamine levels to be elevated during the phase of abrupt withdrawal. The reaction can be treated with either clonidine or propranalol.

Minoxidil has not caused prominent neurologic side effects. One patient, an epileptic receiving phenytoin, developed status epilepticus while receiving minoxidil and intensive diuretic therapy.[67]

Prazosin (Minipress) is a potent antihypertensive medication that may induce severe orthostatic hypotension and dizziness, particularly following the initial dose. This has been called the "first dose phenomenon" and occurs in one percent of patients within 30 to 90 minutes of receiving the initial 2 mg tablet of prazosin.[67] Manifestations of the first dose phenomenon include dizziness, headache, weakness, lassitude and blurred vision, but sudden syncopal collapse may occur, with coma persisting for up to one hour. Patients who have experienced a first dose reaction may tolerate subsequent doses very well even though plasma prazosin levels are rising for several days. In order to avoid the first dose phenomenon, the initial dose should not exceed 1 mg and should be taken at bedtime. Later doses of prazosin may also induce dizziness, vertigo, headache, nervousness, depression, drowsiness, and weakness.

Guanethidine (Ismelin) may cause symptoms of postural and exertional hypotension, aggravated by factors promoting vasodilatation, such as hot weather and the ingestion of alcohol.[68] Such postural hypotension is most severe after a period of bedrest, and typically presents as paroxysmal weakness, dizziness, and syncope.

Hydralazine (Apresoline) may cause headache and dizziness. In addition, a hydralazine-induced peripheral neuropathy is dose-related and may be severe.[69] Hydralazine neuropathy is rare when doses not exceeding 200 mg daily are used, but becomes more common on higher dosage. Manifested by distal paresthesias and numbness of the extremities (with weakness much less common) hydralazine neuropathy is probably due to pyridoxine deficiency and is correctable by the administration of Vitamin B_6. It has been suggested that hydralazine may form a complex with and thus inactivate circulating pyridoxine.

Trimethaphan, a ganglionic blocking agent, when given parenterally in the treatment of hypertensive crisis may cause acute respiratory paralysis, probably due to its curare-like action at the neuromuscular junction.[70] This drug has also been reported to potentiate the action of succinylcholine, leading to post-operative respiratory depression.[71]

Adrenocorticosteroids

When used in the treatment of vasculitis, this group of potent anti-inflammatory agents, may, because of the high dosages often required, exhibit major neuromuscular side effects. Vascular diseases in which steroids commonly are used include polyarteritis, lupus erythematosus, giant cell arteritis and granulomatous angiitis of the central nervous system.[42-44,72] When adrenal steroids are used in the treatment of collagen diseases, the neurologic complications of the administered medication must be distinguished carefully from the neurologic manifestations of the diseases themselves.[73] It is, for example, often difficult to determine whether convulsive seizures or an organic psychotic reaction are caused by the cerebral lesions that have appeared in the natural course of the collagen vascular disease or by the adrenocorticoid therapy.[74] Both seizures and confusional states may be induced by these hormones in the treatment of other diseases which do not predispose to central nervous system lesions, so that clearly the hormones are themselves capable of altering brain function.

A myopathy, preceded by asthenia, is common in patients receiving steroid hormones over a period longer than a few weeks, and is manifested initially by weakness of the hip flexors and deltoid muscles.[75] Before becoming generalized, it may involve only the lower extremities. Steroid myopathy is not due to hypokalemia and does not respond to the administration of potassium. It is often the most disabling side effect of chronic steroid medication. The proximal myopathic weakness may respond to treatment with phenytoin, thus permitting the continuation of the needed steroid dosage.[76] In one such patient, favorable results to phenytoin were obtained with a double-blind crossover method.

Steroid therapy may also cause convulsions, hallucinations and psychosis.[74] These are more likely to be side effects of the medication rather than complications of the disease itself if there are other prominent manifestations of Cushing's syndrome and if the symptoms occur after a sustained period of therapy. Fluid retention and potassium losses may infrequently contribute to these cerebral complications. A rare complication is steroid-induced hypertension with hypertensive encephalopathy, and cerebral hemorrhages may be identified on computerized tomographic scanning of the brain. Adrenocorticosteroid treatment has apparently induced the onset of convulsive seizures in predisposed patients with polyarteritis nodosa, systemic lupus erythematosus and dermatomyositis.[73,77] There is strong evidence that these hormones act to lower the convulsive threshold and to enhance cortical excitability or susceptibility to convulsive seizures. Moreover, both the acute and the chronic administration of adrenal steroids have induced EEG abnormalities and have enhanced bilateral spike-and-wave discharged in epileptic patients independently of any effects upon the serum electrolytes.[77] Death in status epilepticus during steroid hormone treatment has been reported. If, however, a patient is improving on steroid treatments, and convulsive seizures are the only complication of this therapy, it is recommended that the seizures be treated with appropriate anticonvulsant medications such as phenytoin or carbamazepine, while continuing the effective steroid therapy.

As in the case of convulsive seizures, it is difficult to be certain whether abnormal mental states arising in the course of steroid therapy are due to the therapy itself or to the vasculitis under treatment.[74] At least 30 percent of patients with systemic lupus erythematosus will have these cerebral manifestations, which are especially common during acute exacerbations of the disease.[72] Nevertheless, such abnormal mental states are much more frequent in the course of hormonal therapy, and have been reported in up to 60 percent of treated patients.[74] In most series, the incidence of psychotic reaction induced by steroid therapy has ranged from five to 20 percent. Prominent symptoms of steroid psychosis include alterations in mood (more often frank euphoria than depression), grandiose, depressive or paranoid delusions, auditory hallucinations, distortion of the body image, severe agitation, mania, and flight of ideas, pressure of speech, poor judgment, overactivity, hypersexuality, aggressiveness, mutism, catatonia, disorientation and confusion. Identical patterns may be found in patients suffering from Cushing's disease. There may be a loss of contact with reality, poor judgment and the potential of harm to the patient and others. Effects upon mood are particularly common, while disturbed higher mental functions denote a more severe steroid encephalopathy. As in other organic mental syndromes, the pre-existing personality appears to play a major role in determining the direction and specific content of the steroid-induced mental changes.

The psychotic reactions may occur at any time during steroid therapy and often appear to be related to the dosage used, responding to a reduction short of discontinuation of steroid. In the process of withdrawing steroid hormone treatment, similar symptoms of weakness, mental depression and irritability may develop. A slow tapering of the medication is helpful in ameliorating this response. Occasionally, however, psychotic symptoms may persist for over a month following drug discontinuation.[74] An alternate day steroid regimen may be helpful in reducing the frequency of neurologic complications.[78]

A characteristic pattern is for an initial feeling of well being (due to the relief of chronic symptoms) to intensify into a profound euphoria and elation, irritability, insomnia, and aggression. The discontinuation of the steroid hormone therapy generally will result in the clearing of these symptoms within several days, but with the use of sedative agents of the benzodiazepine type, it may be possible to continue the steroid therapy at full and effective dosage. Similarly, steroid mania may respond to the use of lithium carbonate therapy,[79] (generally 300 mg t.i.d. with monitoring of serum lithium levels) while steroid-induced depression may respond quite nicely to tricyclic anti-depressant medication, again permitting the continuation of the needed steroid suppression of the basic disease. Siegal[80] recently reported a dramatic response of steroid induced psychosis to lithium therapy. His patient's symptoms were essentially hypomanic. Subsequently, Falk found lithium prophylaxis to be effective in the prevention of steroid psychosis.[79] Lithium prophylaxis was tried because mood disorder is so prominent a feature of steroid psychosis. In none of 27 patients treated with lithium carbonate did a psychotic reaction occur, in contrast to the 14 percent of a comparable group previously treated with corticotropin who became psychotic.

Further discussion of the neurological side effects of the adrenocorticosteroids can be found in Chapters III and XI in this book.

References

1. Gilbert GJ, Glaser GH: On the nervous system integration of water and salt metabolism. *Arch Neurol* 5:179-196, 1961.
2. Gilbert GJ: Neurologic manifestations of hyponatremia. *New Engl J Med* 274:1153, 1966.
3. Ruby RJ, Burton JR: Acute reversible hemiparesis and hyponatremia. *Lancet* 2:1212, 1977.
4. Faris AA, Poser CM: Experimental production of focal neurologic deficit by systemic hyponatremia. *Neurology* 14:206-210, 1964.
5. Fichman MP et al: Diuretic-induced hyponatremia. *Ann Int Med* 75: 853-863, 1971.
6. Kao I, Gordon AM: Alteration of skeletal muscle cellular structures by potassium depletion. *Neurology* 27:855-860, 1977.
7. Van Horn G, Drori JB, Schwartz FD: Hypokalemic myopathy and elevation of serum enzymes. *Arch Neurol* 22:335-341, 1970.
8. Guyer PB: Stokes-Adams attacks precipitated by hypokalemia. *Brit Med J* 2:427-428, 1964.
9. Malinow KC, Lion JR: Hyperaldosteronism (Conn's disease) presenting as depression. *J Clin Psychiat* 40:358-359, 1979.
10. Editorial-LHN. Digitalis and neurotoxicity. *Conn Med* 28:329-330, 1964.
11. Bresnahan JF, Vlietstra RE: Clinical pharmacology. 3 Digitalis glycosides. *Mayo Clin Proc* 54:675-684, 1979.
12. Church G, Marriott HJL: Digitalis delirium. *Circulation* 20:549-553, 1959.
13. Duroziez P: De delire et du coma digitaliques. *Gaz Hebdo de med et de chir* 11:780, 1974.
14. Douglas EF, White PT, Nelson JW: Three per second spike-wave in digitalis toxicity. Report of a case. *Arch Neurol* 25:373-375, 1971.
15. Petsche H, Tappelsberger P, Prey Z, Suchatzki BU: The epileptogenic effect of ouabain (g-Strophanthin). Its action on the EEG and cortical morphology. *Epilepsia* 14:243-260, 1973.
16. Bernat JL, Sullivan JK: Trigeminal neuralgia from digitalis intoxication. *JAMA* 241:164, 1979.
17. Greenlee JE, Crampton RS, Miller JQ: Transient global amnesia associated with cardiac arrhythmia and digitalis intoxication. *Stroke* 6: 513-516, 1975.
18. Gilbert GJ: Transient global amnesia: Manifestation of medial temporal lobe epilepsy. *Clin EEG* 3:147-152, 1978.
19. Riseman JEF: Current concepts in therapy. The treatment of angina pectoris. II. *N Engl J Med* 261:1126-1129, 1959.
20. The Medical Letter. Oral isosorbide dinitrate for angina. 21:88, 1979.
21. Abrams J: Current concepts: Nitroglycerin and long-acting nitrates. *N Engl J Med* 302:1234-1237, 1980.
22. Fardeau M, Tome FMS, Simon P: Muscle and nerve changes induced by perhexiline maleate in man and mice. *Muscle Nerve* 2:24-36, 1979.
23. Argov Z, Mastaglia FL: Disorders of neuromuscular transmission caused by drugs. *N Engl J Med* 301:409-413, 1979.
24. Kornfeld P, Horowitz S, Gerkins G et al: Myasthenia gravis unmasked by antiarrhythmic agents. *Mt Sinai J Med* 43:10-14, 1976.
25. Gilbert GJ: Quinidine dementia. *Amer J Cardiol* 41:791, 1978.
26. Gilbert GJ: Quinidine dementia. *JAMA* 237:2093-2094, 1977.

27. Yagiela JA, Benoit PW: Skeletal muscle damage from quinidine. *N Engl J Med* **301**:437, 1979.
28. The Medical Letter. Treatment of cardiac arrhythmias. **20**:113-120, 1978.
29. Holland OB, Kaplan NM: Propranolol in the treatment of hypertension. *N Engl J Med* **294**:930-936, 1976.
30. Federman J, Vlietstra RE: Clinical pharmacolog. 2. Antiarrhythmic drug therapy. *Mayo Clin Proc* **54**:531-542, 1979.
31. Usubiaga JE, Wikinski JA, Morales RL et al: Interaction of intravenously administered procaine, lidocaine and succinylcholine in anesthetized subjects. *Anesth Analg* (Cleve) **46**:39-45, 1967.
32. The Medical Letter on Drugs and Therapeutics. Verapamil for Arrhythmias, **23**:29-30, 1981.
33. Drachman DA, Skom JH: Procainamide — a hazard in myasthenia gravis. *Arch Neurol* **13**:316-320, 1965.
34. Herishanu Y, Rosenberg P: Beta-blockers and myasthenia gravis. *Ann Intern Med* **83**:834-835, 1975.
35. Hughes RO, Zacharias FJ: Myasthenic syndrome during treatment with practolol. *Brit Med J* **1**:460-461, 1976.
36. Weisman SJ: Masked myasthenia gravis. *JAMA* **141**:917-918, 1949.
37. Norris FH Jr., Colella J, McFarlin D: Effect of diphenylhydantoin on neuromuscular synapse. *Neurology* **14**:869-876, 1964.
38. Brumlik J, Jacobs RS: Myasthenia gravis associated with diphenylhydantoin therapy for epilepsy. *Can J Neurol Sci* **1**:127-129, 1974.
39. Wells CE, Urrea D: Cerebrovascular accidents in patients receiving anticoagulant drugs. *Arch Neurol* **5**:553-558, 1960.
40. Dooley DM, Perlmutter I: Spontaneous intracranial hematomas in patients receiving anticoagulation therapy. *JAMA* **187**:396-398, 1964.
41. Edwards KR: Hemorrhagic complications of cerebral angiitis. *Arch Neurol* **34**:549-552, 1977.
42. Gilbert GJ: Herpes zoster ophthalmicus and delayed contralateral hemiparesis. Relationship of the syndrome to central nervous system granulomatous angiitis. *JAMA* **229**:302-304, 1974.
43. Gilbert GJ: Evidence of viral cause in granulomatous angiitis. *Neurology* **27**:100-101, 1977.
44. Gilbert GJ: Hemorrhagic complication of cerebral arteritis. *Arch Neurol* **35**:396-397, 1978.
45. Michaels L: Incidence of thromboembolism after stopping anticoagulant therapy. Relationship to hemorrhage at the time of termination. *JAMA* **215**:595-599, 1971.
46. Gilbert GJ: Femoral neuropathy and retroperitoneal hemorrhage. *JAMA* **3**:211, 501, 1970.
47. Gilbert GJ, Laughlin R: Hemorrhagic femoral neuropathy: report of a case due to anticoagulant. *Southern Med J* **60**:170-176, 1967.
48. Gilbert GJ, Laughlin R: Acute femoral neuropathy induced by anticoagulation. *Dis Nerv Syst* **38**:365, 1977.
49. Krasno LR, Kidera GJ: Clofibrate in coronary heart disease. *JAMA* **219**:845-851, 1972.
50. Gabriel R, Pearce JMS: Clofibrate-induced myopathy and neuropathy. *Lancet* **2**:906, 1976.
51. Langer T, Levy RI: Acute muscular syndrome associated with administration of clofibrate. *N Engl J Med* **279**:856-858, 1968.

52. Smals AG, Beex LVAM, Kloppenborg PWC: Clofibrate-induced muscle damage with myoglobinuria and cardiomyopathy. *N Engl J Med* **296**: 942, 1977.
53. Goldberg AP, Applebaum-Bowden DM et al. Increase in lipoprotein lipase during clofibrate treatment of hypertriglyceridemia in patients on hemodialysis. *N Engl J Med* **301**:1073-1076, 1979.
54. Bridgman JF, Rosen SM, Thorp JM: Complications during clofibrate treatment of nephrotic syndrome hyperlipoproteinemia. *Lancet* **1**:506-509, 1972.
55. Pierides AM, Alvarez-Ude F, Kerr DNS: Clofibrate-induced muscle damage in patients with chronic renal failure. *Lancet* **2**:1279-1282, 1975.
56. The Medical Letter. Drugs for Hypertension. **19**:21-24, 1977.
57. Jackson G, Pierscianowski TA, Mahon W, Condon J: Inappropriate antihypertensive therapy in the elderly. *Lancet* **2**:1317-1319, 1976.
58. Kumar GK, Dastoor FC, Robayo JR, Razzaque MA: Side effects of diazoxide. *JAMA* **235**:275-276, 1976.
59. Gilbert GJ: Reserpine for migraine. *Headache* **16**:125-126, 1976.
60. Adler S: Methyldopa-induced decrease in mental activity. *JAMA* **230**: 1428-1429, 1974.
61. Kurtz JB: Methyldopa and forgetfulness. *Lancet* **1**:202-203, 1976.
62. AMA Dept. of Drug. Current status of propanalol hydrochloride (Inderal). *JAMA* **225**:1380-1384, 1973.
63. Koch-Weser J: Drug Therapy: Metroprolol. *N Engl J Med* **301**:698-703, 1979.
64. Lavin P, Alexander CP: Dementia associated with clonidine therapy. *Brit Med J* **1**:628, 1975.
65. Allen RM, Flemenbaum A: Delirium associated with combined fluphenazine-clonidine therapy. *J Clin Psychiat* **40**:236-237, 1979.
66. Dargie HJ, Dollery CT, Daniel J: Minoxidil in resistant hypertension. *Lancet* **1**:515-518, 1977.
67. Kosman MW: Evaluation of a new antihypertensive agent. Prazosin hydrochloride (Minipress). *JAMA* **238**:157-159, 1977.
68. Weinshilboum RM: Clinical Pharmacology. 8. Antihypertensive drugs that alter adrenergic function. *Mayo Clin Proc* **55**:390-402, 1980.
69. Koch-Weser J: Hydralazine. *N Eng J Med* **295**:320-323, 1976.
70. Dale RC, Schroeder ET: Respiratory paralysis during treatment of hypertension with trimethaphan camsylate. *Arch Intern Med* **136**:816-818, 1976.
71. Poulton TJ, James FM, Lockridge O: Prolonged apnea following trimethaphan and succinylcholine. *Anesthesiology* **50**:54-56, 1979.
72. Glaser GH: Neurologic manifestations in collagen diseases. Problems of prognosis and treatment. *Neurology* **5**:751-766, 1955.
73. Soffer LJ, Elster SK, Hamerman DJ: Treatment of acute disseminated lupus with corticotropin and cortisone. *Arch Intern Med* **93**:503-514, 1954.
74. Glaser GH: Psychotic reactions induced by corticotropin (ACTH) and cortisone. *Psychosom Med* **15**:280-291, 1953.
75. Marshall LF, King J, Langfitt TW: The complications of high-dose corticosteroid therapy in neurosurgical patients: a prospective study. *Ann Neurol* **1**:201-203, 1977.

76. Stern LZ, Gruener R, Amundsen P: Diphenylhydantoin for steroid-induced muscle weakness. *JAMA* **223**:1287-1288, 1973.
77. Glaser GH: On the relationship between adrenal cortical activity and the convulsive state. *Epilepsia* **2**:7-14, 1953.
78. The Medical Letter on Drugs and Therapeutics. Alternate-day corticosteroid therapy. **17**:95-96, 1975.
79. Falk WE, Mahnke M, Poskaner DC: Lithium prophylaxis of corticotropin-induced psychosis. *JAMA* **241**:1011-1012, 1979.
80. Siegal FP: Lithium for steroid-induced psychosis. *JAMA* **299**:155-156, 1978.

Chapter III

Neurological Complications of Cancer Chemotherapy

Dean F. Young, M.D.

Introduction

Cytotoxic drugs developed over the past thirty years have had a dramatic impact on cancer therapy. Patients with most forms of cancer now face a significantly better outlook since chemotherapy has been added to the standard treatment modalities — surgery and radiation therapy (RT). In some instances, such combined aggressive therapy has produced cure of tumors not previously curable.

These powerful drugs are not devoid of serious untoward effects. The vast majority of useful chemotherapy agents are cytotoxic not just for tumor cells, but may cause reversible or irreversible damage to normal tissue as well. Rapidly growing tissues — the bone marrow, the gastrointestinal (GI) tract and buccal mucusa, germinal tissues, skin, and hair are the most vulnerable. Frequently, toxicity directed at these tissues is regarded as acceptable if therapeutic effectiveness, relative to the degree of toxicity ("therapeutic index"), is sufficiently high. Toxicity directed against more vital tissues — liver, kidney, cardiac muscle, lung — is generally to be avoided although some degree of hepatic or renal toxicity may be accepted for very effective agents.

Some of these drugs may produce nervous system toxicity which may in turn result in significant functional impairment, rarely even in death. If such toxicity is directed primarily against the peripheral nervous system (PNS), and is largely reversible as is the case with vinca alkaloids, nervous system toxicity may be an acceptable side effect. Irreversible neurotoxicity or any significant central nervous system (CNS) toxicity whether reversible or not is unacceptable and always requires discontinuation of the causative agent. In addition to direct nervous system toxicity, indirect CNS toxicity may be seen as a result of end organ failure attributable to these agents. Such indirect toxicity may be reversible if the end organ failure is reversible (e.g., hepatic encephalopathy), but may also be irreversible if a secondary CNS lesion is structural (e.g., a CNS hemorrhage or infection resulting from bone marrow failure).

The nervous system, particularly the CNS, does enjoy some protection from the toxic effects of these drugs. Some of the reasons are: (1) as noted above, cytotoxic drugs generally damage rapidly growing cells first so that damage to other tissues such as bone marrow or GI tract is "dose limiting"; (2) drugs having substantial nervous system toxicity are usually abandoned as unacceptable after initial trials; (3) given an intact blood-brain barrier, access to cerebrospinal fluid by most chemotherapy agents is sharply limited, so that their potential CNS toxicity is usually never realized. Many clinically non-neurotoxic agents are quite neurotoxic if the barrier is bypassed experimentally such as by intrathecal injection.

Several trends, however, have increased clinical neurotoxicity of the cytotoxic drugs and will continue to do so as therapy becomes more vigorous. They include the following:

1. New extremely *potent drugs* are appearing, many effective against tumors previously regarded as unresponsive to chemotherapy. As a result, chemotherapy is now applied to many forms of cancer for which only radiation and/or surgery had a role previously.

2. Chemotherapy is increasingly given in multi-agent approaches (*combination chemotherapy*), thereby increasing the number of patients exposed to neurotoxic drugs as well as increasing the likehood of additive or synergistic effects.

3. Chemotherapy is also often given as a part of *multi-modality* approach (combined with radiation therapy, surgery, or other newer modalities such as immunotherapy, hyperthermia, etc.), raising the risk of synergistic neurotoxic effects — particularly CNS toxicity arising from combined RT and drug therapy.

4. Chemotherapy drugs are being tried in *innovative* ways. They include administration:

(a) in very high doses — doses allowing significant CNS penetration — often applying various techniques to "rescue" vulnerable tissues, chiefly bone marrow.

(b) directly to the nervous system to treat nervous system cancer — such as by intracarotid infusion, intrathecally, or even directly into tumors.

When neurotoxic drug effects occur, either the peripheral or the central nervous system may be the target depending on the drug and the way it is given. Some primarily affect CNS (e.g., fluorouracil, L-asparaginase), others mainly the PNS (e.g., vinca alkaloids). Still others potentially affect both (e.g., procarbazine, mitotane). With some drugs neurotoxic effects are common and reversible. For example vinca alkaloids produce neurotoxicity in virtually every patient treated. More commonly, neurotoxic effects such as those produced by 5-FU are quite uncommon. Most such effects are reversible but certain forms such as methotrexate leucoencephalopathy are frequently irreversible. Any of these effects may result in major distressing functional impairment which substantially affects the quality of life, particularly if mental function, walking, dexterity, vision, hearing or autonomic function are impaired. Early recognition is important since clinically reversible effects may become irreversible if the responsible drug is continued.

All the neurotoxic side effects of these drugs closely mimic other potential neurological complications of cancer — metastatic complications or nonmetastatic or remote effects.[1] Cerebellar dysfunction from 5-FU may mimic cerebellar metastasis, meningeal tumor, "cerebellar degeneration", or other causes of cerebellar dysfunction, for example, ethanol abuse. It is important for the neurologist to assist the oncologist in determining whether new neurological dysfunction is caused by the primary disease or is a result of treatment. These problems may be quite perplexing to the oncologist who may be ill at ease with new neurological disturbances having many possible etiologies, and also to the neurologist who is relatively unfamiliar with cancer therapy and the effects of chemotherapeutic agents. The purpose of this chapter is to elucidate the clinical neurological problems associated with the use of the more commonly employed agents as well as some of the less commonly used drugs which show promise of more widespread use as well as drugs used infrequently which show prominent established neurotoxicity. Several reviews have treated aspects of this subject previously.[2-5]

Since neurologists and neurosurgeons may be unfamiliar with the principles underlying cancer chemotherapy, we will briefly review some basic cellular and pharmacological principles familiar to oncologists.

Principles of Chemotherapy

The ultimate goal of cancer therapy is cure. Chemotherapy has afforded cure in some patients with certain disseminated tumors, not otherwise curable by surgery and/or radiation therapy (acute leukemia in children, some lymphomas, choriocarcinoma, testicular carcinoma). However, most patients with non-localized tumor cannot yet be cured. Unfortunately, the ultimate tool — "a magic bullet" — a drug able to kill all tumor cells with little or no damage to normal tissues, is surely not achievable. Short of this, the chemotherapist, in order to improve the results of therapy, is willing to risk injury to normal tissues if such injury can be reversed either through the elapse of time or through special techniques designed to carry the patient through the acute phase, such as white cell or platelet transfusions or more recently bone marrow transplantation. Additional techniques have emerged as well to prevent such injury — diuresis with fluid and mannitol to prevent renal damage from cis-platinum, or antagonist drugs (citrovorum factor for methotrexate) designed to limit systemic toxicity without blocking anti-tumor effect. Establishment of maximum tolerated doses for certain drugs has helped to prevent certain systemic toxicities such as daunorubicin-induced cardiomyopathy.

Our ability to cure tumors depends on the potential of reducing tumor cells to a number so small that one's body immune mechanisms can kill the remainder. When that is not possible, the optimal chemotherapy drug is one which most completely reduces the body's tumor burden. The chemotherapy drugs are proportionately more effective in reducing tumor burden when it is small. The initial therapy of many solid tumors therefore uses other modalities — primarily surgery and radiation — to reduce bulk tumor prior to chemotherapy. The initial small tumor bulk is important since most drugs kill cells by first order kinetics, i.e., they will kill 90% (1 log kill) or rarely 99% (2 log kills) of the cells no matter how many are present initially. Thus, if a drug kills 90% of one million tumor cells (reducing the burden to 100,000), it is much less likely to be effective than if only 1,000 cells are present initially since the body's defense mechanism and/or other therapeutic modalities may be able to kill the remaining 100 cells. A second major reason why a small initial tumor is important in chemotherapy lies in the fact that tumor growth tends to follow a so-called Gompertz' curve: growth rate slows as the tumor enlarges.[6] Thus the metabolic processes which the drug affect are less quickly impaired. particularly since many cells are in a resting, non-dividing state during which time many drugs have little cytotoxic effect.

Logical planning of a chemotherapy program for a particular tumor depends on knowledge of the cell kinetics of that tumor being treated and also upon knowledge of the pharmacokinetics of the drug as well as its mechanism of action. Specifically, the cell cycle against which it acts is important. Many drugs are so-called "cell cycle specific" working most often during the S-phase of mitosis during which DNA rapidly divides in preparation for actual cell division (the M-phase). The antimetabolites such as methotrexate and Cytarabine are good examples of phase-specific or cell cycle specific agents. Other drugs are specific mainly for mitotic phases (vinca alkaloids, the M-phase). Other groups of agents appear to act at all phases of the cycle, so-called "cell cycle non-specific" agents, of which the alkylating agents are classic examples. Knowing the kinetics and growth rate of the tumor being treated, how the drug acts, and in which tissues it achieves therapeutic concentrations, allows the chemotherapist to adjust dose and route of administration to maximize anti-tumor effect. Pharmacokinetic data dealing with drug entry into the CSF is obviously of great importance in treating tumors of the CNF — metastatic or primary. If the CNS provides a "sanctuary" for residual tumor cells which interferes with cure as it occurred in the past in acute lymphoblastic leukemia, then using a drug route designed to achieve therapeutic concentrations in the nervous system, i.e., intrathecally, becomes important in successful treatment.

The wide difference in responses of different tumors to single agents emphasizes the fact that cancer is many different diseases. The response of a given tumor to single agents has frequently been improved by multi-agent or combination chemotherapy. Multiple anti-tumor agents may be used simultaneously and/or sequentially in the treatment of cancer. One reason such treatment is often superior to single agent therapy is that different agents act at different sites within the cells, increasing the likelihood of cytotoxic damage. Moreover, they act at different stages in the cell's cycle, a fact enabling cell cycle specific and nonspecific agents to be combined to great advantage. Thus multiple drugs may produce a synergistic clinical effect. Sequential use of multiple drugs may also be logically chosen. Such is the case with acute leukemia, a disease for which high dose multi-drug regimens are used at the time of diagnosis to massively reduce the initial tumor burden (the induction phase) much as surgery and radiation therapy are used for solid tumors. Less intense therapy with other drugs having different properties follows (the consolidation phase), and this in turn is followed by still less intensive lower dose drug therapy designed to hold clinical remission (the maintenance phase). Another major reason why multiple drugs may be more effective than single agents is the apparent heterogeneity of many tumors. One can clone a variety of tumor lines from cell cultures of several animal and human tumors.[7] Human malignant gliomas have recently been shown to be strikingly heterogeneous.[8] Experimentally different tumor lines possess different biochemical properties and presumably also differing pharmacologic susceptibility. Thus one agent may effectively kill some cells from a given tumor and fail against others, which may be more susceptible to a second agent. Use of multiagent chemotherapy increases the likelihood that all cells within a heterogeneous tumor may respond to treatment.

Multi-modality therapy adds the effects of other treatment modes in order to produce additive or synergistic effects. and also to reduce the initial tumor burden. For most tumors chemotherapy is the only current modality useful against disseminated metastases. Radiation therapy combined with chemotherapy may produce synergistic toxicity and examples of this as applied to the nervous system will be subsequently discussed. The neurological side effects of radiation therapy are fully discussed in Chapter V of this book. Immunotherapy for treating cancer is thus far poorly developed and not yet applicable for most tumors, and so will not be discussed.

A new chemotherapy drug ordinarily goes through three clinical trials or testing phases. It is first tested in phase I trials, the first trials of the drug in man. Phase I trials: (1) establish the optimal dose and the maximum tolerated doses for a given schedule and route of administration of the drug; (2) establish toxicity and whether it is reversible, predictable and tolerable, and (3) identify evidence of activity against specific tumors. Patients who have exhausted established chemotherapy for their tumor and have continued evidence for progression are ordinarily those chosen for phase I chemotherapy. Agents without unacceptable toxicity and with some indication for effectiveness are entered into phase II trials, which more systematically define the degree of activity against a specific neoplasm and the nature of adverse vs beneficial effects. Phase II trials may be randomized but frequently are not. Response rates may be gauged against historical controls. Successful phase II agents move on to phase III, in which anti-tumor activity is systematically studied. These studies are controlled and often randomized usually between conventional and experimental treatment groups. With this approach, anti-tumor activity is confirmed. In addition, new toxicities may be defined. The outcome of the phase III trials determines whether the drug will be made generally available for cancer treatment.

Chemotherapy Drugs

Classification systems for the chemotherapy agents vary considerably but all are based primarily on the mechanism of action of the drugs.[9-11] We shall use one such classification (Table I) in the subsequent discussion of the neurotoxicity of the individual agents. The chemotherapy agents can be broadly divided into hormonal and non-hormonal agents. The majority of widely used drugs fall into the latter category.

Non-Hormonal Agents

The two original groups of chemotherapy agents are the alkylating agents and the antimetabolites which respectively represent classic examples of cell cycle non-specific and cell cycle specific agents. In addition to the so-called "classic" alkylating agents, many other cell cycle non-specific agents included in other groups in Table I have mechanisms of action similar to the alkylating agents and are grouped by some authors under that general heading.[10] Such alkylating-like agents include the nitrosoureas, some of the antibiotic anti-neoplastic agents, and several other "miscellaneous" agents, including cis-platinum.

The "Classic" Alkylating Agents

The classic alkylating agents exert their primary effect on cells by alkylating pyrimidine and purine bases (chiefly guanine), producing non-functional bases which prevent replication of DNA and in turn cause cell death. The original agent, nitrogen mustard (mechlorethamine, HN_2), now has limited use but many of the other agents are widely useful. They include: cyclophosphamide (Cytoxan), chlorambucil (Leukeran), melphalan (Alkeran), thiotepa and busulfan (Myleran). The systemic toxicity of these agents is directed largely at bone marrow and the gastrointestinal tract. Common side effects include thrombocytopenia, leukopenia, nausea and vomiting, diarrhea and, with cyclophosphamide, hair loss.

Nitrogen Mustard (mechlorethamine, HN_2)

Anti-tumor properties of nitrogen mustard and its relatives became apparent when gases of the sulfur mustard and nitrogen mustard variety, under investigation as weapons of warfare, were found also to inhibit cell growth, particularly of myeloid and lymphoid tissues. Accordingly, its initial clinical application was in the treatment of lymphomas and leukemias. Newer agents have largely supplanted mechlorethamine although it is still used occasionally in combination with other agents, most commonly vincristine (Oncovin), procarbazine, and prednisone — so-called "MOPP" — in treating advanced Hodgkin's disease and other lymphomas.

Apart from occasional intracavitary use, rapid intravenous injection is the only currently used route of administration. In customary doses, neurological toxicity does not occur. Although non-specific complaints such as headache and drowsiness are sometimes attributed to the drug, only one case of severe cerebral dysfunction has been described following standard use.[12] This patient received two standard intravenous doses of nitrogen mustard for Hodgkin's disease and one week later developed unexplained fever, hemiplegia and coma. Elevated intracranial pressure and cerebrospinal fluid (CSF) pleocytosis (517 white blood cells including 54% polymorphonuclear cells) were noted. After ventricular drainage, the patient rapidly improved. When the patient died of a myocardial infarction four years later, autopsy disclosed multifocal areas of neuronal loss and gliosis but no evidence of tumor. The authors concluded the reaction represented an idiosyncratic reaction of the drug. A causal effect, although likely, seems uncertain.

More clear-cut neurotoxicity can occur when the nervous system is exposed to higher concentrations of the drug. One early use of the drug was to treat brain tumors by administering substantial doses via the intracarotid route. Since patients so treated presumably had an impaired blood-brain barrier, the drug, which ordinarily passes the barrier minimally, undoubtedly achieved relatively high focal brain concentrations.

Table I
Classification of Chemotherapeutic Agents

Non-Hormonal Agents

I. Alkylating Agents ("Classic")

    A. Mechlorethamine (nitrogen mustard, HN_2, Mustargen)
    B. Cyclophosphamide (Cytoxan, CTX)
    C. Chlorambucil (Leukeran)
    D. Thiotepa (Triethylene thiophosphoramide)
    E. Melphalan (Phenylalanine mustard, Alkeran, L-PAM)
    F. Busulfan (Myleran)

II. Antimetabolites

    A. Folic Acid Antagonists
        1. Methotrexate (MTX, formerly amithopterin)
        2. Triazinate* (Baker's antifol, TZT)
    B. Antipyrimidines
        1. 5-Fluorouracil (5-FU)
        2. Ftorafur*
        3. Cytosine arabinosine (Cytarabine, Ara-C, Arabinosyl cytosine, Cytosar)
        4. 5-Azacytidine
    C. Antipurines
        1. 6-Mercaptopurine (6-MP)
        2. Thioguanine (TG, 6-TG)
        3. 8-Azaguanine

III. Plant Alkaloids

    A. Periwinkle Derivatives
        1. Vincristine (Oncovin, VCR)
        2. Vinblastine (Velban, VLB)
        3. Vindesine* (DVA, desacetyl vinblastine amide)
    B. Podophyllotoxins
        1. Epipodophyllotoxin VM-26* (Teniposide)
        2. Epipodophyllotoxin VM-16* (Etoposide)
    C. Others
        1. Maytansine*

IV. Antibiotics

    A. Doxorubicin (Adriamycin)
    B. Bleomycin (Blenoxane)
    C. Dactinomycin (Actinomycin-D)
    D. Daunorubicin (Daunomycin, Cerubidine)
    E. Mithramycin
    F. Mitomycin-C

V. Miscellaneous Synthetic Agents

    A. Nitrosoureas

Continued

      1. BCNU (Carmustine, bischlorethyl nitrosourea)
      2. CCNU (Lomustine, cyclohexyl chlorethyl nitrosourea)
      3. Methyl-CCNU* (Semustine)
      4. Streptozotocin*
  B. Others
      1. Cis-platinum (Cisplatin, DDP, platinum
         cis-diamminedichloroplatinum II)
      2. Galactitol* (Dianhydrogalactitol)
      3. Hexamethylmelamine* (HXM, HMM)
      4. Dacarbazine (DTIC, Dimethyltriazine imidazole carboxamide)
      5. Hydroxyurea (Hydrea)
      6. L-Asparaginase; other enzymes: SAGA
      7. Procarbazine (Methylhydrazine, Matulane, Natulan)
      8. Mitotane (Lysodren, o-p'-DDD)
      9. PALA* (N-Phosphoacetyl L-aspartic acid)
    10. Thymidine* (TdR)
    11. Methyl-GAG* (Methyl-glyoxal-bis-guanylhydrazone)
    12. AMSA*

Hormonal Agents

   I. Adrenocorticosteroids
  II. Estrogens
 III. Progestins
 IV. Androgens
  V. Anti-estrogens

---

*Investigational drug, not commercially available.

Cerebral toxicity with this approach was uncommon, but it was of sufficient severity that given marginal therapeutic success, this technique was abandoned. In several cases focal signs such as hemiplegia, seizures, coma, and even death occurred following intracarotid administration.[13-15] At autopsy one such patient showed diffuse cerebral edema, most prominent on the side ipsilateral to the injection, as well as demyelination and gliosis attributed by the authors to an injection seven weeks previously.[13] Edema and focal hemorrhages have also been noted experimentally in cats and monkeys sacrificed 2 to 3 days after intracarotid injection.[13]

    Peripheral nerve injury has also occurred following unconventional uses of nitrogen mustard. Intra-arterial perfusion techniques designed to produce high tissue concentrations locally to treat limb or pelvic tumors have resulted in clinical evidence of lower motor neuron damage to plexus or peripheral nerve.[16,17]

    High systemic concentrations of the drug resulting from large intravenous doses or from regional intra-arterial perfusions also may produce hearing loss, tinnitus, and vestibulopathy in some patients[18,19] The site of injury is presumably the acoustic and vestibular nerves.

Cyclophosphamide (Cytoxan)

Cyclophosphamide has the widest therapeutic spectrum of any of the alkylating agents. It is usually used in combination with other agents to treat both non-Hodgkin's lymphoma and Hodgkin's disease, adult leukemia, and a number of solid tumors, including breast carcinoma, endometrial carcinoma, and oat cell carcinoma of the lung. Transient symptoms such as facial flushing, pharyngeal tingling, tongue burning, or dizziness or mild intoxication, usually lasting only a few minutes, are noted in a few patients after a standard intravenous bolus of the drug.[20,21] Transient blurring of vision at various intervals after therapy was reported in one series to occur in 5 of 29 children treated with high doses.[22] The etiology was more likely ocular than cerebral. Inappropriate antidiuretic hormone (ADH) secretion has on rare occasions been linked to fairly high doses of Cytoxan.[23] The problem is exacerbated by fluid loading to protect the kidneys when used in high dose regimens. One fatal case has been reported.[24] Fortunately no significant neurological toxicity results from standard oral or intravenous use of the drug, or even for that matter from unconventional high dose schedules.[25] Only minute quantities of the drug or of its active metabolites reach the CSF.

Chlorambucil (Leukeran)

Chlorambucil is a well-tolerated drug with wide antitumor activity. Its major current use is for the long-term maintenance treatment of chronic lymphatic leukemia, but it has also been used to treat ovarian carcinoma, choriocarcinoma, and breast carcinoma as well as lymphoma. Available in a sugar-coated pill, the drug has been ingested in large quantities by two children, resulting in massive overdoses. One developed repetitive seizures and coma, the other irritability, "jerking movements" and ataxia. Both recovered without sequelae.[26,27] In general the drug is not neurotoxic. However, a recent report proposes that seizures may be a complication of chlorambucil given in conventional doses to children with nephrotic syndrome.[28] The seizures reported during therapy in 7 of 91 patients treated were not attributable to metabolic factors, and ceased when the drug was stopped.

Thiotepa (triethylene thiophosphoramide)

Thiotepa has been used systematically to treat breast, ovarian, and bladder carcinoma and Hodgkin's disease. Systemic use is now uncommon since more effective drugs, including other alkylating agents, have been substituted. Topical bladder irrigation with the drug to treat superficial papillary tumors and intracavitary installation to treat serous effusions are the main current uses. It has been tried in the treatment of malignant gliomas, but found ineffective.[29] It is lipid-soluble and is thought to cross the intact blood-brain barrier minimally. Systemic administration of thiotepa causes no neurotoxicity.

Intrathecal administration to treat meningeal tumor holds some therapeutic promise. Thiotepa is one of the few drugs found sufficiently safe experimentally to permit the risk of intrathecal administration in man. The drug rapidly disappears from CSF into the systemic circulation,[30] so one would not expect the agent to be especially effective in the treatment of meningeal tumor. Nevertheless, Gutin et al[31] reported that five of seven patients with meningeal leukemia responded well to intrathecal administration although three with meningeal carcinomatosis did not. Of the 10 patients treated with multiple intrathecal (lumbar) doses of thiotepa, clinical neurological toxicity occurred in two. One developed a lower motor neuron disorder consisting of weakness, back pain, leg pain and areflexia, associated with appropriate EMG changes, after the second dose. The autopsy in that patient revealed demyelination and gliosis in the posterior columns, extending rostally to the medulla. A second patient developed an ascending myelopathy after the eighth dose. This led to respiratory paralysis and death. No autopsy was permitted. Leucoencephalopathy was seen in the brain of a third patient but methotrexate, known to cause such changes, had been given intrathecally as well. Potential brain toxicity is suggested by studies in monkeys given intracisternal doses. Doses of 12 mg/m^2 caused opisthotonos and extensor rigidity and doses of 24 mg/m^2 resulted in neurological deaths.[32]

Melphalan (Alkeran, phenylalanine mustard, L-PAM)

This drug, used primarily to treat multiple myeloma, is nonneurotoxic. Intracarotid administration to treat brain tumors has been abandoned. Such use was noted in one case to cause sudden hemiplegia the day following intracarotid injection.[14]

Busulfan (Myleran)

This drug, an oral agent used almost exclusively to treat myelogenous leukemia, is not neurotoxic. One case, a patient with chronic myelogenous leukemia treated with busulfan, was reported to have developed myasthenia gravis.[33] A causative role is unlikely.

The Antimetabolites

The antimetabolites as a group exert their primary activity during DNA synthesis, the S phase of the cell cycle. These agents are structural analogues of naturally occurring substances, and compete with purines, pyrimidines or their precursors for enzymatic reactions important in

DNA synthesis. These drugs tend to be effective against rapidly growing tumors. Synthesis of purines and pyrimidine bases are blocked, or in some instances ineffective bases are produced.

The antimetabolites are generally divided into three general classes: folic acid antagonists, antipyrimidines, and antipurines.

Folic Acid Antagonists

The only folic acid antagonist now in common clinical usage is methotrexate (MTX). Its anticellular effect is prototypic for all the drugs in this group. Methotrexate tightly binds the enzyme dihydrofolate reductase, thereby preventing the conversion of folic acid to tetrahydrofolic acid and in turn blocking the subsequent conversion of tetrahydrofolic acid to folinic acid. Synthesis of purines is dependent on folic acid. Its metabolites, the synthesis of which is blocked by MTX, are important in donating formyl groups, so that MTX inhibits both purine and thymidylic acid synthesis. Folinic acid (citrovorum factor) given systemically can circumvent the actions of the folic acid antagonists and has been used clinically to reduce adverse effects on normal tissues, chiefly bone marrow (citrovorum "rescue").

Methotrexate: Although nitrogen mustard was investigated earlier, the use of methotrexate and its predecessor, aminopterin, to treat acute leukemia, was perhaps the most important early step in the development of chemotherapy for treatment of malignant disease. Subsequently, MTX demostrated impressive effectiveness in treating a wide variety of tumors including trophoblastic tumors, breast carcinoma, lymphoma, including Burkitt's lymphoma, and mycosis fungoides. MTX cured over 50% of patients with choriocarcinoma, providing the first example of cure of malignant disease by a chemotherapeutic agent. Innovative methods of using the drug evolved subsequently, which have extended greatly its therapeutic potential. These methods include intrathecal injection and, more recently, high dose systemic regimens.

When standard doses of MTX are given orally or intravenously, the drug is toxic to bone marrow and GI tract, producing pancytopenia, diarrhea and stomatitis. Hepatotoxicity occurs, skin and hair follicle toxicity is fairly common, and renal and pulmonary toxicity occur uncommonly.

In ordinary systemic doses, MTX is essentially not neurotoxic. The drug does not reach the CNS in cytotoxic concentrations and the blood-brain barrier (BBB) permits limited passage of the drug so that CSF concentration is less than 10% of that in plasma after conventional oral or parenteral doses.

Methotrexate can be toxic to the nervous system if a sufficient concentration reaches the brain, spinal cord or meninges. Such concentrations are achieved by instilling the drug directly into the subarachnoid space, or by infusing massive systemic doses followed by citrovorum rescue. Methotrexate used in these ways has the capacity to produce not only transient neurological impairment, but structural damage to the CNS. It is the only drug clearly shown to produce structural brain damage when used in currently established protocols. With more widespread use of these techniques, MTX neurotoxicity is becoming an increasingly important clinical problem.

Older methods of using the drug provided early evidence for potential neurotoxicity to brain. The drug has been given by intracarotid administration, a route which usually results only in systemic toxicity. However, a single case has been reported of coma and death following shortly upon infusion of methotrexate into the internal carotid artery for brain tumor treatment.[34] Autopsy disclosed multifocal hemorrhagic infarcts in both cerebral hemispheres. Cortical and leptomeningeal vessels were abnormal, showing prominent fibrinoid degeneration and hyaline thrombosis. Carotid perfusion for brain tumors is not a very effective treatment of MTX and is currently obsolete.

Intratumoral infusion of methotrexate has also been used for the treatment of brain tumors. Clinical neurotoxicity has not been reported, but cerebral edema with some surrounding necrosis and astrocytosis has been noted pathologically.[35]

The neurotoxicity of methotrexate may be either acute or delayed (Table II). The following general types of methotrexate neurotoxicity will be discussed:
1. Transient acute side effects of intrathecal methotrexate.
2. Permanent acute side effects of intrathecal methotrexate.
3. Delayed side effects of MTX:
   a) Methotrexate encephalopathy (leukoencephalopathy).
      1) due to intrathecal methotrexate.
      2) due to systemic administration (high dose) (?conventional doses given with brain irradiation).
   b) other delayed side effects.
4. Acute cerebral dysfunction due to high dose methotrexate.
5. Long-term effects of intrathecal methotrexate.

1. The Transient Acute Side Effects of Intrathecal Methotrexate.

The use of intrathecal methotrexate (IT MTX) was found effective in treating meningeal leukemia in 1958, and this led to its use in treating meningeal lymphomas and meningeal carcinomatosis. In recent years, IT MTX given prophylactically has drastically improved the outlook in childhood leukemia.

The first neurological toxic effect of IT MTX to be recognized and still the most common toxic effect is aseptic meningitis.[36,37] The signs and symptoms include rapidly developing meningismus, with stiff neck, headache, nausea and vomiting, fever and lethargy, associated with a

Table II
Methotrexate Neurotoxicity

Systemic Administration Oral, Intravenous, Intramuscular	Intracarotid	Intravenous
Conventional doses (varies 10-60 mg/m^2/dose)		High-dose with citrovorum rescue (200-20,000 mg/m^2/dose)
?rare leukoencephalopathy (multifocal pontine) (i.v. route)	hemorrhagic cerebral infarction	Delayed: 1) Leukoencephalopathy 2) Acute focal cerebral dysfunction

Brain Tumor Bed

     Focal necrosis, edema

Intrathecal Administration

    Acute
      1. Sterile meningitis
      2. Acute myelopathy
        (transient or permanent)
      3. ?Seizures (rare)

    Chronic
      1. Leukoencephalopathy
      2. Cortical atrophy
      3. ?Myelopathy
      4. ?Cerebellar degeneration
      5. *?Optic atrophy
      6. *?Learning disabilities/
        behavioral abnormalities

*probably require cranial RT.

modest CSF pleocytosis which may include polymorphonuclear cells. The diagnosis is strongly suggested by the temporal relationship of intrathecal methotrexate administration. The symptoms start within a few hours after dosage, usually peak within 6 to 12 hours, but may persist while gradually subsiding for 2 to 3 days. There are no sequelae, and repeated dosage usually does not produce meningismus again. However, in some patients repetitive occurrence is noted and may warrant switching intrathecal drugs to arabinosyl cytosine (Ara-C). The cause is not certain. The frequency of occurrence markedly varies in a pattern suggesting that certain batches of the drug may be more irritative. The reaction has been attributed to the preservatives used, either the benzyl alcohol in the methotrexate solution or the methyl parabens in the lyophilized power, but their presence is not required to produce the reaction.[3,37,38] Most likely it is the drug itself or impurities within it that produce the reaction. The presence of CNS or meningeal disease is not required. It occurs in children with acute lymphoblastic leukemia being treated prophylactically although it appears to be more common in those with active meningeal leukemia.[39,40]

Other transient side effects of methotrexate are usually of little consequence. Evidence of transient radiculopathies primarily limited to radicular pain occurs occasionally after lumbar injection. Most likely there has been partial epidural or subdural injection of the drug in many cases. The symptoms gradually subside usually with no neurological signs developing, allowing one to distinguish the rare occurrence of needle-induced spinal subdural hematoma, which also produces radiculopathy or myelopathy after intrathecal injection.[41]

Intraventricular injection can cause nausea and vomiting immediately but dilution of the drug with 10 or more ml of CSF and gradual injection prevents this minor problem. Seizures have occasionally been attributed to intrathecal methotrexate but a causative role is indefinite. High intrathecal doses can produce seizures in dogs.[42]

2. Permanent Acute Side Effects of Intrathecal Methotrexate.

The only acute permanent side effect of intrathecal drug is the rare occurrence of acute transverse myelopathy associated with paraplegia. While transient paraparesis or paraplegia occurs, most of the reported cases developed permanent weakness. It is quite rare. Only 12 cases have been described, and little pathological correlation is available.[5,43] Autopsy on one patient who died within 30 minutes showed no pathological abnormality of the spinal cord.[44] We have not seen acute transverse myelopathy but we have seen two patients who developed ascending myelopathy after treatment with multiple doses of combined intrathecal methotrexate and Ara-C for meningeal leukemia. Extensive necrosis of the cord was noted at autopsy in one. The reaction is not entirely specific for MTX and has been seen also with Ara-C. In fact, two cases developed transient paraparesis after MTX which improved, only to recur on administration of Ara-C, leaving permanent sequelae.[45,46] The rarity of this reaction suggests it is an idiosyncratic response. It is certainly not dose related. In fact, one child who was inadvertently given ten times the intended intrathecal dosage developed no untoward reaction.[47]

3. Delayed Toxic Effects of Methotrexate.

a) Methotrexate Encephalopathy (Leukoencephalopathy) (see Table III).

Methotrexate leukoencephalopathy occurs as a delayed side effect in some patients following repetitive doses of intrathecal MTX. It also occurs in other patients who have been treated with repeated courses of high-dose systemic administration. Because it is often severe and irreversible, leucoencephalopathy has become the most vexing of all the neurological problems associated with chemotherapy. Although there are some differences in the distribution of the lesions in the cerebral white matter, the clinical and pathological picture of leukoencephalopathy

produced by intrathecal (intralumbar or intraventricular) administration of MTX and that following high-dose systemic administration is similar. The clinical picture is rather variable. Frequently there is progressive personality change, confusion, lethargy and
dementia associated with motor abnormalities including tremor, ataxia,
paresis and occasionally seizures. Progression to coma may occur with
intrathecal administration.[48,49] However, there may be sudden onset of
severe neurological signs which include hemiplegia and coma, and if
progression is fulminant, death may result.[50,51] Pathologically the lesion
is primarily a leukoencephalopathy consisting of multifocal areas of
demyelination. In the center of the lesions there is often coagulative
necrosis and the regional small blood vessels show fribrinoid change
and necrosis.[38,50,51,52] Axonal swelling may be an early change. The
pathology is strikingly similar to that produced by radiation necrosis.

The syndrome was first recognized when the drug was given by the
ventricular route.[50,53] Bresnan's patients had received whole brain radiation and he postulated a synergistic role of radiation.[53] Shapiro et al
described three patients with posterior fossa tumors who developed
severe clinical encephalopathy after receiving repetitive intraventricular
MTX.[50] They emphasized the periventricular distribution of the demyelination and coagulative necrosis outside the port of brain irradiation
and suggested that ventricular obstruction was a critical factor(Fig. 1). It
was assumed that hydrocephalus associated with this obstruction
allowed an increased transependymal absorption of MTX into the periventricular white matter, resulting in cytotoxic drug concentrations in
parenchyma. At about the same time clinical leukoencephalopathy was
observed in children treated with repetitive lumbar injections.[51] Postmortem examination in one case disclosed necrotic areas in temporal and
parietal lobes not confined to periventricular regions. Characteristic
blood vessel changes were also seen. Series presented by Rubinstein[52]
and by Price and Jamieson[38] gave further support to the view that radiation therapy was important in enhancing MTX encephalopathy. Their

Table III
Methotrexate-Induced Leukoencephalopathy

Disorder	Methotrexate Administration	Radiation Therapy
Acute lymph. leukemia	i.t., i.v. or p.o.	+
Meningeal carcinomatosis	i.t.	+
Primary brain tumor	i.t. or high dose i.v.	+
Osteosarcoma	High dose i.v.	—

studies suggested some variability of the pathological change. They described extensive demyelination of the central white matter frequently associated with some axonal swelling (Fig. 2). They also noted a degree of gliosis surrounding the acute lesion in some cases and some evidence for neuronal loss in severe lesions. Diffuse spongy changes may be seen in the white matter.[49] Foci of calcification are frequently seen.

Since the evolution of CT scanning, there has been radiological correlation with these clinical and pathological changes. Computerized brain scan often shows periventricular attenuation or diffuse or multifocal lucencies in the deep cerebral white matter (Fig. 3).[54,55] Some investigators have reported such changes in the absence of neurological signs, suggesting that mild forms of encephalopathy occur.[55,56] The incidence of such CT changes ranged as high as 50% in one study.[54] This data correlates with pathological evidence in children dying of leukemia. Examination of brains in some patients has showed significant changes in the white matter, chiefly gliosis, spongy change as well as some abnormalities of neuronal morphology, even though there was no clini-

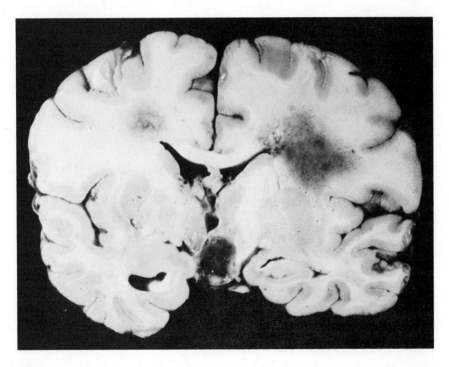

Figure 1. Horizontal section of brain from a patient who received high dose intravenous methotrexate for a soft tissue sarcoma. Note hydrocephalus ex vacuo and a focus of white matter necrosis in the right frontal region.

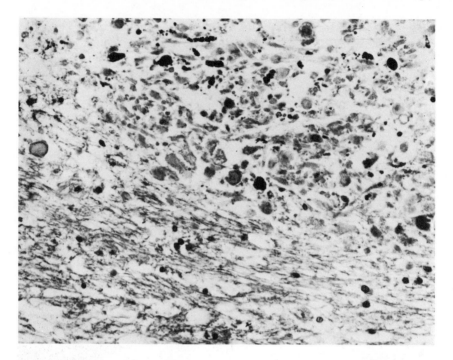

Figure 2. Discrete focus of leukoencephalopathy. Note cluster of axonal swellings and focal mineral deposits (black ovoid bodies). (H&E x 250).

cal history of encephalopathy.[52,57] In addition to white matter attenuation, the CT scans may disclose enlarged ventricles, frequently a concomitant of meningeal seeding by tumor and occasionally cerebral calcifications.[55,58,59] In addition to lucency, focal contrast enhancing lesions have been reported.[49]

Only recently has a similar clinical and pathological picture been associated with the use of high dose intravenous MTX, currently employed to treat several solid tumors, including carcinomas of the head and neck and bone sarcomas. Unlike many patients treated intrathecally, the patients had no prior central nervous system tumor and had not received whole brain radiation therapy (see Table III). Allen and his colleagues described seven patients having various bone and soft tissue sarcomas receiving high dose MTX (HD MTX) with citrovorum factor rescue in addition to MTX.[49] On average, the patients received 11 treatments over a period of 4 to 5 months at doses ranging from 8 to 20 gm/m^2. The CNS syndrome began in the second or third month after initiation of treatment with a peak of severity ranging between 2 and 12

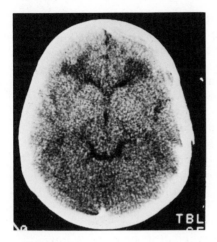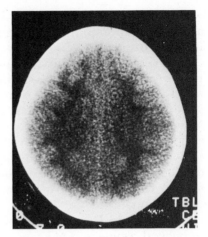

Figure 3. A head CT scan without contrast of a 6-year-old boy with acute lymphoblastic leukemia and active meningeal leukemia who had received 8 courses of intrathecal methotrexate over 3 months during induction chemotherapy. No cranial irradiation was given. The patient was mildly confused and demented at the time of this scan. Diffuse white matter hypodensity is present in the superior cut on the right and periventricular hypodensity is seen anterior to the frontal horn in the inferior cut on the left.

months. All seven patients developed dementia, pseudobulbar palsy and spastic quadriparesis. However, the syndrome was not easily recognized in small children since very subtle personality change, often attributed to the patient's general illness, was often the first sign. Impairment of consciousness progressing to stupor occurred in six, and four had periods of delirium. Despite improvement after discontinuation of the drug, neurological sequelae were severe. CT scans on four patients showed cerebral atrophy. Earliest changes were attenuation of the white matter and slight ventricular enlargement. In addition, one patient developed a focal contrast enhancing lesion, a finding noted in a few other cases produced by intrathecal drug administration. All seven cases had detectable levels of MTX measured from 3 to 9 days after high dose treatment. This correlates with findings of Bleyer which suggests that patients with prolonged elevations of CSF MTX concentrations were those most likely to develop encephalopathy.[40] Hence the CNS may act as a reservoir exposing nervous tissue for prolonged periods to cytotoxic concentrations of the drug. The incidence of the encephalopathy following high dose therapy is less than 2% and these patients resemble those who do not develop the complication.

The course of leukoencephalopathy after intrathecal injection is quite variable. Some patients progress to stupor, coma and death despite withdrawal of the drug, others maintain a persistent vegetative state, but a larger group improve if the drug is withdrawn.[48,50] Even those who improve frequently have devastating neurological sequelae although there is occasionally essentially full recovery.[60] CT scans also may show improvement after drug discontinuation.[61]

The only clearly useful treatment is discontinuation of the drug although some investigators have employed citrovorum factor as well.[51] Monitoring the patient with sequential CT scans would seem advisable, although the clinical dilemma of whether one should discontinue an important part of total antitumor treatment should mild CT changes develop has not been resolved. Since Ara-C has not been clearly shown to cause leukoencephalopathy alone, this drug can be used as an alternative for intrathecal use.

Only a small percentage of patients treated with conventional intrathecal regimens of MTX or with high dose therapy develop clinical encephalopathy. The factors responsible for vulnerability to this complication are not understood. There is a general correlation with total cumulative dose by either route of administration but certain patients are clearly more susceptible. Radiation therapy to the whole brain clearly enhances the reaction.[38,52] Whether radiation promotes MTX toxicity by breaking down blood-brain barrier has been controversial. The presence of ventricular obstruction contraindicates the use of intraventricular drug[50] and it seems likely that leukoencephalopathy is more frequent in patients with active meningeal disease in whom there is frequently a degree of communicating hydrocephalus.[40,62] It is likely that any mechanism which increases the exposure of brain cells to prolonged high concentrations of MTX enhances the likelihood of permanent brain damage from this agent. However, reversible encephalopathy has been reported in a child with no evidence of abnormal CSF retention of MTX,[60] suggesting persistent high CSF concentrations are not always required. Vincristine may contribute to MTX encephalopathy in patients with bone sarcomas treated with high dose MTX. Tejada and Zubrod noted that vincristine given 23 hours after high dose MTX increases the CSF concentration of MTX 2.5 fold.[64]

It is not certain by what mechanism the drug damages the brain, since despite the presence of dihydrofolic acid reductase in the brain, the usual action of MTX requires dividing cells, Astrocytes, endothelial cells and probably oligodendroglia do divide, but neuronal cells do not. The primary target cell of this toxic effect is disputed. The white matter change suggests it may be the oligodendroglia, the vascular changes suggest possible endothelial cell damage, and the early axonal changes raise the question of direct neuronal injury. MTX may well affect the brain by mechanisms as yet poorly understood.[63] Nutritional, neoplastic and infective factors do not seem important.[38]

Although conventional doses of MTX have been regarded as safe for the brain, a recent report suggests that such doses when combined with radiation therapy to the brain can produce CNS damage. Breuer et al[65] reported four cases of progressive brain stem dysfunction marked by quadriparesis and pseudobulbar palsy. All four cases had received posterior fossa irradiation and three had received systemic MTX as well as other drugs. A fourth had received methyl-CCNU. Neuropathological findings included multifocal pontine demyelinative lesions with associated axonal swelling and microvaculolization. Rubenstein had noted two pontine lesions in his report of leukoencephalopathy[52] and we have also subsequently observed such findings in one case having no neurological history.

Other delayed neurotoxic effects in which MTX may have been implicated have been reported. We observed one patient who after repetitive doses of combined MTX and cytosine arabinoside developed progressive disabling cerebellar dysfunction. No residual meningeal leukemia was found at autopsy but extensive loss of cerebellar neurons was present. The patient also had spinal necrosis. Both findings were regarded as secondary to the toxic effects of the combined intrathecal therapy. Optic atrophy associated with blindness has also developed in two patients with leukemia treated with multimodality therapy which combined cranial irradiation with intrathecal methotrexate and cytosine arabinoside as well as systemic vincristine.[66] However, radiation therapy alone also can produce optic neuritis and atrophy.

4. Long-Term Side Effects of Methotrexate Therapy
    a) (Intrathecal or High Dose)
The long-term effects of intrathecal or high dose MTX therapy on patients, especially children, who do not develop overt clinical leukoencephalopathy have not yet been defined. Except for one study suggesting subtle neurological impairment in many patients,[66a] most others have disclosed no such long-term effects.[67-69] In that one report, 12 of 23 leukemic children treated with prophylactic cranial radiation, IT MTX and systemic chemotherapy showed evidence of incoordination, minor motor and gait abnormalities and seizures 10 to 18 months after initial treatment. Motor, language and behavioral abnormalities were said to persist later in some. By contrast, other studies of patients 2 to 5 years after generally similar treatment showed normal neurological and psychometric development, despite CT scan evidence of cerebral atrophy in 25%.[67,68] At Memorial Hospital, where no prophylactic irradiation is added to the IT MTX and systemic chemotherapy, no neurological or psychometric changes were noted in a small number of children studied from 1 to 4 years later. Further studies covering a longer period of follow-up are needed.

5. Transient Cerebral Dysfunction from High Dose MTX.

A quite distinctive type of encephalopathy consisting of sudden onset of focal cerebral dysfunction occurs in 1% to 2% of patients treated with repetitive administrations of high-dose MTX.[70] The patients have been young patients with osteogenic or other sarcomas. The syndrome begins acutely one to two weeks following a prior drug administration, usually after the third or fourth such course. Clinically, the picture is one of a vascular accident with focal cerebral abnormalities consisting primarily of hemiplegia, speech disturbance or focal seizures. The opposite side may become involved within one or two days. The signs frequently fluctuate but finally slowly resolve usually after several days. Ordinarily recovery is complete but occasionally there is mild residual paresis. The etiology of the syndrome is obscure. There is no known pathological basis. Whether vincristine acts synergistically in producing this effect is likewise unclear.

Triazinate: Triazinate or Baker's antifol is an old investigative drug which has received renewed interest. It is included here because it has been used recently to treat brain tumors. It is lipid soluble and enters CNS readily. Systemic toxicity is primarily directed at the gastrointestinal tract and skin. Neurotoxicity is not well established, although it is said occasionally to cause somnolence.[71]

Antipyrimidines

Antipyrimidines are structural analogs of natural pyrimidines and act primarily by competitively inhibiting enzymatic steps necessary for pyrimidine synthesis.

Fluorouracil (5-FU): Fluorouracil is converted to its active product, 5-fluoro-2'deoxyuridine-5'-monophosphate, and this nucleotide product binds thymidylate synthetase, thereby blocking DNA synthesis. 5-FU is given by oral or rapid intravenous infusion for treatment of a variety of solid tumors, chiefly colorectal carcinomas and breast carcinoma (frequently in combination chemotherapy). Bone marrow suppression, mucosal alterations and diarrhea are the dose limiting side effects.

Current treatment regimens produce neurotoxicity only rarely. The most common neurotoxic manifestation is the development of cerebellar ataxia of subacute onset: gait ataxia, ataxia of the extremities with dysmetria, dysarthria, coarse nystagmus and hypotonia. Symptoms occur usually within days after the treatment and in most instances last only a few days.[72] In general the clinical picture is reversible but retreatment with 5-FU may again cause the syndrome.[73] Frequent administration may cause an additive effect which may be prevented by increasing the interval between courses or reducing each dose.[74] In doses higher than those customarily now employed the incidence of cerebellar ataxia ranged as high as 3% to 7% [74-76] although current experience suggests the incidence is less than 1%.[77,78]

Although the cerebellum appears especially susceptible to 5-FU, other central nervous system side effects have been seen, particularly when higher doses have been used. High dose infusions were reported to cause encephalopathy in up to 40% of patients, with symptoms varying from lethargy to coma. Cerebellar symptoms in this group were not prominent.[79,80] Marked slowing of the electroencephalogram occurred and the syndrome reversed within 3 to 4 weeks after drug administration. Extrapyramidal syndromes, including a fairly typical Parkinsonism, have been reported to occur repetitively with each treatment, although in one instance reversibility was incomplete.[81,82] Blurring of vision has been reported and in two reported cases diplopia and extraocular paresis preceded the development of the cerebellar syndrome.[73,83] Cessation of drug led to clearing of the visual symptoms. Pathological changes have occasionally been observed in the cerebellum in patients on the drug but there is poor correlation with clinical toxicity.[72,84] Patients with prominent neurological toxicity have exhibit no pathological abnormality at necropsy.[72]

Intrathecal administration confers no advantage for treating CNS tumors since the drug enters the nervous system readily and CSF levels nearly equal those of plasma within an hour.[85] Experimentally intracarotid and intrathecal administration appear to augment the formation of metabolites, specifically fluoroacetate and fluorocitrate which are toxic to the cerebellum in cats.[84,85] It has also been noted that the active metabolite, 5-fluoro-2'deoxyuridine-5'-monophosphate, concentrates in the cerebellum of mice.[85] As clinically used, fluorouracil is generally a non-neurotoxic drug but these potential effects should be kept in mind should unusual neurological symptoms develop during treatment.

A new combination therapy, thymidine plus 5-FU, clearly sharply increases the incidence of cerebellar dysfunction[86] (see thymidine).

Ftorafur: This drug is a derivative of 5-FU and *in vivo* is slowly hydrolized to 5-FU. Other metabolites, however, may be active as well. It enters the CSF rapidly. Neurological and gastrointestinal side effects are sufficiently dose-limiting that it has not achieved widespread usefulness. Dizziness and ataxia start several days after therapy but are usually transient. Some patients develop lethargy, encephalopathy and headache.[87,88]

Cytarabine (cytosine arabinoside) (arabinosyl cytosine) (Ara-C): Ara-C acts primarily as a false nucleoside thereby competing with natural cytidine nucleotides for enzymes involved in the conversion to deoxycytidine nucleotide and subsequently for conversion into DNA. Its major use is in the induction and maintenance treatment of acute myelogenous leukemia usually in combination chemotherapy. The major systemic side effect is hematopoietic depression followed by nausea and vomiting and stomatitis. The drug is administered intravenously and if given by infusion enters the CSF fairly well. Cytidine deaminase activity is lacking in the CSF and if the drug is given intrathecally it is eliminated very slowly.

The drug is non-neurotoxic when given systemically. It has been used intrathecally to treat meningeal neoplasm, particularly leukemia and lymphoma. It has also been used intrathecally in combination with IT MTX to treat both solid and lymphoid tumors.[62] It also provides a substitute for IT MTX when the latter fails or is poorly tolerated. Although toxic reactions are reported with intrathecal use, aseptic meningitis occurs in a small percentage of cases, probably less than with MTX.[2] The clinical picture is similar. Permanent paraplegia followed the installation of cytosine arabinoside into the lumbar subarachnoid space in three cases, two of which had previously had transient paraparesis following MTX installation.[45,89] Autopsy on the patient who received intrathecal Ara-C alone revealed striking white matter changes consisting of axonal swelling, demyelination and microvacuolization within the spinal cord.[90] Two patients with acute lymphoblastic leukemia treated with whole brain radiation therapy, multi-agent systemic chemotherapy and combination intrathecal Ara-C and MTX developed optic atrophy and blindness much later while receiving only monthly intrathecal Ara-C. Optic nerve biopsy, however, showed changes normally ascribed to radiation damage.[66] Peripheral neuropathies have been reported with systemic Ara-C but the association is not clearly established.[91]

5-Azacytidine: 5-Azacytidine is not a commonly used drug but is discussed here because it produces important neurological toxicity. It is used in man primarily to treat acute myelogenous leukemia and is given by intravenous infusion usually over several days. The drug is largely excluded from entry into CSF. Dose-limiting systemic toxicity is nausea and vomiting and bone marrow suppression.

Neurological side effects have recently come to light. In one series of patients treated with substantial doses for 5 days, 17 of 18 patients developed generalized muscle tenderness, weakness and lethargy associated with an abnormal gait and difficulty rising from a chair. In over half, this was followed by mental status abnormalities, particularly confusion or lethargy.[92] The symptoms usually appeared on day 4 of treatment and were completely reversed within a week. Pain in the tongue, throat and jaw muscles have been noted as well. Hypophosphatemia has recently been noted to correlate temporally with these symptoms and is probably at least in part responsible.[93]

Antipurines

The commonly used antipurines include 6-mercaptopurine (6-MP) used primarily in the treatment of chronic leukemia, and 6-thioguanine (TG), used primarily to treat acute leukemia. These two drugs have no neurological toxicity in conventional usage. Another antipurine, 8-azaguanine, is rarely used but has been regarded as a potential drug for treatment of brain tumors since these tumors lack azaguanine deaminase which is present in normal brain tissue. In fact, treatment directly into brain tumor bed has been attempted. This technique did not cause neurological toxicity but unfortunately yielded no therapeutic benefit.

Plant Alkaloids

The plant alkaloids include the periwinkle derivatives vincristine and vinblastine, both clinically important drugs with well established neurotoxicity. These two compounds derive from the periwinkle plant and a recent new member of this group, desacetyl vinblastineamide (Vindesine, DVA) is a semi-synthetic derivative of vinblastine. Their mode of action is not precisely known. It is believed they interfere with cell division in metaphase although interference with RNA and DNA synthesis is likely as well. The vinca alkaloids are toxic to both central and peripheral nervous systems. Other plant alkaloids are currently experimental and will be given only brief reference.

Periwinkle Derivatives

Vincristine (Table IV): Vincristine is a unique chemotherapeutic agent. It is the only generally available agent whose major and dose-limiting toxicity is directed at the nervous system. It is most toxic to the peripheral nervous system but it also affects cranial nerves, the central nervous system and the autonomic nervous system. A mild degree of sensorimotor peripheral neuropathy occurs in virtually every patient treated with repeated doses. Non-neurological side effects including bone marrow depression are uncommon. The drug is administered by rapid intravenous injection. It does not enter the CNS in appreciable amounts.

Peripheral Neuropathy: The first symptoms of peripheral neuropathy are usually sensory. Paresthesias frequently appear after several weekly doses and affect the hands and feet, not always simultaneously. Despite the early appearance of prominent sensory symptoms, major sensory signs are usually absent.[94] Minor distal threshold changes are commonly observed. Prior to the development of any symptoms, the examiner usually notes absent ankle jerks and diffusely diminished deep tendon reflexes. As cumulative dose increases, all reflexes may disappear.[95] A single dosage has peak depressive effect on the ankle jerk at 17 days.[96]

Distal weakness may occur, usually after sensory complaints are quite apparent. Intrinsic muscles of the hands and feet and the dorsiflex-

Table IV
Vincristine Neurotoxicity

	Peripheral Nervous System	Autonomic Nervous System	Cranial Nerves	Muscle	Central Nervous System
Early Effects (1 day-3 weeks)	↓ AJ, other deep tendon reflexes	Ileus-cramping abdominal pain	Jaw pain	Myositis-"myopathy" (muscle weakness, pain)	—
Intermediate Effects (1-6 weeks)	Diffuse ↓ DTRs Paresthesiae Numbness	Same as chronic	Photophobia	—	Seizures-Inappropriate ADH secretion
Chronic Effects (> 4 weeks)	Distal weakness Mild objective sensory signs	Constipation Impotence Urinary hesitency (rare) Orthostatic hypotension (rare)	Optic atrophy Ptosis VI N. paresis VII N. paresis Vocal cord paresis Dysphagia	—	Same as above

ors of the feet and toes and the everters of the feet, as well as extensors of the wrist and fingers, are prominently affected. Significant weakness is not very common with current dosage regimens of the drug although it appears to be more common in children in whom dosage regimens are relatively higher. In general, weakness is reversible but occasionally slight residual weakness remains and recovery frequently takes many months.[94,96,97]

Electrical studies usually reveal only slight reduction in motor conduction velocities at a time when peripheral neuropathy is quite symptomatic. The values may decrease during therapy but remain within normal limits, especially in younger patients. The distal motor latencies may be prolonged and distal sensory latencies are prolonged and significantly reduced in amplitude and may be unobtainable.[95,97-99] Needle electromyography indicates distal denervation of muscles.[95,97] The H-reflex is usually absent but on occasion remains intact when the ankle jerk is no longer present. This has led to speculation that vincristine may act directly on muscle spindle which is not involved in the H-reflex but is required to produce the ankle jerk.[97] The electrical findings, particularly the minimal slowing of motor conduction velocities, suggest that this neuropathy is secondary to axonal degeneration rather than to demyelination.

Pathological studies support the view that this neuropathy is primarily an axonal neuropathy of the dying-back variety. Biopsied sural nerves before and after vincristine therapy revealed post-treatment Wallerian degeneration without segmental demyelination.[100] Animal studies have produced variable results. Peripheral neuropathy, chiefly axonal, is seen predominently in some animals but in others myopathic change is more prominent.[101-105] Disruption of the myofibrillary elements has been seen in electron microscopy studies in man[97] (see Myopathy below).

The peripheral neurotoxicity of vincristine is dose related and the effect is cumulative if the drug is given in standard weekly doses. Severe neuropathic effects are observed with inadvertent overdoses: one 15-year-old leukemic girl died 33 hours after a 32 mg dosage.[106] However, a number of factors related to the patient may influence the neurotoxicity. It is clear that some individuals are far more sensitive to the neurotoxic effects of the vinca alkaloids than others.[107] Pre-existing neuropathy may enhance the neurotoxicity of vincristine. A patient with a minimal form ("forme fruste") of presumed Charcot-Marie-Tooth, presenting only with pes cavus and bilateral foot drop, died as a result of paraplegia with subsequent bulbar paralysis after receiving only two weekly doses of vincristine.[108] We have observed two similar patients who developed profound neuropathy after one or two doses, but recovered. A patient with myotonic dystrophy worsened significantly while on vincristine.[109] It has not been well established, however, whether the common peripheral neuropathies due to diabetes and alcohol abuse enhance the neuropathic effects of vincristine.[95] Malnutrition does appear to enhance the neuropathy related to vincristine even though thiamine and B-12 administration failed in one study to reverse it.[110] It is said that patients with obstructive liver disease are more susceptible to the drug's toxic effects although this is not established. However, the impaired hepatic function produced by L-asparaginase appears to enhance the effects of vincristine toxicity. If vincristine is given prior to L-asparaginase, no enhancement occurs.[3] The combination of vincristine, L-asparaginase and isoniazide has produced severe neuropathy in three patients.[111]

Compression neuropathies, particularly common peroneal palsy, are rather common with vincristine and appear to be due to a combination of the effects of the drug and the weight loss attendant on the primary illness. In addition, asymmetrical neuropathic symptoms may be seen distal to proximal involvement by tumor so that the first symptoms are brought out by the vincristine on the involved side.

Autonomic Neuropathy: Autonomic neuropathy is seen fairly frequently but is usually less clinically significant. In one large series, constipation was a common problem occurring in about a third of the patients.[94] When we used this drug in combination chemotherapy to treat primary brain tumors, constipation was a special problem for the elderly patient.[112] Occasionally it required discontinuation of the drug. A more acute phenomenon occurs occasionally, primarily in children, rarely in adults, in which the patient develops fairly acute abdominal pain within a few hours or days following a dose of vincristine. The paralytic ileus which causes the syndrome may become sufficiently severe to suggest an "acute abdomen." This complication occurs earlier than that of constipation. Other autonomic complaints include occasional bladder dysfunction, impotence and orthostatic hypotension, all reported in a small percentage of patients.[96,97,113]

Cranial Nerve Impairment: Cranial nerve impairment is uncommon except when there is fairly severe peripheral neuropathy. Bilateral 7th nerve pareses of mild degree occur occasionally, particularly in children, usually associated with foot drop or other signs of sensorimotor neuropathy.[96] The facial weakness, although usually bilateral, may be symmetrical or asymmetrical and so may be confused with meningeal seeding or tumor occurring at the base of the brain. Strictly unilateral weakness would be more likely to be associated with tumor or other causes. A very early side effect which is thought to be cranial nerve in origin is paroxysmal jaw pain or throat pain which occurs within hours of drug administration and subsides within days. In general, this does not recur with later administration of the drug.[114] It is possible this pain relates to muscle injury but its paroxysmal nature suggests it is neuropathic. Extraocular muscle paresis related to 6th or 3rd nerve dysfunction is seen rarely.[96] Ptosis is usually the first sign of 3rd nerve paresis. Ocular findings may precede other signs of neurotoxicity.[115] Lower cranial nerve impairment producing hoarseness and dysphagia associated with vocal cord paresis has been described rarely.[116,117] One report suggests optic atrophy may be caused by vincristine. In the case reported, the patient has been treated with multi-agent chemotherapy but the time course suggested vincristine was the offending agent. Pathology disclosed loss of ganglion cells primarily in the region of the macula.[118] Photosensitivity is occasionally encountered in patients on vincristine.

Myopathy: Clinical evidence of myopathy has been noted primarily in children.[2] Muscle tenderness and pain occur within one week of administration of vincristine and this is followed by weakness in the proximal muscles. The symptoms generally clear within a few days. Muscle necrosis has been described histologically in man.[97] Electromyographic data are lacking.

CNS Side Effects: The brain and spinal cord are protected from the neurotoxic effects of vincristine by its failure to pass the blood-brain barrier. If the drug is injected intrathecally, it causes ascending myelopathy with brainstem dysfunction and death.[119,120] Seizures have been reported secondary to vincristine. Seizures generally result from hyponatremia produced by another side effect of vincristine administration — inappropriate antidiuretic hormone (ADH) secretion. However, in an early series with substantial doses of vincristine, 1% to 4% of patients suffered seizures several days after treatment without clear evidence for metabolic or structural disease.[121-123] It is difficult to be certain that structural illness was not present in these patients, although no recurrence occurred on later administration. Lethargy and hallucinations have also been occasionally described.[94]

Vinblastine (Velban): This drug has been used primarily to treat Hodgkin's disease and testicular carcinoma, usually in combination regimens. Its major toxic side effect is bone marrow depression although it is a fairly well tolerated drug. Vinblastine produces neurotoxicity qualitatively similar to that of vincristine although much less frequently since the hematologic effects are dose limiting. Neurotoxic effects tend to be mild and usually develop with chronic use. They include evidence of peripheral neuropathy including paresthesias, distal sensory loss and weakness, as well as jaw pain, urinary retention, orthostatic hypotension, photosensitivity and vocal cord paralysis.[124-127] In addition, headache and depression have been attributed to this drug.

Vindesine (desacetyl vinblastine amide sulfate) (DVA): This promising agent is a semi-synthetic derivative of vinblastine. It has been used alone or in combination for non-small cell carcinoma of the lung and is said to show activity against other relatively unresponsive cancers such as esophageal carcinoma. In general, its neurotoxicity is similar to that of vincristine. Relative to vincristine, the drug is used in current regimens in considerably higher doses and hence has produced rather significant neurotoxic reactions in many patients. Weakness often seems more severe than sensory complaints as compared with vincristine neuropathy. There frequently is a moderate amount of proximal weakness suggesting there may be a myopathic component although this has not been observed pathologically or electromyographically. In fact, evidence of denervation with prominent fibrillation potentials has been seen in severely affected patients as far proximally as the iliopsoas muscles.[5] The spectrum of neurological toxicities is similar to that of vincristine and includes paresthesias, distal and proximal muscle weakness, constipation, abdominal cramps, paralytic ileus, hoarseness, jaw pain, myalgia, and vertigo.[128-134]

Podophyllotoxins

VM-26 (Teniposide): This agent is still investigational but shows considerable activity against both Hodgkin's and non-Hodgkin's lymphoma as well as pediatric leukemia. It is also effective against bladder cancer and phase II studies suggest some effectiveness in the treatment of malignant gliomas.[135,136] Its access to the CSF is minimal (less than 1%) in the presence of an intact blood-brain barrier but there is suggestion that this is much increased if blood-brain barrier function is impaired.[137] Hematologic toxicity is dose-limiting although this is not a major problem in most current protocols. Hypotension is seen occasionally if the drug is given too rapidly.

Neurological toxicity has not been a problem in our experience in treating brain tumor patients with a weekly dosage of 100-300 mg/m^2. However, earlier phase II studies using slightly high doses indicated that 10-20% of patients developed peripheral neuropathy.[138]

VP-16 (Etoposide): Like VM-26, this drug produces metaphase arrest and also prevents cells from entering mitosis. Effects on DNA, RNA and protein synthesis also appear to contribute to cytotoxic effects. VP-16 demonstrates activity against small cell tumor of the lung and several hematologic malignancies, and is currently in phase I trials. Bone marrow suppression and some degree of gastrointestinal toxicity are the primary side effects. Little drug reaches the CSF and no neurological toxicity has been well documented, though associated paresthesiae and headache have been noted rarely.

Other Plant Alkaloids

Maytansine: This is an experimental agent currently in phase I studies. It has suggested activity in leukemia, lymphoma and several solid tumors including breast carcinomas. The mechanism of action appears similar to that of the podophyllotoxins and the vinca alkaloids. Toxicity is largely gastrointestinal, hepatic and neurological. Higher doses produced profound lethargy which may have been partly related to metabolic encephalopathy.[138a] In addition, repetitive doses produced neurotoxicity similar to vincristine neuropathy. Symptomatically, paresthesias, distal extremity weakness, depressed deep tendon reflexes and jaw pain have been noted.[138,139]

Antibiotic Agents

These drugs are the product of microbial fermentation and usually have anti-infective activity as well. However, their cytotoxic activity precludes their use as antimicrobial agents. The precise mechanisms of action of these drugs are poorly understood. Some appear to act as alkylating agents. Drugs in this group include doxorubicin (Adriamycin), daunorubicin (Daunomycin), bleomycin, dactinomycin (Actinomycin-D), mithramycin (Mithracin), and mitomycin-C.

Nausea and vomiting following these agents is frequently profound and in general gastrointestinal and bone marrow side effects limit the dosage. Doxorubicin and daunorubicin have unique cardiotoxicity resembling cardiomyopathy, which occurs following high cumulative doses. Bleomycin occasionally produces pulmonary fibrosis which is less clearly dose-related. The group as a whole has a broad spectrum of antitumor activity. The newer agents, doxorubicin and bleomycin, are particularly effective against many solid tumors as well as lymphomas. Many of these tumors had been largely unresponsive to earlier agents.

Doxorubicin (Adriamycin)

Doxorubicin is a highly effective agent against many tumors. It has rather profound toxicity directed at bone marrow, GI tract, hair follicles and cardiac muscle. Extravasation produces severe skin necrosis. Its neurotoxicity is interesting even though it does not produce clinical neurotoxicity as currently employed. However, Cho noted that rats receiving 10 mg/kg (a very high relative dose) developed severe posterior limb ataxia and forelimb ataxia approximately 11 days after injection.[140,141] The focus of pathological injury was the dorsal root ganglion which is unprotected by the blood-brain barrier. CNS toxicity was not seen in the rats. As with most of the antibiotics, virtually none crosses the blood-brain barrier. Significant clinical changes similar to those in the rat have not been seen although careful pathological examination of the dorsal root ganglion has not been done routinely. It is of some interest that in another species, the guinea pig, this neurotoxicity is not nearly so prominent as cardiac toxicity, the reverse of that in the rat.

Bleomycin

Bleomycin is the only cell phase specific agent in this group. It inhibits replication of DNA by DNA polymerase and in addition causes breakage of DNA strands. It is a very effective drug, usually in combination chemotherapy against a wide variety of solid and lymphoid tumors. Its most serious toxicity is "bleomycin lung," a problem which is not consistently reversible. When given in combination with other drugs (MTX or cytoxan and 5-FU), reversible disturbances of consciousness and cognition have been noted.[142,143] It has also been alleged to cause peripheral neuropathy but this has not been the general clinical experience. Cochlear damage occurs in animals but there is no clinical evidence for its occurrence in man.[144]

Dactinomycin (Actinomycin-D)

This is a highly effective agent against Wilms' tumor and a variety of other solid tumors, but has been replaced in many instances by newer agents. There is essentially no penetration into the CNS and no significant clinical neurotoxicity has been observed. Animal studies, however, show clearly that it is a very neurotoxic drug. When injected intracranially or directly into the CSF it produces seizures, tremors, myoclonic jerks, encephalopathy and myelopathy in a variety of animal studies. Widespread CNS demyelination and spongy necrosis have been noted pathologically in experimental studies.[145,146]

Other Antibiotics

Daunorubicin, mithramycin and mitomycin-C are not commonly used and are not associated with significant neurological toxicity. The neurological complications of antibiotics are discussed in Chapter I of this book.

Miscellaneous Chemotherapy Agents (Table I)

This category includes a large number of agents having quite variable mechanisms of action. Some, including the nitrosoureas, and several others including cis-platinum, dacarbazine, galactitol and hexamethylmelamine have alkylating properties whereas others such as asparaginase, an enzyme, and procarbazine, a monoamine oxidase inhibitor, act by quite distinct mechanisms.

Nitrosoureas

The nitrosoureas are a group of cell cycle non-specific agents which have alkylating properties and appear to inhibit both DNA and protein synthesis. They are largely lipid soluble compounds and have the capacity to enter CNS readily following systemic administration. Two of these agents, BCNU (carmustine) and CCNU (lomustine), are now commercially available. Methyl-CCNU is widely employed but still not commercially available. Other nitrosoureas include streptozotocin, PCNU, ACNU and DCNU (chlorozotocin). All of these agents show evidence of effectiveness or are being tried in the treatment of primary brain tumor. CCNU and methyl-CCNU are supplied in oral form.

BCNU, the original agent of this group, was first used to treat meningeal leukemia and subsequently has shown activity against a number of solid and hematologic tumors including lung cancer, leukemia, Hodgkin's disease and myeloma. It is now widely accepted as an effective drug in the treatment of malignant glioma.[147] Systemic toxicity consists primarily of early nausea and vomiting and delayed thrombocytopenia and leukopenia. Hepatic dysfunction is seen occasionally and both pulmonary fibrosis and renal failure have been seen very rarely with large cumulative doses.

BCNU is a good example of a drug which is probably non-neurotoxic as conventionally used, but clearly neurotoxic when used in innovative ways. Even in conventional dosage, we and others have raised the issue of whether nitrosoureas may be synergistic with radiation therapy delivered to the whole brain for treatment of malignant glioma in producing insidious dementia associated with cerebral atrophy seen in a small percentage of patients.[5] Another example of such apparent synergistic toxicity was a case reported by Breuer of a child treated for cerebellar malignant glioma with posterior fossa radiation and repeated conventional doses of systemic methyl-CCNU who developed spastic quadriparesis and was found to have multifocal pontine demyelinative lesions at necropsy.[65] The lesions seen were relatively non-specific since similar lesions have been seen with radiation and methotrexate (see methotrexate).

In an effort to increase the amount of drug delivered to brain tumor with less systemic toxicity, several centers have undertaken to treat both primary and metastatic brain tumors with intracarotid injections of BCNU. In one report[148] nine patients with metastatic lung tumors were so treated. Therapeutic efficacy was demonstrated but there were complications. Seven developed orbital, eye, and neck pain at the time of the injection, three developed focal seizures, two developed transient encephalopathy, and two nausea. In our small experience we have seen one patient develop a transient ischemic episode following vertebral artery injection. Another patient had a transient increase in neurological signs. Focal head pain has been seen in the majority of patients. It is not yet clear whether any permanent neurotoxicity will occur with this technique. Experimentally, BCNU has been largely nontoxic to the brain and to the eye when injected into rhesus monkeys although in one report such injection resulted in blindness in dogs.[149,150]

Finally, the experimental use of BCNU in very high doses ranging form 1500 to 3000 mg/m^2/dose (versus a conventional 200 to 240 mg/m^2) followed in one week by autologous bone marrow transplantation to prevent lethal bone marrow toxicity has been attempted at several centers to treat both brain tumors and patients with diffuse metastatic disease, sparing the brain. Three patients so treated developed multifocal neurological abnormalities 3 to 12 weeks after dosage.[151] Pathology in these cases revealed foci of coagulative necrosis. There was also fibrinoid necrosis and an increase in size of the axis cylinders, but no evidence of inflammation. The changes seen were remarkably similar to those produced by radiation necrosis of brain, although these patients had never received brain irradiation. There was no evidence of CT scan or pathologically of brain metastases. The evidence suggested that the drug and not the autologous bone marrow transplant was the responsible factor in producing these lesions. If so, this treatment method provides a second example in addition to MTX leukoencephalopathy of structural brain abnormality resulting from the use of a chemotherapeutic agent.

CCNU has been used for treatment of both primary and metastatic tumors of the brain and several groups have used it in combination chemotherapy for treatment of primary malignant glioma. It also has effectiveness in certain solid and lymphoid tumors. No clear evidence exists for neurotoxicity although the issue of possible potentiation of radiation effects is unsettled.

Methyl-CCNU has also been used to treat brain tumor as well as malignant melanoma. It is discussed above.

Streptozotocin is now in phase III trial in the treatment of primary brain tumors for which it appears to be a modestly effective agent. It is also used for treatment of malignant carcinoid and for islet cell carcinoma. It has the unfortunate side effect of producing rather marked predictable nausea and vomiting which occasionally can limit its use, particularly since it is usually given weekly. It is relatively marrow sparing but has significant potential renal toxicity producing both renal tubular acidosis and a Fanconi-like syndrome in patients given substantial cumulative doses. PCNU, ACNU and DCNU are all in early trials for a variety of tumors. These four drugs have no established neurological toxicity.

Other Agents

Cis-platinum (cis-diamminodichloroplatinum II) (DDP) (Cisplatin): Cis-platinum is the first heavy metal compound to be used as an anti-neoplastic agent. A number of chemical relatives are in early laboratory trials. Its cytotoxic action appears to depend on inhibition of DNA precursors although there is interference as well with protein and RNA synthesis. There is some evidence that it functions in part as an alkylating agent. This drug is used to greatest advantage in treatment of testicular carcinoma but also shows considerable activity againt ovarian carcinoma, carcinoma of the head and neck, lymphoma, some sarcomas, as well as bladder, prostate and breast carcinoma. Hematologic toxicity is mild. Anaphylactic reactions occur occasionally. Its dose-limiting side effect is nephrotoxicity and in addition it possesses significant ototoxicity. Both of these side effects are dose-related and occur most commonly with higher (e.g., 120 mg/m^2) or more frequent individual doses.

The most significant side effect upon the neurosensory system is ototoxicity.[152-154] On occasion this may actually be dose-limiting although, in general, partial deafness is considered a tolerable side effect. In most instances the deafness is transient although some irreversibility has been noted.[155] Diminished auditory acuity is noticed frequently within 3 to 4 days after initial treatment and may be accompanied by tinnitus. It is generally bilateral but there may be a degree of asymmetry. Improvement occurs over the subsequent days and weeks of no further treatment is given, but repeated doses usually produce a cumulative effect. The predominant hearing loss is at high frequencies from 4000 to 8000 Hz. Speech discrimination is usually little affected although profound deafness occasionally affects all frequencies.[152,154] Tinnitus frequently accompanies the deafness. It is generally thought that vestibular function is not disturbed since the target site of toxicity experimentally is the organ of Corti. However, vestibular dysfunction with abnormal electronystagmography has been rarely observed.[156] The ototoxic effects appear more prominent in elderly patients although mild deafness does not generally contraindicate the use of the drug. The combination of slower infusion of the drug and the widespread use of pretreatment with intravenous hydration and mannitol to promote renal excretion has significantly reduced the problem of dose limiting renal toxicity and ototoxicity.[157-159]

An acute reversible encephalopathy and occasional seizures have been noted with cis-platinum administration. Frequently this is related to the severity of the gastrointestinal toxicity, and almost always such cerebral events are associated with significant metabolic alterations associated with renal tubular dysfunction produced by the drug. Many of these patients have been profoundly hypomagnesemic and hyponatremic. Tetany associated with hypomagnesemia and hypocalcemia has been reported in four of eight children with neuroblastoma.[160] A single case was reported of transient cortical blindness followed by generalized seizures developing within 4 hours of cis-platinum infusion given to a patient with disseminated testicular carcinoma but no brain metastases.[161] The etiology of this episode of blindness and seizures was not defined. A notable feature of this case was a CSF platinum level of 7.2 mcg/ml, a level nearly equal that in serum, despite the findings of prior distribution studies showing that the drug is largely excluded from the CNS.

An uncommon but more direct neurological complication is peripheral neuropathy. Neuropathy occurs in a small percentage of treated patients but has been clearly associated with cis-platinum therapy by several groups.[162-167] In general the neuropathy occurs after several courses of cis-platinum, usually high dose regimens. The neuropathy is predominantly a sensory neuropathy which generally manifests as a mild non-disabling problem manifested by paresthesias of the hands and feet and some objective sensory loss. However, a number of patients have progressed to develop a profound disabling ataxia associated with marked paresthesias and dysesthesias and prominent objective sensory loss. One recent report has emphasized that the neuropathy is a pure sensory neuropathy which spares temperature and pin sensation while profoundly affecting posterior column functions, proprioception and vibration.[166] In our experience, the neuropathy has differed significantly from vincristine in producing a much greater degree of objective sensory loss particularly of position and vibration sense. However, all modalities are sometimes affected and occasionally minor distal weakness appears as well. The reversibility of this syndrome is not entirely clear since some cases have persisted long after discontinuation of treatment. If the neuropathy does remain purely sensory, a remote sensory neuropathy of carcinoma is to be distinguished. In additon, meningeal seeding by tumor should be considered, although in that disorder one would expect motor or autonomic complaints to accompany the sensory findings.

One group of investigators provided good pathological evidence that the neuropathy is of a dying-back, axonal variety.[166,168] One prior report[163] had suggested that the lesion was primarily demyelinative. In the more recent study, however, sural nerve biopsy in man showed primarily axonal change and a parallel study in rats showed Wallerian degeneration not only in the peripheral nervous system but axonal alteration and swelling in the spinal cord and optic nerve.[168] In addition, autopsy of one child disclosed fiber loss in the posterior column, a finding which raises the concern that CNS toxicity may eventually result from the use of this drug. Two cases of possible optic nerve toxicity in patients receiving repeated doses of cis-platinum have been reported.[169] One, also on doxorubicin, developed papilledema which disappeared after cis-platinum was stopped. The other patient developed persistent retrobulbar neuritis. In addition there has been one report of paralytic ileus thought to be related to the drug.[167] Whether there is potentiation of neurotoxic effects of other drugs is not clear. The drug is frequently used with vindesine which is highly neurotoxic peripherally but we have not found evidence of synergistic effects. This drug is now commercially available and it is highly useful agent for a wide variety of tumors. Hence, its potential neurotoxicity may become an increasingly important clinical problem.

Galactitol (dianhydrogalactitol): This drug is included because it has recently been employed in a number of studies in the treatment of primary brain tumor as well as a number of other malignancies. It appears chiefly to work as an alkylating agent and at least as currently used is not known to be neurotoxic.

Hexamethylmelamine: There has been suggestion that this agent acts as an alkylating agent since it is structurally similar to an early alkylating agent, triethylene melamine, but others regard it as an antimetabolite. Its precise mechanism of action is not known. It has limited use but has been employed in the treatment of ovarian cancer and shows activity against a number of other cancers. Nausea, vomiting and abdominal cramps are the most common dose limiting toxicities.

This drug demonstrates both central and peripheral neurotoxicity. Conventional dosages of 8 mg/kg/day result in the occurrence of neurological problems in 10% to 20% of patients.[170-172] Encephalopathies with confusion, anxiety, hallucinations and depression as well as ataxia and tremor have been noted. Rarely a Parkinsonian syndrome has been seen. Symptoms tend to develop after prolonged cumulative daily oral doses. Similarly, peripheral neuropathy with hyperreflexia, paresthesias and occasionally distal sensory loss and weakness is more likely to develop the longer a daily dose is continued.[170,171,173] Prior neuropathy induced by vincristine may enhance this occurrence.[173] One report suggests pyridoxine is beneficial in its treatment.[174]

Dacarbazine (DTIC) (dimethyl triazeno imidazole carboxamide): DTIC appears to have activity against malignant melanoma and it has also been used to treat malignant gliomas as well as refractory Hodgkin's disease and certain soft tissue sarcomas. It is sometimes grouped as an alkylating agent but others have suggested anti-metabolic effects. Little drug enters to CSF since it is poorly lipid soluble. Nausea and vomiting are a problematic acute side effect and moderate myelosuppression is a delayed side effect. An unusual manifestation consisting of a flu-like syndrome with fever, malaise and myalgia occurs about 7 days after treatment in a small number of patients. There have been rare reports of CNS reaction including dementia, hemiparesis, seizures and cerebral hemorrhage, but the presence of brain metastases or other potential complicating factors may have been responsible for these symptoms.[4,5] There is no well established neurotoxicity of this drug.

Hydroxyurea: This drug affects the synthesis of DNA without interfering with RNA or protein synthesis. It is generally considered cell cycle specific but its precise mechanism is not clear. It is an oral drug which has been used for many years to treat both acute and chronic phases of chronic myelogenous leukemia. It has occasionally been used to treat other solid tumors and particularly has effectiveness in advanced carcinoma of the prostate. Phase II studies have recently shown that hydroxyurea is effective in the treatment of malignant glioma.[175] This drug readily passes the blood-brain barrier. There have been rare descriptions of headache, dizziness, drowsiness or even hallucinations. but in general the drug is not neurotoxic. We have encountered one patient who received 6000 rads whole brain RT for the treatment of malignant glioma followed by oral hydroxyurea given for 2 years who developed CT scan changes compatible with leukoencephalopathy very similar to that seen with MTX. The patient developed no new neurological signs and symptoms during this period.

The Enzymes

L-Asparaginase: L-asparaginase is an enzyme which hydrolyzes asparagine to aspartic acid and ammonia. Many tumor cells are unable to manufacture asparagine and the drug deprives them of this essential amino acid. Its major use has been in the treatment of acute lymphoblastic leukemia. Systemic side effects are prominent and may be dose limiting. They include nausea and vomiting, bone marrow depression, hepatotoxicity and, much less commonly, hemorrhagic pancreatitis, anaphylaxis, and non-ketotic hyperglycemia.

CNS neurotoxicity of this drug may be dose limiting. This neurotoxicity is characterized by an acute alteration in mental state during the course of treatment. Early trials with the drug employed much larger doses than those currently used. Doses of 1000 to 5000 IU/kg/day caused lethargy and confusion on the first day of administration in as many as 20% to 60% of patients.[176-178] Common current regimens are 200 to 1000 IU/kg/day or 60,000 IU/m^2 twice weekly. With these doses, encephalopathy is less frequent but is still a significant problem requiring discontinuation of the drug in about 15% of cases treated at Memorial Hospital. On a biweekly schedule, encephalopathy usually occurs after the third or fourth dose.

Subtle memory or personality change may precede lethargy and confusion. In general the symptoms are mild and reversible but particularly with higher doses progression to coma occasionally occurs and we have had at least one unexplained death. Delirium with hallucinations has been reported and impairment of recent memory is seen.[179,180] Reversion to normal occurs within a few days after treatment ceases. Ohnuma postulated that a separate disturbance of cerebral function occurred one week after institution of therapy, but it seems likely this was simply related to cumulative dose.[181] In general, a dose-effect relationship applies although the encephalopathy occasionally occurs with low dosage. Focal cerebral dysfunction and seizures have been reported but are rare.[178] During the acute period the EEG is diffusely slow and it changes concomitantly with the patient's state.[182]

This enzyme is a large protein which fails to cross the blood-brain barrier. The etiology of the central neurotoxicity has not been fully defined. There may be multiple factors. This drug alters amino acid and protein metabolism. Specifically, the serum levels of L-aspartate, L-glutamate and ammonia are elevated while those of L-asparagine and L-glutamine are lowered. In addition, significant hepatic dysfunction occurs in up to 50% of patients treated with the drug depending on the dosage. Triphasic delta waves which sometimes accompany hepatic encephalopathy although are not specific, have been reported also in L-asparaginase encephalopathy.[183] This raises the issue that some cases of drug-induced encephalopathy may be primarily due to a heptic dysfunction. Interference with brain protein synthesis has also been postulated. It seems likely the encephalopathy is multifactorial in origin.

Other Enzymes

As an enzyme, L-asparaginase has been in a unique class as an antineoplastic agent. However, other similar agents are now undergoing scrutiny as potential agents. One in particular, SAGA (succinylated acinetobacter glutaminase-asparaginase), has recently shown considerable promise in the treatment of acute leukemia. However, neurotoxicity has proved dose limiting. The encephalopathy it produces is in many ways similar to that seen with L–asparaginase.[184] Clinical trials of several similar enzymatic agents are being planned.

Procarbazine (methylhydrazine, Natulan, Matulane): This drug, a methylhydrazine derivative, is a monoamine oxidase inhibitor with antineoplastic activity. Its chief use has been in the treatment of Hodgkin's disease as well as in non-Hodgkin's lymphoma. However, it has achieved considerable attention in the treatment of malignant glioma in the past several years.[185,186] Its mode of action is unclear. Some of its metabolites appear to be cytotoxic and there is evidence that it inhibits RNA, DNA and protein synthesis. Peripheral side effects are primarily gastrointestinal, chiefly nausea and vomiting, an early side effect, and later hemotologic suppression, chiefly leukopenia. Skin rash, a maculopapular or occasionally vesicular lesion develops in a small percentage of cases and may require discontinuation of the drug. Our impression in treating brain tumor patients is that this skin rash is more common in patients already on phenytoin.[186]

Procarbazine is a neurotoxic drug but its neurotoxicity is no longer a prominent problem. Toxicity is directed at both the central and peripheral nervous systems. Procarbazine passes readily through the blood-brain barrier in both man and animal. In its early usage, intravenous administration was common. This method frequently produced prolonged somnolence[187] and has been largely abandoned. Current oral doses are 100 to 300 mg daily in contrast to doses of 200 to 1000 mg used previously. With the latter dosage, 31% of patients developed some degree of encephalopathy[188] and in slightly lower doses the figure was 14%.[189] In addition to lethargy and somnolence, hallucinations, confusion, depression and mania have been noted.[190-192] Because it is a monoamine oxidase inhibitor, central nervous system effects of phenothiazines, barbiturates and narcotics and possibly alcohol may be enhanced by procarbazine.[5,188,193,194] The precise mechanism of the CNS depression, however, is not clear. Although tyramine-containing foods such as cheese might potentially be expected to cause acute hypertension, this is not a clinical problem. Orthostatic hypotension, however, has been described.[190]

In addition to its central neurotoxic effect, peripheral neuropathy occurs with procarbazine in 10% to 15% of patients treated with relatively high dosages. It is unusual, however, with most current schedules including in our experience in treating brain tumor patients.[186] This drug is administered orally on a daily basis over a given period of time and in general paresthesias appear after about one month on a substantial oral dosage.[188,190] In one series depressed deep tendon reflexes were noted in 17%. In some cases symptoms improved while treatment continued at the same dosage.[190] Ataxia is occasionally seen, probably as a part of the peripheral neuropathy.[189] Muscle weakness distally is seen occasionally and proximal muscle myalgias have also been described.[188,190] A structurally related compound, hydrazine, now largely abandoned in the treatment of cancer patients, causes a primary sensory peripheral neuropathy in most patients treated.[195] Isoniazid is also a relative of hydrazine. Since the neuropathy produced by that drug is reversed by pyridoxal phosphate, pyridoxine has been tried in the treatment of procarbazine but there is little indication that it alters either the encephalopathy or the peripheral neuropathy.[188,196]

Mitotane (o-p'-DDD): The antitumor activity of this drug is limited largely to adrenocorticocarcinoma. Its effect appears directed at the mitochondria of adrenocortical cells. As such, it is sometimes grouped under "hormonal" agents. Although it is a rarely used drug, it is discussed here because it has prominent neurotoxicity. Systemic problems include gastrointestinal disturbances, anorexia, nausea, vomiting and diarrhea in 80%, and skin rashes in 15% to 20%.

Neurotoxicity is described in 35% to 40% of patients treated and the incidence may be even higher.[197,198] The major effects are somnolence, lethargy, vertigo, headache, dizziness and blurred vision. Peripheral neuropathy is also rarely reported to occur. Although the effects are generally reversible, reversibility is said to be rarely incomplete. Reduction of dosage usually permits continuation of the drug.

PALA (N-phosphoacetyl aspartic acid): PALA is an experimental antineoplastic agent which inhibits the enzyme aspartate transcarbamylase, an early step in *de novo* pyrimidine biosynthesis. Systemic toxicity is predominantly directed against the gastrointestinal tract and skin whereas the bone marrow is relatively spared. The drug has shown evidence for clinical activity against bladder, colorectal, lung and breast cancer and is currently in single drug and multidrug trials.

Despite the fact that some preclinical animal studies reported acute neurotoxicity including seizures, ataxia, lethargy and weakness with large intravenous bolus injections in small rodents, clinical neurotoxicity was not expected in the doses employed. Clinical trials at Memorial Hospital in which the drug was given weekly by intravenous infusion induced delayed onset neurotoxicity, seizures, and/or encephalopathy in some patients.[199] Among 77 patients receiving adequate dosage, nine (or 12%) developed multiple seizures after 3 weeks or more of PALA treatment, usually one to two weeks after the last dose. Eight of these patients had multiple seizures and three developed status epilepticus, poorly responsive to anticonvulsants. There was noted to be correlation between the development of seizures and concomitant structural brain disease. Such structural abnormalities were present in seven of nine patients who developed seizures: three had cerebral metastases, three had traumatic or surgical scars, and one had a focally abnormal CT which was not diagnosable. The two patients developing seizures without evidence of focal disease had received a mean dosage 10 times that of those who had focal disease over a much more prolonged period. Thus, although PALA can cause seizures in patients without structural disease, a combination of PALA and a brain lesion carries a very high risk of seizures at low doses.

In addition, seven patients (9%) developed encephalopathy sufficient to require hospitalization. Each of these patients improved after PALA was stopped. The encephalopathy tended to develop between 2 and 6 weeks of cumulative treatment. Several other patients experienced transient symptoms such as perioral anesthesia, lethargy, weakness, and lightheadedness during one infusion. A slower infusion rate prevented these symptoms.

While the degree of neurotoxicity was thought to be sufficient to limit the drug's application, alternate schedules used at other institutions were safer, and additional clinical trials are currently under way.

Thymidine (TdR): This drug has been used with several other cytotoxic drugs. For example, it has been used with methotrexate to partially "rescue" systemic tissues from toxicity. It is used in combination with 5-FU to produce synergistic cytotoxic effects resulting in part form augmented incorporation of 5-FU into abnormal (FU) RNA. In addition, in very high dose infusions, thymidine has cytotoxic activity of its own when used as a single drug. Phase I studies of the drug have been reported in treatment of a variety of tumors including colon, ovary and non-Hodgkins' lymphoma. Reversible encephalopathy has been reported in a number of patients receiving both TdR and 5-FU.[200] This is manifest by confusion and lethargy developing within 48 hours of treatment and subsiding within days after cessation of treatment. More recently Cheng and his colleagues have reported that cerebellar signs typical of fluorouracil are markedly enhanced when combining it with thymidine.[86] A partial explanation may lie in the fact that the half life of fluorouracil is significantly prolonged if it is combined with thymidine. These observations suggest that not only is the cytotoxicity of fluorouracil increased by adding thymidine but also certain of its toxic effects. Encephalopathy manifested by somnolence, headache, memory impairment and visual illusions has also been seen in patients treated with high-dose thymidine infusions alone.[201]

Methyl-GAG (methyl-glyoxal-bis-guanylhydrazone): This drug was used many years ago but abandoned because of gastrointestinal toxicity. However, new dosage schedules are being tried with promising results in the treatment of several solid tumors. The drug appears to act by interfering with certain enzymes involved in synthesizing important polyamines, particularly spermadine, which in turn are involved in the initiation of DNA synthesis. Systemic toxicity includes severe mucositis, pharyngitis and esophagitis, and severe diarrhea. Hematologic suppression is not a major problem.

In older trials, rare occurrences of neuropathy, myopathy and ileus were alleged. As currently being employed, we have seen several patients who developed significant proximal weakness associated with a profound feeling of general malaise appearing several days after each treatment and reversing slowing until the next treatment was given. Muscle enzymes have been normal and EMG studies in two patients showed no evidence for myopathy, although neuropathy was noted in one patient probably secondary to prior chemotherapy.

m-AMSA (Amsacrine) (4'-[9-acridinylamino]-methanesulfon-m-anisidide) (AMSA): AMSA is a synthetic agent which binds DNA at multiple sites and also prevents its synthesis.[202] It is currently in phase I trials for both solid and hematologic tumors. The predominant systemic side effect is leukopenia. Cardiac rhythm abnormalities have also been described after AMSA treatment.[203]

Possible CNS toxicity (generalized seizures in four patients)[203] and PNS toxicity (stocking-glove paresthesiae) have been possibly attributed to AMSA therapy. The causal relationship of the drug has not yet been confirmed.

A summary of the neurotoxicity of non-hormonal agents discussed above is provided in Table V.

Hormonal Agents

Adrenocorticosteroids

The adrenocorticosteroids can be divided into glucocorticoids and adrenally-produced androgens (see sex hormones) depending on their major physiological effect. The glucocorticoids have many uses in patients with cancer. Their dramatic effect in the treatment of cerebral edema associated with brain tumors is well-known to neurologists. In addition, they are used as chemotherapeutic agents for some systemic cancers. For example, glucocorticoids, particularly prednisone, are part of the multidrug regimen used in treating acute lymphoblastic leukemia. They are used also for treatment of chronic lymphocytic leukemia as well as myeloma and both Hodgkin's and non-Hodgkin's lymphomas. Modest daily doses are frequently employed in the treatment of metastatic breast cancer. The mechanism of their antitumor activity is not clear. Glucocorticoids frequently have beneficial effects in relieving bone pain of cancer. They also exert a salutory effect in the treatment of epidural cord compression for metastatic tumor. It is well known that corticosteroids may contribute to a wide range of systemic complications, although most are seen with relatively long-term usage.

The neurological toxic effects of these agents have recently been reviewed by Ehrenkranz and Posner.[205] The effects on mental state are often quite prominent. Patients with cancer have a general feeling of well-being and are often euphoric. A few patients, however, may experience depression or mild agitation. Physiological activity increases: eating improves and patients are more active, although insomnia may be a problem. Patients on substantial doses of steroids (equivalent to 60-80 mg of prednisone) quite frequently have a fine tremor on sustention of the arms. This tremor appears to be an exaggeration of the normal physiological tremor. Frank psychotic episodes are uncommon in cancer patients.

Steroids probably lower the threshold for seizures in man. In fact, high doses of glucocorticoids produce seizures in mice although there is no such direct evidence in man.[206] However, we have seen patients with

Table V
Neurotoxicity of Some Chemotherapeutic Agents

Drug	Route of Administration* Producing Toxicity	Peripheral NS Autonomic NS Muscle	Spinal Cord/Mets Meninges	Brain/Cranial Nerves
Mechlorethamine	high dose iv, intra-arterial including intracarotid	Neuropathy, plexopathy	—	Cerebral necrosis, edema focal cerebral dysfunction
Thiotepa	i.t.	?	Myelopathy, radiculopathy	?
Methotrexate (see Table II)	p.o., i.v. (conventional dose)	—	—	Rare pontine leukoencephalopathy (with cranial RT) Leukoencephalopathy
Methotrexate	i.v. (high dose)	—	—	Leukoencephalopathy
Methotrexate	i.t.	—	Aseptic meningitis Myelopathy (acute) Radiculopathy (transient)	Leukoencephalopathy
5-Fluorouracil	i.v.	—	—	Cerebellar ataxia Rare encephalopathy Extraocular paresis
Ara-C	i.v.	—	Aseptic meningitis Myelopathy	—
5-Azacytidine	i.v.	Painful, weak muscles ("myopathy")	—	Encephalopathy
Vincristine (see Table IV)	i.v., p.o.	Peripheral neuropathy Autonomic neuropathy	—	Seizures Inappropriate ADH secretion Cranial neuropathy

Drug	Route	Neuropathy		Central/other complications
Nitrosourea	i.v., p.o.	—	—	?chronic dementia (with brain RT) / Focal head pain / Seizures / Transient focal cerebral dysfunction
Nitrosourea	intracarotid	—	—	Multifocal cerebral, brainstem dysfunction / Multifocal necrotic and demyelinative lesions
Nitrosourea	high dose i.v. (with autologous bone marrow transplant)	—	—	Ototoxicity
Cis-platinum	i.v.	Neuropathy (predominantly sensory)	—	
Hexamethelamine	p.o.	Neuropathy	—	Encephalopathy / Extrapyramidal symptoms / Jaw pain
L-asparaginase	i.v.	—	—	Encephalopathy
Procarbazine	p.o. (i.v. obsolete)	Neuropathy (rare)	—	Encephalopathy (rare)
Mitotane	p.o.	Neuropathy	—	Encephalopathy / Repetitive seizures
PALA	i.v.	—	—	Encephalopathy
Thymidine	i.v. (alone or with 5-FU)	—	—	Encephalopathy / Cerebellar ataxia (with FU)
Methyl-GAG	i.v.	?"myopathy" ?neuropathy	—	—

brain metastases who appear to develop focal or generalized seizures shortly after institution of steroids. A number of other effects have been described. Patients receiving phenothiazines or tricyclic antidepressants are thought to develop extrapyramidal symptoms more readily if concomitantly given steroids.[207] Pseudotumor cerebri is frequently listed as a side effect of steroid withdrawal, especially in children.[206,208] Exophthalmos has been described in four patients on prolonged doses of steroids.[209] Dependency, both psychological and physical, has been attributed to steroids.[210,211] Occasionally sudden withdrawal or reduction of steroid dosage causes a syndrome marked by severe muscle and joint pain, fever and general malaise often called steroid pseudo-rheumatism.[212]

An unusual side effect of large doses of intravenous dexamethasone which is often now employed in the acute treatment either of rapidly progressing brain tumor or of epidural spinal cord compression is the occurrence during and after injection of intense anogenital burning. The symptom is very alarming and uncomfortable for the patient but will reverse within 2 to 3 minutes and can be minimized by slower injection.[213]

"Steroid myopathy" is surely the most common neurological side effect which interferes with function. Substantial doses of either prednisone or dexamethasone (equivalent to 40 mg or more of prednisone daily) given over 3 to 4 weeks appear to cause a mild degree of steroid myopathy in most patients. Fluorinated compounds are thought to produce myopathy more frequently.[214-216] However, there appears to be rather marked individual variation in the degree of weakness produced. Some patients can tolerate high doses for long periods; others will have major disability after high doses for 4 weeks. The most common complaint is difficulty rising from a low chair or from the toilet or difficulty climbing stairs and, less commonly, difficulty with combing hair. If steroids are reduced or discontinued, steroid myopathy improves rather slowly over weeks or months.[217] Further discussion of steroid neurotoxicity can be found in Chapter II of this book.

Sex Hormones: Androgens and Estrogens

Estrogens, particularly diethylstilbestrol (DES) and ethinylestradiol (Estinyl) are used in the management of hormonally responsive breast carcinoma. In addition, stilbestrol and diethylstilbestrol are common agents employed in the treatment of prostatic carcinoma. Although they produce systemic side effects including feminization and fluid retention, there are no specific neurological side effects. The *progestins* used primarily for treatment of endometrial carcinoma, and for breast and renal carcinoma (Depo-Provera or medroxyprogesterone) and for prostate cancer (norethindrone) are without known neurological toxicity. *Andro-*

gens are used in the hormonal manipulation in treating breat cancer. They also have systemic side effects including masculinization and fluid retention but no neurological side effects.

Anti-estrogens

Tamoxifen is the major anti-estrogen compound available in recent years for the treatment of breast cancer positive for estrogen-binding receptors. Its systemic side effects are minimal although it occasionally causes nausea. In patients with bony disease, hypercalcemia occasionally occurs shortly after starting the drug. In turn this at times leads to confusion and encephalopathy. Retinopathy has been attributed to the use of Tamoxifen.[218] However, there are no specific toxic effects directed against the central or peripheral nervous system.

References

1. Posner JB: Neurological complications of systemic cancer. *Med Clin N Amer* **55**:625-646, 1971.
2. Allen JC: The Effects of cancer therapy on the nervous system. *J Pediat* **93**:903-909, 1978.
3. Weiss HD, Walker MD, Wiernik PH: Neurotoxicity of commonly used antineoplastic agents. *N Engl J Med* **291**:75-81, 127-133, 1974.
4. Sawicka J, Dawson DM, Blum R: Neurologic aspects of the treatment of cancer. In: Tyler HR, ed: *Current Neurology, Vol. 1.* Boston, Houghton Mifflin, 1977, Ch. 13.
5. Young DF, Posner JB: Nervous system toxicity of the chemotherapeutic agents. In: Vinken PJ, Bruyn GW, eds: *Handbook of Clinical Neurology. Vol. 39.* Amsterdam, North-Holland Publishing Co., 1980.
6. Laird AK: Dynamics of tumor growth. *Brit J Cancer* **18**:490-502, 1964.
7. Heppner GH, Dexter DL, DeNucci T, et al: Heterogenicity in drug sensitivity among tumor cell subpopulations of single mammary tumor. *Cancer Res* **38**:3758-3763, 1978.
8. Shapiro WR, Yung WA: Human glioma heterogeneity: karyotypic and phenotypic (chemosensitivity, growth rate) demonstration in dissociated and cloned cells from freshly resected tumors. *Proc Amer Assoc Cancer Res* **588**:147, 1980.
9. Carter SK, Bakowski MT, Hillman K: *Chemotherapy of Cancer.* New York, John Wiley, 1977.
10. Dorr RT, Fritz WL: *Cancer Chemotherapy Handbook.* New York, Elsevier North Holland, Inc., 1980.
11. Silver RT, Lauper RD, Taroski CH: *A Synopsis of Cancer Chemotherapy.* New York, Dun-Donnelly, 1977.
12. Bethlenfalvay NC, Bergin JJ: Severe cerebral toxicity after intravenous nitrogen mustard therapy. *Cancer* **29**:366-369, 1972.
13. French JD, West PM, Van Amerongen FK, Magoun HW: Effects of intracarotid administration of nitrogen mustard on normal brain and brain tumors. *J Neurosurg* **9**:378-389, 1952.
14. Ariel IM: Intra-arterial chemotherapy for metastatic cancer to the brain. *Amer J Surg* **102**:647-650, 1961.

15. Owens G: Chemotherapy of primary gliomas of the brain. *NYS J Med* **64**:1933-1937, 1964.

16. Brunschweig A, Brockunier A: Postoperative rupture of major vessels after pelvic operation. *Amer J Obstet Gynec* **80**:481-484, 1960.

17. Creech O, Ryan RF, Krementz ET: Regional chemotherapy of isolated perfusions in the treatment of melanoma of the extremities. *Plast Reconstr Surg* **28**:333-346, 1961.

18. Conrad ME, Jr, Crosby WH: Massive nitrogen mustard therapy in Hodgkin's disease with protection of bone marrow by tourniquets. *Blood* **16**:1089-1103, 1960.

19. Clifford P, Beecher JL, Harries JR, et al: Nitrogen mustard therapy with aortic occlusion in nasopharyngeal carcinoma. *Brit Med J* **1**: 1256-1260, 1963.

20. Tashima CK: Immediate cerebral symptoms during rapid intravenous administration of cyclophosphamide (NSC-26271). *Cancer Chemother Rep* **59**:441-442, 1975.

21. Arena PJ: Oropharyngeal sensation associated with rapid intravenous administration of cyclophosphamide (NSC-26271). *Cancer Chemother Rep* **56**:779-780, 1972.

22. Kende G, Sirkin SR, Thomas PRM, et al: Blurring of vision. *Cancer* **44**:69-71, 1979.

23. DeFronzo RA, Braine H, Colvin OM, et al: Water intoxication in man after cyclophosphamide therapy. *Ann Intern Med* **78**:861-869, 1973.

24. Harow PJ, DeClerck YA, Shore NA, et al: A fatal case of inappropriate ADH secretion induced by cyclophosphamide therapy. *Cancer* **44**: 896-898, 1979.

25. Allen JC (Personal communication).

26. Wolfson S, Olney MB: Accidental ingestion of a toxic dose of chlorambucil: report of a case in a child. *JAMA* **165**:239-240, 1957.

27. Green AA, Naiman JL: Chlorambucil poisoning. *Amer J Dis Child* **116**:190-191, 1968.

28. Williams SA, Makker SP, Grupe WE: Seizures: a significant side effect of chlorambucil therapy in children. *J Pediatr* **93**:516-518, 1978.

29. Edwards MS, Levin VA, Seager ML, et al: Phase II evaluation of Thiotepa for treatment of central nervous system tumors. *Cancer Treat Rep* **63**:1419-1421, 1979.

30. Blasberg RG, Patlak C, Fenstermacher JD: Intrathecal chemotherapy: brain tissue profiles after ventriculocisternal perfusion. *J Pharmacol Exp Ther* **195**:73-83, 1975.

31. Gutin PH, Levi JA, Wiernik PH, et al: Treatment of malignant meningeal disease with intrathecal Thiotepa: A phase II study. *Cancer Treat Rep* **61**:885-887, 1977.

32. Weiss HD, Walker MD, Wiernik PH, et al: Preclinical and phase I clinical studies of intrathecal N,N', N''-triethylenephosphoramide (Thiotepa-NSC 6396). *Proc Amer Assoc Cancer Res* **15**:65, 1974.

33. Djaldetti M, Pinkhas J, DeVries A, et al: Myasthenia gravis in a patient with chronic myeloid leukemia treated by busulfan. *Blood* **32**:336-340, 1968.

34. Greenhouse A, Neuberger KJ, Bowerman DL: Brain damage after intracarotid infusion of methotrexate. *Arch Neurol (Chicago)* **11**:618-625, 1964.

35. Weiss SR, Raskind R: Pathological findings in brain tumors treated with local methotrexate. *Int Surg* **52**:310-319, 1969.

36. Sullivan MP, Vietti TJ, Fernback DJ, et al: Clinical investigation in

the treatment of meningeal leukemia: radiation therapy vs. conventional intrathecal methotrexate. *Blood* **34**:301-319, 1969.

37. Duttera MJ, Bleyer WA, Pomeroy TC, et al: Irradiation, methotrexate toxicity and the treatment of meningeal leukemia. *Lancet* **II**:703-707, 1973.

38. Price RA, Jamieson PA: The central nervous system in childhood leukemia. II. Subacute leukoencephalopathy. *Cancer* **35**:306-318, 1975.

39. Rosner F, Lee SL, Kazen M, et al: Intrathecal methotrexate. *Lancet* **I**: 249-250, 1970.

40. Bleyer WA, Drake JC, Chabner BA: Neurotoxicity and elevated cerebrospinal fluid-methotrexate concentration in meningeal leukemia. *N Engl J Med* **289**:770-773, 1973.

41. Edelson RN, Chernik NL, Posner JB: Spinal subdural hematomas complicating lumbar puncture. *Arch Neurol* **31**:134-137, 1974.

42. Rall DP, Rieselbach RE, Olliverio V, et al: Pharmacology of folic acid antagonists as related to brain and cerebrospinal fluid. *Cancer Chemother Rep* **16**:187-190, 1962.

43. Gagliano RG, Costanzi JJ: Paraplegia following intrathecal methotrexate. *Cancer* **37**:1663-1668, 1976.

44. Back EH: Death after intrathecal methotrexate. *Lancet* **II**:1005, 1969.

45. Bagshawe KD, Magrath IT, Golding PR: Intrathecal methotrexate. *Lancet* **II**:1258, 1969.

46. Thompson SW, Saiki J, Kornfeld M, et al: Paraplegia following intrathecal antileukemic therapy. *Neurology* **21**:454, 1971.

47. Lampkin BC, Huggins GR, Hammond D: Absence of neurotoxicity following massive intrathecal administration of methotrexate. *Cancer* **20**:1780-1781, 1967.

48. Meadows AT, Evans AE: Effects of chemotherapy on the central nervous system: a study of parenteral methotrexate in long-term survivors of leukemia and lymphoma in childhood. *Cancer* **37**:1079-1085, 1976.

49. Allen JC, Rosen G, Mehta BM, et al: Leukoencephalopathy following high dose IV methotrexate chemotherapy with leucovorin rescue. *Cancer Treat Rep* **64**:1261-1273, 1980.

50. Shapiro WR, Chernik NL, Posner JB: Necrotizing encephalopathy following instillation of methotrexate. *Arch Neurol* **28**:96-102, 1973.

51. Kay HEM, Knapton PJ, O'Sullivan JP, et al: Encephalopathy in acute leukemia associated with methotrexate therapy. *Arch Dis Child* **47**: 344-354, 1972.

52. Rubinstein LJ, Herman MM, Long TF, et al: Disseminated necrotizing leukoencephalopathy: a complication of treated central nervous system leukemia and lymphoma. *Cancer* **35**:291-305, 1975.

53. Bresnan MJ, Gilles FH, Lorenzo AV, et al: Leukoencephalopathy following continued irradiation and intraventricular methotrexate therapy of brain tumors in childhood. *Trans Am Neurol Assoc* **97**:204-206, 1972.

54. Arnold H, Kuhne D, Franke H, et al: Findings in computerized axial tomography after intrathecal methotrexate and radiation. *Neuroradiology* **16**:65-68, 1978.

55. Allen JC, Thaler HT, Deck MDF, Rottenberg DA: Leukoencephalopathy following high dose intravenous methotrexate chemotherapy: quantitative assessment of white matter attenuation using computed tomography. In: Wendon S, ed: *Proceedings of the XI Symposium Neuroradiologicum*. Heidelberg, Springer, 1978.

56. Peylan-Ramu M, Poplack DG, Pizzo PA, et al: Abnormal CT scans of

the brain in asymptomatic children with acute lymphocytic leukemia after prophylactic treatment of the central nervous system with radiation and intrathecal chemotherapy. *N Engl J Med* **298**:815-818, 1978.

57. Hendin B, DeVivo DC, Torack R, et al: Parenchymatous degeneration of the central nervous system in childhood leukemia. *Cancer* **33**:468-482, 1974.
58. Flament-Durant J, Ketelbant-Balsse P, Maurus R, et al: Intracerebral calcifications appearing during the course of acute lymphocytic leukemia with methotrexate and X-ray. *Cancer* **35**:319-325, 1975.
59. Mueller S, Bell W, Seibert J: Cerebral calcifications associated with intrathecal methotrexate therapy in acute lymphocytic leukemia. *Pediatrics* **88**:650-653, 1976.
60. Pizzo PA, Bleyer WA, Poplak DG, et al: Reversible dementia temporally associated with intraventricular therapy with methotrexate in a child with acute myelogenous leukemia. *J Pediatr* **88**:131-133, 1976.
61. Fusner JE, Poplack DG, Pizzo PA, et al: Leukoencephalopathy following chemotherapy for rhabdomyosarcoma: reversibility of cerebral changes demonstrated by computed tomography. *J Pediatr* **91**:77-79, 1977.
62. Shapiro WR, Posner JB, Ushio Y, et al: Treatment of meningeal neoplasms *Cancer Treat Rep.* **61**:733-744, 1977.
63. Shapiro WR, Allen JC, Horten BC: Chronic methotrexate toxicity to the central nervous system. *Clin Bull* **10**:49-52, 1980.
64. Tejada F, Zubrod CG: Vincristine effect on methotrexate cerebrospinal fluid concentration. *Cancer Treat Rep* **63**:143-145, 1979.
65. Breuer AC, Blank NK, Schoene WC: Multifocal pontine lesions in cancer patients treated with chemotherapy and CNS radiotherapy. *Cancer* **41**:2112-2120, 1978.
66. Fishman ML, Bean SC, Cogan DG: Optic atrophy following prophylactic chemotherapy and cranial radiation for acute lymphocytic leukemia. *Amer J Ophthal* **82**:571-576, 1976.
66a. McIntosh S, Klatskin EH, O'Brien RT, et al: Chronic neurologic disturbance in childhood leukemia. *Cancer* **37**:853-857, 1976.
67. Soni S, Martin G, Pitner S: Effect of central nervous system irradiation on neuropsychologic functioning of children with acute lymphatic leukemia. *N Eng J Med* **293**:113-118, 1975.
68. Verzosa M, Aur B, et al: Five years after central nervous system irradiation of children with leukemia. *Int J Radiat Biol* **1**:209-215, 1976.
69. Obetz SW, Smithson WA, Groover RV, et al: Neuropsychologic follow-up study of children with acute lymphocytic leukemia. *Amer J Ped Hematol* **1**:207-213, 1979.
70. Allen JC, Rosen G: Transient cerebral dysfunction following chemotherapy for osteogenic sarcoma. *Ann Neurol* **3**:441-444, 1978.
71. Rodriguez V, Gottlieb J, et al: Phase I studies with Baker's antifol (BAF) (NSC 139, 105). *Cancer* **38**:690-694, 1976.
72. Riehl JL, Brown WJ: Acute cerebellar syndrome secondary to 5FU therapy. *Neurology* **14**:961-967, 1964.
73. Boileau G, Piro AJ, Lahiri SR, et al: Cerebellar ataxia during 5FU (NSC-19893) therapy. *Cancer Chemother Rep* **55**:595-598, 1971.
74. Moertel CG, Rettemeier RJ, Bolton CF, et al: Cerebellar ataxia associated with fluorinated pyrimidine therapy. *Cancer Treat Rep* **41**:15-18, 1964.
75. Horton J, Olson KB, Sullivan J, et al: 5-fluorouracil in cancer: an improved regimen. *Ann Intern Med* **73**:897-900, 1970.

76. Piro AJ, Wilson RE, Hall TC, et al: Toxicity studies of fluorouracil used with adrenalectomy in breast cancer. *Arch Surg* **105**:95-99, 1972.
77. Bateman JR, Pugh RP, Cassidy FR, et al: 5-fluorouracil given once weekly: comparison of intravenous and oral administration. *Cancer* **28**:907-913, 1971.
78. Gailani S, Holland JF, Falkson G, et al: Comparison of treatment of metastatic gastrointestinal cancer with 5-fluorouracil (5-FU) to a combination of 5-FU with cytosine arabinoside. *Cancer* **29**:1308-1313, 1972.
79. Bagley CM: Single IV doses of 5-fluorouracil — a phase I study. *Proc Amer Assoc Cancer Res* **16**:12, 1075.
80. Greenwald ES: Organic mental changes with fluorouracil therapy. *JAMA* **235**:248-249, 1976.
81. Bergevin PR, Patwardhan VC, Weissman J, et al: Neurotoxicity of 5-fluorouracil. *Lancet* **I**:410, 1975.
82. Nichols M, Bergevin PR, Vyas AC, et al: Neurotoxicity from 5FU (NSC-26980). *Cancer Treat Rep* **60**:293-294, 1976.
83. Bixenman WW, Nicholls JVV, Warwick DH: Oculomotor disturbances associated with 5-fluorouracil chemotherapy. *Am J Ophthal* **83**:769-793, 1977.
84. Koenig H, Patel A: Biochemical basis for fluorouracil neurotoxicity. *Arch Neurol* **23**:155-160, 1970.
85. Bourke RS, West CR, Chheda G, et al: Kinetics of entry and distribution of 5FU in cerebrospinal fluid and brain following IV injection in a primate. *Cancer Res* **33**:1735-1746, 1973.
86. Cheng E, Woodcock T, Young C, et al: Enhanced neurotoxicity of 5-fluorouracil (FU) by thymidine. *Amer Soc Clin Oncol (Proc)* **21**:350, 1980.
87. Hall SW, Benjamin RS, Griffin AC, et al: Pharmacokinetics and metabolism of ftorafur in man. *Amer Assoc Cancer Res* **17**:128, 1976.
88. Valdivieso M, Body GP, Gottlieb JA, et al: Clinical evaluation of ftorafur. *Cancer Res* **36**:1821-1824, 1976.
89. Saiki JH, Thompson S, Smith F: Paraplegia following intrathecal chemotherapy. *Cancer* **29**:370-374, 1972.
90. Breuer AC, Pitman SW, Dawson DM, Schoene WC: Paraparesis following intrathecal cytosine arabinoside: a case report with neuropathologic findings. *Cancer* **40**:2817-2822, 1977.
91. Russell JA, Powles RL: Neuropathy due to cytosine arabinoside. *Brit Med J* **2**:652-653, 1974.
92. Levi JA, Wiernik PH: A comparative clinical trial of 5-azacytidine and guanazide in previously treated adults with acute nonlymphocytic leukemia. *Cancer* **38**:36-41, 1976.
93. Ho M, Bear RA, Garvey MB: Symptomatic hypophosphatemia secondary to 5-azacytidine therapy of acute non-lymphocytic leukemia. *Cancer Treat Rep* **60**:1400-1402, 1976.
94. Holland JF, Scharlan C, Gaolani S, et al: Vincristine treatment of advanced cancer: a cooperative study of 392 cases. *Cancer Res* **33**:1258-1264, 1973.
95. Casey EG, Jellife AM, LeQuesne M, Millett Y: Vincristine neuropathy: clinical and electrophysiological observations. *Brain* **96**:69-86, 1973.
96. Sandler SG, Tobin T, Henderson ES: Vincristine-induced neuropathy: a clinical study of fifty leukemic patients. *Neurology* **19**:367-374, 1969.
97. Bradley WG, Lassman LP, Pearce GW, et al: Neuropathy of vincristine in man *J Neurol Sci* **10**:107-131, 1970.

98. Tobin W, Sandler SG: Neurophysiologic alterations induced by vincristine (NSC-67574). *Cancer Chemothr Rep* **52**:519-526, 1968.

99. McLeod JG, Penny R: Vincristine neuropathy: an electrophysiological and histological study. *J Neurol Neurosurg Psychiat* **32**:297-304, 1969.

100. Gottschalk PG, Dyck RJ, Kiely JM: Vinca alkaloid neuropathy: nerve biopsy results in rats and in man. *Neurology* **18**:875-882, 1968.

101. Bradley WG: Neuropathy of vincristine in the guinea pig. An electrophysiological and pathological study. *J Neurol Sci* **10**:133-162, 1970.

102. Slotwiner P, Song SK, Anderson PJ: Spheromembranous degeneration of muscle induced by vincristine. *Arch Neurol* **15**:172-176, 1966.

103. Uy QL, Moens TH, Johns RJ, et al: Vincristine neurotoxicity in rodents. *Johns Hopkins Med J* **121**:349-360, 1967.

104. Journey LJ, Burdman J, Whaley A: Electron microscopic study of spinal ganglia from vincristine-treated mice. *J Natl Cancer Inst* **43**:603-619, 1969.

105. Shelanski ML, Wisniewski H: Neurofibrillary degeneration induced by vincristine therapy. *Arch Neurol* **20**:199-206, 1969.

106. Berenson MP: Recovery after inadvertent massive overdosage of vincristine (NSC-67574). *Cancer Chemother Rep* **55**:525-526, 1971.

107. Mubashir BA, Bart JB: Vincristine neurotoxicity. *N Engl J Med* **287**:517, 1972.

108. Weiden PL, Wright SE: Vincristine neurotoxicity. *N Engl J Med* **286**:1369-1370, 1972.

109. Michalak JC, Dibella NJ: Exacerbation of myotonia dystrophica by vincristine. *N Engl J Med* **295**:283, 1976.

110. Gubisch NJ, Norena D, Perlia CP, et al: Experience with vincristine in solid tumors. *Cancer Chemother Rep* **32**:19-22, 1963.

111. Hildebrand J, Kenis Y: Additive toxicity of vincristine and other drugs for the peripheral nervous system. *Acta Neurol Belg* **71**:486-491, 1971.

112. Shapiro WR, Young DF: Treatment of malignant glioma: a prospective randomized study of chemotherapy and irradiation. *Arch Neurol* **33**:494-500, 1976.

113. Gottlieb RJ, Cuttner J: Vincristine-induced bladder atony. *Cancer* **28**:674-675, 1971.

114. Rosenthal S, Kaufman S: Vincristine neurotoxicity. *Ann Intern Med* **80**:733-734, 1974.

115. Albert DM, Wong VG, Henderson ES: Ocular complications of vincristine therapy. *Arch Ophthal* **78**:709-713, 1967.

115a. Sandler SG, Tobin T, Henderson ES: Vincristine-induced neuropathy: a clinical study of fifty leukemic patients. *Neurology* **19**:367-374, 1969.

116. Bohannon RA, Miller DG, Diamond HD: Vincristine in the treatment of lymphomas and leukemias. *Cancer Res* **23**:613-621, 1963.

117. Whittaker JA, Griffith IP: Recurrent laryngeal nerve paralysis in patients receiving vincristine and vinblastine. *Brit Med J* **1**:1251-1252, 1977.

118. Sanderson DA, Kuwabara T, Cogan DG: Optic neuropathy presumably caused by vincristine therapy. *Amer J Ophthal* **81**:146-150, 1976.

119. Schochet SS, Jr, Lampert PW, Earle KM: Neuronal changes induced by intrathecal vincristine sulfate. *J Neuropathy Exp Neurol* **27**:645-658, 1968.

120. Shepherd DA, Steuber CP, Starling KA, et al: Accidental intrathecal administration of vincristine. *Med Pediatr Oncol* **5**:85-88, 1978.

121. Fine RN, Clarke RR, Shore NA: Hyponatremia and vincristine therapy. *Amer J Dis Child* **112**:256-259, 1966.

122. Cutting HO: Inappropriate secretion of antidiuretic hormone secondary to vincristine therapy. *Amer J Med* **51**:269-271, 1971.

123. Robertson GL, Bhoopalam N, Zelkowitz LJ: Vincristine neurotoxicity and abnormal secretion of antidiuretic hormone. *Arch Intern Med* **132**:717-720, 1973.

124. Breza TS, Halprin KM, Taylor JR: Photosensitivity reaction to vinblastine. *Arch Dermatol* **111**:1168-1179, 1975.

125. Ginsberg SJ, Comis RL, Fitzpatrick AV: Vinblastine and inappropriate ADH secretion (letter). *N Engl J Med* **296**:941, 1978.

126. Frei E, III, Franzino A, Shnider BI, et al: Clinical studies of vinblastine. *Cancer Chemother Rep* **12**:125-129, 1961.

127. Brook J, Schreiber W: Vocal cord paralysis: a toxic reaction to vinblastine (NSC-49842) therapy. *Cancer Chemother Rep* **55**:591-593, 1971.

128. Smith IE, Hedley DW, Powles TJ, et al: Vindesine: a phase II study in the treatment of breast carcinoma, malignant melanoma, and other tumors. *Cancer Treat Rep* **62**:1427-1433, 1978.

129. Casper ES, Gralla RJ, Golbey RB: Vindesine (DVA) and cis-dichlorodiammineplatinum II (DDP) combination chemotherapy in non-small cell lung cancer. *Proc Amer Assoc Cancer Res* **20**:337, 1979.

130. Kelsen DP, Bains M, Golbey R, et al: Vindesine in the treatment of esophageal carcinoma. *Proc Amer Assoc Cancer Res* **20**:338, 1979.

131. Rossof AH, Chandra G, Wolter J, et al: Phase II trial of vindesine (desacetyl vinblastine amide sulfate, VND) in advanced metastatic cancer. *Proc Amer Assoc Cancer Res* **20**:147, 1979.

132. Bayssas M, Gouveia J, DeVassal F, et al: Phase II clinical trials with vindesine for remission induction in leukemias and lymphomas. Apparent absence of cross resistance with vincristine. *Proc Amer Assoc Cancer Res.* **20**:48, 1979.

133. Obrist R, Paravicini U, Hartmann D, et al: Vindesine: a clinical trial with special reference to neurological side effects. *Cancer Chemother Pharmacol* **2**:233-237, 1979.

134. Gralla RJ, Raphael BG, Golbey RB, et al: Phase II evaluation of vindesine in patients with non-small cell carcinoma of the lung. *Cancer Treat Rep* **63**:1343-1346, 1979.

135. Kessinger A, Lemon HM, Foley JF: VM–26 as a second drug in the treatment of brain gliomas. *Proc Amer Assoc Cancer Res* **20**:295, 1979.

136. Sklansky BD, Mann-Kaplan RS, Reynolds AF, et al: 41-demethyl-epipodophyllotoxin-B-D-thenylidene-glucoside (PIG) in the treatment of malignant intracranial neoplasms. *Cancer* **33**:460-467, 1974.

137. Creaven PJ, Allen LM: Clinical pharmacology of the new anticancer drug VM-26. *Clin Pharmacol Ther* **17**:232, 1975. ·

138. Domernowsky P, Nissen ME, Larsen V: Clinical investigation of a new podophyllum derivative, epipodophyllotoxin, 4-demethyl-9-(4,6-0-2-thenylidene-B-D-glucopyranoside) (NSC-122819), in patients with malignant lymphomas and solid tumors. *Cancer Chemother Rep* **56**: 71-82, 1972.

138a. Chabner BA, Levine AS, Johnson BL, et al: Initial clinical trials of maytansine, an antitumor plant alkaloid. *Cancer Treat Rep* **62**:429-433, 1978.

139. Blum RH, Kahlert J: A phase I study of an ansa macrolide with antitumor activity. *Cancer Treat Rep* **62**:435-438, 1978.

140. Cho ES: Toxic effects of adriamycin on the ganglia of the peripheral

nervous system: a neuropathologic study. *J Neuropath Exp Neurol* **36**:907-915, 1977.

141. Cho ES, Schaumberg HH, Spencer PS: Adriamycin produces ganglio-radiculopathy in rats. *J Neuropath Exp Neurol* **36**:597, 1977.

142. Broquet MA, Jacot-Descome E, Montandon A, et al: Traitement des carcinomes epidermoides oropharyngo-larynges par combinaison de methotrexate et de bleomycine. *Schweiz Med Wschr* **104**:18-22, 1974.

143. Fazio M, Cavellero P, Minetto E, et al: Polichemotherapy of advanced head and neck malignancies. *Tumori* **62**:599-608, 1976.

144. Dal I, Edsmyer F, Stahle J: Bleomycin therapy and ototoxicity. *Acta Oto-laryng (Stockh)* **75**:323-324, 1973.

145. Rizzuto N, Gambetti PL: Status spongiosus of rat central nervous system induced by actinomycin D. *Acta Neuropath (Berl)* **36**:21-30, 1976.

146. Taira M, Kohina K, Takeuchi H: A comparative study of the action of actinomycin D and antinomycinic acid on the central nervous system when injected into the cerebrospinal fluid of higher animals. *Epilepsia (Amst)* **13**:649-662, 1972.

147. Walker MD, Alexander E, Jr, Hunt WE, et al: Evaluation of BCNU and/or radiotherapy in the treatment of anaplastic gliomas. A cooperative clinical trial. *J Neurosurg* **49**:333-343, 1978.

148. Yamada K, Bremer AM, West CR, et al: Intra-arterial BCNU therapy in the treatment of metastatic brain tumor from lung carcinoma. *Cancer* **44**:2000-2007, 1979.

149. Crafts DC, Levin VA, Nielsen S: Intracarotid BCNU (NSC-409962): A toxicity study in six rhesus monkeys. *Cancer Treat Rep* **60**:541-545, 1976.

150. Dewys WD, Fowler EH: Vasculitis and blindness after intra-carotid injection of 1,3-Bis (2-chloroethyl)-1-nitrosourea (BCNU) in dogs. *Cancer Chemother Rep* **57**:33-40, 1973.

151. Schold SC, Fay JW: Central nervous system toxicity from high-dose BCNU treatment of systemic cancer. *Neurology* **30**:429, 1980.

152. Piel IJ, Meyer D, Perlia CP, et al: Effects of cis-diamminedichloro-platinum (NSC-119, 875) on hearing function in man. *Cancer Chemother Rep* **58**:871-875, 1974.

153. Rosencweig M, Von Holf DD, Slavik M, et al: Cis-diammine-dichloro-platinum (II). *Ann Intern Med* **86**:803-812, 1977.

154. Hayes DM, Cvitkovic E, Golbey RB, et al: High-dose displatinum diammine dichloride. *Cancer* **39**:1372-1381, 1977.

155. Lippman AJ, Helson C, Helson L, et al: Clinical trials of cis-diam-minedichloroplatinum (NSC-119875). *Cancer Chemother Rep* **57**:191-200, 1973.

156. Glass JP (personal communication).

157. Chary KK, Higby DJ, Henderson ES, et al: Phase I study of high-dose cis-dichlorodiamminoplatinum (II) with forced diuresis. *Cancer Treat Rep* **61**:367-370, 1977.

158. Merrin C: A new method to prevent toxicity with high doses of cis-diamminedichloroplatinum (therapeutic efficacy in previously treated widespread and recurrent testicular tumors). *Amer Soc Clin Oncol* **17**:243, 1976.

159. Hayes DM, Cvitkovic E, Golbey RB, et al: High-dose cis-platinum diamminedichloride. *Cancer* **39**:1372-1371, 1977.

160. Hayes FA, Green AA, Senzer N, et al: Tetany: a complication of cis-

dichlorodiammineplatinum (II) therapy. *Cancer Treat Rep* **63**:547-548, 1979.

161. Berman IJ, Mann MP: Seizures and transient cortical blindness associated with cis-platinum (II) diamminedichloride (PDD) therapy in a thirty-year-old man. *Cancer* **45**:764-766, 1980.

162. Kedar A, Cohen ME, Freeman AI: Peripheral neuropathy as a complication of cis-dichloro-diammineplatinum (II) treatment: a case report. *Cancer Treat Rep* **62**:819-821, 1978.

163. VonHoff DD, Reichert CM, Cuneo R, et al: Demyelination of peripheral nerves associated with cis-diamminedichloroplatinum (II) (DDP) therapy. *AACR Abstracts*, 91, 1979.

164. Hadley D, Herr HW: Peripheral neuropathy associated with cis-dichloro-diammineplatinum (II) treatment. *Cancer* **44**:2026-2028, 1979.

165. Becher R, Schutt P, Osieka R, et al: Peripheral neuropathy and ophthalmologic toxicity after treatment with cis-dichlorodiaminoplatinum II. *J Cancer Res Clin Oncol* **96**:219-221, 1980.

166. Hemphill M, Pestronk A, Walsh T, et al: Sensory neuropathy in cis-platinum chemotherapy. *Neurology* **30**:429, 1980.

167. Bruckner HW, Cohen CC, Deppe G, et al: Chemotherapy of gynecological tumors with platinum II. *J Clin Haemat Oncol* **7**:619-632, 1977.

168. Clark AW, Parhad IM, Griffin JW, et al: Neurotoxicity of cis-platinum pathology of the central and peripheral nervous systems. *Neurology* **30**:429, 1980.

169. Ostrow S, Hahn D, Wiernik PH, et al: Ophthalmologic toxicity after cis-dichlorodiammineplatinum (II) therapy. *Cancer Treat Rep* **62**: 1591-1593, 1978.

170. Sawicka J, Dawson DM, Blum R: Neurologic aspects of the treatment of cancer. In: Tyler HR, ed: *Current Neurology, Vol. 1*. Boston, Houghton Mifflin, 1977, Ch. 13.

171. Stolinsky DC, Bateman JR: Further experience with hexamethylmelamine (NSC-13875) in the treatment of carcinoma of the cervix. *Cancer Chemother Rep* **57**:497-499, 1973.

172. Wilson WL, Bisel HF, Cole D, et al: Prolonged low dosage administration of hexamethylmelamine (NSC-13875). *Cancer* **25**:568-570, 1970.

173. Bergevin PR, Tormey DC, Blom J: Clinical evaluation of hexamethylmelamine (NSC-13875). *Cancer Chemother Rep* **57**:51-58, 1973.

174. Smith JP, Rutledge FN: Random study of hexamethylmelamine, 5-fluorouracil and melphalan in treatment of advanced carcinoma of the ovary. *National Cancer Institute Monograph 42 — Symposium on Ovarian Carcinoma*, 1975, pp 169-172.

175. Lerner HJ: Hydroxyurea and irradiation in the treatment of astrocytomas. *Proc Amer Assoc Cancer Res* **16**:5, 1975.

176. Oettgen HF, Stephenson PA, Schwartz MK, et al: Toxicity of E. coli L-asparaginase in man. *Cancer* **25**:253-278, 1970.

177. Ohnuma T, Holland JF, Freeman A, et al: Biochemical and pharmacological studies with asparaginase in man. *Cancer Res* **30**:2297-2305, 1970.

178. Land VJ, Sutow WW, Fernback DJ, et al: Toxicity of L-asparaginase in children with advanced leukemia. *Cancer* **30**:339-347, 1972.

179. Haskell CM, Canellos GP, Leventhal BG, et al: L-asparaginase: therapeutic and toxic effects in patients with neoplastic disease. *N Engl J Med* **281**:1028-1034, 1969.

180. Zubrod CG: The clinical toxicities of L-asparaginase: in treatment of leukemia and lymphoma. *Pediatrics* **45**:555-559, 1970.
181. Ohnuma T, Holland JF, Freeman A, et al: Biochemical and pharmacological studies with asparaginase in man. *Cancer Res* **30**:2297-2305, 1970.
182. Moure JMB, Whitecare JP, Bodey GP: Electroencephalogram changes secondary to asparaginase. *Arch Neurol* **23**:365-368, 1970.
183. Pratt CB, Choi SI, Holton CP: Low-dosage asparaginase treatment of childhood acute lymphocytic leukemia. *Amer J Dis Child* **121**:406-409, 1971.
184. Warrell RP, Chou T-C, Gordon C, et al: Phase I evaluation of succinylated acinetobacter glutaminase-asparaginase in adults. *Cancer Res* **40**:4546-4551, 1980.
185. Kumar ARV, Renaudin J, Wilson CB, et al: Procarbazine hydrochloride in the treatment of brain tumors. Phase 2 study. *J Neurosurg* **40**:365-371, 1974.
186. Shapiro WR, Young DF: Chemotherapy of malignant glioma with CCNU alone and CCNU combined with vincristine sulfate and procarbazine hydrochloride. (to be published, 1981)
187. Chabner BA, Sponza R, Hubbard S, et al: High-dose intermittent intravenous infusion of procarbazine (NSC-77213). *Cancer Chemother Rep* **57**:361-363, 1973.
188. Brunner KW, Young CW: A methylhydrazine derivative in Hodgkin's disease and toxic effects studied in 51 patients. *Ann Intern Med* **63**:69-86, 1965.
189. Stolinsky DC, Solomon J, Pugh RP, et al: Clinical experience with procarbazine in Hodgkin's disease, reticulum cell sarcoma, and lymphosarcoma. *Cancer* **26**:984-990, 1970.
190. Samuels ML, Leary WB, Alexanian R, et al: Clinical trials with N-isopropyl-a-(2-methylhydrazino)-p-toluamide hydrochloride in malignant lymphoma and other disseminated neoplasia. *Cancer* **20**:1187-1198, 1967.
191. Mann AM, Hutchison JL: Manic reaction associated with procarbazine by hydrochloride therapy of Hodgkin's disease. *Can Med Assoc J* **97**:1350-1353, 1967.
192. Deconti RC: Procarbazine in the management of late Hodgkin's disease. *JAMA* **215**:927-930, 1971.
193. Devita VT, Hahn MA, Oliverio VT: Monoamine oxidase inhibition by a new carcinostatic agent, N-isopropyl-a-(2-methylhydrazino)-p-toluamide (MIH). *Proc Soc Exp Biol Med* **120**:561-565, 1965.
194. Billmeier GJ, Holton CP: Procarbazine hydrochloride in childhood cancer. *J Pediatr* **75**:892-895, 1969.
195. Ochoa M, Wittes RE, Krakoff IH: Trial of hydrazine sulfate (NSC-150014) in patients with cancer. *Cancer Chemother Rep, Pt. 1*, 1975.
196. Falkson G, DeVilliers PC, Falkson HC: N-isoprophyl-x-(2-methyl-hydrazino)-p-toluamide hydrochloride (NSC-77213) for treatment of cancer patients. *Cancer Chemother Rep* **46**:7-26, 1965.
197. Danowski TS, Sarver ME, Moses C, Bonessi JV: O-p'DDD therapy in Cushing's syndrome and in obesity with cushingoid changes. *Amer J Med* **37**:235-250, 1964.

198. Hutter AM, Kayhoe DE: Adrenal cortical carcinoma. *Amer J Med* **41**: 582-592, 1966.
199. Wiley RG, Gralla RJ: Neurotoxicity of a new chemotherapeutic agent, phosphonoacetyl-L-aspartate (PALA): clinical observations and a laboratory model. *Trans Amer Neurol Assoc* **105**:61-63, 1980.
200. Woodcock TM, Martin DS, Damin LAM, et al: Combination clinical trials with thymidine and fluorouracil: a phase I and clinical pharmacologic evaluation. *Cancer* **45**:1135-1143, 1980.
201. Martin DS, Stolfi RL, Sawyer RC, et al: An overview of thymidine. *Cancer* **45**:1117-1128, 1980.
202. Issell BF: Amsacrine (AMSA). *Cancer Treat Rep* **7**:73-83, 1980.
203. Legha SS, Latreille J, McCredie KB, et al: Neurologic and cardiac rhythm abnormalities associated with 4'-(9-acridinylamino) methanesylfon-m-anisidide (AMSA) therapy. *Cancer Treat Rep* **63**:2001-2003, 1979.
204. VanEcho DA, Chiuten DF, Cormley PE, et al: Phase I clinical and pharmacological study of 4'-(9-acridinylamino)-methanesulfon-m-anisidide using an intermittent biweekly schedule. *Cancer Res* **39**:3881-3884, 1979.
205. Ehrenkranz J, Posner JB: Adrenocorticosteroids. In: Gilbert H, Posner JB, Weiss L, eds: *Brain Metastasis*. Boston, G.K. Hall, 1979, Ch. 1.
206. Woodbury DM: Biochemical effects of adrenocortical steroids on the central nervous system. In: *Handbook of Neurochemistry, Vol. VII*. New York, Plenum Press, 1972, pp 255-287.
207. Cooperative Study: *JAMA* p 889, 1973.
208. Byyng RL: Withdrawal from glucocorticoid therapy. *N Engl J Med* **295**: 30-32, 1976.
209. Slansky HH, Kolbert G, Gartner S: Exophthalmos induced by steroids. *Arch Ophthal* **77**:579-581, 1967.
210. Amatruda TT, Hurst MM, D'Esopo ND: Certain endocrine and metabolic facets of the steroid withdrawal syndrome. *J Clin Endocr* **25**: 1207-1217, 1965.
211. Kimball CP: Psychological dependency on steroids *Ann Intern Med* **75**:111-113, 1971.
212. Rotstein J, Good RA: Steroid pseudorheumatism. *Arch Intern Med* **99**:545-555, 1957.
213. Czerwinski AW, Czerwinski AB, Whitsett TL, et al: Effects of a single large intravenous injection of dexamethasone. *Clin Pharmacol Therap* **13**:638-642, 1972.
214. Golding DN, Begg TB: Dexamethasone myopathy. *Brit Med J* **2**:1129-1130, 1960.
215. Afifi AK, Bergman RA, Harvey MC: Steroid myopathy; clinical, histologic and cytologc observations. *Johns Hopkins Med J* **123**:158-173, 1968.
216. Kjellstrand CM: Side effects of steroids and their treatment. *Transplant Proc* **7**:123-129, 1975.
217. Yates DA: Steroid myopathy. *Rheum Phys Med* **11**:28-33, 1971.
218. Kaiser-Kupfer MI, Lippman ME: Tamoxifen retinopathy. *Cancer Treat Rep* **62**:315-320, 1978.

Chapter IV

Neurologic Complications of Vaccines

Peter A. Gross, M.D.,
and Anthony B. Minnefor, M.D.

Introduction

The severity, incidence and type of adverse neurologic reaction to vaccines varies widely from one of these biologicals to another. The vaccines themselves contain viral, bacterial, or other antigens, that are prepared and administered either "live" or inactivated. A given preparation may contain more than one kind of immunizing agent for simultaneous inoculation.

The pathogenesis of the neurologic complications seen with vaccines varies and in some instances is only poorly understood. There are several factors of importance which should be kept in mind when considering this problem. Neurologic "reactions" occur against a background of naturally occurring disease and it may not always be possible to separate causality from coincidence. Components in a vaccine other than the microbial antigen itself, such as substrate for viral replication or seemingly minor variations in manufacturing procedures, may account for differences in the reported incidence of adverse reactions. Since the vast majority of vaccine doses overall are given to infants and children, responses may be age-specific. For example, uncomplicated febrile seizures following non-specific pyrogenic responses to vaccines are common in children and per se are of no more significance than those of other etiology. This is perhaps the most common untoward neurologic response between the ages of 1-5 years and fortunately is considered a benign condition. The occurrence of seizures in this setting, however, usually calls for a subsequent modification of the usual immunization routine.[1,2]

The most clear-cut situation is that in which a live microorganism is given and replication occurs in neural tissue because of an abnormal immune response in the recipient. The clinical sequelae of such incidents varies with the agent given and the hosts' underlying disorder. These serious, occassionally fatal reactions can be avoided if one recognizes that immunodeficiency states and immunosuppressive therapy are contraindications for live vaccine administration.

Among the most feared responses to vaccine administration are those unpredictable, "idosyncratic," neurologic reactions which are considered immunologically mediated and which occur for the most part in normal individuals. These encephalopathies may result in serious long-term sequelae or death. Although fortunately most are rare, they are often the most important consideration in the risk-benefit decision prior to vaccine administration. In this chapter we will concentrate on those immunizing agents which have been clearly recognized as having neurotropism. No attempt will be made to detail anecdotal clinical reports where documentation is not substantial and causality not generally accepted.

Diphtheria–Pertussis–Tetanus (DPT) Vaccine

These agents are generally administered simultaneously to children during primary immunization and may conveniently be considered together. There is overwhelming evidence, however, that the risk of neurologic sequelae is largely confined to the pertussis component. Severe encephalopathies and occassional deaths were reported soon after the initiation of prophylactic pertussis inoculation programs.[3-6] The histologic features noted in the few autopsy specimens available are noteworthy by the absence of inflammatory changes and consistent with a primary, degenerative encephalomyelopathy.

The responsible organism *Bordatella pertussis* contains a variety of biologically active substances that account in some way for the untoward reactions, but the precise mechanism(s) is unknown. Of course, in addition to neurologic reactions, side effects of a less severe nature such as fever, local pain, rashes, etc. are also reported. In the U.S.A., although pertussis vaccines must pass standard tests which include measures of potency and freedom from toxicity in mice, correlation with reactogenicity in humans is incomplete.[7,8] Similarly, there is considerable product variability between manufacturers and from lot to lot. Efficacy rates for pertussis vary between 70-90% in large population studies but may be less after institutional or household exposure. Thus, it is not surprising that the risk-benefit ratio of pertussis immunization has been carefully scrutinized. [9-11]

Since tabulation and reporting of adverse reactions is likely to overestimate the incidence, several attempts have been made to survey large populations in this regard. Strom reviewed the experience in Sweden with DPT during the years 1959-65.[12] There were 167 cases of neurological reactions among over 500,000 triple vaccinees; an incidence of 1:3100.

These included three cases with encephalopathy; other diagnoses included convulsions,[80] hypsarrythmia,[4] shock,[54] uncontrollable screaming[24] and serous meningitis. The author concluded that endotoxin of the pertussis bacteria was responsible since reactions occurring after the first injection were unlikely to be allergic in nature

Another retrospective analysis of the problem was conducted in England, Scotland and Wales.[13] The National Childhood Encephalopathy Study examined the records of every child between the ages of 2 and 36 months admitted to a hospital (1976-79), with a neurologic disorder and reported their data on the first 1,000 cases. Affected children[35] were compared to controls for a variety of variables including pertussis immunization. There was a statistically significant difference (p < 0.001) in the incidence of pertussis immunization in the 7 days prior to illness. Of note, there was no such significant association in those children receiving just diptheria and tetanus vaccine. The authors calculated the risk of serious neurological damage from DPT vaccine to be 1:110,000. This estimate is much lower than the earlier reports which raised questions concerning the continuing use of pertussis containing vaccines.[9,14] Other serious reactions reported in the literature include delirium, shock, coma and permanent, serious neurologic sequelae.[15-17]

In this country, the Pertussis Vaccine project is the first to attempt to determine accurately on a prospective basis the incidence of adverse reactions associated with DPT adsorbed versus DT adsorbed vaccines.[18] Preliminary data from this study once again incriminate the pertussis component in serious reactions. There were no instances of convulsions or collapse in DT recipients versus a 0.2% rate of each for those given DPT. Persistent crying was also more common in the latter group (5.9 to 2.2%). Thus far no cases of encephalopathy have been observed. In most instances, serious reactions occur within 12 hours of injection and are usually, but not always associated with fever. When this project is completed, data on the rates, nature and etiology of adverse reactions relevant to U.S. licensed vaccines will be available for the first time.

The toxoids of diptheria and tetanus are associated with a relatively high incidence of minor side effects (sore arm, swelling at injection sites, itching, occasional fever, etc.).[19] The tetanus component would appear to be mainly responsible.[20] Although very uncommon, neurologic reactions have been reported in some instances without excluding individuals receiving mixed vaccinations. Peripheral neuropathy and transverse myelitis seem to be well documented complications.[21,22] The interval between injection and neurological signs and symptoms varies from hours to days and is often but not always associated with local or general allergic reactions. It is sometimes difficult to distinguish "vaccinogenic" from traumatic nerve injury when findings are anatomically consistent with either.

The syndromes reported have included brachial nerve or brachial plexus palsy, paralysis of the radial nerve, transverse myelitis and acute idiopathic polyneuropathy (Landry-Guillain-Barre'-Strohl syndrome).[22-24] In the latter case, a male patient inadvertantly received three separate injections of tetanus toxoid over a 14-year period, in each instance developing the syndrome. The aforementioned notwithstanding, experience suggests that fear of neurologic sequelae or other adverse side effects should not preclude proper administration of these toxoids.

Smallpox Vaccination

A milestone in the history of medicine was achieved on October, 1977 when the last case of naturally occurring smallpox was diagnosed in Somalia.[25] Thus, except for the potential isolated laboratory accident, this disease is now primarily of historic interest. The eradication of smallpox attests to the success of a world-wide public health program and the efficacy of smallpox vaccine. Routine smallpox vaccination is no longer practiced.

This live virus was given by mulitiple puncture technique. With proper inoculation of potent smallpox vaccine virtually 100% of primary vaccinees developed a Jennerian vesicle or "major reaction" at the vaccination site 6 to 8 days later.[26,27] A variety of complications were noted ranging from a benign erythema multiforme-like rash to generalized vaccinia, vaccinia necrosum, eczema vaccinatum and post-vaccineal encephalitis.[28]

Individuals with post-vaccineal encephalitis were generally healthy pre-vaccination. Clinically the disease is similar to other post-infectious encephalidites. The mortality rate for this complication was in the order of 30%, with 20% of survivors having permanent sequelae.[29,30] Other described neurologic complications included transverse myelitis, convulsions, muscular paralysis, polyneuritis and brachial neuritis.[31-33] Normally post-vaccineal encephalitis developed following a successful vaccination (Jennerian vesicle) but has been reported without any cutaneous reaction.[34] Vaccinia immune globulin (VIG) was not effective once the illness had begun. Steroids and other measures to treat cerebral edema were used with variable success.

BCG (Bacille Calmette-Guerin)

BCG is a live attenuated vaccine prepared from the bovine tubercle bacillus. Vaccination has been carried out all over the world for tuberculosis prophylaxis. In normal individuals employing the doses usually recommended, the vaccine is judged extraordinarily safe considering the millions of doses administered.[35] More recently BCG has been tried as an adjunct in cancer chemotherapy as a result of studies showing tumor regression in animals.[36] For tuberculosis prevention BCG is given intra-dermally by scarification or multiple puncture-tine techniques. It has been shown that BCG spreads via the lymphatics to regional and distant lymph nodes where multiplication occurs and cellular immunity deve-lopes. Paradoxically, despite its action on the immune system, CNS toxicity has not been due to this mechanism and "allergic" or post-vaccination encephalopathies are conspicuously absent. As an immu-notherapeutic agent for human cancer, larger doses of organisms are given, repeatedly, and often directly into the tumor mass itself.[37, 38] Under these conditions large numbers of organisms may more easily gain access to the circulation with the potential for widespread visceral dissemina-tion. There are well documented examples of such occurrences and on rare occasions the CNS has been involved. Although CNS granulomata may be noted coincidentally in patients dying of generalized disease, a primary, neurological presentation is extremely rare. Pedersen et al[39] des-cribed an apparently immunocompetent 6-year-old girl given BCG who developed relentlessly progressive neurologic disease characterized by headache, vomiting, diplopia and ataxic gait. Papilledema and widened sutures developed and the patient died despite antituberculous therapy. At post mortem examination arachnoiditis and granulomata were noted.

Obviously, in the immunosuppressed cancer patient, BCG must be considerd a potentially lethal, investigational tool which is likely to be replaced by better, safer immunomodulating substances. In the patient with suspected or documented dissemination, prompt therapy with standard antituberculous therapy is indicated. The BCG organism is gen-erally sensitive to the action of isoniazid, rifampin, ethambutol, and paraaminosalicylic acid.[38] Finally, BCG can cause activation of old, dor-mant acid-fast infection and stimulate the growth of tumor in some animals.[40] Although highly unlikely, these two undesirable outcomes could eventually involve the CNS in one way or another.

Typhoid-Paratyphoid Vaccine (T.A.B.) and Cholera Vaccine

This preparation is an inactivated, bacterial vaccine which seems relatively effective in the prevention of serious disease due to *Salmonella typhi* and *Salmonella paratypi* A and B. It is often given in conjunction with a similar inactivated bacterial vaccine containing *Vibrio cholerae*. Neurologic complications are not commonly seen but have been reported.[41] These have included radiculitis, polyneuritis, and Landrys' paralysis but are heavily weighted with reactions occurring during the intravenous administration of T.A.B. for artificial fever therapy. Some of the non-neurologic complications such as those involving heart and kidney may even be lethal in debilitated individuals. These have been recently reviewed.[42, 43] On balance, however, the recent experience with these vaccines would indicate that they carry a very low risk of significant neurologic sequelae.

Influenza Virus Vaccines

Prior to 1976 influenza vaccine was rarely associated with neurologic complications and some of those may have been coincidental.

Encephalitic reactions have rarely been reported. Evidence of an etiologic relationship are tenuous. The alleged association is the vaccine was given before the illness or a seroconversion was observed following immunization.[44, 45] In some instances an oil adjuvant was used.[44] The reported reactions began hours to days after vaccination. The relationship between vaccine and subsequent disease has been difficult to verify. Recovery from the illness has been the rule.

In 1976, swine influenza virus, an Hsw1N1 subtype of influenza type A virus, was isolated from army recruits at Fort Dix.[46] Many soldiers in two platoons were infected as documented by serologic studies. One soldier died after an overnight march. Spread of virus beyond Fort Dix was not demonstrated subsequently. The virus, nevertheless, was presumed to have seeded the United States. This virus subtype by serologic archeology — a retrospective method of attempting to demostrate the etiology of past infections — was thought to have caused the devastating influenza pandemic of 1918 which resulted in a world-wide death toll of 20 million with 5 million deaths in the United States alone.

A scientific prognostication of its recurrence had been made. It was expected to reappear in the 1970's or 1980's. Past teachings suggested that the appearance or reappearance of a new subtype (i.e., new H) (Hemagglutinin) or N (Neuraminadase) would be associated with a pandemic. Thus, the chain of events, at Fort Dix plus the epidemiologic past history from 1918 paved the way for the dire forecasts of another influenza pandemic.

This background led to the conclusion that a nationwide immunization campaign was necessary to prevent an epidemic.

When the association between Guillain-Barré syndrome (GBS) and swine influenza vaccine was first suspected, public health authorities were astonished because this association was unexpected. Past reports had rarely linked influenza vaccine with GBS, or other similar neurologic disorders. One case among 1100 cases of GBS had been noted in a 17-year search of the literature.[47] Two cases of polyneuropathy had been observed in patients given vaccine with an oil adjuvant.[44] As more and more millions of doses of vaccine were given in 1976, the number of reported cases of GBS rose. By December 16, 1976, the Center for Disease Control had sufficient evidence to say there was a statistical association between GBS and swine influenza vaccine. The National Influenza Immunization Program was immediately suspended.[48]

Most cases occurred in recipients of the monovalent, influenza A/New Jersey/76 (HswlN1) or the bivalent influenza A/NJ/76 and A/Victoria/75 (H3N2) vaccines. Though a few cases occurred with non-HswlN1 vaccines such as influenza B/Hong Kong/72 and older bivalent influenza vaccines, rates could not be determined for these vaccine groups because the total number immunized was relatively small.[48]

Vaccine-associated cases exhibited an incubation period of 1 to 10 weeks, with most cases occurring 2-3 weeks post-vaccination.

For the 17-year-old and under group, only one case occurred among vaccinees, so the attributable risk for vaccination is insignificant. In the same age group the attributable risk of GBS from viral infections is higher.[48]

In the 18-year-old and above population the attack rate was 7.4 cases per million vaccinees per month or just under one case per 150,000 vaccinees. For those 18 and above who were unvaccinated, the attack rate was 0.97 cases per million persons. Although there were 362 cases of GBS among vaccinated persons and 332 cases among unvaccinated persons, there were approximately seven times as many unvaccinated as those vaccinated. The difference in the denominator accounts for the higher attack rate in vaccinated persons.

The case-fatality rates over 17 years of age were similar in both groups — 6.0% among the vaccinated and 5.7% among those unvaccinated.[48] Significant neurologic residua were observed in another approximately 5% in each group.

The syndrome of Guillain-Barré is usually characterized by an ascending motor paralysis with less prominent sensory symptoms. In this series of cases, associated sensory symptoms, cranial nerve involvement, and chronic illness were significantly more common in the vaccinated group while a history of an acute respiratory or gastrointestinal illness in the past 4 weeks was more likely among the unvaccinated cases.

This latter difference suggested the vaccine may have replaced an acute illness as an immunopathologic trigger of GBS. Similar proportions in each group had respiratory impairment and similar proportions required respirators.[48]

No significant differences in incidence of GBS were noted among the four types of vaccines used or among the vaccine lots.

Since 1976, the CDC has maintained surveillance for influenza vaccine-associated GBS through over 1000 neurologists in the United States. This program has been unable to show a significant statistical association between influenza vaccine and GBS despite the use of 20-25 million doses annually.[49,50]

Why GBS was associated with influenza vaccine in 1976 and not thereafter remains unclear. Perhaps influenza A/New Jersey/76 (Hsw1N1) is immunologically unique for the human host and favors the rare but definite development of an immunopathologic reaction to neurologic tissue. This type of host reaction is clinically and pathologically related to Waksman's animal model of experimental allergic neuritis elicited by injections of peripheral nerve tissue with an adjuvant. The model is related to allergic encephalomyelitis and polyneuritis in man following killed rabies vaccine derived from nervous tissue.[51] Hence, influenza vaccine composed of influenza A/New Jersey/76 should be added to the long list of vaccines, infectious agents and drugs associated with GBS. This list includes live virus vaccines (mumps, rubella, measles), killed virus vaccines (rabies), numerous respiratory and gastrointestinal viruses and cytomegalovirus, chronic illnesses (Hodgkin's disease, other malignancies, systematic lupus erythematosus), surgical procedures and other forms of trauma, drugs (such as organophosphates and metabolic insults).[47-56]

The known risk of GBS following one form of influenza vaccine was one case per 100,000 vaccines. On the other hand, the chance of a high risk person dying from influenza infection is one in 1,000. The risk benefit ratio for immunization is still favorable.[57] In addition, it now appears that GBS is no longer statistically associated with the current influenza vaccine strain.

Poliovirus Vaccines

The control of epidemic poliomyelitis by immunization is one of the great sagas in the annals of preventive medicine.[58] A disease which appears to have been recognized by the Egyptians in 1500 B.C. was placed on the threshold of conquest when Enders, Weller and Robbins isolated the virus in non-neural tissue culture in 1949.[59] Four years later, Salk first reported the successful immunization of human subjects with formalin-inactivated poliovirus vaccine.[60] The incidence of paralytic disease dramatically fell following the licensure of this vaccine in 1955 and further declined after the introduction of Sabin's oral attenuated live virus vaccine in 1962.[61]

Following the successful Francis field trials, inactivated polio vaccine (IPV) was introduced nationwide. In April, 1955, cases of paralytic polio appeared exceeding that expected to be occurring in vaccine recipients. The cases appeared within 4 to 10 days after vaccination.[62-64] The incubation period was less than the 12-day median incubation period commonly accepted for naturally occurring paralytic poliovirus. The epidemologic investigation showed that most cases could be traced to two pools of vaccine manufactured by Cutter Laboratories. These lots contained residual live virulent virus. Once recognized, the vaccine was recalled and the vaccination program temporarily suspended until the problem was resolved.

The virulent type 1 Mahoney virus and the intramuscular injection route probably accounted for the shortened incubation period, the high incidence of bulbar involvement, and the marked tendency for the initial paralysis to localize in the injected arm. The observed acquisition of infection by family and community contacts of vaccinated cases was consistent with previous epidemiologic studies on the spread of wild poliovirus.

Oral poliovirus (OPV) is the vaccine most commonly used in the United States now. Continued use of OPV has been criticized by Salk and Salk because the incidence of paralytic polio from OPV now exceeds that caused by the wild virus.[65] Currently, the risk of paralytic disease in persons vaccinated is one case in a recipient for every 11.5 million persons vaccinated, in household contacts is one case for every 3.9 million persons vaccinated, and in community contacts is one case for every 22.9 million persons vaccinated. The vaccine recipients and community contacts are mostly under 10 years old while the household contacts are mostly parents, between 20 and 40 years of age. If the data is analyzed by vaccine distribution, there is one case in a recipient per 20 million doses distributed, and one case in a contact per 6 million doses distributed.[66] Differences were also noted in the incubation period: 7 to 14 days for recipients and 20-29 days for contacts.

The neurologic disease caused by OPV is typical of naturally occurring polio with asymmetrical onset of weakness, fasciculations and areflexia which progresses rapidly to maximum paralysis in two weeks. Cases of vaccine-associated disease must fit certain criteria.[67] A compatible case has: (1) "onset of illness between 4 and 30 days following feeding of the specific vaccine type in question and with onset of paralysis not sooner than six days after the feeding; (2) significant residual lower-motor-neuron paralysis; (3) laboratory data not inconsistent with respect to multiplication of the vaccine virus fed; (4) no evidence of upper-motor-neuron disease, definite sensory loss, or progression or recurrences of paralytic illness one month or more after onset." The compatible cases were divided into "probable" case: (1) evidence of fever at onset of paralysis; (2) history of systemic illness preceding the development of paralysis; (3) clinical evidence of meningeal involvement manifested either by nuchal ridigity or cerebrospinal fluid cell count greater than 10 cells per cubic milliliter;" and "possible" case when "one or more of these criteria were missing."[67]

Strict adherence to these criteria will avoid confusion with the Guillain-Barré syndrome where fever and meningismus are usually absent, paralysis is symmetrical, sensory loss is more common, paralysis extends for up to two weeks, and spinal fluid pleocytosis is invariably absent.

Ten percent of the paralytic cases in the United States have occurred in congenitally immunodeficient children.[68] Type 2 OPV is most commonly associated. Either B or T cell deficiencies can occur though combined defects carry greater risk.

An atypical chronic progressive neurologic disease has been reported in these immunodeficiency patients. The incubation period is prolonged up to 30-120 days post-vaccination. The illness is also prolonged and may be progressive with paralysis not reaching peak severity for weeks. Chronic meningitis has been reported. Unusual pathologic features are predominance of involvement in the basal ganglion and thalamus with microcytic degeneration. The case fatality rate is high at 40%.[69-71] In the future, an adequate history should preclude vaccine administration in immunodeficient patients.

Whether IPV should be used instead of OPV in the United States is currently a topic of controversy.[66,72] Use of OPV will be continued because it is felt that this vaccine provides protection through herd immunity in a country where barely a majority of persons are immunized. Unless 90% or greater vaccine compliance can be achieved, as occurs in Scandanavian countries with IPV, this vaccine should not be used in the United States as the sole form of vaccine.

Rabies Vaccines

Neurologic reactions to rabies vaccines have been well recognized since Pasteur introduced a vaccine prepared from neural tissue in 1884.[73] The rate of significant neurologic complications has been reported to be as high as one in 600 with a mortality of 10-25% with neural tissue derived vaccines.[74-76] Neurologic reactions are even more prevalent if electroencephalographic studies are performed; up to 14% have abnormalities.[77]

Pasteur's original vaccine was made from a suspension of infected rabbit spinal cord. The final suspension had been serially passed 90 times in rabbits,[78] then was partially inactivated. In 1919, Semple introduced a vaccine fully inactivated by formalin treatment.

The neurotoxic reactions seen with these nerve tissue products clinically and pathologically resembles Waksman's experimental allergic encephalomyelitis,[79] an inflammatory demyelinating disease in animals produced by immunization with myelin basic protein. Central myelin is thought to be involved in this and other types of post-infectious myelitis or encephalomyelitis seen with viral exanthems and viral respiratory infections. In contrast, sensitization with peripheral myelin is hypothesized as crucial to the development of the Guillain-Barré syndrome associated with rabies and other viral infections and vaccines.[80]

In 1955, Peck, Powell, and Culbertson produced an antirabies vaccine in duck-embryo tissue devoid of central myelin.[81] The virus is inactivated by beta-propriolactone. In the 15 years after the vaccine was licensed, six million doses were given to 424,000 persons. Though local reactions at the vaccine site were the rule (60-100%) and constitutional symptoms were common (10-33%), neurologic reactions were rare. Five cases of cranial or peripheral neuropathy, four cases of transverse myelitis, four cases of encephalitis (two fatal) were reported. Overall the incidence of major neurologic reactions following duck-embryo derived vaccine was approximately one in 32,000,[82] considerably lower than one in 600 reported with nerve-tissue derived vaccines.

Major neurologic reactions were defined as occurring within 6 weeks of starting the vaccine series and finding no other apparent cause. The 13 reported complications began within 3 to 16 days.

The peripheral neuropathies were one with bilateral abducens nerve palsy, one with sciatic and median nerve palsy, one with sciatic and facial nerve neuropathy, and two with optic neuritis. They were treated with steroids and antihistamines. All slowly recovered.[82] Peripheral neuropathies appear to be more common in European reports.[83]

The cases of transverse myelitis had painless, flaccid paraplegia, loss of leg reflexes, impairment of bladder and bowel function, sensory level loss, and fever.[82]

Of four cases of encephalitis, the two non-fatal ones began within a week of starting the vaccine series while the two fatal cases began later. These fatalities may in fact have been due to rabies but insufficient studies were done to confirm this possibility.[87]

Guillain-Barré Syndrome has not been reported after the duck embryo vaccine whereas 200 or more such cases have been seen with the nervous-tissue derived vaccines.

Minor neurologic reactions are more common than major ones and were reported in 137 persons. Objective signs last less than 4 days, no laboratory abnormalities in the cerebrospinal fluid or on the electroencephalogram are apparent. Symptoms may include one or more of the following: headache, photophobia, paresthesias, listlessness, malaise, increased fatigueability, or sleepiness and they may last for as long as one year in a few individuals.

Iatrogenic rabies due to inadequately inactivated rabies vaccine has been reported 19 times.[84] This is a more frequent finding in the rabies vaccines used for immunization of dogs becuase the vaccine itself uses an attenuated live virus.[85]

Another type of rabies vaccine thought to be less neurotoxic was a vaccine grown in the brain of suckling mice.[86] At this stage in the animal's development the brain has not been myelinated. The rates of neurologic reactions to this type of vaccine, however, have not been as thoroughly evaluated.

Because of the incomplete immune response elicited by the duck embryo vaccine and occasional reports of failure to protect against rabies, a more potent and safer vaccine was sought.[87-89]

Koprowski and Wiktor developed a vaccine prepared in human diploid tissue culture.[90] Three types of rabies vaccines are now being produced. A split product vaccine where the virus is grown in WI-38 cells, purified and split with tri-n-butyl phosphate; it was licensed in 1980 for use in the United States and is produced by Wyeth. Both vaccines used in Europe are whole virus vaccines where virus is grown in WI-38 cells (produced by Merieux, France) or MRC-5 cells (produced by Behring Werke, West Germany). Virus is then purified and inactivated by beta-propriolactone.[90,91]

These newer vaccines are superior immunogens and have replaced the duck embryo vaccine because higher levels of antibody are stimulated by fewer doses and fewer local and systematic reactions occur. One case of Guillain-Barré syndrome has been reported with the Merieux vaccine; the patient recovered completely.[92] It is still too early to know whether the incidence of major neurologic reactions with the human diploid cell rabies vaccines will be less than the rare occurrence noted following duck embryo rabies vaccine.

Measles

Encephalitis within 30 days of measles vaccination has been reported in approximately one case per one million doses.[93] The association is temporal and no casual relationship has been established. The Centers for Disease Control have stated that "a certain number of cases of encephalitis may be expected to occur in a large childhood population in a defined period of time even when no vaccines are administered,"[93] (see discussion under Mumps).

The natural incidence of encephalitis following infection with wild measles virus is one case per 1,000 reported infections. The benefit-risk ratio is again easily in favor of immunization.[93] Furthermore, cost analysis of an immunization program compared to long-term care of cases of natural measles encephalitis also favors immunization.[94]

Subacute sclerosing panencephalitis (SSPE), a rare, degenerative disease of the central nervous system, has been reported to follow measles vaccination by several years.[95] It occurs in children and young adults, begins with insidious onset of psychologic and intellectual impairment, then progresses over months to years to a decorticate state and death. Persons with SSPE typically have a history of natural measles infection under two years of age.

The incidence of SSPE following natural measles infection is 5-10 cases per million infections. In contrast, the incidence of SSPE in children without a history of measles who received measles vaccine is one case per million doses distributed. The chance of unrecognized natural measles occurring in the first year of life in these cases cannot be entirely eliminated. Nevertheless, the incidence following vaccine is at least 5-10 times less than that following natural infection. The vaccine appears to offer a protective effect, if anything, from acquiring SSPE. The incidence of SSPE has declined dramatically in the United States after the use of measles vaccine became widespread in the late 1960's.[96]

A number of other neurologic complications have rarely been temporally associated with measles vaccine. Guillain-Barré syndrome[97] and optic neuritis.[98] One author reported a high incidence of neurologic complications in Europe but the risk-benefit ratio was still favorable.[99]

Rubella

Polyneuritis is a natural feature of rubella and has also been reported following rubella vaccine. Two syndromes have been associated with the vaccine.[100,101] The "arm syndrome" begins about 39 days (10-62 days range) after vaccine administration. The patient usually is awakened from sleep by paresthesias in the arm and hand. The symptoms may be brief — 30 seconds — or may last for one hour. They may recur several times during the night. The other syndrome, the "catcher's crouch" syndrome, occurs about 45 days (29-70 days range) following immunization and is characterized by difficulty in knee extension due to pain behind the knee. The pain is at its peak in the morning and decreases during the day. Symptoms may last for 1-5 weeks.

Relapses of either syndrome have been reported to occur within a period of 2-3 years.[102,103] Nerve-conduction velocities are decreased in both syndromes. The reported incidence of the two syndromes is 1-22 cases per 10,000 doses.[100] These syndromes have been seen with virus grown in non-human tissue. Experience with the RA27/3 vaccine-live virus grown in human fibroblast cells is more limited.

Though encephalitis (1 case per 5,000 infections) and progressive panencephalitis have been reported to occur following natural rubella infections,[104-106] neither have been associated with rubella vaccine.

Guillain-Barré syndrome has rarely been reported following rubella vaccine.[107] Association with the other virus strains (i.e. measles and mumps) in the trivalent vaccine cannot be eliminated.

Mumps

Encephalitis and other central nervous system (CNS) reactions are very rare following live mumps vaccine. A cause-and-effect relationship is far from clear. Simultaneous administration of measles and rubella vaccine further complicates interpretation.

Reports of such complications are often made to vaccine manufacturers. Twenty-two such reports have been received.[108] In four cases other etiologic agents were established. Two were benign febrile convulsions and two occurred beyond 30 days. Fourteen cases remain in which CNS reactions have been reported within 1 month (range 2-20 days) of vaccination. Ten had meningoencephalitis by clinical or laboratory criteria, one had focal and generalized seizures, two had visual disturbances, and one unilateral deafness.

The reported incidence of encephalitis following natural mumps is difficult to determine precisely as 60% of patients with clinical evidence of mumps (mainly parotitis) have an increase in white blood cells in the cerebrospinal fluid.[109] Distinctions between aseptic meningitis and encephalitis is often arbitrary. The various CNS disorders associated with mumps are often therefore combined together in the category meningoencephalitis. Most CNS disorders following mumps, however, are mild as indicated by the low fatality ratio of 1.4%.[108]

Mumps has always been the most commonly reported type of encephalitis accounting for 36% of all causes.[110] The ratio is approximately 2.6 cases per 1,000 infections or 3.5 per 1,000 if meningitis is included.[108] Some authors report higher ratios for encephalitis[111-113] and much higher rates for meningitis.[114-116] CNS involvement increases with increasing age.[108]

Deafness is another well-recognized CNS complication of natural mumps infection whether or not clinical meningoencephalitis occurs.[117,118] It is usually unilateral and permanent, it is due to demyelination of the auditory portion of the eighth cranial nerve secondary to a labyrinthitis. The incidence is probably underestimated at 1-7 per 100,000 cases of mumps infection.[118,119]

Because of the relatively high incidence of CNS complications from natural mumps (2600 cases of encephalitis per one million cases of mumps), the estimated incidence of 0.9 episodes of CNS disease per million doses of monovalent mumps vaccines represents a risk-benefit ratio strongly in favor of vaccination.

Whether this low incidence of CNS disease following mumps vaccine is truly related to vaccination is another question still. In a survey of young children in New Jersey for encephalitis of unknown etiology, a rate of 2.86 cases of encephalitis per million children age 1-9 years was observed in a 4-week period.[119] A similar survey in the same age group in Florida showed an incidence of 2.28 cases per million in a 4-week period.[108] Reported cases to the CDC for the same age group several years after the above two studies showed an incidence rate of 1.03 cases per million per 4-week period.[120-122] Thus, the reported rate following mumps vaccine is less than that found in these three studies and suggests that attribution of unusual risk of CNS disease to mumps vaccination may be unwarranted.

Yellow Fever Vaccine

The 17D live virus strain of Theiler is the only yellow fever vaccine licensed in the United States. It is used exclusively for travel to certain foreign countries. The vaccine strain was passaged in tissue culture and is prepared in chick embryo to eliminate the viruses inherent neurotropism. Encephalitis is rare. It occurs typically in young infants and usually resolves without sequellae. One death has been reported.[123-125]

In a study of vaccine-associated encephalitis in Brazilian children, the risk of encephalitis with the 17D strain varied depending on the production lot administered and the culture passage of the lot. Neurovirulence of the vaccine strains for monkeys was shown to be a reliable predictor of CNS complications in man.[123] As a result of these studies, master seed lots with the lowest risk have been sequestered for use.

The 17D strain vaccine is heat labile. It must be stored in dessicated form at -25° C and should be used within 1 hour after reconstitution. For mass immunization in tropical countries the Dakar vaccine is more widely used because it is applied by the scratch technique and the virus strain is more stable under adverse environmental conditions.[126]

The Dakar vaccine is made from the mouse brain passaged French neurotropic virus strain. It is definitely encephalitogenic in man. The incidence of encephalitis is approximately 5 cases per 1000 doses. This complication occurs more often in children under 14 years of age. This vaccine is not licensed for use in the United States.

Multiple sclerosis has been reported following yellow fever vaccine and several other vaccines.[127] The association, however, is tenuous.

Other Vaccines

Numerous other viral and a few rickettsial vaccines are commercially available or are being tested. The viral vaccines include adenovirus, type B hepatitis, rhinovirus, parainfluenza, respiratory syncytial, cytomegalovirus, herpes simplex, varicella-zoster, and eastern, western, and Venezualan equine encephalitis viruses.[128-132] The rickettsial vaccines available are for epidemic typhus and Rocky Mountain Spotted Fever.[131,133] Vaccines for mycoplasma (M. pneumoniae) and chlamydia (C. trachomatis) have also been tested.[130,134] Limited experience with all of these vaccines precludes judgement on the risk of neurologic reactions. The same can be said for polyvalent pneumococcal vaccine and the Group A and C meningococcal vaccines.

Serum

Peripheral neuropathies may follow the injection of serum. The reaction is infrequent. Brachial plexus neuropathy is the most common form and presents pari passu with the typical clinical findings of serum sickness. An acute inflammatory necrotizing vasculitis of the neuronal vessels is thought to be responsible.[135,136]

References

1. Melin K-A: Pertussis immunization in children with convulsive disorders. *J Pediatr* **43**:652-654, 1953.
2. Griffith AH: Pertussis vaccine and convulsive disorders of childhood. *Proc Roy Soc Med* **67**:372-374, 1974.
3. Madsen T: Vaccination against whooping cough. *JAMA* **101**:187-188,1933.
4. Byers RK, Moll FC: Encephalopathies following prophylactic pertussis vaccine. *Pediatrics* **1**:437-456, 1948.
5. Globus JH, Kohn JL: Encephalopathy following pertussis vaccine prophylaxis. *JAMA* **141**:507-509, 1949.
6. Berg JM: Neurological complications of pertussis immunization. *Brit Med J* **2**:24-27, 1958.
7. Pittman M: Instability of pertussis vaccine component in quadruple antigen vaccine. *JAMA* **181**:25-30, 1962.
8. Pittman M, Cox CB: Pertussis vaccine testing for freedom-from-toxicity. *Appl Microbiol* **13**:447-456, 1965.
9. Kulenkampff M, Schwartzman JS, Wilson J: Neurological complications of pertussis inoculation. *Arch Dis Child* **49**:46-49, 1974.
10. Dick G: Reactions to routine immunization in childhood. *Proc R Coy Soc Med* **67**:371-372, 1974.

11. Stewart GT: Vaccination against whooping cough. Efficacy versus risks. *Lancet* 1:234-237, 1977.

12. Strom J: Further experience of reactions, especially of a cerebral nature in conjunction with triple vaccination: A study based on vaccinations in Sweden 1959-65. *Brit Med J* 4:320-323, 1967.

13. Miller DL, Ross EM, Alderslade R, et al: Pertussis immunization and serious acute neurological illness in children. *Brit Med J* 282:1595-1599,1981.

14. Editorial. Pertussis vaccine. *Brit Med J* 282:1563-1564, 1981.

15. Toomey JA: Reactions to pertussis vaccine. *JAMA* 139:448-450, 1949.

16. Thursby-Pelham DC, Giles C: Neurological complications of pertussis immunization. *Brit Med J* 2:246, 1958.

17. Melchior JC: Infantile spasms and immunization in the first year of life. *Neuropaediatric* 3:3-10, 1971.

18. Baraff LJ, Cherry JD: Nature and rates of adverse reactions associated with pertussis immunization. *International Symposium on Pertussis*, 3d, N.I.H, 1978, Bethesda, DHEW/NIH, 1979, p 291-296.

19. Middaugh JP: Side effects of Diphtheria-Tetanus toxoid in adults. *AJPH* 69:246-249, 1979.

20. Relyveld EH, Henocq E, Bizzini B: Studies on untoward reactions to diphtheria and tetanus toxoids. *International Symposium on Immunizations: Benefit versus risk factors*, Brussels, 1978. *Develop Biol Standard* 43:33-37, 1979.

21. Baust W, Meyer D, Wachsmuth W: Peripheral neuropathy after administration of tetanus toxoid. *J Neurol* 222:131-133, 1979.

22. Whittle E, Robertson NR: Transverse myelitis after diphtheria, tetanus and polio immunization. *Brit Med J* 1:1450, 1977.

23. Schlenska, GK: Unusual neurologic complications following tetanus toxoid administration. *J Neurol* 215:299-302, 1977.

24. Pollard JD, Selby G: Relapsing neuropathy due to tetanus toxoid. Report of a case. *J Neurol Sci* 37:113-125, 1978.

25. The global eradication of smallpox: Final reports of the Global Commission for the Certification of Smallpox eradication, Geneva, December 1979. Geneva: World Health Organization, 1980:122.

26. Espmark JA: Smallpox vaccination studies with serial dilutions of vaccine: I. Primary vaccination and revaccination in human adults. *Acta Pathol Microbiol Scand* 63:97-115, 1965.

27. Espmark JA, Ralso E: Smallpox vaccination studies with serial dilutions of vaccine: III. Comparison of take rates in two age groups of infants. *Acta Paediatr Scand* 54:149-154, 1965.

28. Goldstein JA et al: Smallpox Vaccination reactions, prophylaxis, and therapy of complications. *Pediatrics* 55:342-347, 1975.

29. Lane JM, Ruben FL, Neff JM, et al: Complications of smallpox vaccination, 1968. *N Engl J Med* 281:1201-1208, 1969.

30. Neff JM, Lane JM, Pert JH, et al: Complications of smallpox vaccination I. National survey in the United States, 1963. *N Engl J Med* 276:125-137, 1967.

31. Neff JM, Levine RH, Lane JM, et al: Complications of vaccination, United States, 1963:II. Results obtained, by four statewide surveys. *Pediatrics* 39:916-923, 1967.

32. de Vries E: *Postvaccinial Verivenous Encephalitis*. Amsterdam, Elsevier Publishing Co., 1959.

33. Spillance JD, Wells CDC: The neurology of Jennerian vaccination: A clinical account of the neurological complications which occurred during the smallpox epidemic in South Wales in 1962. *Brain* **87**:1-44, 1964.

34. Rockoff A, Spigland I, Lorenstein B, et al: Post vaccinial encephalomyelitis without cutaneous vaccination reaction. *Ann Neurol* **5**:99-101, 1979.

35. Lotte A, Wasz-Höckert O, Lert F, et al: International Symposium on Immunization: Benefit versus risk factors, Brussels, 1978. *Develop Biol Standard* **43**:111-119, 1979.

36. Zbar B, Tanoka T: Immunotherapy of cancer: Regression of tumors after intralesional injection of living mycobacterium bovis. *Science* **172**:271-273, 1971.

37. Sparks FC: Hazards and complications of BCG immunotherapy. *Med Clin N Amer* **60**:499-509, 1976.

38. Aungst CW, Sokal JE, Jager BV: Complications of BCG vaccination in neoplastic disease. *Ann Intern Med* **82**:666-669, 1975.

39. Pedersen FK, Engbaek HC, Hertz H, et al: Fatal BCG infection in an immunocompetent girl: *Acta Paediatrica Scand* **67**:519-523, 1978.

40. Old LJ, Benacerraf B, Clarke DA, et al: The role of the reticuloendothelial system in the host reaction of neoplasia. *Cancer Res* **21**:1281, 1961.

41. Miller HG, Stanton JB: Neurological sequelae of prophylactic inoculation. *Quart J Med* **23**:1-27, 1954.

42. Mittermayer MC: Lethal complications of typhoid-cholera vaccination. *Beitr Path Bd* **158**:212-214, 1976.

43. Eisinger AJ, Smith JG: Acute renal failure after TAB and cholera vaccination *Brit Med J* **1**:381-382, 1979.

44. Wells CEC: A neurological note on vaccination against influenza. *Brit Med J* **3**:755-756, 1971.

45. Gross WL, Ravens KG, Hansen HW: Meningoencephalitis syndrome following influenza vaccination. *J Neurol* **217**:219-222, 1978.

46. Hodder RA, Gaydos JC, Allen RG, et al: Swine influenza A at Fort Dix, New Jersey (January-February 1976). III. Extent of spread and duration of the outbreak. *J Infect Dis* **136**:S369-S375, 1977.

47. Leneman F: The Guillain-Barré syndrome. *Arch Intern Med* **118**:139-144, 1966.

48. Schonberger LB, Bregman DJ, Sullivan-Bolyai JZ, et al: Guillain-Barré syndrome following vaccination in the national influenza immunization program, United States, 1976-1977. *Amer J Epidem* **110**:105-123, 1979.

49. Guillain-Barré Syndrome Surveillance Report Summary Jan 1978-Mar 1979 Center for Disease Control, issued October 1980.

50. Hurwitz ES, Schoenberger LB, Melsan DB, Holman RC: Guillain-Barré syndrome and the 1978-1979 influenza vaccine. *N Eng J Med* **304**:1557-1561, 1981.

51. Waksman BH: Experimental allergic encephalomyelitis and the "auto-allergic" disease. *Int Arch Allergy Appl Immunol* **14** (suppl):1, 1959.

52. Dowling PC, Menonna JP, Cook SD: Guillain-Barré syndrome in greater New York-New Jersey. *JAMA* **238**:317-318, 1977.

53. Froelich CJ, Searles RP, Davis LE, Goodwin JS: A case of Guillain-Barré syndrome with immunologic abnormalities. *Ann Intern Med* **93**:563-565, 1980.

54. Kennedy RH, Danielson MA, Mulder DW, Kurland LT: Guillain-Barré syndrome. A 42-year epidemiologic and clinical study. *Mayo Clin Proc* **53**:93-99, 1978.

55. Fisher JR: Guillain-Barré syndrome following organophosphate poisoning. *JAMA* **238**:1950, 1977.
56. Dowling P, Menonna J, Cook S: Cytomegalovirus complement fixation antibody in Guillain-Barré syndrome. *Neurology* **27**:1153-1156, 1977.
57. Conference on influenza A/USSR/77 (H1N1). Department of Health Education & Welfare, Washington, DC, January 30, 1978, p 26.
58. Paul JR: *A History of Poliomyelitis*. New Haven, Yale University Press, 1971.
59. Enders JF, Weller TH, Robbins FC: Cultivation of the Lansing strain of poliomyelitis virus in cultures of various human embryonic tissues. *Science* **109**:85, 1949.
60. Salk JE, Bennett BL, Lewis LJ, et al: Studies in human subjects on active immunization against poliomyelitis. I. A preliminary report of experiments in progress. *JAMA* **151**:1081-1098, 1953.
61. Live Poliovirus Vaccines. First and Second International Conferences on Live Poliovirus Vaccines. Washington, DC, World Health Organization, 1959, 1960.
62. Nathanson N, Langmuir AD: The Cutter incident. Poliomyelitis following formaldehyde-inactivated poliovirus vaccination in the United States during the spring of 1955. I. Background. *Amer J Hyg* **78**:16-28, 1963.
63. Nathanson N, Langmuir AD: The Cutter incident. Poliomyelitis following formaldehyde-inactivated poliovirus vaccination in the United States during the spring of 1955. II. Relationship of poliomyelitis to Cutter vaccine. *Amer J Hyg* **78**:29-60, 1963.
64. Nathanson N, Langmuir AD: The Cutter incident. Poliomyelitis following formaldehyde-inactivated poliovirus vaccination in the United States during the spring of 1955. III. Comparison of the clinical character of vaccinated and contact cases occurring after use of high rate lots of Cutter vaccine. *Amer J Hyg* **78**:61-81, 1963.
65. Salk J, Salk D: Control of influenza and poliomyelitis with killed virus vaccines. *Science* **195**:834-847, 1977.
66. Nightingale EO: Recommendations for a national policy on poliomyelitis vaccination. *N Engl J Med* **297**:249-253, 1977.
67. Henderson DA, Witte JJ, Morris L, Langmuir AD: Paralytic disease associated with oral polio vaccines. *JAMA* **190**:153-167, 1964.
68. Annual Poliomyelitis Summary 1973, Neurotropic Disease Surveillance. Center for Disease Control, issued February, 1975.
69. Davis LE, Bodian D, Price D, et al: Chronic progressive poliomyelitis secondary to vaccination of an immunodeficient child. *N Engl J Med* **297**:241-245. 1977.
70. Wright PF. Hatch MH, Kasselberg AG, et al: Vaccine-associated poliomyelitis in a child with sex-linked agammaglobulinemia. *J Pediatr* **91**:408-412, 1977.
71. Wyatt HV: Poliomyelitis in hypogammaglobulinemics. *J Infect Dis* **128**:802-869, 1973.
72. Nathanson N, Martin JR: The epidemiology of poliomyelitis: enigmas surrounding its appearance, epidemicity, and disappearance. *Am J Epidemiol* **110**:672-692, 1979.
73. Pasteur L: Methode pour prevenir la rage après morsure. *C R Acad Sci (Paris)* **101**:765-774, 1885.
74. Rubin RH, Gregg MB, Sikes RK: Rabies in citizens of the United States,

1963-1968: epidemiology, treatment, and complications of treatment. *J Infect Dis* **120**:268-273, 1969.

75. Applebaum E, Greenberg M, Nelson J: Neurological complications following antirabies vaccination. *JAMA* **151**:188-191, 1953.

76. Blatt NH, Lepper MH: Reactions following antirabies prophylaxis: Report on 16 patients. *Amer J Dis Child* **86**:395-402, 1953.

77. Gibbs FA, Gibbs EL, Carpenter PR: Comparison of rabies vaccines grown on duck embryo and on nervous tissue. An electroencephalographic study. *N Engl J Med* **265**:1002-1003. 1961.

78. Meyer HM: Rabies Vaccine. *J Infect Dis* **142**:287-289, 1980.

79. Waksman BH: Experimental allergic encephalomyelitis and the "autoallergic" disease. *Int Arch Allergy Appl Immunol* 14(Suppl):1, 1959.

80. Griffin DE, Johnson RT: Encephalitis, myelitis, and neuritis. In: Mandell GL, Douglas RG Jr, Bennett JE, eds: *Principles and Practice of Infectious Diseases*. New York, John Wiley & Sons,1979, pp 769-779.

81. Peck FB Jr, Powell HM, Culbertson CG: A new antirabies vaccine for human use. Clinical and laboratory results using rabies vaccine made from embryonated duck eggs. *J Lab Clin Med* **45**:679-683, 1955.

82. Rubin RH, Hattwick MAW, Jones S, et al: Adverse reactions to duck embryo rabies vaccine. *Ann Intern Med* **78**:643-649, 1973.

83. Cremieux G, Dor JF, Mongin M: Peripheral facial paralysis and post-antirabies-vaccination polyneuroradiculitis (French). *Acta Neurol Belg* **78**(5):279-300, 1978.

84. Para M: An outbreak of post-vaccinal rabies (rage de laboratoire) in Fortaleza, Brazil, in 1960. Residual fixed virus as the etiological agent. *Bull WHO* **33**:177-182, 1965.

85. Vaccine-induced canine rabies - California. *MMWR* **27**:224-225. 1978.

86. Fuenzalida E, Palacios R: Rabies vaccine prepared from brains of infected suckling mice. *Boletino Instituto Bacteriologico Chile* **8**:3-10, 1955.

87. Anderson JA, Daly FT Jr, Kidd JC: Human rabies after antiserum and vaccine postexposure treatment. Case report and review. *Ann Intern Med* **64**:1297-1302, 1966.

88. Dehner LP: Human rabies encephalitis in Vietnam. *Ann Intern Med* **72**: 375-378, 1970.

89. Corey L, Hattwick MAW, Baer GM, Smith JS: Serum neutralizing antibody after rabies postexposure prophylaxis. *Ann Intern Med* **85**:170-176, 1976.

90. Wiktor TJ, Koprowski H: Successful immunization of primates with rabbies vaccine prepared in human diploid cell strain WI-38. *Proc Soc Exp Biol Med* **118**:1069-1073, 1965.

91. Plotkin SA: Rabies vaccine prepared in human cell cultures: progress and perspective. *Rev Infect Dis* **2**:433-448, 1980.

92. Adverse reactions to human diploid cell rabies vaccine. *MMWR*: **29**:609-610, 1980.

93. Federal Register. Department of Health, Education, and Welfare. Part II Food & Drug Administration. April 1980. Viral and Rickettsial Vaccines; proposed implementation of efficacy review. FR 45: no. 74.

94. Kogan BA, Murray RA, Hanes B, et al: Mass measles immunization in Los Angeles County. *Amer J Publ Health* **58**:1883-1890, 1968.

95. Modlin JF, Jabbour JT, Witte JJ, Halsey NA: Epidemiologic studies of measles, measles vaccine and subacute sclerosing panencephalitis, *Pediatrics* **59**:505-512, 1977.

96. Modlin JF, Halsey NA, Eddins DL: Epidemiology of subacute sclerosing panencephalitis. *J Pediatr* **94**:231-236, 1979.
97. Grose C, Spigland I: Guillain-Barré syndrome following administration of live measles vaccine. *Amer J Med* **60**:441-444, 1976.
98. Kazarian EL, Gager WE: Optic neuritis complicating measles, mumps, and rubella vaccination. *Amer J Ophthal* **86**:544-547, 1978.
99. Allerdist H: Neurological complications following measles vaccination. *Develop Biol Standard* **43**:259-264, 1979.
100. Schaffner W, Fleet WF, Kilroy AW, et al: Polyneuropathy following rubella immunization. A follow-up study and review of the problem. *Amer J Dis Child* **127**:684-688, 1974.
101. Gilmartin RC, Jabbour JT, Duenas DA: Rubella vaccine myeloradiculoneuritis. *J Pediatr* **80**:406-412, 1972.
102. Kilroy AW, Schaffner W, Fleet WF, et al: Two syndromes following rubella immunization. Clinical observations and epidemiological studies. *JAMA* **214**:2287-2292, 1970.
103. Spruance SL, Metcalf R, Smith CB, et al: Chronic arthropathy associated with rubella vaccination. *Arthritis Rheum* **20**:741-747, 1977.
104. Heggie AD, Robbins FC: Natural rubella acquired after birth. *Amer J Dis Child* **118**:12-17, 1969.
105. Sherman FE, Michaels RH, Kenny FM: Acute encephalopathy (encephalitis) complicating rubella. *JAMA* **192**:675-681, 1965.
106. Wolinsky JS, Dau PC, Buimovici-Klein E, et al: Progressive Rubella Panencephalitis: Immunovirological studies and results of isoprinosine therapy. *Clin Exp Immunol* **35**(3):397-404, 1979.
107. Gunderman JR: Guillain-Barré syndrome. *Amer J Dis Child* **125**:834-835, 1973.
108. *Center for Disease Control: Mumps Surveillance. July 1974-December, 1976.* Issued July, 1978.
109. Bang HO, Bang J: Involvement of the central nervous system in mumps. *Bull Hyg* **19**:503-504, 1944.
110. *Center For Disease Control: Encephalitis Surveillance Report, Annual Summary 1975.* Issued May 1977.
111. Strusberg S, Winter S, Friedman A, et al: Notes on mumps meningoencephalitis; some features of 199 cases in children. *Clin Pediat* **8**:373-374, 1969.
112. Philip RN, Reinhard KB, Lackman DB: Observations on a mumps epidemic in a "virgin" population. *Amer J Hyg* **69**:91-111, 1959.
113. Bjorvatin B, Wolontis S: Mumps meningoencephalitis in Stockholm November 1964-July 1971. I. Analysis of hospitalized study group. *Scand J Infect Dis* **5**:253-260, 1973.
114. Lennette EH, Mayoffin NL, Knowf EG: Viral central nervous system disease. *JAMA* **179**:687-695, 1962.
115. Adair CU, Gaulf RL, Smadel JE: Aseptic meningitis, a disease of diverse etiology: Clinical and etiologic studies on 854 cases. *Ann Intern Med* **39**:675-704, 1953.
116. Young NA: Chickenpox, measles, and mumps. In: Remington JJ, Klein JO, eds: *Infectious Disease of the Fetus and Newborn Infant.* Philadelphia, WB Saunders Co, 1976, p 573.
117. Prasud LW: Complete bilateral deafness following mumps. *J Laryngol* **77**:809-811, 1963.
118. Everberg G: Deafness following mumps. *Acta Otolaryngol* **48**:397-403,

1957.
119. Nader PR, Warren RJ: Reported neurologic disorders following live measles vaccine. *Pediatrics* 41:998-1001, 1968.
120. Center for Disease Control: Encephalitis Surveillance Report, Annual Summary 1973, Issued December 1975.
121. Center for Disease Control: Encephalitis Surveillance Report, Annual Summary 1974. Issued August 1976.
122. Center for Disease Control: Encephalitis Surveillance Report, Annual Summary 1975. Issued May 1977.
123. Fox JP, Penna HA: Behavior of 17D yellow fever virus in rhesus monkeys; relation to substrain. Dose, and neural or extraneural inoculation. *Amer J Hyg* 38:152-172, 1943.
124. Fox JP, Lennette EH, Manso C, Souza Aguiar JR: Encephalitis in man following vaccination with 17D yellow fever virus. *Amer J Hyg* 36:117-142, 1942.
125. Viral and Rickettsial Vaccines: *Federal Register* April 15, 1980, pp 25652-25758.
126. Smithburn KC: Yellow fever vaccination. Geneva, World Health Organization, 1956.
127. Miller H, Cendrowski W, Schapira K: Multiple sclerosis and vaccination. *Brit Med J* 2:210-213, 1967.
128. Hilleman MR: Adenovirus vaccine: development, field evaluation and appraisal of the need for vaccination in military and civilian population. *Arch Intern Med* 101:47-53, 1958.
129. McAuliffe VJ, Purcell RH, Gerin JL: Type B Hepatitis; A review of current prospects for a safe and effective vaccine. *Rev Infect Dis* 2:470-492, 1980.
130. Dudgeon JA: Immunization in times ancient and modern. *J Roy Soc Med* 73:581-586, 1980.
131. Viral and Rickettsial Vaccines; proposed implementation of efficacy review. *Federal Register* April 15, 1980.
132. Russell PK: Alphavirus (eastern, western, and Venezuelan equine encephalitis). In: Mandell GL, Douglas RG Jr, Bennett JE, eds: *Principles and Practice of Infectious Diseases.* New York, John Wiley & Sons, 1979, pp 1243-1247.
133. DuPont HL, Hornick RB, Dawkins AT, et al: Rocky mountain spotted fever. A comparative study of the active immunity induced by inactivated and viable pathogenic rickettsia rickettsii. *J Infect Dis* 128:340-344, 1973.
134. National Institutes of Health. Report of a workshop: disease accentuation after immunization with inactivated microbial vaccines. *J Infect Dis* 131:749-754, 1975.
135. Dyck PJ: Diseases of the peripheral nervous system. In: Beeson PB, McDermott W, Wyngaarden JB, eds: Cecil Textbook of Medicine, 15th Ed. Philadelphia, WB Saunders Co, 1979, pp 899-913.
136. Hughes RR: Neurological complications of serum and vaccine therapy. *Lancet* 2:464-467, 1944.

Chapter V

Neurological Complications of Radiotherapy

Paul S. Berger, M.D.

Introduction

Normal tissue injury is a risk of any course of radiation in the therapeutic dose range. Indeed, with the exception of a few highly sensitive tumors, it is normal tissue tolerance that determines the final dose that a patient receives. Attention to identification and management of these injuries is then of interest for several reasons. Understanding of sites of injury and the details of the radiation there can help identify especially sensitive (or resistant) tissues. The clinical diagnosis that radiation necrosis has occurred is critical, both because in some cases effective therapy is available, and because the injury can mimic tumor recurrence. In the latter case, re-irradiation can be catastrophic.

The sequence of injury to normal tissue is dependent in part upon the relative radiosensitivity of the parenchymal tissue and the supporting vasculature and stroma.[1] Organs with a rapidly renewing parenchymal compartment may suffer severe acute damage. Whether or not such injury heals depends upon the ability of the reserve component to repopulate the parenchyma as well as the integrity of the supporting compartment. Organs in which the parenchyma renews slowly will have a fate largely determined by effects upon the stromal tissue.

Rubin and Casarett[1] divide the time course of radiation-related events into four arbitrary but useful periods: acute (up to 6 months), subacute, chronic (2-5 years), and late. The acute phase is characterized by dose and sensitivity dependent organ damage which need not be clinically apparent and which may be completely repaired. In the subacute phase, recovery from the acute damage and delayed injury become manifest. In the chronic and late periods, there may appear further evidence of injuries. These delayed, irreversible lesions have as their etiology ischemia with deterioration of the organ vasculature and increase in its

137

connective tissue component. Carcinogenesis may also become apparent in the late period. The sequence is summarized in Figure 1.

Radiation injury to the nervous system is a specific case of the above general outline, and the different phases can be identified with varying clarity. This chapter considers the injuries to the compartments of the nervous system that may be caused by radiation and will attempt to identify the clinical circumstances in which such injury is likely to occur. It should be remembered, however, that radiation necrosis is not a specific

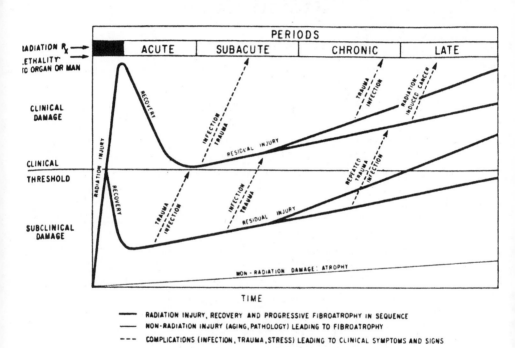

Clinicopathologic course: general scheme.

Figure 1. This diagram illustrates generally, with respect to clinical periods, the waxing and waning (vertically) of organ damage with time (horizontally) in the sequence of acute damage, recovery from acute damage and persistence or progression of residual damage. The heavy continuous lines depict radiation damage of different degrees or after radiation doses of different size. The lighter continuous line indicates the accumulation of organ damage with time or "aging," as a result of causes other than the radiation in question, that may be additive to radiation damage in its effect or consequence. The rising broken arrows indicate precipitation of damage from subclinical or clinical levels to clinically significant or even lethal levels, as a result of complications such as trauma or infection or of deterioration of the vasculature and failure of blood circulation. No precise values or relationships are intended for the slopes or shapes of the graph lines. From: Rubin P, Casarett GW: *Clinical Radiation Pathology*, WB Saunders Co., Philadelphia, 1968, with permission.

entity and that it can be mimicked or modified by a multitude of processes. Familiarity with the syndromes and a healthy index of suspicion may suggest the diagnosis, but confirmation will require biopsy or, as is often the case, remain as a diagnosis by exclusion.

Radiation Damage To The Brain

Radiation injury to the central nervous system[2-5] and to the brain[6] has been well reviewed. It is clear that multiple factors must be considered in analyzing the phenomenon. These include:

(1) *Dose.* The risk is proportional to the dose. There is no absolute threshold, but rather a percentage risk of damage that varies directly with the total dose.

(2) *Individual fraction size.* The larger the size of the individual fraction, the greater the risk of damage. Thus 5000 rads can be given to the whole brain in five weeks with little risk of complication, if the usual fractionation of 200 rads, five times a week is used. If, however, the same dose were given in single, weekly, 1000 rad fractions, the results would be catastrophic.

(3) *Overall time of treatment.* A certain dose will be more likely to cause complications if given over a shorter period of time.

The aforementioned three factors — dose, fraction size, and overall treatment size — have been incorporated by Ellis[7] into a single formula to determine the nominal standard dose (NSD):

$$NSD = D \times N^{-.24} \times T^{-.11}$$

where D is the total dose, N is the number of fractions, and T is the treatment time in days.

The Ellis formula was calculated using retrospective data to determine the tolerance of normal connective tissue. However, experimental spinal cord data[8] indicates that fraction size is more important than overall time, leading to a proposed modification of the formula for neurological damage.

$$Neurets = D \times N^{-.44} \times T^{-.06}$$

That these data are approximate is shown by the fact that others[9] have calculated the proper N exponent to be minus .33. Analysis of data for injury of the brain by several groups[10-12] has derived exponents for N of between $-.377$ to $-.45$ and for T of $-.02$ to $-.058$. All point to the fact that for nervous tissue, as compared to connective tissue, individual treatment fraction size is more important, while overall treatment time is less. And, in spite of the uncertainty of the specific values, the formula emphasizes the importance of including all these variables in describing a course of radiotherapy. The typical statement that a patient received a dose of 6000 rads conveys no more information than saying that the patient drank a quart of whiskey. Without information as to the period of time over which the whiskey was drunk and the amount taken at each sitting, no conclusion concerning biologic effect can be drawn.

(4) *Volume irradiated.* The larger the irradiated volume, the greater will be the sensitivity to irradiation. Indeed, the mechanism of damage may differ for small versus larger volumes.[2]

(5) *Modifying factors.* Multiple variables can affect this complex process, including the status of the vasculature and hence oxygen supply and the type of radiation used.

Early Reaction

Freeman et al[13] reported on somnolence after prophylactic cranial irradiation of children with acute lymphoblastic leukemia. In this series, 28 children received either craniospinal radiation (7 patients) or cranial and reduced spinal irradiation with intrathecal methotrexate. The dose was 2400 rads in 28 days (except only 1000 rads in five days to those patients receiving reduced spinal radiation). Twenty-two children (79%) developed a syndrome characterized predominantly by somnolence, preceded and followed by several days of anorexia and irritability. In 11 children the symptoms were severe, with the patient sleeping up to 20 hours a day, and in 11 they were mild. The symptoms appeared between 24 and 56 days after the completion of radiation and lasted 10 to 38 days. Symptoms were independent of the type of treatment, although younger patients were more severely affected. No consistent CSF findings were identified. In all cases, systems resolved spontaneously and completely. The authors attribute the syndrome to a transient radiation-induced disturbance of myelination.

That the somnolence is not a reflection of underlying CNS disease is indicated by the earlier report of Druckmann[14], who reported similar somnolence in children after scalp irradiation for ringworm.

Rider[15] reported on three patients with tumors in and around the middle ear who received 5500 rads in one month in 16, 20, and 27 fractions with Cobalt 60. About 10 weeks after completion of the therapy, they developed nausea and vomiting, followed by ataxia, dysarthria, and dysphagia. Physical examination revealed gross cerebellar ataxia, horizontal nystagmus, and Romberg's sign in all three. Two of the patients made a complete recovery in six to eight weeks, but one patient died four weeks after the onset of symptoms. Autopsy in this patient revealed patchy, disseminated demyelination indistinguishable from disseminated sclerosis except that the plaques were confined to the irradiated volume. Blood vessel damage was minimal.

Boldrey and Sheline[16] reported 13 cases in which clinical deterioration occurred about two months after completion of high-dose (approximately 5000 rads) radiotherapy. The symptoms lasted for a few days to weeks and resolved spontaneously. Their syndrome differed from the above in that children showed less predisposition for the entity and in that all patients had an intracranial neoplasm. The authors attribute the symptoms to an effect on brain adjacent to a neoplasm or which has been disturbed surgically.

Munro and Mair[17] reported the autopsy findings on a man who died 14 weeks after completion of a course of pituitary gland irradiation, and after six weeks of neurological symptoms felt to be related to his treatment. Pathologically, the lesion was predominantly in the white matter with loss of myelin and oligodendioglia and presence of giant astrocytes. Vascular changes were minimal.

Lampert and Davis[18] and Almquist et al[19] report early cases as well, with similar pathological changes.

A final early reaction to nervous system irradiation, mentioned primarily for purposes of exclusion, is acute irradiation-induced edema. While transient edema may occur, it is usually mild and easily controlled by steroids and symptomatic therapy. As emphasized by Kramer,[2] the shrinkage of sensitive tumors will exceed volume increase of edema. Thus the practice of starting a treatment course with small fractions and gradually raising it to full fraction size only serves to delay the delivery of adequate doses, and therapy is best initiated with full daily fractions. Two hundred rad daily fractions have been delivered to the 7000-8000 rad range without significant immediate sequelae.[20]

Delayed Reactions

The complication of nervous system irradiation that most commonly confronts the clinician is that which is delayed by at least several months from treatment. Numerous series have reported this complication[18,21-25] as a consequence of treatment of benign diseases,[26] extracranial tumors,[27-38] intracranial tumors,[39-42] and tumors in the region of the pituitary.[19,43-49]

The incidence of the late necrosis is hard to estimate, since many patients receive radiotherapy for tumors in and around the brain, but the complication is rarely reported. In a survey of neurosurgeons, Raskind[50] reported that 188 of 295 responders had never encountered a case of central nervous system complication resulting from X-ray therapy. Including his own cases, only 104 cases were reported. In a review of the world literature, Kramer[2] identified only 57 cases of bona fide delayed radionecrosis of the brain.

As a percentage of treated cases, meaningful data is also hard to come by. Of 112 patients treated with high doses for carcinoma of the nasopharynx,[29] four developed necrosis, which was fatal in three cases. The incidence of necrosis may be larger in patients treated for intracranial tumors, the normal brain tissue having been compromised by the presence of neoplasm. Burger et al[41] report necrosis of normal tissue in four of 17 patients who received between 5000-6000 rads. Marsa et al[40] reported the results of irradiation of 256 patients with various tumors of central nervous system, in whom clinical necrosis was diagnosed on eight occasions. At 66 autopsies performed, pathologic evidence of necrosis was seen ten times, but this had been clinically apparent in only two of the ten cases. Thus pathologic studies clearly overestimate the incidence of necrosis as a clinically significant entity.

The location of the primary tumor for which treatment is given can vary. They are listed in Table I as reported by two large reviews. No predisposing site would seem to exist. However, a difference between the irradiation of extracranial and intracranial damage lies in the fact that, in the former case, the underlying brain is presumably normal and better able to withstand a course of irradiation.

The clinical syndrome has been well described. The patient may present from three months to 12 years after radiotherapy, although most will present at one to three years. Signs and symptoms are those of intracranial space-occupying mass. Rottenberg et al[37] reviewed the clinical and laboratory presentation of 25 patients with necrosis due to irradiation of extracranial lesions (six of their own and 19 from review of the literature) and summarized the findings (Table II). There is rarely a means of distinguishing necrosis from tumor recurrence or other entities such as abscess. Specifically, the presence of increased intracranial pressure does not mean that tumor recurrence is present, since it is clearly common as well, in the case of necrosis.

Laboratory findings can include elevated CSF pressure and/or protein. The electroencephalogram will usually show focal slowing lateralized to the affected side.

Table I
Location of Tumors for Which Radiotherapy Was Given in Patients Who Developed Brain Necrosis

Reference	Extra-cranial	Pituitary or Parasellar	Other Intra-cranial	Total
Sheline[6]	32	22	29	83
Kramer[2]	19	31	7	57

Table II
Clinical and Laboratory Findings in 29 Patients with Cerebral Radiation Necrosis

Manifestation	Number
Seizures	12
Headache	12
Personality change	10
Focal motor weakness	18
Papilledema	9
Dysphasia	6
Impaired consciousness	5
Lumbar puncture	
Pressure 160 mm CSF	4/10*
Protein 50 mg/dl	7/10
Brain scan — focal uptake	7/8
EEG — focal slowing	13/15
Angiography — avascular mass	15/16

* Denomintor is the number of patients in whom data is available.
From Rottenberg DA, et al: Cerebral necrosis following radiotherapy of extracranial neoplasm *Ann Neurol* 1:339-357, 1977, with permission.

Radiographic findings are consistent, but not specific. Plain films of the skull are generally not contributory. Although lytic or sclerotic changes may be seen, they cannot be distinguished from changes due to tumor invasion, infection, or post-surgical demineralization. Brain scan is usually positive, but the peripheral location of the focal activity often requires a complementary bone scan to rule out a calvarial lesion. Angiography reveals an avascular mass without diagnostic characteristics.

Wilson et al[39] reviewed the pneumo-encephalographic films of 40 patients who had received irradiation to the brain and found atrophy in 17.

The advent of computerized axial tomography, however, has largely rendered such invasive procedures as pneumo-encephalography obsolete in the diagnosis of radiation necrosis. The CAT scan is usually positive in cases of necrosis. Mikhael[25] reported four cases of histologically confirmed necrosis, and all had similar findings. Before contrast medium injection, there was a mass lesion with low density, and after contrast medium injection there was enhancement. The enhancement was irregular in distribution, sometimes peripheral and sometimes central, and the CAT criteria alone were not sufficient to distinguish necrosis from tumor recurrence. However, the areas of necrosis on CAT scan could be correlated with the areas of maximal radiation dose when dosimetry was reconstructed; necrosis was seen in brain volumes that had received 6000 rads or more. The association of these radiographic findings with an area of high dose should serve to raise the physician's level of suspicion that necrosis is, in fact, present. Brismar et al[51] described similar findings and emphasized the usefulness of CAT scan in ruling out entities such as hemorrhage or shunt dysfunction.

Carella et al[52] recommend routine CAT scan before and after the irradiation of intracerebral tumor, feeling that correlation of multiple studies offers the best guide.

The management of cerebral radionecrosis is sometimes surgical, and resection of the necrotic mass can be life-saving. At surgery, the necrotic area often resembles a glioma,[22,32,35] so that the diagnostic dilemma often persists even at this late stage of intervention. Multiple authors[22,24,25,27,28] report excellent results with such therapy. The role of corticosteroids in management is unclear. While in many situations, the use of steroids is not mentioned, in others it is important to the outcome. The patients of Littman et al[36] required postoperative steroids for three months before they could be tapered without clinical deterioration, and that of Eyster et al[33] required steroids apparently indefinitely. The patient of Querroz and Neto[35] required progressively larger doses of steroids postoperatively to prevent clinical decline, and he eventually died of a gastrointestinal hemorrhage. Thus, while some patients can do well after only surgery, there is clearly a population in whom steroids are essential, presumably as a means of reducing cerebral edema.

The pathology of cerebral radionecrosis has also been well reviewed.[53-55] Early delayed effects, as described above, consist of multiple punched-out areas of demyelination that resemble multiple sclerosis. In cases of late delayed necrosis, the involved area grossly appears as an ill-defined, firm, space-occupying mass that resembles a glioma on inspection and palpation. The white matter is the area of primary damage, although the border between white and gray matter is obscured. The affinity for white matter is, however, a characteristic feature of the injury.

Microscopically, multiple pictures may be seen. One may see areas in which demyelination is the most prominent feature with loss of oligodendroglial cells and myelin sheaths. This is accompanied by a marked macrophagic reaction and perivascular infiltration of inflammatory cells.

The most striking and often emphasized findings are the vascular changes. Rubinstein[53] emphasizes the varying chronicity of the alterations. The "most characteristic and virtually diagnostic" change is fibrinoid necrosis of the blood vessel wall, which is accompanied by extravasated fibrinoid material and recent parenchymatous hemorrhages. In vessels where the changes are older, proliferation is seen of the vascular endothelium and periadventitial fibroblasts. More chronic lesions include hyaline thickening of the vessel walls with occlusion and focal calcifications. Other changes that are described include amyloid deposition,[56,57] telangiectasia, and changes in the neuroglia. The last consist of hypertrophy of the astrocytes, whose nucleii show irregularity and hyperchromatism, and formation of multinucleated giant cells.

Although the appearance of radiation necrosis is generally agreed upon, the mechanism of the injury is a matter of debate. Various observers consider the pathogenesis to be primarily: (1) injury to the neural elements,[58] (2) injury to the vasculature,[22,59] or (3) immunological.[43] In the first case, vascular changes are considered secondary to parenchymal damage. According to the second hypothesis, the primary injury is to the vascular endothelium, and vascular alterations lead to parenchymal necrosis. However, neither of these is satisfactory in explaining the delay in the onset of the necrosis or the variable age of the lesions. For this reason the third hypothesis is advanced. Crompton and Layton[43] emphasize the profuse fibrinous exudate, the presence of fibrin or fibrinoid change in the vessel wall, and the large number of eosinophilic leucocytes they observed in one case, and propose an allergic mechanism. The antigen they propose might be either an altered protein of the cells themselves or a new protein produced as a result of radiation-induced mutation. Berge, et al[60] and Hopewell and Wright[61] feel that the vascular etiology is most important at lower dose levels while primary neuronal damage is apparent in the higher dose range. Although agreement is by no means universal, interference with the blood supply is considered most likely to be the dominant mechanism of radiation necrosis when the usual clinical volume is irradiated.[2]

Having described the syndrome, recommendations are in order as to what dose represents a reasonable risk to the nervous system. It must be kept in mind that, as is usually the case in radiation therapy, one is balancing the risk of damage to the normal tissues with the need to control a potentially lethal disease. Furthermore, there is no absolute threshold for radiation necrosis, but rather a risk that increases with dose. Thus no absolute guidelines are possible. Clinical judgment is needed to expose the patient to a risk that is in keeping with his illness.

Experimental studies are not of much value, because of the use of doses that are not relevant to the clinical situation. Caveness[62,63] irradiated monkeys to 4000, 6000, and 8000 rads in four, six, and eight weeks respectively, using two hundred rad fractions five times weekly. The group reported minimal damage at 4000 rads and severe changes at 8000 rads. At 6000 rads, which is within the clinical range, multiple small necrotic lesions were seen at six months, most of which had calcified by 12 months and been replaced by widespread areas of capillary dilatation and telangiectasia.

Boden[21] calculated the tolerance of the normal brain at 4500 R in 17 days for small fields and 3500 R in 17 days for large fields (greater than 100 cm^2), using orthovoltage X-rays. Using standard fractionation, Verity[4] and Fletcher and Million[29] gave 5000 rads in five weeks (NSD = 1570 rets) as a safe dose. Indeed, this dose is used widely clinically[64,65] without untoward effects. Lindgren[42] carefully analyzed his data and drew curves to describe the risk of necrosis at various treatment doses and times. He calculates 4500-5000 rads over five weeks to be the lowest dose level at which necrosis can be expected to be found. Rottenberg, et al[37] feel tolerance is greater and that absorbed doses below 1700 rets are well tolerated by the normal brain. Kramer[2] states that the normal brain will ordinarily tolerate 6500-7000 rads in 6½ to 8 weeks, using five daily fractions per week and supervoltage equipment. Sheline[6] has carefully calculated the dose characteristics of 83 patients who developed brain necrosis and for whom precise information is available (see Table III). Forty-five of the 83 cases occurred in patients who received over 6000 rads. Only eight cases are reported below 4500 rads, and of these, in only

Table III
Summary of Radiation Doses Associated with Brain Necrosis

Dose to Lesion (R or rads)	Lesion Treated*				
	Skin	Extra-cranial Nonskin	Pituitary Region	Intracranial Non-pituitary	Total
2,000- 2,500	3 (1,1,3)	0	0	0	3
2,501- 3,500	2 (1,1)	0	0	1†(10)	3
3,501- 4,499	0	0	1(13)	1(20)	2
4,500- 5,000	2 (10,22)	3(13,15,15)	9(15-25)	0	14
5,001- 6,000	2	6	2	4 + 2†	16
6,001- 7,000	3	6	9	6 + 2†	26
7,001- 8,000	1	1	1	7	10
8,001- 9,000	0	2	0	5	7
9,001-11,000	0	0	0	1	1
18,000	1	0	0	0	1
Total	14	18	22	24 + 5†	83

* Parentheses indicate number of fractions.
† Radiation therapy plus multicycle/multidrug chemotherapy.
From Sheline GE: Irradiation injury of the human brain: a review of clinical experience. In: Gilbert HA, Kagen AR, eds: Radiation Damage to the Nervous System. New York, Raven Press, 1980, with permission.

one case was the individual dose kept at below 225 rads. Even in the 4500-5000 rad dose range, eight of the 14 patients received individual fractions of greater than 250 rads.

Most authorities would agree that 5000 rads in five weeks is a safe dose for treatment of the brain. Higher doses, however, are routinely used when tumor control warrants it. It is not at all uncommon to treat patients to 6000 to 7000 rads for control of craniopharyngioma or glioma.[3]

Fraction size is an important variable. If significant patient longevity is anticipated, it is well worth the inconvenience of more treatment sessions of smaller individual doses to avoid late sequelae. On the other hand, high doses and even retreatment of previously irradiated areas can provide significant palliation in cases where that is the goal,[66,67] and this can be done with acceptable (although significant) sequelae.

Other Effects

Investigators in the Soviet Union report physiological alterations at low doses on the order of one rad. However, no consistent alterations in behavior or physiology below a dose of several hundred rads can be demonstrated.[68]

Samaan et al[69] reported on 15 patients, aged 15 to 79 years, irradiated for carcinoma of the nasopharynx and disease-free at least five years later. Of these, 14 had evidence of endocrine deficiency. Twelve patients had evidence of hypothalmic dysfunction, seven developed primary pituitary hormone deficiencies, and three developed primary hypothryoidism. This suggests that pituitary and/or hypothalmic injury may be a not uncommon sequela of high-dose irradiation to these areas.

Spinal Cord

Radiation myelitis is among the most devastating of complications of radiotherapy, since the patient will usually have been cured of the malignancy (most recurrences would have occurred during the latency period), but is left in such condition that it is debatable whether any benefit has been achieved. As in the case of the brain, acute and chronic spinal cord syndromes occur. The syndromes have been classified by Reagan et al[70] (Table IV).

| Table IV |
| Classification of Radiation Myelopathies |

1. Acute, transient
2. Lower motor neuron syndrome
3. Acute, progressive myelopathy
4. Chronic, progressive myelopathy

From Reagan TJ, Thomas JE, Colby MY, Jr: Chronic progressive radiation myelopathy. *JAMA* **203**:128-132, 1968, with permission.

Acute Transient Myelopathy

Acute transient myelopathy was described by Boden[71] in four of the ten patients in his series. Dynes and Smedal[72] stated that patients receiving a dose of 4800 rads in 5½ weeks "not uncommonly" experienced these symptoms. Jones'[73] classic article describes the cases of seven patients who received external irradiation for upper respiratory tract neoplasms and whose treatments to potential lymph node metastases-bearing areas required inclusion of the cervical spine. Typically, within a few weeks of radiation, the patient complains of numbness or paresthesias radiating from the neck to the spine and legs. Characteristically, neck flexion precipitates a feeling of an electric shock (Lhermitte's sign), at various levels below the neck, usually confined to the lumbosacral segments. No objective neurological signs can be elicited, and the patients do not complain of motor deficits or impairment of sphincter control. Although the symptoms usually resolve over a period of three to five months, the significance of the syndrome is in dispute. Those patients in Jones' and Dynes and Smedal's series all had complete return to normal sensation without sequelae, and some reviewers[74] do not feel that it is related to subsequent neurologic difficulty. In several reports[71,75,76] on the other hand, electrical paresthesias were the first manifestation of a course that progressed to chronicity with severe disability and death. Clearly Lhermitte's sign per se is a benign entity, but patients who have electrical paresthesias after radiation must be followed closely, since the sign does not indicate the upper level of dose to which the cord was exposed, and late signs may appear.

The pathogenesis of the symptoms described by Lhermitte was suspected by him after observing them in cases of trauma and disseminated sclerosis. He reasoned that recent demyelination would render these fibers sensitive to stimuli, such as neck flexion. Since tissue samples are not available in such irradiated patients, one must turn to experimental data. Mastaglia et al[77] sacrificed rabbits shortly after single radiation doses to the spinal cord. They describe changes occurring as early as two weeks after exposure to between 500 and 6000 rads. Findings included breakdown of paranodal myelin and nodal widening, which increased in frequency with dose and time in the first two months after irradiation. After three months, increasing numbers of thinly myelinated fibers were seen, suggesting that the paranodal demyelination was followed by remyelination. This time course corresponds nicely to the time course of acute transient radiation myelopathy and lends credence to the concept of demyelination as its etiology.

Lower Motor Neuron Syndrome

The lower motor neuron syndrome is a rare entity first reported by Greenfield and Stark[78] and rarely since then.[79,81] The cases are summarized in Table V. Also, many of the patients in the series published by Maier et al[82] probably belong to this group.

After a latency period of 3 to 26 months, patients note muscular weakness of the lower extremities. The process progresses to muscle atrophy, weakness, depressed deep reflexes, and fasciculation. The findings are usually symmetrical, although two cases of unilateral leg involvement are reported.[80] Only one case of sphincter involvement was reported by Greenfield and Stark,[78] although their remaining two patients also had bladder atony cystometrically. Objective sensory findings are absent. Myelography does not show any abnormalities, and laboratory study are within normal limits, except for the occasional finding of mildly elevated protein level in the cerebrospinal fluid. The symptoms usually stabilize after a period of advancement, and it is important to note that the prognosis with this syndrome is better than with the other chronic radiation myelopathies.

The pathogenisis presumably involves damage to the anterior horn cells, resulting in the motor findings and absence of sensory ones. Many of the patients with this syndrome (8 of 11) were irradiated for testicular tumors, involving only exposure to the lumbar spine, accounting for the level of the injury. The other three, however, were presumably irradiated to the entire spinal cord, and the development of this unusual deficit is harder to explain in these cases.

Finally, in spite of the rarity of this syndrome, the incidence was three cases out of 180 treated (1.7%) in the experience of Greenfield and Stark.[78] In view of the large number of patients receiving irradiation to the lumbar spine, the symptoms may be more frequent than is realized. And as extended field radiation of the para-aortic lymph node chain is attempted more often in the treatment of gynecologic and gastrointestinal malignancies, one can expect to see this complication more frequently.

Table V
Lower Motor Neuron Syndrome

Reference	Age at Diagnosis of Tumor	Radiotherapy (rads/days)	Latency Period months	Course
Greenfield[78]	24	6480/44	7½	alive with stable deficit
	20	5400/90	5	alive with stable deficit
	28	5488/84	4	alive with stable deficit
Sadowsky[79]	15	4763/31	11	alive with stable deficit
Schiødt[80]	31	1670 CRE	23	alive with stable deficit
	35	1670 CRE	26	alive with stable deficit
	33	1670 CRE	12	alive with stable deficit
	24	1670 CRE	10	gradual improvement
	25	1608 CRE	14	gradual worsening
Hildebrand[81]	45	6200/3 courses over 4½ years	23	alive
	27	4000/29	3½	alive

Acute Progressive Myelopathy

Acute progressive myelopathy is another rare manifestation of radiation-induced spinal cord damage. It is characterized by acutely developing paraplegia or quadriplegia in which progression from the asymptomatic state to full-blown manifestation of the syndrome occurs within days. Phillips and Buschke[83] have described two patients in whom complete paraplegia developed after a sudden beginning, evolving to the final state within two weeks.

The presumed mechanism is arterial occlusion which occurs suddenly and produces dramatic events. DeChiro and Herdt[84] described one patient with radiation-induced myelomalacia in whom angiography demonstrated occlusion of the radiculomedullary and anterior spinal arteries which had not been present before treatment.

Chronic Progressive Myelopathy

Chronic progressive myelopathy is the most common form of serious complication of spinal cord irradiation. This often devastating occurrence has been described on numerous occasions.[4,23,65-67,70-72,75,77,78,80-98] The reported cases are listed in Tables VI-VIII.

Symptoms can occur from four months to 13 years after treatment, but onset is usually within a year. Sensory symptoms predominate early in the course, consisting of numbness, paresthesias (often burning), and diminished sensitivity to pain and temperature. Occasionally,[86] motor weakness predominates. Findings are mainly in the lower extremities, although pain and/or burning in the irradiated segments of the neck are not uncommon complaints. Weakness and spasticity then appear. Sensory findings ascend in level and, if initially unilateral, spread to the other side. Eventually the clinical situation will often evolve to a high sensory level with long tract involvement of sensory and motor pathways. Sphincter impairment is common and is considered an ominous prognostic sign.[85] A partial Brown-Séquard syndrome may develop with motor weakness and pyramidal signs in one lower extremity and change in sensory perception, especially of pain and temperature, in the other. As often as not, this is a transient state, and the patient will eventually develop paraplegia or quadriplegia, depending upon the level of the injury. Hemiparesis also may be seen.[23,72]

Pallis et al[85] established criteria for the diagnosis of radiation-induced myelitis: (1) that the spinal cord be included within the irradiated field; (2) that the main neurological damage be within the segments exposed; and (3) that myelography exclude metastases. Laboratory data is usually unrevealing. The cerebrospinal fluid may have a slightly elevated protein content. Myelography usually shows the spinal cord to be normal or occasionally reduced in volume.[70] Notable exceptions occur. Lechevalier, et al[93] reported five cases in all of whom the cord was enlarged even to the point of producing a block in one case. Although this situation is unusual, both swelling[75] and block[91] have been observed by others.

The clinical course is unpredictable. Most authors describe a period of progression over several months, followed by stabilization, although considerable individual variability exists. Once established, deficits are not considered apt to regress, and the long-term outlook is grim, as indicated by the high percentage of mortality seen in the pertinent

Table VI
Cervical Myelopathy

Reference	Material	Dose Description dose/fx/days	1^0	Latency (months)	Course
Boden[71]	6	1) 2000/1/1	pharynx	11	died
		2) 2222/1/1	pharynx	4	died
		3) 5200/?/17	pharynx	10	died
		4) 3936/?/17	lymphosarcoma	12	Brown-Sequard
		5) 4210/?/17	Hodgkin's disease	15	died
		6) 4320/?/17	Hodgkin's disease	11	died
Malamud[23]	1	5000/?/20	nasopharynx	12	died
Dynes[72]	3	1) 4500/?/51	nasopharynx	7	spasticity
		2) 6000/?/68	pharynx	24	died
		3) 6000/?/52	parotid	25	died
Pallis[85]	3	1) 8700/?/35	pharynx	15	slow progression
		2) 4000/?/42	pharynx	18	died
		3) 3680/?/39 & 1700/?/27	thyroid	8	paraplegia
Kristensson[87]	5	1) 5100/?/27	all-hypo-	40	paraparesis
		2) 5100/?/26	pharynx	7	quadriparesis
		3) 5100/?/44		13	hemiparesis
		4) 4000/?/31 (at least)		20	quadriparesis
		5) 4500/?/29		15	paraparesis
Reagan[70]	8	1) 4000/?/10	esophagus	5	died
		2) 5100/?/4 years	Hodgkin's disease	10	died
		3) 5400/?/51	nasopharynx	30	Brown-Sequard
		4) 5450/?/56	tongue-base	26	died
		5) 6000/?/56	nasal cavity	15	died
		6) 6000/?/31	esophagus	12	died
		7) 6400/?/47	ear	16	died
		8) 6900/?/43	pharynx	9	unknown
Black[97]	2	1) 6000/?/?		9	died
		2) 2000 and 4000/?/3 split course	phrynx	12	died
Solheim[90]	5	1) 4700/?/19 3200 after 7 months	1) hypopharynx	1) 19	1-4) considerable improvement
		2) 5000/?/13	2) thyroid	2) 15	1) 9 years
		3) 4800/?/28	3) nasopharynx	3) 5	2) 6 years

Table VI cont.

Reference	Material	Dose Description dose/fx/days	1⁰	Latency (months)	Course
		4) 5000/?/22		4) 6	3) 4 years
		5) less than 12,500/?/12 months	5) Hodgkin's disease	5) 11	4) 7 years 5) no improvement over 3 years
Palmer[91]	3	1) 4170/16/29 2) 5510/44/59 3) 3040/8/10	1) tonsil 2) nasopharynx 3) lympho-sarcoma	1) 19 2) 48 3) 17	1) died 2) died 3) died
Yaar[92]	2	1) 9700 over 2 years (2 courses) 2) 9000/3 months (2 courses)	1) Cylindroma 2) Nasopharynx	1) 31 2) 12 months	1) alive and progressing 2) alive with quadri-paresis
Lechevalier[93]	5	1) 5400/18/38 2) 5940/18/44 3) 7000/14/42 4) 2700/9/18 2700/9/18 4&5) split course 97 days overall 5) 5400/18/38	1) base of tongue 2) tongue 3) reticulum cell sarcoma 4) pyriform sinus 5) vallecula		
Baekmark[94]	8		Hodgkin's disease		
Godwin-Austen[75]	2	1) 6000/?/5 weeks 2) 5250/?/21	1) fibrosarcoma 2) tonsil	1) 5 2) 8	1) died 2) died
Wara[95]	3	1) 3750/23/27 2) 4860/27/38 3) 5000/25/42			
Abbatucci[96]	12	1) 5400/18/42 (5) 2) 5400/18/44 3) 5400/18/46 4) 5400/18/48 5) 5110/18/42 6) 5940/18/46 7) 6000/18/44 8) 10,000/3 courses			

Table VII
Thoracic Myelopathy

Reference	Material	Dose Description dose/fx/days	1°	Latency (Months)	Course
Dynes[72]	7	1) 2500/?/18 (overlap?)	lymphoma	11	paraplegia
		2) 6000/?/51	metastases	24	paraplegia
		3) 6000/?/57	nasopharynx	13	spasticity
		4) 1000/?/15 ⎫95 5000/?/36 ⎭	lung	50	paraplegia
		5) 2000/?/? ⎫app. 120 6000/?/49 ⎭	lung	33	died
		6) 6000/?/54	lung	24	died
		7) 6000/?/49	lung	20	died
Pallis[85]	2	1) 7000/?/32	pharynx	7	died
		2) 4410/?/28	lung	7	slow progression
Locksmith[88]	6	1) 3870/15/21	all lung	21	died
		2) 3890/15/18		16	Brown-Sequard
		3) 4850/19/27		35	died
		4) 3950/16/21		14	Brown-Sequard
		5) 4070/16/21		12	Brown-Sequard
		6) 4370/13/23		12	paraplegia
Reagan[70]	2	1) 4730/?/40	breast	5½	paraparesis
		2) 6000/?/30	lung	9	died
Coy[89]	3	1) 4200/8/29	mediastinal	12	died
		2) 4200/8/25	lung	11	paraplegia
		3) 4200/8/23	lung	9	died

Palmer[91]	4	1) 4090/8/51	lymphoma	13	died
		2) 4250/14/30	lung	12	died
		3) 3740/10/26	esophagus	6	died
		4) 3530/30/41 } overlap 1700/14/18 }	testicle	17	died
Yaar[92]	2	1) 4300/?/?	breast	48	progressive

		2) 4800/24/42 int. mammary
		   3300/11/ } 6 months to
		   2000/10/ } supraclavicular
			breast	12	improved

Goodwin-Austen[75]	1	1) 5500/15/19	esophagus	5	
Wara[95]	6	1) 3300/6/23			
		2) 4350/6/24			
		3) 7000/26/61			
		4) 6700/37/55			
		5) 6700/37/59			
		6) 6753/36/55			
Dische[98]	9	1) 4977/20/29	all lung	7	All died
		2) 3452/6/18		34	in 13 to
		3) 3373/6/18		18	44 months
		4) 3375/6/18		25	
		5) 3526/6/20		22	
		6) 3427/6/22		10	
		7) 3453/6/18		9	
		8) 3450/6/22		14	
		9) 3426/6/22		8	

Table VIII
Myelopathy - Other

Reference	Material	Dose Description dose/fx/days		1^0	Latency (months)	Course
Atkins[86]	14	1) 1900/2/7		breast	10	died
		2) 1900/2/7		breast	29	paraplegia
		3) 1900/2/7		breast	19	paraplegia
		4) 1900/2/7		breast	15	paraplegia
		5) 3480/10/21		breast	9	paraplegia
		6) 3800/12/26		breast	21	paresthesias
		7) 4000/12/25		breast	12	died
		8) 5200/26/32		trachea	7	paraplegia
		9) 830-2850/3/14		esophagus	29	died
		10) 2370/2/7		lung	10	died
		11) 2370/2/7		base of tongue	9½	died
		12) 2960/3/14		lung	15	died
		13) 4550/15/35		lung	6	mild changes
		14) 2040/10/13 1520/2/7		Hodgkin's disease	8	paraplegia
Maier[82]	15	1) 4653/?/72		all	64	paralysis
		2) 3810/?/29		testicle	27	paralysis
		3) 4810/?/72			15	paralysis
		4) 4150/?/32			7	paresis
		5) 4701/?/68			156	paresis
		6) 4558/?/50			12	died
		7) 3719/?/79			12	palsy
		8) 5060/?/83			13	paraplegia
		9) 4420/?/64			12	died
		10) 3690/?/24			12	foot drop
		11) 4800/?/85			6	died
		12) 5680/?/56			12	died
		13) 3710/?/28			9	leg weakness
		14) 5310/?/39			4	died
		15) 5400/?/87			12	leg weakness

tables. Two authors, however, have reported a total of five cases with symptomatic improvement. Yaar et al[92] presented one patient with carcinoma of the breast, and Solheim[90] reported on four patients with head and neck tumors whose myelopathy improved with time. In the latter report, however, only two patients underwent myelography, and in one case it showed severe arachnoiditis. Thus some doubt is cast upon the accuracy of the diagnosis of myelitis in the first place. Certainly, resolution of symptoms once established is the exception. Godwin-Austen et al[75] reported on two patients who had significant improvement in their symptoms upon administration of corticosteroids with deterioration upon their withdrawal. These patients are among that group that also had swollen spinal cords, and the diminution in edema presumably accounts for the therapeutic benefits of steroids in their particular situation.

The pathologic changes that occur involve both vascular and parenchymal elements, and some debate regarding the relative importance of each exists, as in the case of brain necrosis. The white matter clearly is more affected than the gray, and some report this effect to be the major one.[83] Demyelination is reported to involve, in decreasing order of severity, the lateral, posterior, and anterior columns.[23] Most observers favor a vascular etiology.[87,91] Morphologically, changes include acute and chronic vasculitis with thickening and hyalinization of small blood vessels, fibrinoid necrosis of blood vessels with extravasation of the fibrinoid material into the perivascular spaces, and telangiectasia. Palmer[91] emphasized that the hemorrhagic necrosis of the dorsolateral white matter that he observed was always associated with extensive vascular damage. However, he did see patchy demyelination independent of the vascular changes, as well as Wallerian degeneration above and below the irradiated segments.

The incidence of myelopathy is difficult to estimate with confidence. Most reports are of the complication without mention of the total population in which it occurred. Even where the total patient population is known in numbers, the risk of myelitis could only be measured if one could match patients for treatment characteristics, rather than merely the primary site of the treated tumor. It is interesting to speculate, however, whether the radiation effects are more common than reported. Palmer[91] reported 12 cases, only seven of which had been diagnosed clinically before autopsy. These additional cases may have become manifest had the patients survived.

Important factors in determining the risk of damage include the total dose, the fractionation (dose per treatment and overall treatment time), and the size of the field irradiated. Recommended dose levels in the literature are listed in Table IX. As can be seen, the recommended dose level varies almost by a factor of two. There are certain situations in which myelitis is obviously more apt to occur. These include repeated courses of treatment to the same area, overlap at the junction of two treatment portals, and dose miscalculation. These injuries can be prevented by proper awareness of the risk of treatment and the institution of precautions that make sense in the particular set of circumstances. Excluding such cases, the remainder of reported cases was reviewed. These cases were excerpted where the total dose per fraction and overall time are given, and the area of injury is clear. These were divided into cervical and thoracic cord for two reasons. First, there is a feeling that the thoracic cord is more susceptible to myelitis due to its

Table IX
Recommended Safe Levels of Spinal Cord Irradiation

Author and Reference	Recommendation Limit
Boden[71]	3500 rads/17 days (large fields) 4500 rads/17 days (small fields)
Pallis[85]	3300 rads/42 days (large fields) 4300 rads/42 days (small fields)
Abbatucci[96]	4500 rads/5 weeks (large fields) 5000 rads/5 weeks (small fields)
Palmer[91]	as per Pallis
Wara[95]	5000 rads/5 weeks
Coy[89]	3750 rads/4 weeks
Phillips[83]	1300 rads/2 fractions 3000 rads/10 fractions 5000 rads/25 fractions 6000 rads/35 fractions
Atkins[86]	4750 rads/25 fractions/35 days
Maier[82]	4000 rads/20 fractions/28 days
Verity[4]	6000-6500 rads/"suitably protracted and fractionated"
Fletcher[29]	5000 rads/ 5 weeks
Kramer[2]	5000 rads/5-6 weeks (cervical cord) 4500 rads/ 4½ weeks (thoracic cord)

more tenous vascular supply. Dynes and Smedal[72] and Coy et al[89] emphasize this, the latter noting that lesions tend to occur in the "watershed area," between the supply of the neck vessels to the upper thoracic segments and of the dorsal radicular vessels to lower segments. Secondly, the length of cord irradiated is usually greater in the thoracic area. The primary tumor is usually lung, esophagus, or breast in these cases, where long segments of spinal tissue are exposed. The cervical cord, on the other hand, is usually exposed during the irradiation of head and neck tumors where fields are smaller and more precisely shaped and where limited lengths of the cord receive a substantial dose. The importance of consideration of the irradiated volume was acknowledged by Boden[71] and Pallis et al[85] in their guidelines and mentioned as important by Abbatucci et al.[96] In all, 60 cases were studied to establish the relationship between myelitis on the one hand and NSD and dose per fraction on the other.

(1) *NSD* — As can be seen, no cases are listed below 1200 rets (Tables X and XI). However, Maier et al[82] have two cases below this level (1069 and 1197), but the dose per fraction and level of injury (thoracic or lumbar) are not clear. Only five cases are listed below 1400 rets. Four of these are from the series of Atkins and Tretter[86] who received unusually large single doses (950 rads per treatment, twice, one week apart). The fifth patient, reported by Wara et al[95] received a low dose at a slow rate and must be considered the victim of an idiosyncratic reaction. Phillips and Buschke[83] accept 1500 rets as a safe dose, while Abbatucci et al[96] allow 1570 rets to limited fields.

Table X

Cervical Myelopathy Dose (in Rets)	Correlation with NSD Number of Cases
< 1200	0
1201-1300	1
1301-1400	0
1401-1500	4
1501-1600	1
1601-1700	1
1701-1800	8
1801-1900	3
1901-2000	2
> 2000	3
	23

Table XI
Correlation of Thoracic Myelopathy with NSD

Thoracic Myelopathy Dose (in Rets)	Correlation with NSD Number of Cases
< 1200	0
1201-1300	4
1301-1400	0
1401-1500	6
1501-1600	9
1601-1700	9
1701-1800	4
1801-1900	3
1901-2000	1
> 2000	2
	38

(2) Dose per fraction – Many of the reported patients were treated with atypical schedules delivering large individual doses. These are listed in Tables XII and XIII. Only eight of the 61 cases occurred in patients receiving less than 250 rads per fraction. This information is of great importance, since the typical course of radiotherapy involves 175-200 rads daily fractions given five times weekly. One is often tempted to accelerate the course to avoid undue inconvenience to a patient with a limited life expectancy, and in such cases, rapid treatment is certainly indicated. However, the risk of myelitis must be always in mind in the case of patients who are likely to survive the latency period. Short-term convenience may demand a grievous price at a later date.

Table XII

Cervical Myelopathy Dose (Rads per day)	Correlation with Dose per Fraction Number of Cases
< 175	2
175-200	2
201-250	0
251-300	12
301-400	4
401-500	1
> 500	2
	23

Table XIII
Correlation of Thoracic Myelopathy with Daily Fraction Size

Thoracic Myelopathy Dose (Rads per Fraction)	Correlation with Dose per Fraction Number of Cases
175-200	3
201-250	1
251-300	6
301-400	8
401-500	0
501-600	13
601-700	0
701-800	1
801-900	0
901-1000	5
1001-1100	0
1101-1200	1
	38

The NSD concept, as discussed above, was introduced to equate various fractionation schedules using a single biological end point, namely the tolerance of normal connective tissue. It is probable that this measurement is not well suited for consideration of damage to the central nervous system. In Figures 2 and 3, the NSD is plotted against dose per fraction for the cervical and thoracic cords. No pattern is discernible for the cervical cord, in part due to the clustering of cases in the 300-330 rad dose range and the paucity of data elsewhere. The data for the thoracic cord would seem to indicate, however, that the NSD is not a stable indicator since it rises with decreasing fraction size. Thus all four cases observed at less than 1400 rets received large single fractions. With doses of less than 200 rads per fraction, however, myelitis is not seen until almost 1800 rets. To account for the apparent importance of fraction size in causation of myelitis, some authors[9-12,95] have recommended variations in the Ellis equation to increase the emphasis of fraction size and which produce a value of greater clinical applicability.

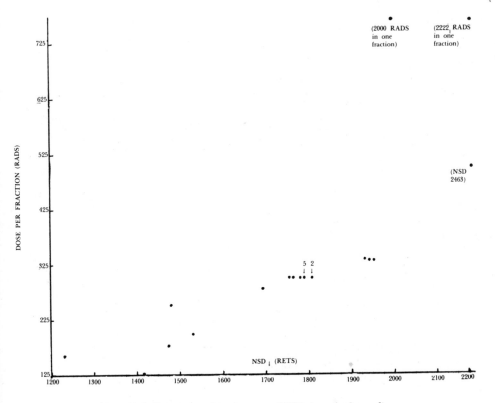

Figure 2. Dose per fraction vs. NSD (cervical cord).

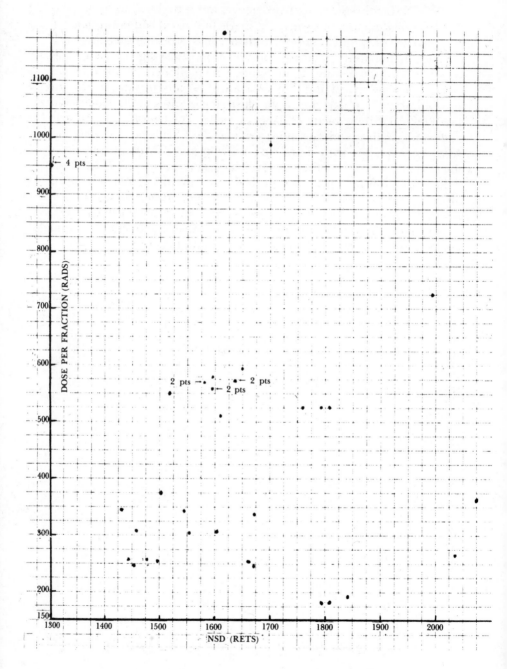

Figure 3. Dose per fraction vs. NSD (thoracic cord).

Finally, there are two other factors which may be considerations in preventing myelitis in individual cases. Abbatucci et al[96] emphasize the role of homogeneity of the dose across the entire cord in causing injury. They point out that if only part of the cord is irradiated to a peak dose, tolerance will increase. Such precise beam localization may be of value in head and neck cases where such precision is not uncommonly indicated. Secondly, Locksmith and Powers[88] noted severe dysphagia in three of their six patients who developed myelitis, and in two cases it was severe enough to require esophageal dilation. While moderate dysphagia is the rule in treating carcinoma of the lung (which these patients had), such severe symptoms are most uncommon. Since the authors ruled out dose error, these patients may have had individual sensitivity to radiation which was first manifest in the esophagus and later in the spinal cord. They all received over 1400 rets (and two received over 1600), so that the complication cannot be totally unexpected. Nevertheless, unusually severe acute reactions during therapy do warrant close attention and consideration that this patient may be prone to long-term sequelae.

Modifying Factors

The production of central nervous system necrosis is the result of a complicated interaction of host and treatment related factors. Modification of any of these can be as important in affecting the risk of sequelae as can adjustment of more obvious elements, such as dose. Possible variables that affect the results of a course of radiotherapy will be discussed so that they may be included in estimation of treatment risk.

High LET Radiation – Oxygen is a powerful radiosensitizer, probably acting by "fixing" a radiation effect that might otherwise be reversible. It has been known for over a quarter of a century that tumors of a diameter above 200 micra will have a hypoxic component to their viable population. Hypoxic cells are 2.5–3 times more resistant to ionizing radiation in the X- and gamma ray range, and these cells serve as a nucleus of subsequent recurrence. For that reason, much effort has been made to develop methods to overcome this problem. In the forefront is the so-called high LET (linear energy transfer) radiation. These are particles (rather than electromagnetic radiation like X-rays) whose deposition of energy in tissue occurs in a more dense pattern. This density apparently reduces the radioresistance of the hypoxic cells and brings them more into line with well-oxygenated cells. Glioblastoma multiforme is a common area of inquiry into the efficacy of these therapies, because necrosis (and by extension, hypoxia) is a common pathologic finding and because current standard therapy of this tumor is singularly ineffective. However, the tolerance of normal tissue to such radiation is not yet well understood. Thus it is anticipated that, as such therapies are brought into more widespread use, the chances will increase that the practicing neurologist will encounter patients thus treated.

The particle used most commonly is the fast neutron.[99-101] To date, no survival advantage is observed for the neutrons over X-rays, but at autopsy, considerably greater antitumor effect is seen with neutrons as compared to what is usually observed after X-ray therapy. Thus, Catterall, et al[101] found minimal or no tumor in 11 of 16 patients in whom tissue was obtained after neutron beam therapy. Unfortunately, diffuse damage to the normal brain is also seen, which correlates with a syndrome of progressive dementia and obtundation without localizing signs. In two series[100,101] patients were irradiated two or three times weekly with a neutron beam with penetrating characteristics comparable to Cobalt[60] to between about 800 and 1800 rads, and subsequent examination revealed more damage to both normal and tumor tissues than was expected. Ornitz et al[102] observed two cases of chronic progressive cervical myelitis at a dose of 1543 rads/28 fractions/7 weeks, which he felt corresponded to an equivalent cord dose of 4821 rads/24 fractions/34 days with X-rays, certainly not an excessive dose. They also saw two cases of brain necrosis at higher equivalent doses (6371 rads/32 fractions/45 days and 5471 rad/27 fractions/38 days) and two cases of Lhermitte's syndrome. They emphasize the uncertainty of estimating the Relative Biological Effectiveness (RBE) of the neutrons because severe late effects were not preceded by unusually severe acute toxicity and tended to occur earlier than with conventional radiotherapy. Bradley et al[103] recently compared neutrons with Cobalt[60] irradiation of canine brain and calculated an RBE of 4 for neutrons. Van der Kogel and Barendsen,[8] using damage to the rat spinal cord as an end point, calculate an RBE of 1.1 for single fraction courses and 1.7 for five fractions.

The obvious uncertainty of the true strength of neutrons used to irradiate nervous tissue, combined with the demonstrated capability to destroy both tumor and normal tissue, means that complications can be expected as this modality is pursued as a potentially effective treatment modality.

Other high LET particles, such as Neon[20] have also been studied for more exotic purposes[104]; they are used as a model for estimation of the effectiveness of cosmic-ray particles in producing nervous tissue damage during space flight. Although the space shuttle program promises to introduce more widespread space travel and although even SST (Concorde) travel could produce very high exposure levels in a solar flare, this topic remains too esoteric for general concern, other than to be aware that it exists.

Another high LET particle used clinically is the proton beam for treatment of acromegaly.[105] The advantage of these particles in this circumstance lies in the sharpness of the edge of the beam and the concentration of the radiation in the end of the path — called the Bragg peak. In following 14 patients, Kjellberg noted three cases of transient diplopia (presumably due to oculomotor nerve exposure), one case of anterior pituitary insufficiency, and headache. In the experience of others,[106,107] however, proton beam therapy carries with it a high risk of long-term injury, including cranial nerve palsy, chiasmatic injury, vertigo, and seizures. Morphologically, injury can be caused to adjacent sites, including the medial temporal lobe and the ventral hypothalamus.[108] In these cases, the injury is similar to that caused by other types of radiation.

Negative pi-mesons is another type of particle being investigated for therapeutic efficacy. Mesons, which are intermediate in size between electrons and protons and which serve as mediators of strong nuclear interactions, also have as a characteristic the ability to deposit their energy at depth while sparing overlying tissues. Studies with these particles[109] indicate that they are more effective than X-rays in causing myelitis, by a factor of 1.3 to 3.2, the ratio increasing with increasing meson fractionation. Of particular concern is the fact that the mesons seem particularly potent in causing neurological injury so that, should these particles develop into part of the radiotherapeutic armamentarium, neurological complications can be expected to occur.

Oxygen – For reasons similar to those causing interest in high LET radiations, hyperbaric oxygen is also an area of inquiry. It is hoped that under oxygen tension of about 3–4 atmospheres, hypoxic cells may be rendered sensitive to irradiation. The question is whether the normal tissues will also react more severely under these circumstances. Theoretically, normal tissue, being well oxygenated, would not be affected by higher O_2 tension, but experience indicates that this may not, in fact, be the case. Three of the 14 patients with radiation myelopathy reported by Atkins and Trotter[86] were irradiated under conditions of hyperbaric oxygen. Van den Brenk[110] reviewed 239 cases of patients with head and neck tumors who survived at least nine months and found 21 cases of myelitis. However, he could not state that this was a higher incidence than might have been expected using conventional radiotherapy. Coy and Dolman[111] found three cases of myelopathy among 17 patients irradiated under hyperbaric oxygen conditions. When they compared the doses that caused myelitis in these cases, as compared to their experience under the usual conditions,[89] they concluded that the spinal cord suffered injury at lower doses in the presence of hyperbaric oxygen. Luk, et al[112] confirmed this observation experimentally when they found that hyperbaric oxygen increased the risk of injury to the rat spinal cord caused by 250kVp X-rays.

Hypertension – If vascular occlusion is the primary culprit in chronic radiation injury, then it stands to reason that patients whose vasculature is compromised before treatment starts will be more susceptible to late sequelae. Hopewell and Wright[61] irradiated the brains of hypertensive and normotensive rats. They found that, at their lower dose range, where vascular damage is probably the most important etiologic factor, hypertension accelerated the injury. At higher dose levels, where parenchymal damage to the white matter occurs independent of vascular changes, hypertension did not have such an effect.

Endocrine Factors – Aristizabal et al[113] noted that of 14 patients who developed damage to the brain or optic nerve after only moderate doses of radiotherapy, seven had Cushing's disease. Since less than 5% of patients who receive pituitary irradiation have Cushing's disease, these patients would seem to be at high risk for complication. The authors could not determine whether hypercorticism, hypertension, or tumor pressure upon the optic nerves and chiasm contributed to the incidence.

Chemotherapy – As multimodality therapy of cancer becomes more commonplace, concern exists that the interaction of various therapies may augment each other's toxicity. Antibiotic chemotherapeutic agents augment radiation injury regularly, but have not been implicated to do so in the central nervous system. The drug most commonly implicated is methotrexate, when combined with cranial irradiation for childhood leukemia.[114,115] However, the role of the radiotherapy is not clear, as the changes may represent simply underlying methotrexate injury.[116] Byfield[117] reported on a child who developed myelitis after a moderate dose of radiation and implicates vincristine as a possible synergistic agent in producing neurotoxicity. A more detailed discussion of the neurologic effects of chemotherapy can be found in Chapter III of this book.

Cranial Nerve Injury

Cranial nerve injury is a rarely reported sequela of radiation therapy. As discussed above, it appears to be a particularly common complication of proton beam pituitary ablation. Reports after conventional radiotherapy are few and are summarized in Table XIV. Forty nine palsies are listed after head and neck irradiation of a mixed group of patients, with the twelfth nerve involved in more than half. The tenth and eleventh nerves are also often injured. In the largest series,[118] the interval between treatment and onset of the palsy could be correlated inversely with the NSD. Kogelnik, et al[119] reviewed the status of 1163 patients who had no evidence of tumor at least five years after treatment and who were alive without evidence of tumor. They found ten palsies

Table XIV
Radiation-Induced Cranial Nerve Palsies

Author and Reference	No. of Nerve Palsies	Nerves Involved	Dose	Latency	Primary Tumor
Berger[118]	35	XII-19 X-9 XI-5 V-1 II-1	6250 rads/41 days to 10000 rads/43 days	12-172 months	head and neck
Kogelnik[119]	10	XII-5 XI-3 X-2		up to 13 years	head and neck
Harris[121]	5	II-5	4500 rads/26 days to 7000 rads/45 days	3-36 months	pituitary adenoma and craniopharyngioma
Cheng[120]	4	XII-4	6000 rads/30 days to 8000 rads/47 days	3 years to 8 years and 10 months	head and neck
Shukovsky[122]	3	II-3	7000-7500 rads/ 39-43 days	4-5 years	ethmoid series and nasal cavity
Westbrook[123]	2	X-2	5000 rads	29 and 98 months	breast
Atkins[86]	2	X-2			breast

in nine patients, an incidence of 0.8%. Cranial nerves are quite resistant to clinical levels of radiation exposure, and cranial nerve palsy is presumably caused by perineural fibrosis. While Berger and Bataini[118] did not note excessive fibrosis clinically, Cheng and Schulz[120] did. The latter reported four cases with hypoglossal nerve damage. In three cases fibrosis preceded the demonstration of the nerve injury, while in the fourth, fibrosis was not recorded. Cranial nerve palsy generally is caused by recurrent tumor, so the importance of identifying a relatively benign sequela of therapy is obvious. Unfortunately, no diagnostic modality can categorically distinguish the two. However, the etiology of the palsy can often be inferred from the latency period to its appearance, and follow-up over time can confirm the clinical impression.

Two series report optic nerve damage due to radiotherapy (one case is also included in the series of Berger and Bataini). Harris and Levene[121] reported on five patients who suffered visual loss out of 55 treated for pituitary adenoma or craniopharyngioma. They noted that no patient who had received less than 250 rads per day developed such loss, and they concluded that, within the dose range used on these patients, fraction size was the most important determinant. Shukovsky and Fletcher[122] saw three cases of optic nerve atrophy in 30 patients treated for tumors of the ethmoid sinus and nasal cavity. They calculated a tolerance dose to the optic nerve of 6800 rads in six weeks (or an NSD of 2000 rets).

Vocal cord paralysis due to recurrent laryngeal nerve paralysis has been reported after irradiation for breast cancer.[86,123] Westbrook et al[123] reviewed 37 cases of breast cancer and vocal cord paralysis and found it to be due to metastatic cancer in 32, radiation fibrosis in two, and miscellaneous causes in three. To distinguish benign from malignant etiologies, it is useful to search for other indications of the specific process. Malignant recurrence is usually accompanied by other evidence of tumor, usually in the neck nodes, on the chest wall, or within the thorax. Both patients with radiation-induced vocal cord paralysis had evidence of scarring and induration within the irradiated fields.

Vocal cord paresis due to recurrent laryngeal nerve has also been reported after administration of I[131]. Craswell[124] reported on a patient treated for hyperthyroidism who developed paresis two days after treatment. The problem was transient, however, and his voice returned to normal after two months.

Peripheral Nerve Injury

Peripheral nerves are extremely resistant to radiation injury, which is observed only at very high dose levels.[125] The most common injury described is brachial plexus injury. This is usually seen after irradiation of carcinoma of the breast,[126-131] but is also described after irradiation of Hodgkin's Disease,[132] melanoma,[130] and sarcomas.[130,131] The plexus lesions usually begin with sensory changes of pain, numbness, or paresthesis. The sensory findings predominate, but motor findings develop also, ranging from mild paresis to paralysis. The difficult differential diagnosis that exists in these cases is to determine whether the plexopathy is produced by radiation or by malignant infiltration. This is particularly important in view of the effectiveness of radiation in controlling the pain of malignant plexopathy in most cases.[133] Thomas and Colby[131] compared the two syndromes at their institution. The only difference they found was with respect to pain. Six of their 14 patients with radiation-induced plexopathy had little or no pain, whereas tumor infiltration always produced early, severe pain. Kori et al[134] reviewed 100 cases of brachial plexopathy. Seventy-eight patients had tumors (34 had received previous irradiation) and 22 had radiation injury. They confirm the association of tumor infiltration with the presence of pain, whereas radiation plexopathy can be relatively pain-free. They further correlated injury to the upper plexus (C_{5-6}) and lymphedema with radiation injury and injury to the lower plexus ($C_7 - T_1$) and Horner's syndrome with tumor infiltration. Nevertheless, the distinction is usually unclear, and many[128-131] mention the need for surgical exploration of the brachial plexus for definitive diagnosis. The breast cancer cases are summarized in Table XV.

Table XV
Brachial Plexus Injury After Postoperative Irradiation
for Carcinoma of Breast

Reference	Patients	Dose	Latent Period
Mumenthaler[126]	8	1680-5000 rads	15-135 months
Stoll[127]	37	5100-5500 rads/ 11-12 fractions 25-28 days	4-30 months
Steiner[128]	6	8000-11000 rads in 5-8 weeks	6 months to 9 years
Westling[129]	31	5400 rads +/- 1000 rads/ 23 days	1 to 5 years
Spiess[130]	23	3200-8100 rads	1 to 13 years
Thomas[131]	14	4000-8000 rads	5 months to 20 years

The incidence of neuropathy is dose-dependent. Thomas and Colby[131] had 14 cases out of 1202 reviewed; the patients received 4000-8000 rads, but the details of the therapy are unavailable. Stoll and Andrews[127] had an incidence of 73% (24 of 33 patients) after 5500 rads but only 15% (13 out of 84) after 5100 rads, using the same fractionation. Thomas and Colby could not correlate dose with latency periods, but Westling et al[129] found that longer latency could be associated with milder paresis of the involved arm. Kori et al[134] found that, for symptoms within one year of a radiation dose of over 6000 rads, radiation injury is usually the cause.

When the lesion is seen surgically, severe perineural fibrosis is the inevitable finding.[126,127,131] Mumenthaler[125] recommends early surgical lysis of the adhesions, in contrast to Spiess[130] who recommends it only in "exceptional cases." Westling et al[129] found that surgery could provide some relief of pain, but that sensory and motor signs remained unaffected.

The prognosis for brachial plexopathy is guarded. It may stabilize, but often progresses to a point at which the extremity is useless. Regression is not seen.

Rarely, other peripheral nerves can be damaged as well. In a review of iatrogenic peripheral nerve injury, Mumenthaler[135] mentions radiation-induced injury of the ilioinguinal and femoral nerves. Schiødt and Kristenson[80] also described two cases of femoral nerve damage after pelvic radiation for malignant testicular tumors. Spiess[130] reported four cases of injury to the lumbosacral plexus (2), femoral (1), and ulnar nerves (1) after irradiation for miscellaneous neoplasms; these were seen, however, only after intense local doses.

Large Vessel Injury

In contrast to the typically observed small vessel injury after radiotherapy, large vessel damage is a curiosity. The production of neurological symptoms due to spinal artery occlusion was discussed above,[84] and Shukovsky and Fletcher[122] saw two cases of central retinal artery thrombosis in their series.

Occlusion or narrowing of the large vessels of the carotid system is the subject of isolated case reports. It is a rare finding. In a review of 7000 carotid angiograms, Momose and New[136] found 140 cases of nonatheromatoris stenosis and occlusion of the internal carotid artery and its branches. Only one of these was due to radiation therapy, in the case of a woman who received two courses for a pituitary adenoma to a total dose of 7500 rads and who subsequently was found to have occlusion of the carotid system. Darmody et al[137] similarly described a patient who developed progressive stenosis and then occlusion of the middle cerebral artery three years after re-irradiation for a pituitary tumor. Hayward[138] described a man who received six 608 rad fractions over a month and a half for hyperthyroidism, and six more smaller doses (57 rads x 3 and 456 rads x 3) over the next year. He estimated a total dose to each carotid artery of 4127 rads (in 12 fractions over 355 days) and an NSD of 1200 rets. He returned 27 years later with severe atherosclerosis in the neck vessels in the absence of evidence of atherosclerotic disease elsewhere. Glick[139] reported on a patient who received an estimated carotid dose of 6076 rads over 46 days during treatment of a vocal cord tumor. She died 16 years later and at autopsy was found to have bilateral common carotid artery occlusion by atheromatous plaques. The vessels were uniformly involved, and the findings were sharply confined to the treatment portals as indicated by the overlying skin changes. The case of Conomy and Kellermeyer[140] was a young woman who died of a stroke eight months after completing radiotherapy for Hodgkin's disease. Autopsy showed complete occlusion of the left internal carotid artery. The location of the occlusion was in an area that had received a high dose of radiation (7200 rads).

The mechanism of these injuries is not agreed upon, and there appear to be two. The patients with a long delay between treatment and presentation with vascular disease (16 and 27 years) are presumed to have had atherosclerosis accelerated by the radiation. The patient of Darmody et al[137] on the other hand, was found at surgery to have thickening and fibrosis of the vessel wall with marked endothelial proliferation. The authors felt that these changes were compatible with the usual vascular injury attributed to radiation. Similarly, while Conomy and Kellermeyer describe thrombotic occlusion of the internal carotid artery, atheromatous lesions were not seen. Subintimal fibrosis and hypertrophy were seen in areas corresponding to the radiation portals. Thus it would seem that those occlusions that appeared soon after high-dose irradiation were mediated through a more direct vascular injury rather than atherosclerosis. Nevertheless, it should be emphasized that these lesions are extremely rare ones, indicating that individual susceptibility may have played a role. Certainly, concern for this complication cannot be a major concern in planning treatment for a patient with malignant disease of predictable morbidity.

Childhood Nervous System

Radiation damage to nervous system of the child is of special concern, since the still developing system is expected to be more susceptible to injury. When combined with the long life expectancy of the patient should cure be achieved, the consideration merits close scrutiny of relevant effects to permit a meaningful choice between benefit and risk.

The recent development of efficacious therapies for childhood acute lymphocytic leukemia is one of the brighter sides of contemporary neoplastic disease treatment. Effective combinations of chemotherapeutic agents have converted a rapidly lethal disease into one in which a remission, often long-term, can be achieved in most cases. However, as remissions were induced, it became apparent that the central nervous system was functioning as a sanctuary site and serving as a common site of recurrence. For this reason, therapy to the central nervous system, usually a combination of whole brain irradiation and intrathecal methotrexate, is given once remission is achieved. The therapy has had gratifying results, reducing the incidence of meningial leukemia from 50–70% to 5–10%. However, important sequelae are also observed.

Symptoms during irradiation are usually mild. However, a serious toxicity may develop in patients treated with radiotherapy and concomitant intrathecal methotrexate for overt meningical leukemia.[141] A rapid neurological deterioration occurs, characterized by signs of increased intracranial pressure developing within a day or two of initiation of treatment. The mechanism for the toxicity is not known.

The somnolence that may develop subacutely has been described above.[13]

The most serious complication is a delayed one. It is chiefly a complication of methotrexate and consists of a progressive leucoencephalopathy. Several papers have appeared in recent years, describing this entity,[114,115,142-154] which consists of a diffuse multifocal coagulation necrosis with axonal dystrophy, demyelination of the white matter, and variable amounts of mineralized cellular debris. All the patients reported to date have received either intrathecal or systemic methotrexate, with or without radiotherapy or other intrathecal medications. Most patients have received intrathecal and systemic methotrexate plus cranial irradiation. The syndrome is characterized by confusion, ataxia, dementia, spasticity, seizures, coma, and death. The role of radiotherapy may be to alter the blood-brain barrier and thereby allow a greater amount of systemically administered drug to reach the central nervous system. Thus Aur et al[115] limit to 40 mg/M^2 the individual dosage of methotrexate given after irradiation. Pizzo et al[141] have described five patients with this syndrome who had detectable lesions on CAT scan of the brain, suggesting that such scanning may be useful in monitoring effects of methotrexate therapy. This is especially important because they also observed three patients in whom the leucoencephalopathy was partially reversible when methotrexate was discontinued, accompanied in one case by anatomic improvement on serial CAT scans.

Another possible complication of prophylactic central nervous system treatment for acute leukemia is cerebral atrophy. Peylan-Ramu, et al[145] reviewed serial CAT scans of 32 patients treated with 2400 rads of cranial irradiation and intrathecal chemotherapy with either methotrexate or cytosine arabinoside. Seventeen patients (53%) showed abnormalities. These included dilatation of the ventricles in eight patients and widening of the subarachnoid space in nine. Four patients showed decreased attenuation coefficients and one showed intracerebral calcification; these lesions have been described as part of methotrexate leucoencephalopathy and, in this series, occurred only in patients who received intrathecal methotrexate. Mild central nervous system dysfunction was detected in seven patients, but did not correlate with the radiographic findings, so that the clinical significance of these changes is at present speculative.

Other neurologic sequelae of childhood irradiation includes intracranial calcification. Flament-Durand et al[146] described a child with leukemia who had received radiotherapy and X-rays and who at autopsy had bilateral calcifications in the cerebral and cerebellar cortex. Harwood-Nash and Reilly[147] reported two cases of calcification of the basal ganglia after radiotherapy. One patient had a glioblastoma multiforma and the other histiocytosis of the skull, and they developed the finding three and nine years, respectively, after exposure. The authors speculate that local hypoxia secondary to radiation-induced vascular injury is the cause of this finding.

Major concern exists about the late functional and hormonal sequelae of high-dose irradiation to the nervous system at a young age. Bamford et al[148] studied 30 long-term survivors of cranial or craniospinal irradiation. Of these, only six (20%) had no residual problems, and six others were profoundly disabled. No child treated before he was 11 years old had a height greater than the tenth percentile for his age. While this incidence of side effects is higher than given in some other series, it may be due to the long follow-up these patients had to allow late clinical findings to appear. The age of the patient at the time of treatment is important. Broadbent et al[149] studied eight patients who were long-term survivors after treatment for medulloblastoma. While all showed some residual problems, five had only minimal disabilities and were leading active lives. Of the three patients with severe deficits, two had been treated before the age of two years. All eight showed a shortened spine, four had lower than expected centile height, and three had significant undergrowth of the mandible. The three most severely affected showed frank mental retardation.

Spunberg et al[150] reviewed the experience of 38 children less than two years of age treated for primary intracranial tumors and studied 14 long-term survivors. They found eight to be essentially normal, 11 within the educable range on intelligence testing, and 12 with Karnofsky performance scores of 70 or above.

Shalet, et al[151,152] examined pituitary function after radiotherapy of intracranial tumors in childhood and found that many had an impaired growth hormone response, a finding not confirmed by Broadbent et al.[149] This could account for the short stature noted, although other etiologies such as the effect of chemotherapy or direct irradiation to the vertebral column (as in the case of medulloblastoma) must also be considered. The deficit appeared to be progressive over time. They also noted a significantly greater basal thyroid-stimulating hormone level and response to thyrotropin-releasing hormone. Spunberg, et al[150] found endocrine changes limited to patients receiving at least 3600 rads to the hypothalamic-pituitary region.

Intracranial occlusive vasculopathy has also been seen after childhood irradiation. Painter et al[153] described four patients who presented with stroke-like symptoms between two and 22 years after radiotherapy for medulloblastoma (2), retinoblastoma (1), and optic glioma (1). Two of the patients underwent angiography which showed narrowing of the intracranial branches of the internal carotid artery. Similarly, Wright and Bresnan[154] described a neonate treated for an orbital hemangioma in whom angiography at age six showed a hypoplastic left carotid artery with occlusion of the anterior and middle cerebral arteries, with collateral vessels bypassing the narrowed segment. These reports indicate that the large vessels of the child are susceptible to two types of radiation injury — hypoplasia due to impaired development of the vessel, and accelerated atherosclerosis which may produce symptoms of occlusive disease prematurely, although after a long latency period. Wright and Bresnan feel, in addition, that the vulnerability of the internal carotid artery is greater in a younger patient.

Induction of Malignancy

Radiation is a well-known carcinogenic agent. Most reported cases deal with risk of low-dose exposure such as militarily (e.g. Hiroshima, Nagasaki) or occupationally (e.g. radium dial painters, pitchblend miners). Diagnostic x-rays also can produce malignancies as indicated, for example, by the increased incidence of breast cancer in patients fluoroscoped for tuberculosis. Similarly, radiotherapy for benign diseases, such as ankylosing spondylitis, is followed by an incidence of neoplasia that is higher than expected. The nervous system, not surprisingly, does not escape this effect. Saenger et al[155] studied 1644 individuals irradiated in childhood for benign diseases and matched them with 3777 unirradiated sibling controls. They found one case of glioblastoma multiforma in a boy treated for cervical adenitis. However, no increased incidence of central nervous system neoplasia was detected in the irradiated children as compared to the controls. Modan et al[156] studied 10,905 children irradiated for scalp ringworm and compared them with two control groups, one of unirradiated siblings and another of a matched population of unirradiated children. They found an increase in brain tumors in the irradiated children.

Malignant neoplasms have also been reported after therapeutic irradiation of intracranial tumors (see Table XVI). The most common pattern is the development of fibrosarcoma after the irradiation of a pituitary tumor.[157-162] This area had been complicated by earlier confusion about the histologic criteria for diagnosing pituitary adenoma versus sarcoma. However, in 1959 Terry et al[157] described three patients who developed fibrosarcoma five to 12 years after multiple courses of radiotherapy to high doses for chromophobe adenoma. The multiple courses were indicated by the persistent recurrence of the neoplasm. While these tumors behaved as benign tumors in the sense that no metastases were demonstrated, they had malignant features histologically. The causal relationship was proposed because of the rarity of pituitary sarcomas. The patients of Terry et al[157] and Goldberg et al[159] all had multiple courses of radiotherapy with a high total dose. Greenhouse[160] and Waltz and Brownell[161] reported cases after single courses to moderate doses. Latency period in these series ranged from five to 20 years. Noetzli and Malamud[158] presented a case of fibrosarcoma developing after irradiation of a medulloblastoma. This case is particularly interesting because the fibrosarcoma was anatomically separate from the original neoplasm, excluding the possibility that the sarcoma represents a malignant transformation of the original neoplasm. Proton beam advocates for pituitary therapy have pointed to the smaller total volume exposed during this kind of treatment, suggesting that there would be less likelihood of carcinogenesis. However, Coppeto and Roberts[162] reported a case of sarcoma developing after proton beam pituitary ablation for acromegaly. Although fibrosarcoma is the usual tumor described after pituitary irradiation, malignant fibrous histiocytoma has also been reported,[163] as have anaplastic carcinoma of the middle ear and paranasal sinus and hemangioendothelioma.[159] Other miscellaneous reports include meningiomas after treatment of optic nerve glioma[164] or medulloblastoma[165] (in this case, multiple meningiomas). Malignant astrocytomas have been described after irradiation of craniopharyngioma,[166] medulloblastoma,[167] as well as after prophylactic cranial irradiation and intrathecal methotrexate for acute lymphocytic leukemia.[168]

Table XVI
Second Neoplasms After Radiotherapy

Paper	Patients	Primary Tumor	Radiation Dose	Age at 1st RT	Latency After RT	Second Tumor
Mann[164]	1	optic nerve glioma	8000 rads over 9 months	4	6 years	meningioma
Terry[157]	3	chromophobe adenoma in all	1) 7500 rads in 5 courses over 6½ years	1) 47	1) 2 months (8 yrs.)	pituitary fibrosarcoma in all
			2) 11400 rads in 3 courses over 34 months	2) 43	2) 6 months (5 yrs.)	
			3) 6500 rads in 4 courses over 7 years	3) 26	3) 5½ years (12 yrs.)	
Noetzli[158]	1	medulloblastoma	1) 4500 rads/ 45 days	10	8 years	fibrosarcoma
Goldberg[159]	4	pituitary adenoma with acromegaly	1) multiple courses over 20 years	1) 22	1) 10 years (30 yrs.)	1) anaplastic carcinoma of sinus or middle ear
			2) at least 2325 rads in 3 courses over 3 years	2) 30	2) 16 years (19 yrs.)	2) hemangia endothelioma
			3) 3940 rads in 2 courses, 6 months apart	3) 18	3) 10 years	3) fibrosarcoma
			4) 6000 rads in 3 short courses over 110 days	4) 31	4) 20 years	4) sarcoma

Greenhouse[160]	1	pituitary adenoma	1) 4000 rads/ 23 days and then 4000 rads/ 26 days seven years later	24	1) 2 months (7 yrs.)	1) sarcoma
Waltz[161]	2	chromophobe adenoma	1) 3500 rads 21 fractions 3½ weeks 2) 4000 rads 24 fractions 4 weeks	1) 38 2) 42	1) 8 years 2) 5 years	fibrosarcoma
Gonzalez-Vitale[163]	1	chromophobe	3600 rads (11 years later 1400 rads)	26	11 years	malignant fibrosis histiocytoma
Sogg[166]	1	craniopharyngioma	6000 rads/ 46 days	9	5½ years	malignant astro-cytoma
Coppeto[166]	1	pituitary adenoma with acromegaly	10000 rads with protons (4800 rads/ 40 days after 7 years)	46	7 years	fibrosarcoma
Iacono[165]	1	medulloblastoma	5000 rads	3	27 years	2 meningiomas
Cohen[167]	1	medulloblastoma	3500 rads	4	14 years	astrocytoma
Chung[168]	1	acute lymphocytic leukemia	2400 rads 2½ weeks	2	5 years	glioblastoma multiforme

Taken together, however, the reports of tumor induction are so few as to constitute a curiosity. In view of the great benefits that have accrued to the thousands of patients irradiated for their neoplasms, concern for secondary tumors should not be a contraindication to radiotherapy.

References

1. Rubin P, Caserett GW: *Clinical Radiation Pathology* W.B. Saunders Co., Philadelphia, 1968.
2. Kramer S: The hazards of therapeutic irradiation of the central nervous system. *Clin Neurosurg* 15:301-318, 1968.
3. Kramer S, Lee KF: Complications of radiation therapy: The central nervous system. *Semin Roentgenol* 9:75-83, 1974.
4. Verity GL: Tissue tolerance: Central nervous system. *Radiology* 91: 1221-1225, 1968.
5. Wigg DR, Koschel K, Hodgson GS: Tolerance of the mature human central nervous system to photon irradiation. *Brit J Radiol* 54:787-798, 1981.
6. Sheline GE: Irradiation injury of the human brain: A review of clinical experience. In: *Radiation Damage to the Nervous System*. Gilbert HA, Kagan AR, eds. Raven Press, New York, 1980.
7. Ellis F: Dose, time, and fractionation: A clinical hypothesis. *Clin Radiol* 20:1-7, 1969.
8. Van der Kogel AJ, Barendsen GW: Late effects of spinal cord irradiation with 300 KV x-rays and 15 MeV neutrons. *Brit J Radiol* 47:393-398, 1974.
9. Hornsey S, White A: Isoeffect curve for radiation myelopathy. *Brit J Radiol* 53:168-169, 1980.
10. Marks JE, Baglan RJ, Prasad SC, et al: Cerebral radionecrosis: Incidence and risk in relation to dose, time, fractionation and volume. *Int J Radiation Oncol Biol Phys* 7:243-252, 1981.
11. Penzer RD, Archambeau JO: Brain Tolerance Unit: A method to estimate risk of radiation brain injury for various dose schedules. *Int J Radiation Oncol Biol Phys* 7:397-402, 1981.
12. Hornsey S, Morris CC, Myers R: The relationship between fractionation and total dose for X-ray induced brain damage. *Int J Radiation Oncol Biol Phys* 7:393-396, 1981.
13. Freeman JE, Johnston FJB, Voke JM: Somnolence after prophylactic cranial irradiation in children with acute lymphoblastic leukemia. *Brit Med J* 4:523-525, 1973.
14. Druckmann A: Schlafsucht als folge der röntgenbestrahlung. Beitrag zur strahlenemphfindlichkeit des gehirns. *Strahlentherapie* 33:382-4, 1929.
15. Rider WD: Radiation damage to the brain — A new syndrome. *J Can Assoc Radiol* 14:67-69, 1963.
16. Boldrey E, Sheline G: Delayed transitory clinical manifestations after radiation treatments of intracranial tumors. *Acta Radiologica (Therapy)* 5:5-10, 1966.
17. Munro P, Mair WGP: Radiation effects on the human central nervous

system 14 weeks after x-radiation. *Acta Neuropathologica* 11:267-274, 1968.

18. Lampert PW, Davis RL: Delayed effects of radiation on the human central nervous system — "Early" and "Late" delayed reactions. *Neurology* 14:912-917, 1964.

19. Almquist S, Dahlgren S, Notter G, et al: Brain necrosis after irradiation of the hypophysis in Cushing's disease. *Acta Radiologica (Therapy)* 2:179-188, 1964.

20. Salazar OM, Rubin P, Mc Donald JV, et al: High dose radiation therapy in the treatment of glioblastoma multiforme: A preliminary report. *Int J Radiation Oncol Biol Phys* 1:717-727, 1976.

21. Boden G: Radiation myelitis of the brainstem. *J Fac Radiol* 2:79-94, 1950.

22. Pennybacker J, Russell DS: Necrosis of the brain due to radiation therapy. *J Neurol Neurosurg Psychiat* 11:183-198, 1948.

23. Malamud N, Boldrey EB, Welch WK, et al: Necrosis of brain and spinal cord following X-ray therapy. *J Neurosurg* 11:353-362, 1954.

24. Martins AN, Johnston JS, Henry JM, et al: Delayed radition necrosis of the brain. *J Neurosurg* 47:336-345, 1977.

25. Mikhael MA: Radiation necrosis of the brain: Correlation between computed tomography, pathology, and dose distribution. *J Comp Assit Tomography* 2:71-80, 1978.

26. Scholz W, Hsü YK: Late damage from roentgen irradiation of the human brain. *Arch Neurol Psychiat* 40:928-936, 1938.

27. Foltz EL, Holyoke JB, Heyl HL: Brain necrosis following X-ray therapy. *J Neurosurg* 10:423-429, 1953.

28. Dugger GS, Stratford JG, Bouchard J: Necrosis of the brain following roentgen irradiation. *Am J Roentgen* 72:953-960, 1954.

29. Fletcher GH, Million RR: Malignant tumors of the nasopharynx. *Am J Roentgen* 93:44-55, 1965.

30. Marra A, Givffrè R: Late cerebral radionecrosis. *Europ Neurol* 1:234-246, 1968.

31. Krayenbühl H, Rüttner Röntgenspätschäden des schläfenhirns nach hochvoltbestrahlung maligner tumoren des epipharynx. *Schweiz med Wschr* 103:225-231, 1973.

32. Diengdoh JV, Booth AE: Postirradiation necrosis of the temporal lobe presenting as a glioma. *J Neurosurg* 44:732-734, 1976.

33. Eyster EF, Nielsen SL, Sheline GE, Wilson CB: Cerebral radiation necrosis simulating a brain tumor. *J Neurosurg* 40:267-271, 1974.

34. Kusske JA, Williams JP, Garcia JH, et al: Radiation necrosis of the brain following radiotherapy of extracerebral neoplasms. *Surg Neurol* 6:15-20, 1976.

35. Queiroz L, Neto JN: Late pseudotumoral brain necrosis following irradiation of a scalp neoplasm. *J Neurosurg* 45:581-584, 1976.

36. Littman P, James H, Zimmerman R, et al: Radionecrosis of the brain presenting as a mass lesion: a case report. *J Neurol Neurosurg Psychiat* 40:827-829, 1977.

37. Rottenberg DA, Chernik NL, Deck MDF, et al: Cerebral necrosis following radiotherapy of extracranial neoplasms. *Ann Neurol* 1:339-357, 1977.

38. Matsumura H, Ross ER: Delayed cerebral radionecrosis following treatment of carcinoma of the scalp: Clinicopathologic and ultrastructural study. *Surg Neurol* 12:193-204, 1979.

39. Wilson GH, Byfield J, Hanafee WN: Atrophy following radiation therapy

for central nervous system neoplasms. *Acta Radiologica (Therapy)* 11: 361-368, 1972.

40. Marsa GW, Goffinet DR, Rubinstein LJ, et al: Megavoltage irradiation in the treatment of gliomas of the brain and spinal cord. *Cancer* 36: 1681-1689, 1975.

41. Burger PC, Mahaley MS, Jr, Dudka L, et al: The morphologic effects of radiation administered therapeutically for intracranial gliomas. *Cancer* 44:1256-1272, 1979.

42. Lindgren M: On tolerance of brain tissue and sensitivity of brain tumors to irradiation. *Acta Radiologica* (Suppl) 170:1-73, 1958.

43. Crompton MR, Layton DD: Delayed radionecrosis of the brain following therapeutic X-radiation of the pituitary. *Brain* 84:85-101, 1961.

44. Peck FC, Jr, Mc Govern ER: Radiation necrosis of the brain in acromegaly. *J Neurosurg* 25:536-542, 1966.

45. Kramer S, Southard M, Mansfield CM: Radiotherapy in the management of craniopharyngiomas. *AM J Roentgen* 103:44-52, 1968.

46. Ghatak NR, White BE: Delayed radiation necrosis of the hypothalamus. *Arch Neurol* 21:425-430, 1969.

47. Holdorff B, Schiffter R: Strahlenspätnekrosen des Hirnstammes, einschliesslich Hypothalamus nach Bestrahlung mit ultraharten Röntgenstrahlen und schnellen Elektronen. *Acta Neurochirurgica* 25:37-56, 1971.

48. Neetens A, Martin J, Rubbens MC: Iatrogenic roentgen encephalopathy. *Bull Soc Belge Opthalmol* 178:87-99, 1977.

49. Sterman A, Protass LM: An atypical case of delayed radiation necrosis of the brain. *Arch Neurol* 36:655-656, 1979.

50. Raskind R: Central nervous system damage after radiation therapy. *Int Surg* 48:430-441, 1967.

51. Brismar J, Roberson GH, Davis HR: Radiation necrosis of the brain: Neuroradiological considerations with computed tomography. *Neuroradiology* 12:109-113, 1976.

52. Carella RJ, Pay N, Newall J, et al: Tomography in the serial study of cerebral tumors treated by radiation. *Cancer* 37:2719-2728, 1976.

53. Rubinstein LJ: Radiation changes in intracranial neoplasms and the adjacent brain. In: *Atlas of Tumor Pathology*, Fascicle 6, "Tumors of the Central Nervous System" pp 349-360, Armed Forces Inst of Pathology, Washington, D.C., 1972.

54. De Reuck J, Vander Eecken H: The anatomy of the late radiation encephalopathy. *Europ Neurol* 13:481-494, 1975.

55. Husain MM, Garcia JH: Cerebral "radiation necrosis": Vascular and glial features. *Acta Neuropath* (Berl) 36:381-385, 1976.

56. Lowenberg-Schrenberg K, Bassett RC: Amyloid degeneration of the human brain following X-ray therapy. *J Neuropath Exp Neurol* 9: 93-102, 1950.

57. Mandybur TI, Gore I: Amyloid in late postirradiation necrosis of brain. *Neurology* 19:983-992, 1969.

58. Arnold A, Bailey P, Harvey RA, et al: Changes in the central nervous system following irradiation with 23-MeV X-rays from the betagron. *Radiology* 62:37-46, 1954.

59. Mc Donald LW, Hayes RL: The role of capillaries in the pathogenesis of delayed radionecrosis of brain. *Am J Path* 50:745-764, 1967.

60. Berge G, Brun A, Hakansson CH, et al: Sensitivity to irradiation of the brain stem. *Cancer* 33:1263-1268, 1974.

61. Hopewell JW, Wright EA: The nature of latent cerebral irradiation damage and its modification by hypertension. *Brit J Radiol* 43:161-167, 1970.
62. Caveness WF: Pathology of radiation damage to the normal brain of the monkey. *Natl Cancer Inst Monogr* 46:57-76, 1977.
63. Nakagaki H, Brunhart G, Kemper TL, et al: Monkey brain damage from radiation in the therapeutic range. *J Neurosurg* 44:3-11, 1976.
64. Reagan TJ, Bisel HF, Childs DS, Jr, et al: Controlled study of CCNU and radiation therapy in malignant astrocytoma. *J Neurosurg* 44:186-190, 1976.
65. Sheline GE: Radiation therapy of the brain tumors. *Cancer* 39:873-881, 1977.
66. Horns J, Webber MM: Retreatment of brain tumors. *Radiology* 88:322-325, 1967.
67. Dritschilo A, Bruckman JE, Cassady JR, et al: Tolerance of brain to multiple courses of radiation therapy. *Brit J Radiol* 54:782-786, 1981.
68. Furchtgott E: Behavioral effects of ionizing radiations. *Psychological Bulletin* 60:157-199, 1963.
69. Samaan NA, Bakdash MM, Caderao JB, et al: Hypopituitarism after external irradiation. *Ann Int Med* 83:771-777, 1975.
70. Reagan TJ, Thomas JE, Colby MY: Chronic progressive radiation myelopathy. *JAMA* 203:128-132, 1968.
71. Boden G: Radiation myelitis of the cervical spinal cord. *Brit J Radiol* 21:464-469, 1948.
72. Dynes JB, Smedal MI: Radiation myelitis. *Am J Roentgen* 83:78-87, 1960.
73. Jones A: Transient radiation myelopathy. *Brit J Radiol* 37:727-744, 1964.
74. Bloomer WD, Hellman S: Normal tissue responses to radiation therapy. *N Engl J Med* 293:80-82, 1975.
75. Godwin-Austen RB, Howell DA, Worthington B: Observations on radiation myelopathy. *Brain* 98:557-568, 1975.
76. Fishman RA: Letter to the editor. *N Engl J Med* 293:669, 1975.
77. Mastaglia FL, Mc Donald WI, Watson JV, et al: Effects of X-radiation in the spinal cord: An experimental study of the morphological changes in central nerve fibers. *Brain* 99:101-122, 1976.
78. Greenfield MM, Stark FM: Post-irradiation neuropathy. *Am J Roentgen* 60:617-622, 1948.
79. Sadowsky CH, Sachs E, Jr, Ochoa J: Postradiation motor neuron syndrome. *Arch Neurol* 33:786-787, 1976.
80. Schiødt AV, Kristensen O: Neurologic complications after irradiation of malignant tumors of the testis. *Acta Radiologica* (Therapy) 17:369-378, 1978.
81. Hildebrand J: *Lesions of the Nervous System in Cancer Patients.* Raven Press, New York, 1978.
82. Maier JG, Perry RH, Saylor W, et al: Radiation myelitis of the dorsolumbar spinal cord. *Radiology* 93:153-160, 1969.
83. Phillips TL, Buschke F: Radiation tolerance of the thoracic spinal cord. *Am J Roentgen* 105:659-664, 1969.
84. Di Chiro G, Herdt JR: Angiographic demonstration of spinal cord arterial occlusion in postradiation myelomalacia. *Radiology* 106:317-319, 1973.
85. Pallis CA, Louis S, Morgan RL: Radiation myelopathy. *Brain* 84:460-479,

1961.
86. Atkins HL, Tretter P: Time-dose considerations in radiation myelo-
    pathy. *Acta Radiologica* (Therapy) 5:79-94, 1966.
87. Kristensson K, Molin B, Sourander P: Delayed radiation lesions of the
    human spinal cord. *Acta Neuropathologica* 9:34-44, 1967.
88. Locksmith JP, Powers WE: Permanent radiation myelopathy. *Am J
    Roentgen* 102:916-926, 1968.
89. Coy P, Baker S, Dolman CL: Progressive myelopathy due to radiation.
    Can Med Assoc J 100:1129-1133, 1969.
90. Solheim φP: Radiation injury of the spinal cord. *Acta Radiologica*
    (Therapy) 10:474-480, 1971.
91. Palmer JJ: Radiation myelopathy. *Brain* 95:109-122, 1972.
92. Yaar I, Herishanu Y, Lavy S: Radiation myelopathy. *Europ Neurol* 10:
    83-88, 1973.
93. Lechevalier B, Humeau F, Houttenville JP: Myélopathies radiothéra-
    piques "hypertrophiantes." *Revue Neurologique*, Paris 129:119-132, 1973.
94. Baekmark UB: Neurologic complications after irradiation of the cer-
    vical spinal cord for malignant tumors of the head and neck. *Acta Ra-
    diologica* (Therapy) 14:33-41, 1975.
95. Wara WM, Phillips TL, Sheline GE, et al: Radiation tolerance of the
    spinal cord. *Cancer* 35:1558-1562, 1975.
96. Abbatucci JS, Delozier T, Quint R, et al: Radiation myelopathy of the
    cervical spinal cord: Time, dose, and volume factors. *Int J Radiation
    Oncol Biol Phys* 4:239-248, 1978.
97. Black MJ, Motaghedi B, Robitaille Y: Transverse myelitis. *The Laryngo-
    scope* 90:847-852, 1980.
98. Dische S, Martin WMC, Anderson P: Radiation myelopathy in patients
    treated for carcinoma of bronchus using a six fraction regime of radio-
    therapy. *Brit J Radiol* 54:29-35, 1981.
99. Parker RG, Berry HC, Gerdes AJ, et al: Fast neutron beam radiothera-
    py of glioblastoma multiforme. *Am J Roentgen* 127:331-335, 1976.
100. Shaw CM, Sumi SM, Alvord EC, Jr, et al: Fast neutron irradiation of
     glioblastoma multiforme neuropathological analysis. *J Neurosurg* 49:
     1-12, 1978.
101. Catterall M, Bloom HJG, Ash DV, et al: Fast neutrons compared with
     megavoltage X-rays in the treatment of patients with supratentorial
     glioblastoma: A controlled pilot study. *Int J Radiation Oncol Biol Phys*
     6:261-266, 1980.
102. Ornitz RD, Bradley EW, Mossman KL, et al: Clinical observations of
     early and late normal tissue injury in patients receiving fast neutron
     irradiation. *Int J Radiation Oncol Biol Phys* 6:273-279, 1980.
103. Bradley EW, Davis DO, Gaskill JW, et al: The effects of fractionated
     doses of fast neutrons or photons on the canine brain: Evoked response
     recording. *Int J Radiation Oncol Biol Phys* 6:1685-1691, 1980.
104. Kraft LM, Kelly MA, Johnson JE, Jr, et al: Effects of high-LET neon
     (^{20}Ne) particle radiation on the brain, eyes, and other head structures
     of the pocket mouse: a histological study. *Int J Radiation Biology* 35:
     33-61, 1979.
105. Kjellberg RN, Shintani A, Frantz AG, et al: Proton-beam therapy in
     acromegaly. *N Engl J Med* 278:689-695, 1968.
106. Dawson DM, Dingman JF: Hazards of proton-beam pituitary irradia-
     tion. *N Engl J Med* 282:1434, 1970.
107. Braunstein GD, Loriaux DL: Proton-beam therapy. *N Engl J Med* 284:

332-333, 1971.
108. Nielsen SL, Kjellberg RN, Asbury AK, et al: Neuropathologic effects of proton-beam irradiation in man. *Acta Neuropath* **21**:76-82, 1972.
109. Amols HI, Yuhas YM: Induction of spinal cord paralysis by negative pi-mesons. *Brit J Radiol* **54**: 602-605, 1981.
110. Van den Brenk HAS: Hyperbaric oxygen in radiation therapy. *Am J Roentgen* **102**:8-26, 1968.
111. Coy P, Dolman CL: Radition myelopathy in relation to oxygen level. *Brit J Radiol* **44**:705-707, 1971.
112. Luk KH, Baker DG, Fellows CF: Hyperbaric oxygen after radiation and its effect on the production of radiation myelitis. *Int J Radiation Oncol Biol Phys* **4**:457-459, 1978..
113. Aristizabal SA, Boone MLM, Laguna JF: Endocrine factors influencing radiation injury to central nervous tissue. *Int J Radiation Oncol Biol Phys* **5**:349-353, 1979.
114. Price RA, Jamieson PA: The central nervous system in childhood leukemia II. Subacute leukoencephalopathy. *Cancer* **35**:306-318, 1975.
115. Aur RJA, Simone JV, Verzosa MS, et al: Childhood acute lymphocytic leukemia — Study VIII. *Cancer* **42**:2123-2134, 1978.
116. Phillips TL, Fu KK: Quantification of combined radiation therapy and chemotherapy effects on critical normal tissues. *Cancer* **37**:1186-1200, 1976.
117. Byfield JE: Ionizing Radiation and Vincristine: Possible Neurotoxic Synergism. *Radiol Clin Biol* **41**:129-138, 1972.
118. Berger PS, Bataini JP: Radiation–induced cranial nerve palsy. *Cancer* **40**:152-155, 1977.
119. Kogelnik HD, Fletcher GH, Jesse RH: Clinical course of patients with squamous cell carcinoma of the upper respiratory and digestive tracts with no evidence of disease 5 years after initial treatment. *Radiology* **115**:423-427, 1975.
120. Cheng VST, Schulz MD: Unilateral hypoglossal nerve atrophy as a late complication of radiation therapy of head and neck carcinoma. *Cancer* **35**:1537-1544, 1975.
121. Harris JR, Levene MB: Visual complications following irradiation for pituitary adenomas and craniopharyngiomas. *Radiology* **120**:167-171, 1976.
122. Shukovsky LJ, Fletcher GH: Retinal and optic nerve complications in a high dose irradiation technique of ethmoid sinus and nasal cavity. *Radiology* **104**:629-634, 1972.
123. Westbrook KC, Ballantyne AJ, Eckles NE, et al: Breast cancer and vocal cord paralysis. *Southern Med J* **67**:805-807, 1974.
124. Craswell PWT: Vocal cord paresis following radioactive iodine therapy. *Brit J Clin Prac* **26**:571-572, 1972.
125. Janzen AH, Warren S: Effect of roentgen rays on the peripheral nerve of the rat. *Radiology* **38**:333-337, 1942.
126. Mumenthaler M. Armplexusparesen in Aschluss an Röntgenbestrahlung. *Schweiz Med Wschr* **94**:1069-1075, 1964.
127. Stoll BA, Andrews JT, Radiation-Induced Peripheral Neuropathy. *Brit Med J* **1**:834-837, 1966.
128. Steiner C, Fallet GH, Moody JF, et al: Lésions du plexus brachial survenant après radiotherapie pour cancer du sein. *Schweiz Med Wschr* **101**:1846-1848, 1971.
129. Westling P, Svensson H, Hele P: Cervical plexus lesions following post-

operative radiation therapy of mammary carcinoma. *Acta Radiologica* (Therapy) 11:209-216, 1972.

130. Spiess H: Die Schädigung des Nervensystems durch Ionisierende *Strahlen Therapeutische Umschau* 27:379-386, 1970.

131. Thomas JE, Colby MY, Jr: Radiation–induced or metastatic brachial plexopathy: *JAMA* 222:1392-1395, 1972.

132. Maruyama Y, Mylrea MM, Logothetis J: Neuropathy following irradiation. *Am J Roentgen* 101:216-219, 1967.

133. Son YH: Effectiveness of Irradiation Therapy in Peripheral Neuropathy Caused by Malignant Disease. *Cancer* 20:1447-1451, 1967.

134. Kori SH, Foley KM, Posner JB: Brachial Plexus Lesions in Patients with Cancer: 100 Cases. *Neurology* 31:45-50, 1981.

135. Mumenthaler M: Mechanische lasionen peripherer nerven durch "ärztliche. *Eingriffe Therapeutische Umschau* 27:365-368, 1970.

136. Momose KJ, New PFJ: Non-Atheromatous Stenosis and Occlusion of the Internal Carotid Artery and its Main Branches. *Am J Roentgen* 118:550-566, 1973.

137. Darmody WR, Thomas LM, Gurdjian ES: Postirradiation vascular insufficiency syndrome. *Neurology* 17:1190-1192, 1967.

138. Hayward RH: Arteriosclerosis induced by radiation. *Surg Clin N Amer* 52:359-366, 1972.

139. Glick B: Bilateral carotid occlusive disease following irradiation for carcinoma of the vocal cords. *Arch Path* 93:352-355, 1972.

140. Conomy JP, Kellermeyer R: Delayed cerebrovascular consequences of therapeutic radiation. *Neurology* 24:394, 1974.

141. Pizzo PA, Poplack DG, Bleyer WA: Neurotoxicities of Current Leukemia Therapy. *Am J of Pediatric Hematol Oncol* 1:127-140, 1979.

142. Hendin B, De Vivo DC, Torack R, et al: Parenchymatous degeneration of the central nervous system in childhood leukemia. *Cancer* 33:468-482, 1974.

143. Rubinstein LJ, Herman MM, Long TF, et al: Disseminated necrotizing leukoencephalopathy: A complication of treated central nervous system leukemia and lymphoma. *Cancer* 35:291-305, 1975.

144. Breuer AC, Blank NK, Schoene WC: Multifocal pontine lesions in cancer patients treated with chemotherapy and CNS radiotherapy. *Cancer* 41: 2112-2120, 1978.

145. Peylan-Ramu N, Poplack DG, Pizzo PA, et al: Abnormal CT Scans of the brain in asymptomatic children with acute lymphocytic leukemia after prophylactic treatment of the central nervous system with radiation and intrathecal chemotherapy. *N Engl J Med* 298:815-818, 1978.

146. Flament-Durand J, Ketelbant-Balasse P, Maurus R, et al: Intracerebral calcifications appearing during the course of acute lymphocytic leukemia treated with methotrexate and X-rays. *Cancer* 35:319-325, 1975.

147. Harwood-Nash DCF, Reilly BJ: Calcification of the basal ganglia following radiation therapy. *Am J Roentgen* 108:392-395, 1970.

148. Bamford FN, Morris-Jones P, Pearson D, et al: Residual Disabilities in children treated for intracranial space-occupying lesions. *Cancer* 37: 1149-1151, 1976.

149. Broadbent VA, Barnes ND, Wheeler TK: Medulloblastoma in childhood: Long-term results of treatment. *Cancer* 48:26-30, 1981.

150. Spunberg JJ, Chang CH, Goldman M, et al: Quality of long-term survival following irradiation for intracranial tumors in children under

the age of two. *Int J Radiation Oncol Biol Phys* 7:727-736, 1981.
151. Shalet SM, Beardwell CG, Morris-Jones P, et al: Pituitary function after treatment of intracranial tumors in children. *Lancet* 2:104-111, 1975.
152. Shalet SM, Beardwell CG, Morris-Jones P, et al: Growth hormone deficiency in children with brain tumors. *Cancer* 37:1144-1148, 1976.
153. Painter MJ, Chutorian AM, Hilal SK: Cerebrovasculopathy following irradiation in childhood. *Neurology* 25:189-194, 1975.
154. Wright TL, Bresnan MJ: Radiation–induced cerebrovascular disease in children. *Neurology* 26:540-543, 1976.
155. Saenger EL, Silverman FN, Sterling TD, et al: Neoplasia following therapeutic irradiation for benign conditions in childhood. *Radiology* 74:889-904, 1960.
156. Modan B, Baidatz D, Mart H, et al: Radiation-induced head and neck tumours. *Lancet* 1:277-279, 1974.
157. Terry RD, Hyams VJ, Davidoff LM: Combined nonmetastasizing fibrosarcoma and chromophobe tumor of the pituitary. *Cancer* 12:791-798, 1959.
158. Noetzli M, Malamud N: Postirradiation fibrosarcoma of the brain. *Cancer* 15:617-622, 1962.
159. Goldberg MB, Sheline GE, Malamud N: Malignant intracranial neoplasms following radiation therapy for acromegaly. *Radiology* 80:465-470, 1963.
160. Greenhouse AH: Pituitary sarcoma. *JAMA* 190:269-273, 1964.
161. Waltz TA, Brownell B: Sarcoma: A possible late result of effective radiation therapy for pituitary adenoma. *J Neurosurg* 24:901-907, 1966.
162. Coppeto JR, Roberts M: Fibrosarcoma after proton-beam pituitary ablation. *Arch Neurol* 36:380-381, 1979.
163. Gonzalez-Vitale JC, Slavin RE, Mc Queen JD: Radiation-induced intracranial malignant fibrous histiocytoma. *Cancer* 37:2960-2963, 1976.
164. Mann I, Yates PC, Ainslie JP: Unusual case of double primary orbital tumour. *Brit J Ophthal* 37:758-762, 1953.
165. Iocono RP, Apuzzo MLJ, Davis RL, et al: Multiple meningiomas following radiation therapy for medulloblastoma. *J Neurosurg* 55:282-286, 1981.
166. Sogg RL, Donaldson SS, Yorke CH: Malignant astrocytoma following radiotherapy of a craniopharyngioma. *J Neurosurg* 48:622-627, 1978.
167. Cohen MS, Kushner MJ, Dell S: Frontal lobe astrocytoma following radiotherapy for medulloblastoma. *Neurology* 31:616-619, 1981.
168. Chung CK, Stryker JA, Cruse R, et al: Glioblastoma multiforme following prophylactic cranial irradiation and intrathecal methotrexate in a child with acute lymphocytic leukemia. *Cancer* 47:2563-2566, 1981.

Chapter VI

Neurotoxicity of Tranquilizers and Hypnosedatives

Christopher G. Goetz, M.D., and
Harold L. Klawans, M.D.

Introduction

Tranquilizers and hypnosedatives are ubiquitous medications in Western society, and it is estimated that from 10-20% of adults ingest drugs on a reasonably regular basis to treat tension.[1] The major tranquilizers are neuroleptic agents usually prescribed for psychosis where tranquilization and antipsychotic activity are needed simultaneously. Minor tranquilizers are used to treat the more common and widespread symptom of anxiety. Hypnosedative agents technically are prescribed for insomnia, although they are used widely as antianxiety agents as well.[2,3] Modern society has been accused by some authorities of being overmedicated, overtranquilized, and hence escapist because of these drugs. Others maintain that such agents are relatively inexpensive and affective means of contending with inevitable and normal stress and its accompanying discomfort and misery. The toxicity of tranquilizers and hypnosedatives is important to discuss because of the frequency with which these agents are ingested, and the variety and severity of drug effects and inter-drug relations.

Neuroleptic Agents

The neuroleptic agents or major tranquilizers include the phenothiazine drugs and the butyrophenone, haloperidol. Their antipsychotic activity is felt to relate to blockade of dopaminergic receptors, possibly at the level of the limbic system.[4] As a class, they are associated with a variety of important neurologic complications. These include sedative and autonomic effects, acute dystonic reactions, akathisia, parkinsonism and the late complication of tardive dyskinesia.

Sedation can be profound with initiation of therapy, although since there is only minimal respiratory depression, these drugs are relatively safe. Toxic confusional states may occur, especially in the elderly, an effect probably related to the anticholinergic effects of these drugs.[5] Autonomic changes include alterations in body temperature and mild anticholinergic signs. These drugs are felt to lower the seizure threshold and have been associated with exacerbation of pre-existing epilepsy as well as the appearance of seizures *de novo*. The less potent, more sedative agents (i.e., the aliphatic group, chloropromazine), are more likely to be associated with this phenomenon than the piperazine drugs or haloperidol.[6]

Acute neuroleptic-induced dystonias are seen early in the course of neuroleptic therapy, and are often seen following a single parenteral dose of phenothiazine or haloperidol. The manifestations can be quite diverse although the most common clinical signs involve the eyes and neck. Patients with oculogyric crisis often complain of inability to move their eyes in the vertical plane as well as double vision, blurred vision and, rarely, pain on attempted gaze. Most often the eyes maintain a sustained upward gaze. The severe dystonic displacement of the eyes may itself be painful, as may other severe acute contorting dystonias. The abnormal postures of the head and neck, including opisthotonos, in which the head and neck are in a retrocollic position, give the patient a bizarre appearance. Other muscles may be involved in the acute drug-induced dystonias but these are much less common.[7]

The incidence of dystonia with different neuroleptics seems to parallel the differential incidence of drug-induced parkinsonism, the piperazine agents being the most hazardous.[8] Agents with a high incidence of parkinsonism have a high incidence of drug-induced dystonia, while those with a low incidence of parkinsonism have a low incidence of dystonia. The simultaneous administration of anticholinergic agents is felt to decrease the incidence of neuroleptic-induced dystonia, and the acute administration of anticholinergic agents almost invariably reverses these dystonias. Physiologically, acute neuroleptic-induced dystonia is felt to represent a sudden disruption of basal ganglia function in some way related to dopamine. This alteration is most probably acute dopaminergic receptor blockade since all offending agents are capable of blocking striatal dopamine receptors. The ability of anticholinergic agents to prevent and ameliorate these dystonias suggests that dopamine-acetylcholine balance is involved in these events. Acute therapy involves intravenous or intramuscular injection of an anticholinergic agent. This treatment will ameliorate the dystonia within minutes, but since the anticholinergic effect is short-lived, oral anticholinergic agents should be prescribed for the next 24-48 hours. If the patient's psychosis requires continued neuroleptic therapy, he should be placed on maintenance anticholinergic treatment for several weeks or switched to another neuroleptic (e.g., thioridazine) with a lower propensity to cause dystonia.

The ability of neuroleptics to elicit dystonia disappears to a great extent as the duration of therapy is extended. New dystonias are rare after the first few weeks, and dystonias which occur in the acute phase are usually no longer present after months of therapy. As a result, the anticholinergic agents used to treat and/or prevent dystonia can be decreased and withdrawn in most patients after 1-2 months of use. Drug-induced dystonias are most common in younger patients given prochlorperazine for vomiting and in young adults (especially between the ages of 20 and 40) being started on chronic neuroleptic therapy.

Akathisia is a severe restlessness, subjectively associated with a feeling of intense anxiety. This neuroleptic side effect usually occurs within the first days of therapy and, similarly to the dystonias, anticholinergic treatment rapidly reverses the syndrome. A less common late onset of akathisia has been described, and is not responsive to conventional anticholinergic treatment. The pathophysiology of the condition is not understood, but may relate to acute imbalances between the dopaminergic-cholinergic systems.[5]

Parkinsonism is a frequent side effect of neuroleptic agents. These agents block striatal dopamine receptors so that drug-induced parkinsonism is descriptively indistinguishable from Parkinson's disease. Usually this effect begins within the 2nd to the 4th week of neuroleptic therapy, and rigidity, resting tremor, bradykinesia and postural reflex abnormalities may all be seen. Because of slow clearance of phenothiazines, the syndrome may persist for up to three months after discontinuation of therapy.[9] Generally older patients are more susceptible to the parkinsonian effect of neuroleptics.

Tardive dyskinesias are abnormal, involuntary, choreatic movements that are associated with chronic neuroleptic therapy. The movements usually begin in the face and tongue (lingual-facial-buccal masticatory syndrome) and progress to involve the trunk and extremities. In some cases the diaphragm may be involved, and breathing becomes irregular with grunting, gasping sounds.[10] The pathophysiology of tardive dyskinesia is felt to relate to chronic dopamine receptor site blockade by the neuroleptics, with resultant striatal denervation hypersensitivity. The abnormal movements often are first noticed when the neuroleptic dose is decreased, presumably because the hypersensitive receptors are now no longer blocked, and are therefore exposed to new concentrations of dopamine.[7] Treatment focuses on attempts to diminish dopaminergic activity so that less neurotransmitter will activate the hypersensitive receptors. Reserpine, which depletes presynaptic dopamine, norepinephrine and serotonin stores, has been moderately successful in doses of 1-5 mg/day. The use of cholinergic agonists, choline chloride and lecithin remains experimental. Judicious use of neuroleptic agents in the lowest possible doses, with frequent "drug holidays" where patients receive no medication, may help to decrease the incidence of this drug-induced condition.[11] Treatment of tardive dyskinesia with neuroleptics themselves is clearly treatment with the presumed offending agent, and should be avoided. This short-sighted therapy may temporarily abate the pathophysiology of the condition, but serves to aggravate its pathogenesis.

No consistent neuropathologic changes are seen in these patients, although the possibility remains that ultrastructural receptor site alterations occur.[12] Initially, following neuroleptic withdrawal, tardive dyskinesias may worsen because of better access of dopamine to striatal receptors. This exacerbation, however, is usually only a short-term effect. Tardive dyskinesias in fact are often reversible and may spontaneously remit following neuroleptic withdrawal. Large series with prolonged follow-up after the withdrawal of anti-psychotic drugs have shown that patients can improve for up to two years after drug cessation, and that mildly affected patients are more likely to remit completely. While the syndrome may be reversible in some patients, residual or even progressive chorea can be seen in over half the patients with tardive dyskinesias.[13]

Meprobamate

This drug was introduced as an antianxiety agent in 1955 and although its specific antianxiety affects are equivocal, it is still a widely prescribed compound. It depresses polysynaptic reflexes in the spinal cord, an effect thought to contribute to its muscle relaxant properties. Additionally, it is a mild analgesic and enhances the analgesia effected by other drugs.[2]

The major toxicity of meprobamate relates to sedation and ataxia. Doses of 1600 mg are associated with considerable learning impairment and slowed reaction time. Sedation is enhanced when meprobamate is consumed along with other drugs, including tricyclic antidepressants, monoamine oxidase inhibitors and possibly ethanol. In these instances, or when mild overdosage occurs (blood concentrations of 30-100 mcg/cc), toxic signs include broadbased stumbling gait, slurred speech, vertigo, and drowsiness which may progress to prolonged sleep. Blood levels of 100-200 mcg/cc are associated with hypotension, respiratory depression, and coma. The lethal dose of meprobamate is generally in excess of 40 grams, although an anecdote of death after 12 grams has been reported. Hemodialysis has been advocated for rapid detoxification and elimination can be enhanced with saline-furosemide therapy. In man, meprobamate ingestion has been associated with exacerbation of grand mal and myoclonic epilepsies.

Systemic side effects include hypotension, urticaria, and exacerbation of acute intermittent porphyria (AIP).[3]

Benzodiazepines

These drugs are currently popular anxiolytic agents, and include diazepam (Valium), chlordiazepoxide (Librium) and oxazepam (Serax). Flurazepam (Dalmane) belongs to this class of agents as well but is used primarily as a hypnosedative. Diazepam is additionally used in conjunction with hydantoin to treat status epilepticus. The general mechanism of action of benzodiazepines appears to relate to depression of multisynaptic reflexes throughout the central nervous system.[14] They act as muscle relaxants on the basis of central mechanisms.[15] These drugs are known to effect neurochemical alterations as well, increasing brain GABA levels and decreasing norepinephrine and serotonin.[16]

Although the therapeutic index of benzodiazepines is 10-30 times that of the barbiturates and hence their absolute toxicity is less, adverse reactions are seven times more frequent with benzodiazepines. This statistic apparently relates to the vast number of patients consuming these anxiolytic agents.[17] Adverse reactions are primarily psychiatric and not purely of a traditional neurologic nature. The most frequent toxic symptoms are increased drowsiness or paradoxical excitation. After large doses, exacerbation of neurotic depression has been reported and antisocial behavior, outbursts of temper, and hypnagogic hallucinations may occur.[18] Withdrawal seizures have been reported as well.[19] A peculiar appetite stimulation has been observed at therapeutic and toxic levels of these agents and may relate to hypothalamic alterations.[20]

Hypnosedative Agents: Barbiturates

Barbiturate toxicity is a frequent and hazardous complication of drug ingestion, and is associated with death in 0.5 to 12% of toxic cases.[3] Most of these cases are the result of deliberate attempts at suicide, but many are accidental poisonings in children or in drug abusers, especially those using more than one drug. One peculiar toxic effect that may relate to the high incidence of lethal toxicity has been termed "drug automatism."[21] The patient fails to sleep after ingesting one or two doses of a barbiturate, but becomes confused and unknowingly overdoses himself. In presumed cases of attempted suicide where patients deny intentional overdosage, some investigators feel this denial is of psychogenic origin, although Jansson investigated almost 500 cases of barbiturate intoxication and estimated that one-quarter could be explained as drug automatisms.[22]

A variety of other neurologic signs and symptoms are seen in patients with moderate barbiturate overdose. These often resemble alcoholic inebriation. Early agitation followed by somnalence and difficulty walking with slurred speech is characteristic. In severe intoxication, patients are comatose and the pupils may be constricted. If the patient becomes hypoxic, however, pupillary dilitation will be seen. The EEG may show a characteristic burst suppression pattern with brief episodes of electrical silence with barbiturate coma. Because of barbiturate effects on the brain stem respiratory system, breathing abnormalities are seen early.

Chronic forms of barbiturate intoxication may result from cumulative effects. The resultant signs and symptoms depend upon the amount administered as well as upon individual sensitivity to the drug and variation in the rate of drug metabolism.

Patients with chronic toxic exposure to barbiturates show ataxic gait, slurred speech, periods of intermittent agitation, but generally depressed affect. Tremors and confusion are also characteristic. Ocular symptoms, including diplopia and blindness along with signs such as ptosis and nystagmus have also been reported.[3]

The wide variety of short, medium, and long-acting barbiturates are all associated with the above neurologic syndromes. The onset of action and duration of toxicity differs according to the half life of each drug.[23,24] Further discussion of barbiturate neurotoxicity can be found in Chapter XIII in this book.

Ethchlorvynol (Placidyl)

This agent is a hypnosedative with a rapid onset and short duration of action. In addition, it has anticonvulsant and muscle relaxant properties. As with the barbiturates, the hypnotic effect of this agent is greatly amplified by concomittant alcohol ingestion.[25] The most common side effects associated with ethchlorvynol use is a strange mint-like aftertaste, dizziness, nausea, vomiting, and facial paresthesias. These latter effects may be associated with hyperventilation. Some patients complain of mild mental confusion or "hang over" effects after consuming the drug.[26] Profound hypnosis, weakness, and syncope unrelated to hypotension have been reported. Idiosyncratic reactions, characterized by marked excitement and histrionic behavior, have been seen when the drug was ingested and a delirium may result when the drug is ingested along with antidepressants. The drug is clearly contraindicated in patients with acute intermittent porphyria. Severe intoxication induces deep coma, respiratory depression, bradycardia and hypotension. Death has occurred with a blood concentration of 4 mg/dl.[26]

Chronic abuse of the drug results in both tolerance and physical dependence. Such chronic patients may appear similar to chronic barbiturate patients and be incoordinated, ataxic with slurred speech, confused with nystagmus and again have visual complaints that include scotomas, amblyopia or diplopia. Withdrawal symptoms mostly resemble those seen in delirium tremens and may be especially severe in elderly patients.

Methaqualone

While all 2,3 — disubstituted quinazolines possess hypnotic activity, only methaqualone is available legally. The drug has antitussive activity comparable to that of codeine, although it lacks independent analgesic properties.[3] The drug may possess tranquilizing properties distinct from its sedative effects, but this has not been fully established. In hypnotic doses, numerous neurologic side effects have been reported.[27] Transient or persisting paresthesias and other signs of peripheral neuropathy that may last months to years after the cessation of drug ingestion have been reported, although in such patients multiple drugs were usually ingested. Paradoxical restlessness and anxiety instead of sedation and sleep are also reported with this drug. Excessive dreaming and somnabolism may also occur. As with many of the drugs already mentioned, there is an additive sedating effect of methaqualone with alcohol.[25] Other drug interactions include an enhanced effect of MAO inhibitors and tricyclic antidepressants, and when the drug is ingested along with phenothiazines or tricyclics, epistaxis and menstrual irregularities have been reported in a higher frequency. Unlike many of the drugs already discussed, this drug has been used without difficulty in patients with intermittent porphyria. In overdosage, restlessness and excitement occur followed by delirium and marked myoclonus. Most lethal cases have been in patients who have ingested multiple drugs or methaqualone with alcohol. Treatment of severe overdosage is primarily supportive. Hemodialysis and peritoneal dialysis have not proven markedly effective.

Methaqualone has become a widely abused substance, presumably based on the popular view that it has aphrodisiac activity. Drug culturists have reported that it induces its "high" without drowsiness as seen with barbiturates.[3] Chronic abusers may employ doses ranging to 2 grams per day. Severe generalized seizures have been seen with abrupt withdrawal from such high doses.

Chloral Hydrate

Following oral ingestion, chloral hydrate is rapidly absorbed from the intestinal tract. It is detoxified in the liver, but part is excreted in the urine. Chloral hydrate has been combined with alcohol to produce the well-known "Mickey Finn."[28] There is a wide variation in individual response to chloral hydrate. It is estimated that 10 grams or more is needed to produce acute intoxication, but death may result with as little as 4 grams. Some degree of tolerance may develop, and habitual users have consumed as much as 92 grams without fatal outcome.

The initial toxic symptoms are nausea and vomiting, followed by ataxia and stupor. The medullary centers are often depressed, with a resultant drop in blood pressure, slowing of respiration, and cyanosis. General vasodilatation is frequently marked, causing a slight diminution in body temperature. There may be conjunctivitis and lacrimation with swelling of the eyelids. Pupillary constriction suggestive of morphine poisoning and diplopia may be seen. Aberrations of vision and partial blindness may result from congestion of the optic nerve.[29] In fatal cases death usually occurs within 5 to 10 hours. In some instances, fatal relapse may occur after apparent recovery. Respiratory paralysis is the most frequent cause of death, but cardiac deaths have been reported.

Chronic chloral hydrate intoxication is rare in the United States, but in India, where chloral hydrate addiction is common, chronic toxicity is frequent. In chronic poisoning the face becomes deep red to purple in color. The icteric skin and sclerae are evidence of hepatic damage. Dermatoses of erythematous, urticarial, or purpuric types are frequent. Gastrointestinal disorders are common and, together with hepatic damage and poor nutrition, contribute to the emaciation usually seen in chloral hydrate addicts. Fatigue and sensations of intense cold and faintness are usual. Loss of libido and urinary and menstrual disorders also occur, as well as joint pains, increased sensitivity to cutaneous stimuli, weakness of the legs, and facial palsies.[30] Treatment is symptomatic with attention to respiratory support and maintenance of electrolyte balance.

Glutethimide

Although claimed to be a non-barbiturate hypnotic, glutethimide (Doriden) is closely related to phenobarbital in structure. Since its introduction in 1964, it has become a remarkably popular prescription sedative. As a result, acute poisoning is not unusual.[31] Clinically, the symptoms resemble those of barbiturate overdosage and treatment involves the same supportive measures.[2] Glutethimide has additional strong anticholinergic properties so that in the case of overdosage, pupillary and other anticholinergic effects are evident. The drug may remain in the gastrointestinal tract for extensive periods of time so that gastric lavage may be particularly efficacious in preventing more extensive toxicity.

Bromides

Medicinal bromides, available as inorganic salts or organic compounds, have been used historically in the treatment of epilepsy and various psychoneuroses. The mechanism of action of bromides remains unknown, but may well relate to a general effect on neuronal membranes rather than a selective alteration of enzyme systems.[32] Abuse or inadvertant intoxication has become less common in the United States since proprietary bromide was removed from the market in 1971. Currently, triple bromide, containing potassium, sodium and chloride salts, is available in the U.S. by prescription.

Following ingestion, bromides are rapidly absorbed into the bloodstream and are distributed to all body organs with only minimal amounts reaching the brain. Bromides appear in all secretions and are present in breast milk in sufficient amounts to affect a nursing infant. Acute poisoning is distinctly uncommon, since doses sufficient to cause acute toxicity induce nausea and vomiting with expulsion of the irritant. Chronic intoxication with bromides, however, is frequently observed and the clinical manifestations of poisoning may be divided into: (1) excessive sedation, 30%, (2) delirium, 65%, and (3) hallucinosis, 5%. Excessive sedation begins at blood bromide levels above 150 mg/dl, and is an accentuation of the medicinal effect. A mild drowsiness develops, associated with loss of concentration and occasional insomnia. In bromide delirium, the patient becomes disoriented, with mood disturbances, delusions and possibly hallucinations. The hallucinatory type of toxicity differs from the delirium in that the hallucinations are experienced in an otherwise lucid setting.[33]

Neurologic findings are present in aproximately 60% of intoxicated patients and are commonly fluctuating. Tremor, ataxia, autonomic disturbances and eye abnormalities appear as the most frequent abnormalities. The tremor is a fine postural one and frequently involves the tongue on extension. As intoxication progresses, speech becomes slurred and gait ataxic, although unlike barbiturate intoxication, limb and trunkal coordination are less compromised.[34] Autonomic disturbances with unexplained fever and cardiac arrhythmias are also common, and eye signs have been a frequent source of diagnostic error. Anisocoria, extraocular palsies and dilated pupils with light/near disassociation are reported and, on occasion, small irregular pupils suggest neurosyphilis.[32] Furred tongue, headache, constipation, digestive disturbances, palpitations, fatigue, masked facies and insomnia have also been attributed to bromide toxicity; however, they cannot be reproduced by experimental intoxication.

Two other non-neurologic characteristics seem common in patients with bromide toxicity and may help to suggest the diagnosis in confusing cases. The first is a state of general cachexia suggesting some form of chronic disease, neoplasm or vitamin deficiency. The physiologic basis of this picture is unclear, but when evaluation does not reveal an explainable cause for the cachexia, bromide toxicity should be considered. Secondly, skin involvement is present in approximately one-third of cases, usually manifested as an acneiform eruption over the face, arms and upper trunk. Folliculitis or pemphigoid blisters may also appear.[35] Treatment involves the removal of all bromide substances, and the institution of hydration to promote diuresis. Sodium chloride 30-90 grams /day may aid in rapid bromide elimination.

References

1. Greenblatt DJ, Shader RI: Pharmacotherapy of anxiety. In: Lipton MA, DiMascio A, Killam KF, eds: *Psycho-Pharmacology: A Generation of Progress.* New York, Raven Press, 1978.
2. Gilbert MM, Koepke HH: Relief of musculoskeletal and psychopathological symptoms with meprobamate. *Curr Ther Res* 15:820-832, 1973.
3. Harvey SC: Hypnotics and sedatives. In: Goodman LS, Gilman A, eds: *Pharmacologic Basis of Therapeutics, 6th Ed.* New York, MacMillan, 1980.
4. Van Rossum JM: Significance of dopamine receptor blockade for mechanism of action of neuroleptic drugs. *Arch Int Pharmacol Ther* 160: 492-494, 1966.
5. Simpson GM, Amuso D, Blair JH, Farkas T: Phenothiazine-produced extrapyramidal system disturbance. *Arch Gen Psychiat* 10:199-208. 1964.
6. Goodman LS, Gilman A: Pharmacologic Basis of Therapeutics, London, MacMillan Co., 1971.
7. Klawans HL, Weiner WJ, Nausieda PA: A Textbook of Clinical Neuropharmacology. New York, Raven Press.
8. Ayd FJ: Neuroleptics and extrapyramidal reactions in psychiatric patients. *Rev Can Biol* 20:451-456, 1961.
9. Simpson GM: Neutotoxicity of major tranquilizers. In: Roisin L, Shiraki H, Grcevic N, eds: *Neurotoxicology*, p. 1-7, New York, Raven Press, 1977.
10. Weiner WJ, Goetz CG, Nausieda PA, Klawans HL: Respiratory dyskinesia, extrapyramidal dysfunction and dyspnea. *Ann Intern Med* 88:327-331, 1978.
11. Klawans HL, Goetz CG, Perlik S: Tardive dyskinesia: review and re-update. *Am J Psych* 137:900-908, 1980.
12. Jellinger K: Neuropathologic findings after neuroleptic long term therapy. In: Roisin L, Shiraki H, Grcevic N, eds: *Neurotoxicology*. New York, Raven Press, 1977.

13. Hersohn HL, Kennedy PF, McGuire RJ: Persistance of extrapyramidal disorders and psychiatric relapse after long term phenothiazine therapy. *Br J Psychiat* **120**:41-50, 1972.
14. Ban TA, Amin M: Hypnotics, minor tranquilizers and sedatives. In: Vinken PJ, Bruyn GW, eds: Handbook of Clinical Neurology Vol 37. Amsterdam, North-Holland Publishing Co., 1979, pp 347-365.
15. Cohen IM: Benzodiazepines. In: Ayd FJ, Blackwell B, eds: *Discoveries in Biological Psychiatry.* Philadelphia , Lippincott, 1970, p 130.
16. Cook L, Seginwald J: Behavioral analysis of effect and mechanism of action of benzodiazepines. In: Costa E, Greengard P, eds: *Mechanism of Action of Benzodiazepines.* New York, Raven Press, 1975.
17. Goth A: *Medical Pharmacology.* St. Louis, C.V. Mosby, 1972.
18. Greenblatt DJ, Shrader RI: *Benzodiazepines. N Engl J Med* **291**:1011, 1974.
19. Hollister LE,, Motzenbecker FP, Degan RO: Withdrawal reactions from chlordiazepoxide. *Psychopharmacology* **2**:63, 1961.
20. Jarvik ME: Benzodiazepines. In: Goodman LS, Gilman A, eds: *Pharmacologic Basis of Therapeutics.* London, MacMillan Co., 1970.
21. Aitken RCB, Proudfoot AJ: Barbiturate automatism — Myth or malady. *Postgrad Med J* **45**:612-616, 1969.
22. Jansson B: Drug automatism as a cause of pseudosuicide. *Postgrad Med J* **30**:A34-A40, 1961.
23. Mann JB, Sandberg DH: Therapy of sedative overdosage. *Ped Clin N Amer* **17**:617-628, 1970.
24. Matthew H, ed: *Acute Barbiturate Poisoning.* Amsterdam, Excerpta Medica, 1970.
25. Breimer DD: Clinical pharmacokinetics of hypnotics. *Clin Pharmacokin* **2**:93-109, 1977.
26. Cummings LM, Martin YC, Scherfling EE: Serum and urine levels of ethchlorvynol in man. *J Pharmacol* **60**:261-263, 1971.
27. Marriott PF: Methaqualone with psychotrophic drugs: Adverse interaction. *Med J Aust* **1**:412-418, 1976.
28. Adams WL: The toxicity of chloral alcoholate. *J Pharmacol Exp Ther* **69**:273, 1940.
29. Lewin L: Phantastica, Narcotic, and Stimulating Drugs: Their Uses and Abuse. London, K. Paul, French, Trubner & Co., Ltd. 1931.
30. Stalker NE, Gambertoglio JG, Fukumitsu CJ: Acute massive chloral hydrate intoxication treated with hemodialysis. *J Clin Pharmacol* **18**: 136-142, 1978.
31. Nover R: Persistent neuropathy following chronic use of glutethimide. *Clin Pharmacol Ther* **8**:283, 1967.
32. Moses H, Klawans HL: Bromide intoxication. In: Vinken PJ, Bruyn GW, eds: *Handbook of Clinical Neurology.* Vol 36. Amsterdam, North-Holland Publishing Co., 1979, pp 291-318.
33. Levin M: Transitory schizophrenia produced by bromide intoxication. *Amer J Psychiat* **103**:229-240, 1946.
34. Moore M, Sohler T, Alexander L: Bromide intoxication. Confin. *Neurol* **3**:1-18, 1940.
35. Greenblatt M, Levin S, Schegloff B: EEG findings in cases of bromide intoxication. *Arch Neurol Psychiat* **53**:431-433, 1945.

Chapter VII

Neurologic Complications of Anesthesia

E. Jane Woolley, M.D.

Introduction

Modern anesthetic techniques have made it possible to perform surgical procedures that are nearly unlimited in scope and duration, and to provide a safe and pain-free operation for the patient. "An outstanding feature of anesthesia, as ordinarily seen, is the fact that removal of the anesthetic from the blood restores the nervous system to its original activity without any appreciable damage," wrote Henderson and Haggard in 1927.[1] Although a wide range of extraordinary conditions may prevent the return of the nervous system to its original activity, neurologic complications of anesthesia are infrequent events. The number of anesthetics given in the United States in one year approximates 20,623,000,[2] and for these, the reported incidence of serious neurologic complications is less than 0.05 percent.[3] These unfortunate situations, in which damage to the nervous system occurs, range in spectrum from minor, transient aches to fatal cerebral anoxia and may involve the brain, spinal cord, or the peripheral nerves.

Physicians caring for the anesthetized patient are responsible for protecting the patient from injury during the course of anesthesia. Postanesthetic neurologic complications frequently result in malpractice litigation. The more severe hypoxic injuries, in which patients suffer postoperative brain damage, have resulted in enormous awards being bestowed upon the plaintiff. A Florida jury recently awarded a 26-year-old cancer patient with postoperative brain damage $6.7 million.[4] This is the largest malpractice verdict ever reached in that state. With a precedent of this magnitude, future awards may exceed this amount; however, there is no amount of money that can compensate for the tragedy of brain damage for the patient, his family, or his physician.

Many neurologic injuries during anesthesia are preventable. A recent study from the United Kingdom[5] analyzed the anesthetic accidents reported from 1970-1977. Of 602 cases reported, 60% involved cerebral hypoxia and death, and 47% of these were due to faulty technique. One-third were due to esophageal intubation. Other causes were aspiration, hypotension, misuse of ventilators, and inattention by the attending anesthesiologist. Seventy percent of these major catastrophies of death or brain damage during anesthesia were caused by physician error. These are summarized in Table I. Dripps, et al, reported 80 deaths from anesthesia and attributed 87% to human error;[6] Clifton and Hatten, 65% of 52 deaths; and Edwards, et al, 83% of 589 deaths.[7]

Prevention is the best treatment for any potential neurologic injury to a patient during his anesthetic course. Awareness of possible injuries with appropriate prophylactic measures, meticulous attention to detail during the administration of anesthesia, and careful and complete recordkeeping will reduce the incidence of complications in patients as well as decrease the physician's susceptibility to malpractice litigation.

This chapter will deal with etiology, clinical cause, and possible treatment of neurologic complications from hypoxia (either from reduced arterial oxygenation or from hypotension), techniques of anes-

Table I
Major Catastrophies:
Causes of Death and Cerebral Damage Treated Together

	Number of Cases	Percent
Faulty technique	163	46.8
Coexisting disease	37	10.6
Unknown	36	10.3
Failure of postoperative care	33	9.5
Drug overdose	18	5.2
Drug sensitivity	16	4.6
Halothane hepatic failure	12	3.4
Hyperthermia	8	2.9
Blood loss	6	1.7
Failure of preoperative assessment	5	1.4
Drug error	5	1.4
Anesthesiologist failure	5	1.4
Embolism	3	0.9
Clot in bypass	1	0.3
Total	348	

From Utting JE, Gray TC, Shelley FC: Human misadventure in anesthesia. *Can Anaesth Soc J* **26**:472, 1979, with permission.

thesia (i.e., dural puncture, nerve blocks), positioning of patients, neurotoxic effects and adverse reactions to anesthetic agents, and patient variations.

Hypoxia

Cerebral Hypoxia

Hypoxia causes central nervous system damage. It may be caused by decreased blood pressure, decreased vascular patency, or decreased arterial oxygen saturation. Table II lists the causes of inadequate oxygenation to the central nervous system.

The neurons of the brain require a continuous supply of oxygen. Total oxygen deprivation for 3 to 5 minutes may produce permanent

---

Table II
Causes of Inadequate Oxygenation of the Central Nervous System

Decreased Blood Pressure
    Hypovolemia
    Shock of any etiology
    Air embolism (acting on the heart)
    Depressant actions on anesthetic agents on the myocardium and peripheral
        vascular tone
    Cardiac disease
    Circulatory arrest
Decreased Vascular Patency or Tone
    Thrombosis
    Air embolism (in cerebral vessels)
    Stasis (from hypoxic capillary dilation)
Decreased Arterial Oxygen Saturation
    Inadequate respiratory exchange
        Depression from anesthetic agents or muscle relaxants
        Airway obstruction
    Inadequate oxygen content of respired gases
        Altitude
    Obesity
    Obstructive lung disease
    Restrictive lung disease
    Thoracic cage injuries or deformities
    Inadequate oxygen-carrying capacity of the blood
        Anemia
        Carbon monoxide poisoning
        Hemorrhage with hemodilutions

From Hunter CR, Dornette WHL: Neurologic injuries in the unconscious patient. *Clin Anesth* **18**:351-367, 1972, with permission.

neurologic damage. Partial deprivation of oxygen for longer periods can produce equally hazardous results.[8,9] The higher, more uniquely developed neurons — those dealing with intellect, memory, and perception — are more sensitive to oxygen lack than the lower centers of the brain; and so they are more readily injured. The oxygen reaching the brain must have adequate partial pressure for utilization. Since partial pressure of oxygen is determined by the arterial saturation and the arterial blood pressure, any cause of reduced blood pressure or arterial oxygen saturation will interfere with cerebral oxygenation. Hypoxia of cerebral capillaries causes capillary dilation, which further reduces blood flow and increases hypoxia. This stasis and hypoxia result in cerebral vascular damage and edema.[10]

Brain Metabolism

The brain derives its energy from glucose, which is metabolized to pyruvate. Five to eight percent of pyruvate is anaerobically converted to lactate, and the remainder enters the Krebs cycle, being metabolized to CO_2 and H_2O. The Krebs cycle utilizes oxygen and produces energy in the form of high energy phosphate at a rapid rate. The production of high energy phosphate from lactate (anaerobic) metabolism produces inadequate energy to maintain normal cerebral function.[11,12]

In mild cerebral hypoxia, lactate production increases in the brain and is reflected by increased lactate levels in CSF and cerebral venous blood. Glucose consumption increases; however, measurable cerebral oxygen consumption is unchanged.[13] High energy phosphate levels are maintained. In extreme hypoxia, cerebral oxygen consumption decreases because high energy phosphate stores in the brain are depleted; EEG slowing occurs at a P_aO_2 of 35 torr, or when cerebral blood flow is 40% of normal due to ischemia. An isolectric EEG implies severe hypoxic damage to the brain cells.[14]

Causes of Hypoxia

Cardiac Arrest

Clinically, total cerebral hypoxia results from cardiac arrest. Energy stores in the brain under these circumstances will be depleted within 3 to 5 minutes, reflecting high lactate levels. Resuscitation of neurons is possible after 8 minutes of hypoxia; however, longer periods of ischemia result in irreversible damage. Total ischemia is aggravated by capillary microthrombi and by perivascular swelling.[15]

Incomplete Ischemia

Incomplete cerebral ischemia may result from vascular occlusion, increased intracranial pressure, arterial hypotension, arterial spasm, air embolus, or reduced arterial oxygenation.

Mild oxygen deprivation may cause personality changes, apathy, convulsions, tinnitus, and headaches that may be transient or permanent. Severe oxygen deprivation may lead to permanent neurologic injury or death. It is difficult to predict the end result in patients with partial oxygen deprivation, particularly prolonged hypotension. Total oxygen deprivation for more than three minutes results in irreversible brain damage with a vegetative organism — spastic, convulsing, and out of touch with his environment; and this can be predicted without equivocation.

Hypotension

Hypotension may also result in focal injury, especially to the occipital cortex resulting in cortical blindness. Areas of the cortex requiring the greatest arterial pressure for perfusion are most susceptible to hypotension.[16] Patients with arteriosclerotic plaques of the cerebral vessels tolerate cerebral hypotension poorly.[17] They already may have borderline perfusion to oxygen-sensitive cortical areas. Regions farthest from the circle of Willis are the first to suffer damage in cerebral hypotension.[16] Echenhoff et al found that healthy volunteers tolerated marked hypotension of 50 torr for a mean of 39 minutes with no apparent neurologic deficit.[18]

Arterial Hypoxemia

In patients with arterial hypoxemia (anemia, decreased arterial oxygen saturation) cerebral blood flow increases so as to deliver adequate O_2 to the brain. This condition is rather well tolerated if the patient is normotensive. If hypotension occurs, rapid deterioration will occur.

Venous Air Embolism

Venous air is a complication of the sitting position for neurosurgical procedures. It has been reported to occur in as few as 1.6% to as many as 93% of patients in the sitting position.[19,20] Neurologic damage may result from cardiac arrest secondary to a massive air embolus in the heart (total cerebral ischemia), or from occlusion of multiple cerebral capillaries from tiny air bubbles (incomplete cerebral ischemia). Mortality rates in reports in the literature range from 0 to 73%,[20] and postoperative complications depend upon the amounts of air absorbed.

Air enters venous channels because of subatmospheric pressure in open veins. The usual sources are the suboccipital veins, dural sinuses, diploic veins, veins in the tumor being operated upon,[21] and burr holes.[20] Infusion of air is usually slow, and so it may be unrecognized until disaster strikes.

Obesity Supine Death Syndrome

Markedly obese patients present a difficult problem in management of anesthesia and are at great risk of compromised cerebral oxygenation. These patients have a reduction in the total respiratory system compliance , which results from abnormal compliance of the chest wall and the lungs, along with increased oxygen consumption, cardiac output, and blood volume.[22] Many of these patients hypoventilate. The resulting low functional residual capacity leads to abnormal ventilation to perfusion ratios.[23] Many morbidly obese patients are in chronic congestive heart failure, and this adds to the dimished lung compliance. Severe hypoxia and hypercapnia added to the increase in cardiac output that occurs in the obese patient in the supine position frequently leads to cardiac collapse and death.[24]

Successful anesthetic management of the morbidly obese patient can be accomplished with adequate oxygenation and controlled mechanical ventilation to relieve the work of breathing.

Prevention of Hypoxia

Prevention of hypoxia is so basic to providing safe anesthesia that it is almost too elementary to discuss; however, since 65 to 85% of reported cases of cerebral hypoxia are caused by physician error, this is where the risk occurs, and preventive measures should be taken to assure adequate oxygenation of the patient.

Monitoring of the patient undergoing anesthesia should include blood pressure, stethoscope, EKG, oxygen analyzer, and temperature — even on simple cases. The more sophisticated monitoring devices of arterial lines for direct blood pressure and arterial blood gases should be used in high-risk surgery, in the critically ill, or when excessive blood loss is anticipated. Swan Ganz catheter, central venous lines, and Dopplers are useful in special circumstances. These monitors are adjuncts to proper anesthesia and do not obviate careful evaluation of the patient. It is important to know the patient's history, physical examination, past surgical and anesthetic experiences, allergies, and medications. Intra-operative evaluation of the patient includes clinical evaluation along with monitoring devices to assist in evaluating the total picture.

Blood Pressure and Pulse

One of the early signs of hypoxia and/or hypercarbia is increase in blood pressure and pulse. Light anesthesia causes similar changes. Evaluation of the patient for signs of cyanosis or hypoventilation will help to determine the proper cause of action.

EKG

Evidence of myocardial ischemia in surgery when only one lead is being used is most readily noted by using the bipolar CM5 lead (central maniburium 5th interspace in the left axillary line). It is the best available method using a single lead to detect T-wave and ST-segment changes during ischemic episodes.[25]

Temperature

Slight increases noted in body temperature during induction of anesthesia will aid in the early diagnosis of malignant hyperthermia.

Oxygen Analyzer

The Joint Commission of Accreditation of the American Hospital Association requires oxygen analyzers on all anesthesia machines.[26] Use of "low flow" anesthesia mandates the use of an oxygen analyzer for adequate delivery of oxygen to the patient. Central oxygen supplies in hospitals, oxygen analyzers, and "fail safe" alarms in anesthesia machines should eliminate the accidental delivery of 100% N_2O to an anesthetized patient.

Stethoscope

Either a precordial or esophageal stethoscope will enable one to listen to heart and breath sounds.

Arterial Lines

Arterial lines are extremely useful for patients in whom rapid changes in blood pressure are anticipated and for the critically ill who require frequent blood gas determinations as well as careful monitoring. This procedure is not without risk of arterial occlusion and should not be used indiscriminately. Excellent non-invasive blood pressure monitors are available for routine anesthesia.

Central Venous Lines

Central venous lines are useful for central venous pressure measurements, as a long-term site for intravenous therapy and for aspiration of air in patients having air embolus.

Doppler

Dopplers are useful for patients in whom air embolus may occur during anesthesia.

Swan Ganz Catheters[25]

The triple lumen Swan Ganz catheter measures right heart function by giving accurate values of stroke volume, right atrial pressure and mean pulmonary arterial pressure.

Treatment of Hypoxia

Treatment of cerebral hypoxia attempts to reduce cerebral metabolic rate, reduce cerebral hypertension, decrease cerebral edema, and improve oxygenation.

Hypothermia

Hypothermia has been used for protection of the brain during surgical procedures in which reduced cerebral circulation was anticipated and to protect a brain from cerebral edema following an ischemic insult.[27] Protection with hypothermia may extend safe periods of cerebral circulatory arrest from 4 minutes at 37°C to 35 minutes at 17°C.[28] This protection probably results from a decrease in cerebral oxygen consumption, as well as a leftward shift of the O_2 dissociation curve.

Recent techniques have been developed in the Rhesus monkey to selectively cool the brain to temperatures of 5-8°C without evidence of neurologic deterioration. This technique of selective hypothermia may prove to be useful in preventing brain death after episodes of cerebral anoxia.[29]

Hyperventilation

Hyperventilation has been used to produce hypocapnea and thus lower cerebral blood flow by cerebral vasoconstriction. This has been advocated to protect patients undergoing carotid endarterectomy by producing less ischemia distal to the carotid clamp. In practice, this has not appeared to be helpful, and in fact some patients seem worse from hyperventilation.

Barbiturate Coma

Barbiturates have been in use to treat cerebral insults for 15 years. It is especially useful in treating patients with cerebral ischemia, increased intracranial pressure, and encephalopathies.[30]

The mechanism by which barbiturates act to protect the brain is that barbiturates decrease cerebral oxygen consumption (C MR_o) up to 50% and slow the rate of depletion of high energy phosphate. This probably reflects decreased cerebral function. Barbiturates are also potent cerebral vasoconstrictors. Cerebral edema is also reduced in barbiturate coma, and capillary flow is less impaired.[31,32]

It has also been suggested that barbiturates are free radical scavengers and prevent the build up of material destructive to lipid membranes.[28] A direct membrane stabilizing effect has also been postulated. Finally, Frost et al have shown that barbiturates act on the pulmonary vasculature to decrease ventilation-perfusion inequities in hypoxia, and thus improve oxygenation.[30]

Barbiturate coma is carried out in an intensive care unit, and requires a specialized team consisting of critical care physicians, ICU nurse, respiratory therapist, and physiotherapist. It is not a treatment to be undertaken in a small community hospital. Patients are intubated, and on respiratory control with a volume ventilator. Monitoring includes arterial pressure, blood gases, temperature, EEG and serum barbiturate levels.

Serious complications may accompany barbiturate coma. These include hypotension, hypoventilation, lung infections, hypothermia, pressure sores, urinary tract infections, phlebitis, vitamin K deficiency, and prolonged coma.[30,32]

Iatrogenic barbiturate coma has proved useful in the treatment of increased intracranial pressure and encephalophathies. The results after cerebral anoxia following cardiac arrest are not encouraging; however, controlled studies are not yet available to determine its long range effectiveness.

Steroids

High doses of steroids are being used, and this too will require future evaluation.

Prophylaxis and Treatment of Air Embolism

A Doppler ultrasound monitor is a very sensitive way to detect air infusion into the heart. Changes in heart sounds occur at a rate of 0.05 ml air/kg/min. Changes heard by an esophageal stethoscope occur at a rate of 1.7 ml/kg/min. Central venous pressure (0.4 ml/kg/min) and EKG changes (peaking of P waves) are also less sensitive than a Doppler. Two ml air/kg/min is usually fatal.

A "chirp" heard on the Doppler is characteristic of air embolism. Immediate treatment, important for a positive outcome, involves flooding the operative field with saline, use of bone wax, pressure on the jugular vein, increasing central venous pressure with positive end expiratory pressure, and aspirating air through the right atrial catheter.

Slow leaks of air may go unnoticed if adequate monitoring is not used, and the results in this case will be diagnosed as prolonged hypotension, which may be blamed erroneously on the anesthesia. The complication of air embolism is well recognized in modern anesthesia, and with proper monitoring and early treatment the patient will be unharmed.[32-34]

Post Anoxic (Delayed) Encephalopathy

Delayed post anoxic encephalopathy has been reported following cardiac arrest, anesthesia, and carbon monoxide poisoning. It occurs in less than 1 per 1000 cases of anoxia. After a period of anoxia, there is apparent full recovery for a period of 2 to 21 days, after which signs of encephalopathy·begin to occur. The lucid interval is followed by irritability, apathy, confusion, skeletal muscle spasticity with rigidity, leading to coma and death. The EEG shows non-focal abnormalities. At postmortem, these brains are found to have diffuse, demyelination of the cerebral white matter. Infarction of the basal ganglia may be seen. The cause of demyelination is unclear, but it seems to be related to early ambulation followed by cerebral edema and vasculitis. Patients recovering from anoxic episodes must be treated with sedation, bed rest, and measures to decrease cerebral edema until there is no evidence of neurologic damage.[35]

Nerve Injuries

Nerve injuries that occur during anesthesia and that are not caused by surgical damage most commonly result from pressure, stretching or ischemia. Other causes may be chemical from extravasation of drugs or solutions, thermal injuries, either by hypothermia or cautery (electrical burns.) Postoperatively patients may present neurologic lesions from previously unrecognized metabolic disorders, tumors, infections, or neurologic disease.[36]

Any postoperative patient with a nerve injury requires a careful work-up to determine the etiology of injury so that effective therapy can be instituted, as well as for medicolegal reasons for responsibility.

The electromyogram is useful in the differential diagnosis of recent versus pre-existing nerve injury. Neuron degeneration requires at least 18 to 21 days for typical EMG changes to be demonstrated. A patient with nerve injury in the immediate postoperative period with neuron degeneration diagnosed by EMG had nerve damage before surgery.

The most common postoperative neurologic complication, other than surgical interruption of a nerve, is caused by faulty position of the patient during anesthesia. The anesthesiologist is charged with protecting the unconscious patient from nerve injuries by careful positioning and padding where necessary.

Nerves with long anatomic courses in the body are more prone to injury than shorter ones. Nerves in ischemic areas are more susceptible to injury than those with normal blood supply, and malnourished nerves are more susceptible than normal ones. Mild stretching of a nerve will rupture epineural vessels and cause ischemic patches in the nerve. Forceful stretching causes hematomas that may necrose nerve fibers.

Postoperative nerve injuries may be mild with temporary paresis to complete fibrous replacement of the nerve with permanent disability.[37]

Peripheral neuropathies have been reported in many nerves, and nearly every peripheral nerve may be injured under certain circumstances. The injuries most commonly seen postoperatively are those of the brachial plexus, the ulnar nerve, and the common peroneal nerve. It is interesting that these are also nerves that are easily protected from injury if proper positioning and padding are used.

Pressure from arm boards, operating table, or tourniquet pressure may cause injuries that are related to the duration and intensity of the pressure.

The following discussion of specific nerve injuries is classified as to anatomic location and not to reported incidence of injuries.

Nerves of the Head and Neck

Cranial Nerves

Cranial nerves are subject to injury for several reasons. Injury to the nerve trunk is caused by stretching or pressure; the nucleus of the nerve is injured primarily by hypoxia.

I. *Olfactory Nerve*

Damage of the olfactory nerve results from cerebral hypoxia and has not been reported as an isolated complication.

II. *Optic Nerve*

Optic neuropathy has been reported as a postoperative complication of cataract extractions following both local or general anesthesia.

Injection of local anesthetic to produce retrobulbar anesthesia may cause ischemia of the optic nerve due to unrecognized hemorrhage or to toxic effect of the drug on the nerve.

Digital pressure on the eye to enhance the retrobulbar block has also been considered as the cause of ischemic optic neuropathy.

Patients having postoperative optic neuropathy after general anesthesia may have had hypotensive episodes to cause neuropathy or a coincidental ischemic episode unrelated to surgery and anesthesia. Cataract patients frequently have arteriosclerotic heart disease and are more likely to suffer vascular accidents than the younger patient.[38]

Postoperative ocular symptoms due to pressure on the eye, either from the anesthetic mask or the prone position are reported in about 4% of patients. The symptoms resulting from prolonged decreased intraocular pressure due to external pressure on the eye were blurred vision and ocular pain lasting up to 6 hours. A combination of pressure on the eyeball and hypotension may cause retinal artery thrombosis and blindness.[39]

III. *Oculomotor Nerve*

Damage to this nerve is usually the result of hypoxia to the brainstem.

IV. *Trochlear Nerve*

Injury of the trochlear nerve is similar to injuries of the oculomotor. It is caused by cerebral hypoxia.

V. *Trigeminal Nerve*

Terminal branches of the trigeminal nerve are injured by pressure on the bony structures of the orbit and nose.

A. *Supraorbital Nerve*

Paresis of the supraorbital nerve results in photophobia, numbness of forehead, and pain in the eye. This injury has been reported from pressure due to metal endotracheal tube adaptors or pressure from a Hudson's harness to hold the endotracheal tube. Permanent supraorbital paralysis has not been reported. Recovery occurs within one to three weeks of surgery.[40]

B. *Infraorbital, Supratrochlear, and Infratrochlear Nerves*

The infraorbital, supratrochlear, and infratrochlear nerves are injured on the face adjacent to the orbit or the nose by excessive pressure from a mask. The injury results in sensory loss of the skin innervated by the affected nerve. This injury is temporary and disappears within two to three weeks.

C. Trichloethelyne injuries to the nerve will be discussed under anesthetic agents.

VI. *Abducens Nerve*

This nerve is not damaged by pressure during anesthesia. Complications after spinal anesthesia are discussed under spinal anesthesia.

VII. *Facial Nerve*

Injuries to the facial nerve, with resultant paralysis, have occurred from unusual forward pressure of the jaw to maintain an airway or too tight head straps during anesthesia. Symptoms are numbness of the tongue and loss of taste sensation or weakness of the muscle around the mouth or eyes. This injury is due to trauma to the lingual and accompanying chorda tympani nerves from pressure on them by the lateral and medial pterygoid muscles where the joined nerves pass between them. Symptoms will usually disappear within one to two weeks.[41,42]

VIII. *Auditory Nerve*

This is extremely sensitive to hypoxia. Postoperative damage has followed a hypotensive or hypoxic episode causing symptoms of tinnitus and deafness.

IX. *Glossopharyngeal Nerve*

This nerve is very resistant to injury.

X. *Vagus Nerve*

Injury to the recurrent laryngeal branch of the vagus will be discussed under Vocal Cord injuries. Central injuries are secondary to hypoxia.

XI. *Spinal Accessory Nerve*

It is not injured.

XII. *Hypoglossal Nerve*

During carotid artery dissection for carotid endarterectomy surgery, the hypoglossal nerve is retracted and palsy of the hypoglossal nerve may occur. This is complicated only by deviation of the tongue to the ipsilateral side. If, however, a carotid endarterectomy is performed on the second side before the opposite hypoglossal function has returned, a bilateral hypoglossal paralysis may occur causing the patient to have postoperative difficulty immediately with speaking, swallowing, and maintaining a patent airway while in the supine position. The latter problem can be a hazard in the recovery room, if not recognized. Airway obstruction is relieved if the patient is in the sitting position.[43]

Cervical Spinal Roots

Injuries of the cervical spinal nerve roots reported after anesthesia result from injury at the exit of the nerves between the vertebrae. The cervical spine is mobile at the base of the skull and between the first and second, and the second and third vertebrae. These nerves are most susceptible to injury. The other stress points are C5-6 and C6-7.

Occipital neuralgia occurs from hyperextension of the head pressing the posterior ramus of the second cervical nerve (greater occipital nerve) between the arches of the first and second cervical vertebrae; this results in severe occipital headache.

Brachial Plexus (Figs. 1-6)

The most common neurologic injury after anesthesia related to the body position during surgery is injury to the brachial plexus. This condition was first reported in 1894 by Budinger as a toxic reaction to chloroform.[44] In 1899 Horsely found microscopic evidence of trauma after stretching the brachial plexuses of cadavers.[45] Halstead in 1908 concluded that the injury resulted from compression of the plexus between the clavicle and the transverse processes of the cervical vertebrae or the clavical and the first rib.[46] Dhuner studied 30,000 patients and found 31 with post-anesthesia nerve injuries — 26 of these involved the upper extremities; 11 had brachial plexus injuries. Stretching of the nerves appears to be the mechanism of injury.[47]

The nerves of the brachial plexus are fixed in the neck to the transverse processes of the spinal vertebrae by the prevertebral fascia and in the arm by the axillary fascia. Abduction of the arm, hyperextension,

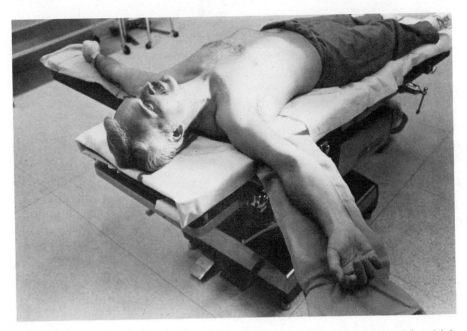

Figure 1. * Arms abducted more than 90° causes excessive stretching of brachial plexus around the humeral head.

and external rotation all place unusual stresses on the nerves by stretching them between their fixed points. The addition of shoulder braces compounds the stresses. Anatomic structures in the neck and shoulder area, such as the scalene muscles, the coracoid process of the scapula and the head of the humerus, add to the possibilities of stretching the nerves. This results in microscopic damage, hemorrhage, and ischemia resulting in palsies.[42]

Positions of the arm that cause unusual stress to the brachial plexus are five:

1. Flexion of the head to one side with downward or backward displacement of the shoulder.

2. Hyperabduction of the arm stretches the nerves around the humeral head.

3. Abduction of the arm, external rotation, and dorsal extension press the nerves between the clavicle and the first rib.

4. Lateral position with the upper arm hanging freely over chest allowing the clavicle to compress the plexus against the first rib.

5. Prone position with arms abducted 90° and elbows flexed 90°, if

* Photography (Figures 1-10) by William Widmayer, Verdugo Hills Hospital.

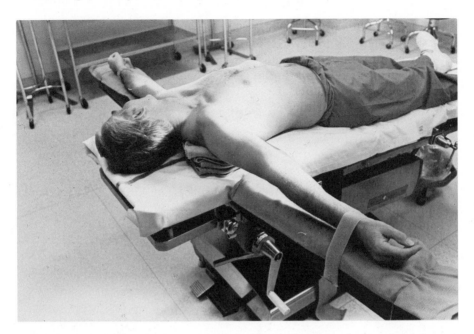

Figure 2. Arms abducted 90° with block under shoulder and head turned stretches the brachial plexus.

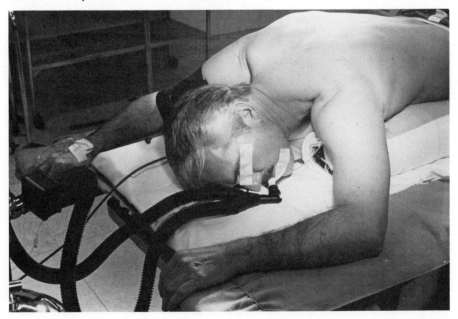

Figure 3. Large rolls cause shoulders to fall forward compressing brachial plexus between clavicle and coracoid process.

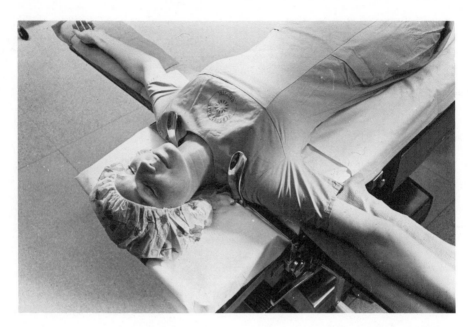

Figure 4. Shoulder braces with arms abducted 90° cause direct pressure on the brachial plexus.

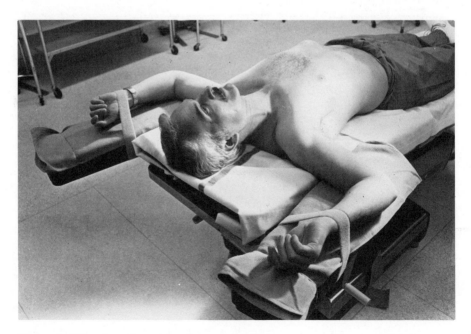

Figure 5. "Hands up" position for sternotomy causes excessive stretching by external rotation.

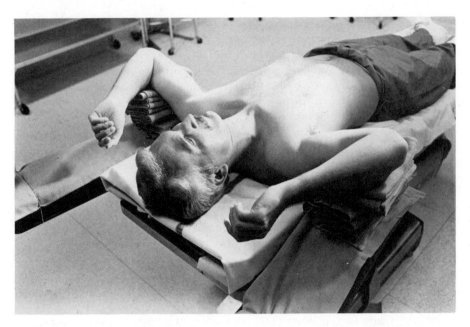

Figure 6. Support of elbows in "hands up" position relieves tension on brachial plexus.

chest rolls are too large and if head is not properly supported, will allow greater abduction than 90° with stretching of the plexus.

Jackson and Keats[48] studied 15 adult cadavers in which they placed the upper extremity in various positions to determine the effect on the brachial plexus. They found that (1) the head-down position with shoulder braces and (2) abduction of the arm to more than 90° caused prominent stretch. There was no more stretching with both arms abducted than with one. They also studied the "hands up" position used in open heart surgery and median sternotomy. In this position the upper arms are abducted 90°-135° toward the head with elbows flexed. Three postoperative palsies have been reported following this position.[48] The position with one arm abducted and the head resting on the palm of the hand has also caused paralysis from stretching.

Postoperative nerve palsies have been reported to be unilateral, bilateral, motor, mixed motor, and sensory. They may last for 21 weeks to one year. No permanent injuries have been reported. Erbs palsy (upper brachial plexus), including damage to long thoracic nerve with resultant serratus anticus paralysis is most common. Klumpke's paralysis (lower brachial plexus roots) occurs one tenth as often as Erbs.

During recovery, sensory loss returns first, followed by lower motor neuron, and finally upper motor neuron recovery occurs.[49]

Costoclavicular syndrome may occur in the sitting position causing pressure on the brachial plexus which may occur with certain movements of the shoulder (backward and downward thrust). This causes pain, numbness, congestion in the hands, and weakness of the arms. Patel et al report a case of costoclavicular syndrome in a two-year-old after anesthesia in a sitting position.[50]

Radial pulses should be checked in patients in the sitting position to assure that the neurovascular bundle is not compromised in the unconscious patient.

In Jackson's series of 34 brachial plexus injuries, three also had Horner's syndrome on the side of injury unrelated to the surgical procedure.[48]

Injuries to the brachial plexus are preventable by proper positioning of the patient during surgery. The anesthesiologist must watch during surgery for change of position that may cause stretching or compression.

In the "hands up" position, stretching is eliminated by raising the elbows 6 inches off the table. In any position, abduction greater than 90° may result in injury; however, abduction accompanied by rotation has caused injury with as little as 60° abduction. The use of steep Trendelenburg and shoulder braces and abduction of the arms should be avoided.[48]

Treatment

Physiotherapy and support of the arm with a sling should be started immediately after a careful neurologic examination is carried out. B-complex vitamins are recommended to improve the nutrition of the nerve.

Circumflex Nerve

A case of circumflex nerve injury following laproscopy was reported by Ellul resulting from pressure upon the patient's shoulder. This patient exibited complete paralysis of the deltoid muscle and loss of sensation over the lower part of deltoid. This was treated with physiotherapy with partial return of function. Residual atrophy of post deltoid muscle persisted.[51]

Radial Nerve

Paresis of the radial nerve has been reported and is probably caused by pressure of a sharp edge of the table or arm board against the area of arm where the radial nerve wraps around the humerus. Paresis of the dorsal antebrachial cutaneous branch of the radial nerve has been reported to occur within as short a surgical time as 45 minutes.

Radial nerve injuries occur in the anesthetized patient from external pressure from improperly padded operating arm boards or Mayo stands, from tourniquet pressure used for orthopedic procedures, or from accidental injections of drugs into the nerve. Wrist drop and loss of sensation of the skin of the dorsal part of the radial two-thirds of the hand are evidence of radial nerve injury.[8,47]

Ulnar Nerve (Figs. 7 and 8)

Ulnar nerve paresis after anesthesia is caused by pressure on the elbow, causing cubital tunnel syndrome. Many of these patients also have tenderness near the ulnar epicondyle. Very little pressure may cause damage to the ulnar nerve as it passes through the ulnar groove. It may be caused by immobilization of the forearm in a flexed, prone position or from prolonged elbow flexion. The forearm in a supinated position with adequate padding during surgery is optimal.

Postoperative patients who are heavily sedated may exert pressure on the ulnar nerve and should be moved frequently to avoid this. An anesthesiologist colleague who had gastric surgery developed an ulnar paresis in the postoperative period, which he attributes to prolonged pressure from lying on his arm on the nerve while he was sedated for pain.

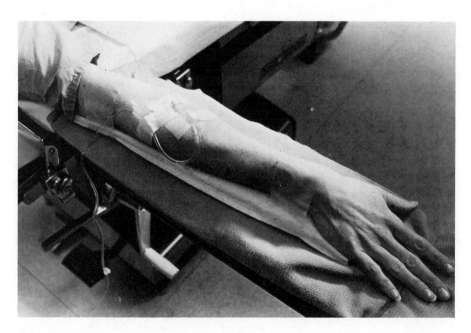

Figure 7. Improper position of arm — Rotation of forearm into pronated position may cause pressure on the ulnar nerve.

The most common cause of ulnar neuropathy at the elbow is the cubital tunnel syndrome with progressive signs of ulnar compression under the aponeurosis connecting the two heads of the flexorcarpiulnerus.[52]

Predisposing factors of instability of the ulnar nerve and constitutional disorders, such as diabetes mellitus, alcoholism, vitamin deficiency, and malignancy, may render the patient especially susceptible to cubital tunnel compression syndrome.[53]

Signs and symptoms of ulnar nerve paresis are sensory loss of the 5th finger, the ulnar half of the 4th finger, and ulnar third of the hand, along with muscle weakness and contracture of the muscles of the 4th and 5th fingers (clawhand). There is delayed nerve conduction at the elbow. This condition may require surgical neurolysis of the nerve with partial resection of the lateral epicondyle of the humerus. Initial symptoms of numbness of the ulnar distribution of the affected hand is usually noted upon awakening from anesthesia and sometimes pain in the forearm is also present. The pain may be transient, lasting only a few months, but the paresthesia, numbness, pins and needles sensation, and tingling have been reported to last from 6 to 96 months postoperatively. There was no correlation between the severity of the neurologic deficit

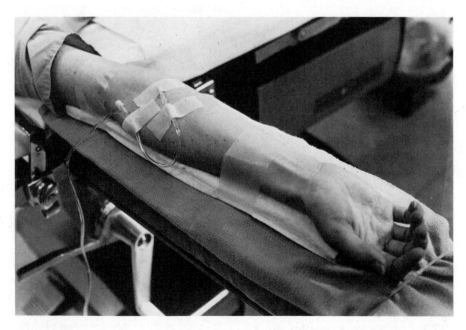

Figure 8. Supinated position prevents pressure on ulnar nerve at the elbow.

and the length of type of operation. Arm position appears to be the factor in producing cubital tunnel syndrome, since the nerve is especially at risk in the pronated position. Position of the arm in the supinated position or with protective padding is extremely important, particularly in patients with pre-existing or potential nerve disease. Tourniquet compression probably causes damage because of direct mechanical compression rather than ischemia. Contact with the metal edge of the operating table or steel rails must be avoided.

These injuries are avoidable by carefully padding prominences during anesthesia.

Median Nerve

The median nerve may be injured in the anticubital fossa or the carpal tunnel region. Puncture of the nerve when attempting venipuncture or extravasation of intravenous fluids are the cause of injuries. The signs of median nerve injury are sensory loss of the skin of the radial two-thirds of the palm and dorsum of 2nd and 3rd fingers and inability to oppose thumb and little finger or flex thumb and two radial fingers.[54]

Further discussion of direct nerve injuries from needle puncture is presented in Chapter XVIII of this book.

Vocal Cord Paralysis

Endotracheal intubation is an excellent way to control the patient's airway during anesthesia. Complications resulting from endotracheal intubation have been reported, and these include arytenoid dislocation, laryngeal laceration, pseudo-membrane formation and vocal cord paralysis. Unilateral vocal cord paralysis is a rare but annoying complication of endotracheal anesthesia. Ellis and Pallister[55] have suggested that the cause is indirect pressure to the recurrent laryngeal nerve by the inflated cuff of the endotracheal tube. These authors suggest a possible anatomic mechanism for indirect trauma to the recurrent laryngeal nerve from an endotracheal tube cuff. They showed by cadaver dissection that an endotracheal tube with cuff inflated within the larynx compresses the anterior branch of the nerve between the cuff and the thyroid lamina and may cause postoperative vocal cord paralysis.

The left cord is affected two times as often as the right. Bilateral post-endotracheal intubation vocal cord paralysis does occur as well. Males are affected seven times more frequently than females. Paralysis has also occurred after the use of non-cuffed tubes in pediatric patients and has even occurred after mask anesthesia and spinal anesthesia.[55]

Ellis and Pallister[55] also postulated that edema resulting from endotracheal intubation may aggravate hoarseness in patients who have unrecognized preoperative unilateral vocal cord paralysis.

Other factors that have been implicated as causing vocal cord paralysis during anesthesia are excessive stretching of the neck, turning or bending the neck, toxic reactions to drugs, and metabolic or viral neuropathies.[56-58]

Soft tissue injuries to the trachea along with pressure of the cuff seems to be the cause of vocal cord paralysis.

Miscellaneous Nerve Injuries

Ankle clonus is a reflex irregular contraction of muscles produced by forcible dorsiflexion of the ankle when there is increased tone in the posterior calf muscles. This has been reported in patients in reverse Trendelenberg position during surgery when the patient's feet are supported by a foot board. This is prevented by careful positioning.[59]

Deep Peroneal Nerve and Posterior Tibial Nerve

The deep peroneal nerve and the posterior tibial nerve may be injured from pressure on the posterior aspect of the leg from improper positioning of the patient's knee on stirrups or the break of the table. (Fig. 9) It has been reported after prolonged lithotomy position resulting in nerve compression that was secondary to severe edema of the legs. Patients with injury of the deep peroneal nerve have a foot drop, inabil-

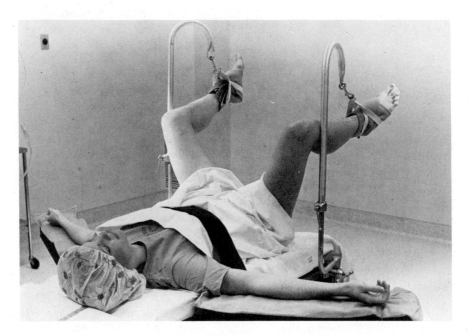

Figure 9. Pressure on the superficial peroneal nerve from careless positioning of the legs in lithomy position.

ity to invert the foot, and sensory loss over the great and second toe. Those with injury to the posterior tibial nerve have atrophy of the small muscles of the foot and sensory loss of the plantar surface of the foot.[8,37]

Sural Nerve and Superficial Peroneal Nerve

Injury to the sural nerve occurs at the posterolateral aspect of the ankle. The superficial peroneal nerve is injured at the dorsum of the foot. These nerves are injured simultaneously when a patient is anesthetized with his legs crossed (Fig. 10). Many patients climb onto the operating table and cross their legs. A very simple pre-anesthetic check by the anesthesiologist or circulating nurse will prevent this injury.[8]

Common Peroneal Nerve

The common peroneal nerve is vulnerable to pressure injury near the point of bifurcation where it winds around the head of the fibula. Metal stirrups used for lithotomy position must be kept from contacting the legs in the region of the fibular head. Pressure from stirrups in the region of the upper outer aspect of the calf may injure the saphenous nerve.[8,37]

Lateral Femoral Cutaneous Nerve

The lateral femoral cutaneous nerve may be injured at the inferior

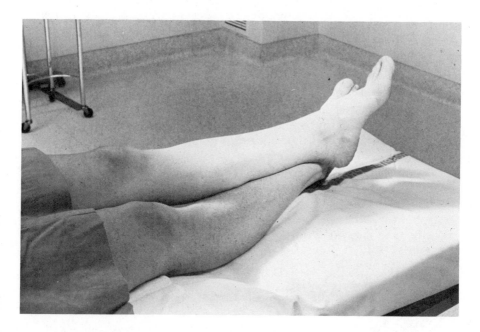

Figure 10. Sural nerve palsies are caused by patient crossing legs.

border of the inguinal ligament. This has been seen postoperatively in patients lying prone with the operating table broken at the level of the hips with thighs flexed on the trunk. I have also seen this in a patient after surgery in the lithotomy position in which her thighs were acutely flexed on the trunk. The patient complains of sensory loss over the anterior thigh. This injury disappears within 2 to 3 months.[8,37]

Sciatic Nerve

The sciatic nerve is injured mainly by injection of irritating substances in the region of the sciatic foramen during intramuscular injections. The sign of a foot drop with anesthesia over the skin of foot and leg will be seen. This injury is best treated with physiotherapy.

Nerve Injuries from Orthopedic Fracture Table

Two cases of unusual nerve palsies resulting from the use of the orthopedic fracture table have been reported. One patient had nerve paralysis from pressure of table over the lateral portion of the sciatic nerve where it leaves the pelvis. Another patient suffered loss of penile sensation following traction of legs against poorly padded orthopedic post, causing pressure on the pudendal nerves against the ischial tuberosities.

The fracture table must be well padded and great care exercised during positioning. Many of the patients who are placed on the fracture table for surgery have systemic disease, such as arteriosclerosis or diabetes, and are at greater risk of nerve damage than a normal patient.[37]

The neuropathies produced during surgery are also discussed in Chapter VIII in this book.

Paraplegia

Paraplegia after general anesthesia is extremely rare and has been reported following hypotensive episodes. Newberry[60] reports a case of spontaneous subdural hemorrhage during anesthesia resulting in paraplegia postoperatively, in which there were no unusual circumstances in the case that may have explained the possible cause. Anesthesia and surgery for a ureteral calculus were uneventful. The patient was supine on the table with no wedges or tilts used. Arterial pressure was normotensive throughout the course of anesthesia. Postoperative paralysis occurred and burr holes three days after initial surgery revealed subdural hemotoma.[60]

Complications of Local Anesthesia

Administration of local anesthesia to a patient may be followed by minor and transient complications. These are rather common. Serious neurologic complications occur approximately 1 in 11,000 anesthesias.[61] The neurologic complications that occur during regional or conduction anesthesia are those related directly to the agents that are administered, as well as supplemental agents, such as the vasoconstrictors, complications related directly to the technique that is used, and to the sterilization equipment and drugs used for sterilization. Complications may result from the physiologic phenomena that occur due to the specific technique that is used, and complications due to other factors, such as the patient's pre-existing disease. Systemic effects directly related to the drug may be due to actual sensitivity to the drug, an allergic type of reaction. Drug sensitivity has been reported following the use of the ester type of local anesthetic. (These are piperocaine, chloroprocaine, procaine, and tetracaine.) Patients who state they have an allergic reaction to a local anesthetic drug should be skin-tested if an ester type of drug is to be used. There are no clearly documented cases of allergy to the amide group of local anesthetic drugs (lidocaine, mepivacaine, prilocaine, and bupivacaine). Tissue reaction to both types of local anesthetic drugs is minimal and has not been demonstrated either in the laboratory or in the clinical practice in the concentrations of anesthetic agents that are in use today.[63] Table III summarizes the two types of local anesthetics.

Systemic Effects

Moore[64] and Bridenbaugh[65] have reported the incidence of CNS reactions after conduction anesthesia to be 1.5%. Two percent of the reactions were thought to be allergic in origin; the remaining 98% were considered to be due to the toxic effect of local anesthetic agent.[64] The degree of toxicity depends upon the blood level of the drug, and this is dependent upon (1) the dosage, (2) the presence or absence of vasoconstrictors, (3) the type of the drug used, and (4) the site of injection.

Table III
Classification of Commonly Used Local Anesthetic Agents

Ester Type	Amide Type
I. Benzoic Acid Piperocaine (metycaine)	Lidocaine (Xylocaine, Lignocaine) Mepivacaine (Carbocaine)

II. Para-aminobenzoic Acid
     Chloroprocaine (Nesacaine)
     Procaine (Novocain)
     Tetracaine (Pontocaine,
       Amethocaine)
	Prilocaine (Citanest)
	 Bupivacaine (Marcain)

The absorption and subsequent blood level of the local anesthetic drugs is related to the uptake of the drug and its removal from the circulatory system. The rate of absorption is decreased by the addition of vaso-constrictors to the local anesthetic drugs. Other factors influencing the uptake of the drugs include their solubility, the degree of ionization, and their protein binding. The toxic effects of local anesthetic agents is determined by the concentration of the drug that reaches the brain.

Inadvertant intra-arterial or intravenous injections, or overdosage will result in the same symptoms, depending on the concentration of the drug. Low drug concentrations cause CNS effects of sedation and anal-gesia. Progressive sensations experienced by the patient at higher concentrations include lightheadedness, dizziness, numbness, nausea, sleepiness, and disorientation. They may also include euphoria, nystag-mus, sweating, and vomiting. As the concentration of the drug increases, more irritability is exhibited; and twitching, fasiculations, and clonic convulsions may occur. Convulsions lead to depression of the central nervous system with coma or death due to respiratory arrest. Cardiovascular depression may be observed prior to respiratory arrest.[65] Tables IV and V present information related to dosage of various local anesthetic agents.

Treatment of Reactions to Local Anesthetic Drugs

Treatment of toxicity to local anesthetic drugs includes the follow-ing: (1) establishment of clear airway and administration of oxygen; (2) intravenous barbiturate or diazepam to stop convulsions; (3) vaso-pressor drugs as necessary; and (4) management of cardiac arrest with standard resuscitative procedures. Allergic reactions, if they occur, should be treated with antihistamines, steroids, and artificial ventila-tion. Convulsions resulting from toxicity to local anesthetic drugs cause

Table IV
Suggested Maximal Doses of Local Anesthetic Agents

Drug	ml/kl per body wt.
1. Procaine	14
2. Prilocaine	10
3. Tetracaine	1.5
4. Lidocaine	7
5. Mepivacaine	7
6. Bupivacaine	3
7. Cocaine (topical)	4
8. Etidocaine	4

Table V
Anesthetic Agents and Toxic Doses

Local Anesthetic Agent	Type	Minimum Toxic IV Dose (mg/kg)	Estimated Intra-arterial Toxic Dose (mg)
Procaine	Ester	19.2	43.2
Tetracaine	Ester	2.5	5.6
Lidocaine	Amide	6.4	14.4
Bupivacaine	Amide	1.6	3.6

no change in the EEG reading, so that using the EEG reading as a method in predicting possible seizure is impractical.[66] Subtoxic doses of local anesthetic drugs produce anticonvulsant effects. It is believed that local anesthetics inhibit neuronal activity and that excitatory pathways are more resistant than inhibitory pathways, so that at subtoxic doses they act as anticonvulsants and at higher concentration they act as convulsants because the excitatory pathways are unopposed.

It is difficult to determine the exact toxic dose for a specific local anesthetic drug.[67,68] There are many factors involved, including individual susceptibility to the drug. Also, it is dependent upon the mode of administration, the site of administration, whether or not the drug has been absorbed into the vascular system (either arterial or venous), and lipoid solubility and acid base balance of the drug. When a local anesthetic drug is administered into vascular area, absorption is more rapid. This can be slowed by the addition of epinephrine. Epinephrine is a vasoconstrictor drug and so reduces the speed with which the local anesthetic drug is absorbed. Rapid absorption of local occurs when it is administered into the tracheobroncheal tree and also after administration of paracervical blocks because of the vascularity in these regions.

Plasma protein binding capacity of local anesthetic drugs also influences the seizure threshold. When local anesthetic drugs are administered in combination with drugs that bind proteins, the dose can be remarkably increased. Patients on such drugs as meperidine and diphenylhydantoin tolerate larger doses of local anesthesia than those on no medication.

The administration of barbiturates probably causes a decreased seizure threshold of local anesthetic drugs. Diazepam is becoming more popular as a prophylatic anticonvulsant.[69-73]

The rate of enzymatic hydrolysis also alters the toxicity. The ester group of local anesthetics is rapidly hydrolized by plasma cholinesterase.

The amide group is metabolized at a slower rate. Patients with congenital atypical plasma cholinesterase are less tolerant to the ester type of local anesthetic drugs.[74]

Alterations in acid-base balance will also effect the toxicity of the drugs. Increasing CO_2 level and lowering the pH increases cerebral blood flow, and this in turn causes more of the toxic drug to reach the brain with increased seizure threshold. In determining the anesthetic toxicity, it is found that arterial blood levels correlate best with the toxicity of the drug. Anesthetic potency of the drug is a less important determinant, although there is a relationship between anesthetic potency and toxicity.[75]

Brain levels do not correlate well with toxic reactions. Because the arterial blood level is the determinate factor in toxicity, very small amounts inadvertantly injected into the arterial system, particularly in the region of the head and neck and upper extremity, can be mainlined to the brain.[65] Korevaar, et al reported tonic-clonic seizures immediately after the injection of 1.5 ml of 0.5% bupivacaine for a stellate block. This was in essence a test dose, but it was enough to cause a seizure when injected intra-arterially.[76] Antiarrythmic drugs used for cardiac patients are chemically related to local anesthetic agents and may compound the convulsive properties of local anesthetics.[77]

It is imperative that material for resuscitation be readily available when blocks are being done. Barbiturates have been considered to be effective prophylactically to prevent seizures when doing blocks: however, Aldrete and Daniel found that they are ineffective prophylatically.[77a] Barbiturates have been used to treat convulsions and may add to the depression of vital centers caused by the local anesthetics. Diazepam is a better agent for treating and for prophylactic prevention of seizures. It has been found that pre-treatment with diazepam can essentially double the dose of local anesthetic necessary to cause seizure activity.[70-73] This has an advantage over barbiturates in that it does not depress the cardiovascular system. Succinylcholine will abolish muscular activity and will permit artificial ventilation. This may be necessary as a means of preventing hypoxia during convulsions.

Convulsions are infrequent complications of nerve blocks. They occur immediately, or up to 5 minutes post block, and the reported incidence is 0.018 to 0.09%.[78,79]

Drug-Induced Parkinsonism

Local anesthetic drugs may induce Parkinsonism. Gjerris reports a case of procaine-induced Parkinsonism and postulates that it is due to a blocking effect on the synapses of the dopaminergic system.[80]

This is another case of anesthesia unmasking neurologic problems that may already exist but have not been diagnosed.

Paracervical Anesthesia

Complications of paracervical block may affect the mother and fetus. Maternal systemic toxic reactions occur and may be avoided by careful aspiration and the use of small doses of anesthetic agents. The effect on the fetus may be more significant. Fetal bradycardia and acidosis occur in 7-70% of cases and may last as long as 30 minutes.[81] The mechanism of fetal distress may be related to decreased uterine blood flow from vasoconstriction and from high fetal blood levels of the local anesthetic drug.[82]

Ester-type local anesthetics result in low plasma concentrations because of rapid hydrolysis by plasma cholinesterase and the amide type in high levels in both fetal and maternal blood. These are slowly metabolized in the liver by microsomal enzymes unlike other amide type drugs. Bupivacaine is highly protein-bound and does not cause high plasma levels in the fetus.

Local anesthetics cross the placenta in a process of simple diffusion, and the drug reaches the fetal circulation within minutes after it appears in the maternal circulation. Local anesthetic toxicity of the neonate is most commonly seen as fetal depression, which is shown by low Apgar scores. Seizures, tonic, clonic or tonic-clonic, mydriasis, loss of oculocephalic reflexes, and apnea may occur.[83,84]

There are reports of seizures, coma, or death following direct injection into the fetal scalp during attempted paracervical blocks.

Treatment of fetal toxicity to local anesthetic drugs consists of exchange transfusions and gastric lavage.

The overall incidence of reported fetal depression after paracervical block is 10-30%.

Complications of Spinal Anesthesia

Neurologic complications of spinal anesthesia may be classified as immediate or delayed. Immediate complications result from high spinal anesthesia ("total spinal") causing paralysis of respiratory muscles and high sympathetic block, which may lead to cardiac arrest. Total respiratory paralysis requires immediate support of the respiration with oxygen via mask or endotracheal tube. Hypotension and bradycardia from high sympathetic block are treated with vasopressors and intravenous fluids. Placing the patient in a Trendelenburg position will aid venous return and help to alleviate hypotension. These supportive measures must continue until the block has worn off and the patient has regained normal cardiorespiratory control.

Delayed neurologic complications of spinal anesthesia have been noted since spinal was first used in 1899, by August Bier.[84a] He noted at that time that some of his patients suffered from cranial nerve palsies and headaches. Headache after spinal anesthesia continues to be the most common and most annoying complication of spinal anesthesia. Rare complications that have been reported are transverse myelitis, adhesive arachnoiditis, and cauda equina syndrome.

Headache

Dripps and Vandam described the incidence of headache at 11% of 10,098 blocks.[85] Moore and Bridenbaugh reported headaches in 1.4% of 11,574 patients who received spinal anesthesia.[85a] Post-spinal blockade is due to leakage of the cerebrospinal fluid causing traction on pain sensitive structures, particularly vascular and meningeal. A typical spinal headache begins on the 2nd or 3rd day after the lumbar puncture. It is generally over the calvarium, throbbing in nature and aggravated by the upright positon. It usually will disappear while the patient is lying supine at bedrest. The headache lasts generally until the 7th post-spinal day; however, they have been reported to last several weeks.[86]

The normal volume of cerebrospinal fluid in the spinal subarachnoid space varies from 25 to 35 ml. It has been shown that the removal of up to 12 ml of CSF does not effect the frequency of spinal headache. The incidence of spinal headache can be significantly altered by the size of the needle used for the lumbar puncture. The incidence of headache has been reported to be as low as 1.2% and as high as 20%. The smaller the needle used, the lower incidence.[87,88]

Obstetric patients suffer post-spinal headache twice as frequently as surgical patients — females more than males, and young patients more than old patients. It is unusual for a patient over 50 to complain of post-spinal headache. This has been attributed to an elevated pain threshold in older patients, as well as to a decrease in elasticity of cerebral vascular structures.[89]

Within two weeks, 80% of the patients recover spontaneously from post-spinal headache. The mechanism of post-spinal headache is continuing loss of CSF through the needle hole in the dura that is faster than the manufacture of CSF in the choroid plexus. The resulting fall in CSF pressure causes the brain to sag while the patient is upright. This places traction on the pain sensitive structures of the brain and causes headache. Painful stimuli arising from the superior surface of the tentorium and above are transmitted by the 5th cranial nerve and are referred to the anterior half of the head. Pain from below the tentorium is transmitted via the 9th and the 10th cranial nerves and is referred to the posterior half of the head and the neck.

In an effort to compensate for fluid loss, there is a secondary vasodilitation, and so there is an added vascular component to the headache.

Prevention and Treatment

The routine use of a 25-gauge spinal needle reduces the overall incidence of post-spinal headache to 1.2-2%, compared to up to 20% in some series with the use of large needles. This technique is not much more difficult to learn than use of a 22-gauge needle and should be routine for spinal anesthesia, especially in obstetric patients.[86]

Adequate hydration during and following delivery or surgery with intravenous fluids is helpful. Oral fluids should be started and encouraged as soon as the patient can tolerate it.

Many techniques have been tried for the treatment of post-spinal headache. They have aimed primarily at increasing the production of fluid and decreasing the fluid loss. Adequate hydration is essential for increased production of CSF. Three liters of intravenous fluid should be given per day for three days. Many times this alone will be adequate to treat the patient. Patients should be encouraged to force fluids orally. IV alcohol has been suggested to stimulate the production of CSF. Pitressin has also been advocated with some favorable results. This consists of the administration of 1,000 ml of 5% dextrose and saline within a 2-hour period post partum. Following this infusion, an ampule of pitressin is given intra-muscularly, and intravenous hydration is continued with 1,000 ml of 5% dextrose and water. Others have advocated the use of nicotinic acid 100 mg/1,000 cc of intravenous fluids.[87]

Because of the leakage of CSF through the dural hole, as the etiology of spinal headache, it has been advocated that patients be kept recumbant for 24 to 48 hours post spinal. This has caused considerable controversy; and in fact some authors have reported a decrease in headaches with early ambulation. Others have found that the incidence was not significantly altered, and others report a significant reduction in headaches with various periods of recumbancy.[88-90] Jones[91] studied 1,134 patients with post-spinal headaches who were kept recumbant for various periods of from 5 to 12 hours. There was no predictable pattern relating to the time spent recumbant and to the occurrence of headaches. However, once the headache occurs, recumbancy aids in pain relief. It is recommended that early ambulation, as soon as motor function permits, results in better patient tolerance to the procedure.[91]

Sikh and Agarwal[92] treated post-spinal headache patients with inhalation of carbon dioxide. They suggest that carbon dioxide dialates the cerebral vessels and increases the production of CSF in the choroid plexus and that this may be an effective way for treating spinal headaches. Forty patients in their series of 52 obtained some relief from this technique.[92]

Abdominal binders have been used to increase the CSF pressure as a treatment of post-spinal headaches.

Nelson described a technique of closing a dural hole by inserting a fibrin plug through the lumbar puncture needle and leaving it in place.[93] This reduced the incidence of headache from 17.4% to 4.9%. However, one-half of his patients complained of cauda equina syndrome, with pain in the neck, popliteal region, and posterior thigh muscles.

Ozdil and Powell[94] recommended the prophylactic injection of 2½ ml of blood into the spinal canal as the spinal needle is being withdrawn. This technique will plug the hole itself and deposit a small amount of clot in the epidural space and also help to close the puncture site. These authors described no headaches after their series of 100 patients. Epidural saline injections (40 to 100 ml) have been advocated by many investigators; and while this technique is effective, it is transient and a significant number of recurrences occur.[94]

Epidural Blood Patch

Epidural blood patch was introduced by Gormly (1960) for the treatment of post-lumbar puncture headaches.[95] This has proved to be a valuable technique, in that it closes the subarachnoid epidural fistula by a fibrin deposit. Epidural blood patch is a safe method of treating headaches with an overall success rate is 96.5%.[96] Some of the theoretical disadvantages to EBP are (1) infection, (2) adhesive arachnoiditis, (3) radiculitis, and (4) possibility of obliterating the epidural space. Most clinicians feel that while epidural blood patch is a very effective treatment of post-spinal headache, it should only be used where the headaches are incapacitating and conservative measures have failed to solve the problem and the headache has lasted more than five days. Presence of infection, fever, use of anticoagulants, or patient refusal are contraindications to EBP.[98-102]

If, during the procedure, bleeding occurs injuring an epidural blood vessel, no blood patch is performed. EBP is perfomed under strict aseptic technique at the site of the previous lumbar puncture. The epidural needle is inserted into the epidural space, and the patient's blood, which has been removed from the anti-cubital vein, is injected slowly, 1 ml per 2 seconds. The total volume injected is between 6 to 10 ml. The patients sometimes complain of backache or neckache during the injection. After treatment, the patient is kept recumbant for one hour and then asked to walk around to evaluate the result. If inadvertant subdural puncture occurs when treating the patient with EBP, the tip of the needle should be withdrawn to the epidural space and then the blood injected very slowly. Increased body temperature following EBP is benign and temporary and does not usually result in any problem.[103-105]

Post-Spinal Anesthesia Nerve Palsies

Cranial nerve palsies occur after lumbar puncture. Venus first described abducens and oculomotor nerve palsies in 1907.[106] Dripps and Vandam reported 8 cases of abducens nerve palsy following 10,098 spinal anesthetics.[85] Moore and Brindenbaugh reported one case in their series of 11,574.[78]

All reported cases of cranial nerve palsies follow headache and are often accompanied by stiff neck and nausea. The etiology is the same as for headache — leakage of CSF with resuting low pressure. The brain sags without its fluid cushion. The abducens nerve, being relatively fixed in the cranium, and the trochlear nerve, the most slender with the longest intracranial course, are especially sensitive to stretching from lowered pressure with resulting paralysis. These patients complain of blurring of vision, double vision, and spots before the eyes.

Paresis of all cranial nerves following spinal anesthesia have been reported except olfactory, glosso-pharyngeal, and the vagus. The abducens (VI) nerve is most frequently involved; oculomotor (III), trochlear (IV), facial (VII), and auditory (VIII) less frequently; and the trigeminal (V) rarely.[107,108] They occur from the 3rd to 15th postoperative day, but may last for several months. Treatment of cranial nerve palsies is the same as for headache.

Cerebral Hemorrhage

Cerebral hemorrhage and subdural hematomas are rare complications of lumbar dural puncture and are easily misdiagnosed as "spinal headache."

Edelman and Wingard reported a case of post-lumbar puncture cephalgia of 38 days duration treated with epidural blood patch who died of respiratory arrest before accurate diagnosis of subdural hematoma was made.[109]

Reduction of CSF volume and pressure after dural leak causes traction on the blood vessels and dura. Tearing of dural vessels from traction may lead to subdural hematoma. This is a rare complication.

Exacerbation of Neurologic Disease

Dripps and Vandam reported 12 patients in their series of exacerbation of neurologic disease after spinal anesthesia. These problems were reappearance of backache, sciatica, leg weakness, and two cases of spinal cord compression syndrome caused by tumor.[85]

Alfery, et al reported a case of headache and 6th cranial nerve palsy following spinal anesthesia which was actually caused by a hypothalamic tumor.[110]

Although headache and cranial nerve palsies are well recognized complications of spinal anesthesia, patients with unusual symptoms or refractory cases must be carefully investigated for underlying neurologic disease. A fundoscopic examination is a simple way to begin and should be part of the workup for patients having post-spinal neurologic sequelae.

Patients with increased intracranial pressure contraindicate the use of spinal anesthesia. Any patient with papilledema should be excluded from spinal anesthesia. Herniation of the tentorium and cerebellum associated with an olfactory groove meningioma has been reported after spinal anesthesia.[111]

Aseptic Meningitis

This is a rare complication of spinal anesthesia. (No case of meningitis was reported in the series of 10,440 patients by Phillips,[87] or by Dripps and Vandam.[85])

Symptoms are fever, headache, nuchal rigidity, and photophobia occurring within 2 hours of the spinal tap. Lumbar puncture reveals cloudy CSF, under increased pressure, with a leucocytosis usually polymorphonuclear, with raised protein and normal sugar. Cultures are negative and no organisms are found. The symptoms usually subside within a week without specific treatment. Prognosis is good.[112]

The etiology is indefinite. It may result from breakdown in technique, direct contamination, faulty equipment, or direct infection from the patient. It has also been suggested that the local anesthetic agents are toxic to the spinal cord. However, this is unlikely. High concentrations of procaine can cause permanent paralysis in dogs and cats, but only in concentrations far above those used clinically in man.

The possibility of a chemical contaminent has been suggested by many authors. Goldman and Sanford blame the disinfecting solutions used for needles.[113] Winkelman et al implicate detergents; however, these authors describe adhesive arachnoiditis and not aseptic meningitis. The use of disposable spinal sets eliminates this possibility.[114]

Viral meningitis cannot be ruled out as a possible cause of post-spinal meningitis.

DiGiovannni and Lathrop have reported 30 cases of aseptic meningitis which they attribute to pyrogens or endotoxins that may not be destroyed by autoclaving.[115]

Blood from a punctured small vessel may act as a foreign protein in the subdural space, causing scarring and neurologic symptoms.[116]

Prophylaxis and Treatment

When administering a spinal anesthetic, the following precautions are recommended to prevent any possible contamination, either chemical, viral, or bacterial:

1. The use of disposable spinal trays that are well within the expiration date.

2. Meticulous technique with checking of sterilization, wearing of gloves, and careful cleansing and preparation of the patient's skin.

3. The use of an intraducer to allow the spinal needle to enter the subdural space without touching the skin.

Treatment is symptomatic, and the patient will recover within 5 to 7 days.

Recurrence of Spinal Headache

Post-lumbar puncture headache may recur after treatment if a leak persists and may require additional treatment. In rare instances, surgical closure of the dura was required for successful therapy.[117]

Mulroy reported a case of a patient treated successfully with epidural blood patch who had recurrence of headache when traveling by air 12 days after lumbar puncture. It may be suggested to patients who had post-spinal headache treated with epidural blood patch to avoid air travel for several weeks.[118]

Transient Global Amnesia

Transient global amnesia after spinal anesthesia is a syndrome characterized by abrupt onset of transient amnesia lasting less than 24 hours. There is usually a period of mild confusion, with some retrograde amnesia. The etiology is unclear, but this syndrome presents a picture identical to concussion. It is a self-limited condition and does not recur, and it is not related to serious neurologic disease.[119]

Prophylactic Blood Patch

Prophylactic blood patch does not prevent headache and should not be used.[105]

Complications of Epidural Anesthesia

Epidural anesthesia is a very popular anesthetic for labor and delivery and has been considered to be extremely safe and free of complications. In 1969, Massey and Dawkins reviewed reports of 32,000 epidural blocks and found 48 cases of transient and 7 cases of permanent paralysis.[120]

Neurologic complications parallel those of spinal anesthesia. Inadvertent dural puncture occurs in 0.5-3% of attempted epidural anesthetics. Of these, 76% result in headaches and 0.2% result in total spinal anesthesia.[102] The incidence of headache is high because a large bore 17 gauge needle is usually used. The technique for performing epidural block includes repeated aspiration to assure that the subdural space has not been entered. Failure to aspirate spinal fluid, however, is not a positive diagnostic measure. A small test dose of local anesthetic injected through the epidural catheter causes immediate anesthesia if the subdural space has been entered and usually will be inadequate to produce total spinal. This is not an absolute safeguard, however. Total spinal anesthesia after a test dose has been reported in which 2.5 ml of 2% chlorprocaine was administered with the patient in head up position resulting in total spinal block and hemicranial palsy.[121] The agent used has a specific gravity at body temperature of 1.0100 and is a hypobaric solution. Test doses of hypobaric local anesthetic agents should be administered with patient in the head down position. In this instance, inadvertent dural puncture would merely produce anesthesia of the lower extremities and perineum.

Total spinal block is indicated by hypotension, paralysis, apnea dilated pupils, and unconsciousness, and it may lead to cardiac arrest. Immediate treatment to support the blood pressure and respiration must begin — oxygen and control of respiration, along with vasopressors and intravenous fluids.[122]

The presence of blood on epidural or subdural puncture is not a problem. Epidural blood patch (EBP) is used to treat headaches and has a low incidence of complications. The suggestion that inadvertent lumbar dural puncture be treated prophylactically with EBP to prevent headaches is invalid since the incidence of headaches has not been reduced by this technique.

Headaches

Headaches occurring after epidural anesthesia may be classified as "post-spinal" headaches caused by accidental dural puncture by the epidural needle or catheter. In reported series, migration of the tip of the epidural catheter to cause dural tap occurs in 0.5-1% of epidurals.[1]

These headaches are treated as spinal headaches. Headaches have also been reported to occur immediately after injection and subside in several hours. Abram and Cherwenks documented 8 headaches in 604 patients who were treated for chronic pain with epidural injections of steroids and local anesthesia.[123] They suggest that air introduced into the subdural space with the patient sitting in the upright position causes the cephalgia. Inhalation of 100% oxygen reduced the duration of headache by facilitating the uptake of nitrogen from the air bubble.

As with spinal anesthesia, post-epidural headache may represent underlying neurologic disease that is assumed to be a complication of the epidural. Famewo reported a case of a patient with post-anesthetic frontal and occipital headache treated with analgesics and diazepam, which was actually caused by intracerebral hemorrhage.[124] Any patient who has a persistent headache after epidural anesthesia requires a careful neurologic workup to rule out significant neurologic disease.

Cerebral Subdural Hematoma

A significant number of cerebral subdural hematomas after lumbar epidural puncture are reported in the literature.[125] A cause-and-effect relationship cannot be established; however, hypertension during labor and delivery may contribute to it.[126]

Spinal Epidural, Subdural, and Subarachnoid Hematomata

Patients on anticoagulant therapy, or those with known bleeding disorders, are not candidates for either spinal or epidural anesthesia. The risk of prolonged bleeding from epidural veins may cause epidural, spinal subdural, or subarachnoid hematoma. Bonica reported cauda equina syndrome after a spinal anesthetic, from a subarachnoid hematoma in a patient with a blood dyscrasia.[127] Thirty cases of spinal subdural hematomata have been reported in the literature; 19 of these occurred in patients with bleeding disorders and one in a patient receiving aspirin.[128] A detailed discussion of the neurologic complications of anticoagulant therapy is presented in Chapter XIV in this book.

Treatment

Therapy of epidural, subdural, or subarachnoid clots is immediate surgical evacuation.

Epidural Abscess

Epidural abscess after epidural anesthesia occurs rarely. It has also been reported as a spontaneous incident following vaginal delivery in patients who did not have spinal or epidural anesthesia. It results from hematogenous dissemination of bacteria. They are almost always caused by penicillin resistant, coagulase-positive *Staphylacoccus aureus* from foci of infection in the skin, respiratory, or urinary tracts. The presence of a small epidural hematoma serves as a culture medium for the hematoglous bacteria.

This entity, because of back pain and neck pain, and meningismus may be confused with aseptic meningitis. Signs of cord compression distinguish it from aseptic meningitis. Epidural abscess requires immediate surgical drainage.[129]

Cauda Equina Syndrome

Cauda equina compression has been reported following epidural injection of local anesthesia with steroids for control of sciatic pain, as well as following epidural hematoma.[130] Patients having persistent saddle parasthesia, bowel discomfort, and anesthesia along the lateral margin of the foot after epidural injections must be worked up for cauda equina compression and treated surgically.[131]

Anterior Spinal Artery Syndrome

Permanent nerve damage following epidural anesthesia is rare but a tragic complication.

An incidence of 0.02% is found in the literature. Eight cases of paraplegia following epidural were reported by Harrison[132] and Urquhart.[133] These cases were found, at post-mortem, to have anterior spinal artery syndromes. Davies et al first reported this syndrome following epidural anesthesia and postulated the possible causes.[134]

Interference with the blood supply appears to be the most likely explanation. In the cases reported, hypotension was produced and was maintained for the operation. In addition, epinephrine, a local vasoconstrictor, was used in 2 of 3 cases. The anterior spinal artery is an end artery, so that reduced perfusion may lead to ischemia.

Spiller first described and named the syndrome. It may be caused by various entities, such as vascular spasm, trauma, compression due to disc or tumor, arteriosclerosis, thrombosis, syphilitic thrombosis, aneurysm, and coarctation.[135]

Other possible causes of post-epidural neurologic defect may be direct trauma by the needle causing nerve damage or hematoma formation, or a direct toxic effect of the local anesthetic solutions.

Lund[136] reported a case of partial paralysis from inadvertant subarachnoidal block with 2% cyclaine. This is an irritating drug, and it is no longer in use. Commonly used local anesthetic agents have not been found to have neurotoxic properties.[136]

Chemical contamination, infection, disc prolapse and accidental spinal have all been considered.

Patients receiving epidural anesthesia should be selected with this in mind, and the role of induced arterial hypotension considered. Any patient with cardiovascular disease tolerates hypotension poorly and is at increased risk of inadequate end artery profusion from hypotension.

Back Pain

Postoperative back pain occurs in 2-3% of cases. (Foldes, et al reported 3%;[137] Bonica and co-workers, 2.41%;[138] Lund et al, 2%.[139]) Back pain is also a common complaint of patients who received general anesthesia.

Etiology of back pain following spinal or epidural anesthesia has been debated and is probably caused by several factors.

Intravertebral disc collapse has been noted in rare cases from needle puncture of disc. The injection of fluid into the interspinous ligaments is another possibility.

Muscle relaxation produced by the anesthesia allows for abnormal stretching of ligaments and joint capsules and may cause pain. Lithotomy position causes a higher incidence of back pain than the supine and also causes more stretching of ligaments. Other factors influencing the incidence of postoperative back pain are age (higher in older age groups), sex (females have higher incidence), and length of operation.

Treatment

Patients tend to blame the "needle" for backache that may occur after a regional anesthetic, even though backaches occur after general anesthesia. They need reassurance that this is not a permanent problem. Symptomatic treatment consisting of mild analgesics, heat and massage is helpful.

Steroids may be injected epidurally for persistent back pain with symptomatic improvement. Delany et al studied the effects of steroids on cats' spinal cords and found no evidence of tissue damage.[140]

Neurologic disease may be coincidental to anesthesia. Neumark et al reported a case of viral meningoencephalitis following epidural anesthesia that was unrelated to the procedure.[141]

Up to 70% of parturient patients receive spinal or epidural blocks for delivery. These are young, healthy patients who are highly motivated to return home to care for their new infants, and psychosomatic complaints are not the rule.

Postoperative neurologic complications must be evaluated for cause. Although infrequent, unsuspected tumors, abscesses, hematomas, and nerve damage do occur, prompt diagnosis and treatment can prevent an unfortunate result.

Equipment Problems

Epidural needles and catheters may break or migrate causing trauma or hemorrhage. All equipment should be checked for possible defects before using it for a block.

Reactions to Local Anesthetic Agents

Seizures and cardiac and respiratory arrest are all reported after epidural block and are caused by rapid absorption or inadvertant intravenous injection of the local anesthetic agent. Diazepam and artificial ventilation vasopressors are used to treat these problems.[142,143]

Horner's Syndrome

Horner's syndrome (ptosis, myosis, warm dry skin on involved side of face) is an unusual, but benign complication of epidural anesthesia. It occurs from paralysis of the preganglionic sympathetic fibers of the first-second thoracic spinal segments, or the postganglionic fibers in the cervical ganglion or cervical sympathetic chain. Hypotension will require treatment with vasopressors. If hypotension is not present, the condition is benign.

Extensive paravertebral spread from increased epidural pressure during labor may explain this unusual complication.[144,145]

Epidural Injections

Injection of local anesthetic and steroids into the lumbar epidural or subdural space has been used for the treatment of patients with low back pain. There are reports of complications following subdural injection of these agents. Delany et al conducted animal experiments using 2% lidocaine and triamcinolone. Examination of the nerve tissues and meningial tissues in cats 30 to 120 days after injection showed that there was very little reaction and the conclusion was that this is apparently a safe technique.[140]

Reports of complications following subdural injection showed cases of adhesive arachnoiditis and sciatica. Sclerosing spinal pachymeningitis has been reported in a patient with multiple sclerosis following injections of methyl prednisone.[130]

Peripheral Nerve Injuries from Local Anesthesia

Peripheral nerve blocks are usually performed by eliciting parethesias and then injecting the local anesthetic into the region of the parethesia to insure a successful block.

In reviewing persistent post-anesthesic parethesias in patients who had brachial plexus blocks, Woolley and Vandam suggested that injecting a drug into the nerve bundle was potentially hazardous.[146] Recently, Selander and co-workers have presented evidence to corroborate this hypothesis.[147] They studied 290 patients in whom parethesia was sought and 243 in the non-parethesia group. Eight patients in the parethesia group had symptoms; two in the non-parethesia group had symptoms. Symptoms varied from mild to moderate and lasted a few weeks to over one year. They also studied the effect of bupivacaine on the sciatic nerve of rabbits. Topical application to the nerve caused no injury, while intrafasicular injection resulted in axonal degeneration and damaged the blood nerve barrier.[148]

Physiologic saline injected intrafasicularly had the same effect as 0.5% bupivacaine. Increasing the concentration of bupivacaine and the addition of epinephrine (5 g/ml) increased the injury.

The type of needle used also affected the degree of injury — flat beveled needles (45°) were less traumatic than steep beveled ones (14°). The sharper bevels cut small nerve fibers. Turning the bevel to run parallel to nerve fibers is also less traumatic.

Infraorbital Nerve Block

Tic douloureux involving the infraorbital nerve has been treated successfully with alcohol injection of the infraorbital nerve. Complications of this procedure include extraocular muscle paresis, paralysis of the ciliary ganglion resulting in an atonic pupil, and blindness probably as a result of occlusion of the central retinal artery. These complications are permanent since the initial alcohol block was to be a permanent neurotoxic type of block. Patients who are to have this procedure must be fully aware of these potential injuries.[149]

Retrobulbar Block

Complications of retrobulbar block were included with injuries of the peripheral nerves.

Mandibular Nerve Block

Amaurosis, both transient and permanent, has been reported after local anesthesia for dental extraction. Several possible mechanisms have been postulated for this unusual complication of dental anesthesia. Some authors believe that local anesthetic may reach the retina via the anastamosis between the internal and external carotid arteries. Others have blamed fat embolism causing central artery occlusion. Temporary reflex arterial spasm has also been implicated.

Direct injection of local anesthesia into the orbit through the inferior orbital fissure is another possible etiology.[150-152]

Trigeminal Nerve Block

Inadvertant blocking of adjacent nerves in peripheral nerve blocks is a frequent complication of therapeutic or diagnostic nerve block. Abducens nerve block has been noted after therapeutic block of the trigeminal nerve.[153] Symptoms of abducens nerve block are double vision, blurring, spots before the eyes, and trouble focusing.

Subarachnoid injection may also occur during trigeminal nerve block.[153,154]

Brachial Plexus Block

Horner's syndrome and hoarseness from recurrent laryngeal nerve paralysis may follow brachial plexus block.[155] Other complications of the supraclavicular approach are phrenic paralysis and subarachnoid injection with total spinal. These are complications of the supraclavicular and interscalene approaches. They do not occur during the axillary technique. Permanent neurologic sequelae result from intraneural injection of local anesthetic agents causing damage to the axon. These symptoms vary from light parasthesias and ache to pain and paresis lasting for more than one year.[146]

Persistent parathesias have not been noted when a "non-parathesia" technique is used for brachial plexus block.

Intercostal Nerve Block

This block may be extremely hazardous. Neurologic complications reported include total spinal anesthesia, air embolism and transverse myelitis if long-acting neurolytic agents are used.

Intraoperative intercostal nerve block with bupivacaine is widely used to control postoperative pain after thoracotomy. Total spinal anesthesia following this procedure may occur from injection of anesthesia into dural cuffs.[156]

This complication requires pharmacological support of the cardiovascular system and mechanical support of respiration.

Moore and his group have not seen these complications and attribute it to site of injection. They inject 3 to 5 ml bupivacaine 6 to 7.5 cm lateral to the spinous processes of the vertebrae and use a needle with a 2 mm bevel.[157]

Inferior Dental Nerve Block

Immediate and delayed paralysis of the facial nerve has been reported following inferior dental block.[154] Other complications of dental anesthesia include block of cranial nerves 3, 4, and 6. The mechanism of the complications has been explained as intra-arterial injection into the inferior dental artery or to superior alveolar artery.[154]

Stellate Ganglion Block

Stellate ganglion block is actually a block of the upper four thoracic sympathetic ganglia, the middle cervical ganglion, the stellate ganglion and the sympathetic cords that connect them. It causes unilateral cervico-thoracic-sympathetic nerve paralysis. Complications of this procedure include high spinal anesthesia, epidural anesthesia, intravascular injections with toxic reactions to the drug and recurrent laryngeal nerve paralysis.[158,159]

Phenol has been used as a neurotoxic agent for selective neural damage. Complications of phenolic injection of the stellate ganglion have been reported to cause hemiplegia, respiratory arrest, and hoarseness.[160]

Coeliac Plexus Block

Paraplegia has been reported as a complication of phenol injection of the coeliac plexus.[161]

Complications of General Anesthesia

General anesthetics act by depressing CNS function. This function, by necessity, is totally reversible in anesthetic practice. Even with relative overdose, the pharmacologic effects of general anesthetic agents, while longer lasting and more profound, are nonetheless reversible. The general anesthetic agents currently in common use are barbiturates, ketamine, and narcotics used intravenously; inhalation agents are halothane, enflurane, methoxyflourane, and trichloroethelyne. Diethylether and cyclopropane are no longer used because of their flammability. Current monitoring and electrocautery equipment used routinely in surgical suites prohibit the use of flammable agents.

Winters[161a] classifies general anesthetic agents as those acting by CNS depression, such as halothane, short-acting barbiturates, and diethylether, and those acting by "cataleptoid CNS excitation," such as N_2O, enflurane, trichlorethylene, and ketamine. Domino and co-workers,[162] studying CNS electrical activity, found that all inhalation anesthetics, as well as the barbiturates, caused spike-like EEG activity at certain levels of anesthesia. Ketamine may induce rhythmic muscle contractions, usually of the upper and lower extremities, which are thought to be extrapyramidal in origin and not associated with EEG change.

The General Anesthetic Agents

Ketamine

Ketamine is an injectable anesthetic agent chemically designated 2-(o-chlorophenyl)-2-(methylamino) cyclohexone. It is a rapidly acting general anesthetic agent causing analgesia, normal pharyngeal and laryngeal reflexes, normal or enhanced muscle tone, and cardiorespiratory stimulation. Its action appears to interrupt association pathways of the brain producing sensory blockade. Ketamine significantly increases cerebral blood flow but has little effect on brain oxygen consumption.

Neurologic side effects in some patients may involve clonic and tonic movements resembling seizures and postoperative hallucinations. Ketamine is reported to cause unpleasant dreams and dilirium in 17-21% of adult patients. Diazepam, 0.17 mg/kg preoperatively will decrease the incidence of hallucinations to 3-0%.[182] Emergence disturbances with ketamine occur up to three weeks postoperatively. Dilirium and hallucinations from ketamine are seen infrequently in children. However, recent reports indicate that long lasting flashbacks and irrational behavior following ketamine anesthesia occur in children as well. The incidence of postoperative hallucinations in children is less than 3%, but they have been noted to last for several months and occur in children as young as three years of age.[183]

Winters noted that epileptic seizure activity and EEG patterns under ketamine anesthesia in cats resemble other drug-induced seizure discharges and postulates that the unconsciousness of ketamine anesthesia in humans is similar to the unconsciousness that is produced from petit mal seizures;[187] however, many investigators dispute this idea.

Corssen et al studied normal and epileptic human volunteers and found no indication of seizure discharge on EEG. Epileptic patients with normal EEG patterns showed no change in their EEG under ketamine anesthesia. Patients with epileptic EEG patterns preoperatively also showed no change with ketamine anesthesia. Patients with focal brain disease, either traumatic or from tumors, showed no worsening with ketamine anesthesia. Four patients in his series did show some change, but it was unpredictable and not uniform. Two patients had improvement of their epileptic EEG patterns and two showed some worsening.[184]

A series of epileptic patients with depth electrode recordings, who were anesthetized with ketamine, 2-4 mg/kg, showed seizure patterns that developed in the limbic and thalamic areas and were accompanied by tonic and clonic motor actions. EEG changes were consistent with intermittent paroxysmal epileptic discharge.[184] Rhythmic, muscular contractions seen with ketamine are not associated with EEG changes and are considered to be extrapyramidal in origin.

CNS excitatory activity has also been seen with halothane and enfurane anesthesia, indicating that perhaps all anesthetic agents are capable of producing spike-like EEG activity at certain levels of anesthesia. Most investigators advise that caution be used during anesthesia for all epileptic patients.

Fine et al reported three cases of transient blindness lasting an average of 25 minutes. This disturbance disappeared with no sequelae. Pupils reacted to light so that the involved area must be distal to the efferent limb of the light reflex and the visual pathway, and probably is the lateral geniculate body, the optic radiations or the visual cortex.[185]

Crumrine et al studied 26 children with hydrocephalus who were given either IM or IV ketamine as anesthesia for neurosurgery or neuro-diagnostic procedures. In all cases, VFP increased regardless of premedication or route of administration of ketamine. These acute rises of VFP may affect marginal areas of CBF and may risk herniation of brain tissue.[186]

Postoperative psychosis after ketamine has been reported in isolated cases. It resembles LSD-induced psychosis and does not appear to be related to pre-existing psychological disturbance.[188]

Methohexital

Methohexital is an ultra-short-acting barbiturate used for short operations in which rapid emergence is desired.

It has been reported to cause muscle twitching, convulsive movements, restlessness, and anxiety.

One percent solutions are used with doses of 1 to 2 mg/kg. The incidence of muscular hyperactivity is increased with the rapidity of injection. A continuous drip method of infusion to administer methohexital will usually prevent this effect.

Extravascular injection of the barbiturates cause pain, ulceration, and necrosis of tissues, including nerves. Intra-arterial injection may result in gangrene.

Narcotics

Narcotics are used routinely as premedicants before surgery and to provide analgesia after surgery. Opiates have been used for centuries for relief of pain during surgery in the form of soporific sponges. In the 19th century, morphine was used subcutaneously, alone, or in combination with scopolamine for complete anesthesia for surgery. Large doses were required for adequate anesthesia and many deaths occurred, so that in the early 20th century doses of morphine and scopolamine were greatly reduced and were used only as premedication for inhalation anesthetics.

Loewenstein reintroduced morphine as a complete anesthetic in 1969 for cardiac patients. Meperidine and fentanyl have also been used as complete anesthetics. Because of prolonged respiratory depression and incomplete anesthesia with narcotics alone, balanced anesthesia (combinations of narcotics with nitrous oxide and muscle relaxants) has become a popular technique in wide use today.[185]

Analgesia is the major pharmologic property of narcotics. Amnesia is not always produced so that narcotics are not truly complete anesthetics. Doses large enough to produce amnesia frequently result in hypotension from vasodilation or in prolonged recovery.

Narcosis following balanced anesthesia is a known complication. When caused by an overdose of narcotic, it is usually readily reversed by narcotic antagonist (naloxone). If the narcotic is not reversed, the narcosis resolves in several hours; however, cases of extremely prolonged recovery have been reported requiring repeated doses of naloxone. Recovery may take as long as 5 days and does not appear to be related to the dose of narcotic.

Prolonged recovery from narcotic anesthetic can be explained by high serum narcotic concentration. This may result from excessive dosages, or in patients with faulty metabolism, faulty excretion, or plasma binding by the narcotic. Narcotics may also be sequestrated in the brain, so that serum concentration would not reflect the retention of morphine.

Recent evidence tends to indicate that narcotics act on the brain by direct stimulation of pain-inhibiting centers that are in the area of the 3rd and 4th ventricles. Brain tissues are known to contain endorphins (*endo*genous mor*phine*-like substance) that have opiate-like effects. Stimulation of the pain-inhibiting receptors can be accomplished with narcotics, endorphins and electrical stimulation. Naloxone blocks analgesia from endorphins. Naloxone has also been found to block the narcosis caused by drugs unrelated to narcotics, and these include diazepam, pentobarbital, halothane, enflurane, cyclopropane, and nitrous oxide. It also blocks the analgesia produced by electrical stimulation of the brain or by acupuncture.[186]

The physiologic roles of opiate receptors and endorphins are presently unknown.

Supportive measures to assure normal cardiorespiratory function are essential in patients with prolonged narcosis. Narcotics desensitize the respiratory center to the stimulating effects of CO_2, causing an increase in the CO_2 threshold and a shift of the pCO_2 alveolar ventilation curve to the right. Large doses of narcotic will result in cessation of involuntary breathing. In patients with prolonged narcosis after narcotics, mechanical ventilation may be necessary to maintain normal blood gases.

Hypotension, bradycardia, hypertension, and tachycardia have all been reported. Hypotension is secondary to vasodilation from direct effect on the blood vessels or secondary to histamine release and from bradycardia due to vagal stimulation.

Acute CNS complications of narcotic anesthesia or analgesia are secondary to reduced cerebral blood flow or reduced cerebral arterial oxygen saturation, causing cerebral hypoxia.

Narcotic-Induced Neuropathy

Weller and Perry[187] reported two cases of neurologic dysfunction in patients who abused morphine, cocaine, and heroin.

One patient developed bilateral anesthesia and motor paralysis in his legs. EMG showed total denervation of both medial and lateral popliteal nerves. Sural nerve biopsy showed total acute axonal degeneration.

Another patient developed weakness of both legs and patchy sensory loss over his back, face, arms and perineal area.

This is a problem that may become more evident as the number of drug abusers in our society increases. Cocaine is rapidly becoming the favorite "recreational" drug in our young adult population. Patients presenting with bizarre, patchy neurologic dysfuction may indeed be drug abusers. A careful history will reveal the cause of these random neuropathies.

Nitrous Oxide

Nitrous oxide was first noted to have anesthetic properties in 1800 by Humphrey Davey. Toward the later part of the 19th century, it was used clinically with inadequate oxygen. Cyanosis was a common, but little understood, problem associated with nitrous oxide anesthesia. Frequently, the end result of nitrous oxide anesthesia was asphyxia. In 1939, Courville[188] studied the brains of a series of patients who failed to regain consciousness after nitrous oxide anesthesia. He pointed out that the chronic oxygen deprivation of nitrous oxide caused respiratory and circulatory collapse, and he described the gross and microscopic changes of the hypoxic brain. Since that time, hypoxic nitrous oxide anesthesia is an accident resulting from improper attention to detail.

Many safeguards are built into modern anesthesia machines, so that this tragedy will not occur.

Pin indexing of anesthetic gas supplies prevents installing the wrong gas on the anesthesia machine. "Fail safe" alarms indicate that oxygen pressure is inadequate, and oxygen analyzers warn of low oxygen concentrations being delivered. Even these safeguards may fail, however, as seen in a new California surgical suite several years ago. The workman had crossed the oxygen and nitrous oxide supply hoses from the central supply of gases.

Nitrous oxide, when used with adequate oxygen, is a safe anesthetic agent. Neurologic complications from anesthetic use are minor. Hearing loss has been reported from changes in middle ear pressure resulting from the differential solubility of nitrous oxide and nitrogen.[189]

Chronic Neuropathy from Nitrous Oxide Abuse

Chronic exposure of nitrous oxide has been reported to cause central and peripheral nerve damage in 15 dentists who abused the drug.[190] They showed numbness, tingling of the hands and feet, patchy at first and then symmetrical, unsteady gait to inability to walk, Lhermitte's electric sign (shock down the back and legs on flexion of the neck), impotence, impaired sphincter control, depression, and impaired memory and reason. Physical examination showed blunting of touch and vibration in the extremities, decreased tendon reflexes and later hyperactive reflexes showing spinal cord involvement and ataxic gait. Electrophysical studies suggest lower motor neuron involvement of peripheral and sensory nerves, and posterior and lateral column involvement of the spinal cord.

This syndrome does not act like hypoxic damage, but rather like a metabolic defect, perhaps of vitamin B_{12} metabolism.

Neurologic symptoms appeared 3 months to 5 years after chronic abuse of nitrous oxide began and disappeared partly or completely after exposure ceased.[190]

Meningitis after General Anesthesia

Kitabata et al[191] report a case of meningitis after anesthesia in a patient who has a skull fracture. Positive pressure respiration with a mask during induction forced nasal contaminants into the cerebral spinal fluid. Awake intubation in patients with skull fracture will avoid this problem. Treatment with antibiotics cured the patient.

Trichloroethylene

TCE was first described by Fischer (1864) and has been widely used in industry as a grease solvent. By 1915, Plessner described toxic actions, especially analgesia of the trigeminal nerve, and thus tricholoroethylene came to be used as an analgesic agent for short operations in the 1930's.[163]

It is a colorless, volatile liquid, manufactured under the names "Trelene" and "Trimar." Concentrations of 10.3-64.5% in O_2 will ignite. It decomposes rapidly, and in the presence of soda lime forms dichloracetylene. This product is responsible for 5th and 7th cranial nerve palsies, as well as those of cranial nerves 3, 4, 6, 10, and 12. Headache and encephalitis are other problems associated with breakdown of products of trichloroethylene. This drug is used infrequently today as an anesthetic agent.

It is of interest to note that the sensory loss in these patients with TCE toxicity is a concentric or an "onion-peel" arrangement centering on the nose, which is indicative of segmental or nuclear trigeminal lesions and which may result from the lipoid solvent effect of TCE on peripheral myelin sheaths. Return in function is gradual and begins with the larger fibers.[164]

Methoxyflurane

Methoxyflurane is 2,2-dichloro-1, 1-difluoroethyl methyl ether. It causes anesthesia or analgesia and is used in conjunction with O_2 and N_2O. It has potent muscle relaxing properties.

Biotransformation in man results in the formation of metabolites of inorganic fluoride — methoxydifluroacetic acid, dichloroacetic acid, and oxalic acid. These metabolites may cause renal failure from oxalite crystals plugging renal tubules.

Neurologic problems reported have been prolonged emergence delirium and postoperative headaches.

Elder et al report a case of nurse anesthetist who developed myasthenia gravis during administration of methyoxyflurane anesthesia. Ptosis of right eyelid, generalized weakness and fatigue persisted 2 to 3 hours after anesthesia; and when an adequate gas-scavenger system was installed, she had no more symptoms.[165]

Halothane (Fluothane)

Halothane is a volatile inhalation anesthetic agent: 2-bromo-2-chloro-1,1,1-trifluoroethane. It is a pleasant non-irritating, non-flammable agent that is used clinically mixed with O_2 and N_2O.

Induction and recovery are rapid. Depth of anesthesia is easily controllable, and with increasing depth of anesthesia, pharyngeal and laryngeal reflexes are obtunded. Apnea results from deep anesthesia, along with reduction in blood pressure and pulse rate. Halothane increases CSF pressure. It causes moderate muscle relaxation. It sensitizes the heart to epinephrine and norepinephrine and may cause cardiac arrythmias. Hyperpyrexia has been reported.

In vivo studies of halothane on mitochondrial metabolism has shown that halothane alters electron transfer and decreases mitochondrial respiratory control in the liver but not in brain mitochondria, so that a direct toxic effect of halothane on the brain at the mitochondrial level has not been demonstrated.[166]

There is, however, a dissociation of cerebral metabolism and cerebral blood flow that is dose related with the administration of halothane and other volatile anesthetic agents (enflurane, isoflurane, methoxyflurane). Cerebral oxygen consumption (CMRO$_2$) decreases with halothane anesthesia; cerebral blood flow increases.

This has the effect of delivering extra O_2 to the brain with a decrease in O_2 requirements. At clinical concentrations of anesthetics, brain lactate levels are unaltered with higher concentrations of agents; brain energy stores are decreased in spite of adequate O_2 concentration, demonstrating a direct toxic effect on the brain.

Volatile agents then do not protect the ischemic brain, as do barbiturates, but rather add to the effect of hypoxia.

In animal experiments with middle cerebral artery ligation, dogs were given barbiturates, halothane, and no anesthesia. Barbiturates had the fewest infarctions. Halothane treated animals had highest incidences of infarctions. This effect may be related to increased CBF with increased intracranial pressure, or to a direct toxic effect on the brain.

Chang et al have demonstrated vacuolation of Golgi complex progressing to the collapse of rough endoplasmic reticulum in the brains of rats exposed to chronic exposure of low doses of halothane, and conclude that the biological membrane system is a prime target of the action of halothane.[167]

Headaches from Halothane

Bromide, a breakdown product of halothane, will cause headaches, ataxia, and lethargy, as well as diffuse EEG changes. It has also been postulated that these symptoms may result from the direct action of halothane on the brain. Bruce[167a] reports that exposure to subanesthetic concentrations (.001% of halothane) have been demonstrated to cause impaired memory, psychomotor activity, and alterance in behavior. Anesthesiologists frequently suffer from headaches after administration of halothane.[168]

Tyrrell and Feldman[169] reported an incidence of postoperative halothane headache in 44% of patients who had controlled respirations and 60% in those with spontaneous respirations during anesthesia. Characteristic halothane headache is frontal, above or between the eyes, and throbbing. The usual duration is 2 to 8 hours.

Zohairy[170] reported giddiness in 75% of patients receiving halothane and headache and vomiting in 50%. Patients treated preoperatively with promethazine and meperidine were less sensitive to headaches.

Other investigators were unable to duplicate this work, but found that subanesthetic concentrations (0.1%) caused mental impairment.[168]

Convulsions from Halothane

Convulsions[171] and tetany[172] have been reported during halothane anesthesia. Explanations of these phenomena have been hypoxia, hypocarbia, and hyperprexia.

Treatment is O_2, barbiturates, succinylcholine for ventilation, and $CaCl_2$ for hypocalcemia.

Halothane Ingestion

Curelaru, et al[173] reported two cases of coma following ingestion of 25 ml halothane. Coma in one patient lasted 36 hours; the other, 72 hours. Both patients had a complete recovery without neurologic deficit.

Enflurane (Ethrane)

Enflurane is a halogenated ether that features rapid induction and emergence, minimal gastrointestinal disturbance, and limited biotransformation. It has a potential for excitation of the CNS, characterized by high amplitude spikes and spike wave complexes with burst suppression on the EEG. EEG abnormalities and seizures have been reported in the presence of respiratory alkalosis. Two cases of delayed seizure activity have been reported. One occurred 6 days postoperatively and lasted four days. The other patient developed visual disturbances on the 6th day, and on the 8th day general motor seizures. EEG showed left parietal occipital disturbances. The first patient had a family history of seizures but was not epileptic; the second patient was on birth control pills.[174-176]

Two to four percent of enflurane is biotransformed to fluorinated metabolites (0.5% inorganic fluorines) and 1.9% organic fluorine; and these are excreted in urine up to 17 days post-anesthesia.

Patients with a history of seizures, intracranial masses, space occupying lesions, and increased intracranial pressure should have alternate methods of anesthesia.

Thiopental during light enflurane will exascerbate spike activity of the EEG, and at greater depth will suppress spike activity. Abolition of myoclonus in dogs receiving enflurane, was reported when given with thiopentone.[176,177]

Enflurane seizures appear to resemble minor motor seizures (i.e, petit mal), characterized by 2 to 3 cycles per second, EEG hypersynchrony, and brief myoclonic movements of facial and neck musculature. Seizures are activited by hyperventilation.

Diazepam and thiopentone augment seizure activity. Diazepam lowers seizure threshold to an enflurane challenge. Hypocarbic techniques also enhance seizure activity and should preclude the use of enflurane.

Treatment for Enflurane Seizures

The treatment for seizures is to correct hypocarbia and eliminate enflurane. Other measures are the same as the treatment of convulsions after local anesthesia.

Thiopental Sodium (Pentothal)

Thiopental sodium is an injectable ultra short acting hypnotic with chemical formula 5-ethyl-5-(1-methylbutyl)-2-thiobarbiturate. It produces anesthesia but not analgesia and is used in clinical anesthesia for pleasant and rapid induction of unconsciousness. It produces hypnosis in 30 to 40 seconds after injection. Recovery is rapid, but repeated doses result in longer recovery because barbiturates are stored in fatty tissues and are released slowly. Shivering and muscle twitches may occur after thiopental sodium.

Prolonged Neuromuscular Blockade

Antibiotics

Prolonged neuromuscular blockade is a well-known adverse effect following administration of antibiotics of the aminogycoside group. These include bekanamycin, dibekacin, dihydrostreptomycin, kanamycin, neomycin, ribostamycin, streptomycin, amikacin, and tobramycin. The main pharmacological mechanism of the neuromuscular block by aminoglycoside group of antibiotics is inhibition of the release of acetylcholine from nerve endings by blocking the inflex of calcium ions, an effect similar to low calcium or high magnesium levels. Neuromuscular blockade by this group of compounds is reversible with calcium and with neostigmine.[192] This problem has been discussed in greater detail in Chapter I in this book.

Disturbances in consciousness has been reported, along with the apnea of antibiotic-induced neuromuscular blockade. The unconsciousness is not related to apnea since artificial ventilation does not alter consciousness. Low serum calcium levels correlate with increased serum levels of aminoglycoside antibiotics. Neostigmine and calcium gluconate are effective in restoring consciousness. Calcium therapy should continue until the serum calcium level is normal.[193]

Neuromuscular Blocking Agents

In clinical anesthesia, neuromuscular blocking agents are used for skeletal muscle paralysis to afford optimal conditions for surgical relaxation and for intubation of the trachea, and they act by their effect on the neuromuscular junction.

Depolarizing agents act at the neuromuscular junction by competing with acetylcholine for the cholinergic receptors at the end plate. Succinylcholine causes depolarization of the postsynaptic membrane, followed by a transient muscle contraction or fasciculation. Pseudocholinesterase hydrolyzes succinylcholine to succinylmonocholine (a weak depolarizing agent) and then to succinic acid and choline. This reaction, after a single dose, lasts about 5 to 10 minutes, after which muscle activity returns to normal. Succinylcholine is rapid acting and is widely used in a single dose for intubation of the trachea or for treatment of laryngospasm. It is also administered as an intravenous drip for longer procedures.

Non-depolarizing neuromuscular blocking agents (i.e, d tubocurarine, pancurium) act at the myoneural junction by increasing the threshold to acetylcholine. It blocks the depolarizing effect of acetylcholine. The membrane potential is unchanged.

Neuromuscular block, with either depolarizing or non-depolarizing agents, is potentiated by inhalation anesthetics, carcinoma, quinine, hypokalemia, and antibiotics (neomycin, streptomycin, kanamycin, gentamycin and bacitracin).

The neuromuscular block of non-depolarizing agent may be reversed by anticholinesterase agents (neostigmine, pyridostigmine). These drugs act by inhibiting the destruction of acetylcholine by cholinesterase.

Support of respiration may be needed in cases of prolonged block not completely reversed by the anticholinesterase.

Pseudocholinesterase Deficiency

When a normal nerve impulse reaches the myoneural junction, acetylcholine, which is present in tiny vesicles, is released into the space between the motor end plate and the muscle fiber. Acetylcholine binds to the cholingergic receptor on the motor end plate, causing an increase in membrane permeability to Na^+ ions. When a certain decrease in resting potential is achieved, extracellular Na^+ enters the cells, depolarization occurs, and the muscle fiber contracts.

Acetylcholinesterase, which is present in the myoneural space, rapidly hydrolyzes acetylcholine, and repolarization occurs.

Neuromuscular blocking agents act by interfering with this enzyme system. Depolarizing agents (succinylcholine) cause muscle paralysis by competing with acetylcholine and maintain the motor end plate in a state of depolarization. Non-depolarization agents (d tubocurare, pancuronium) act by blocking the cholinergic receptor.

Normal neuromuscular activity returns after hydrolysis or diffusion from the end plate of neuromuscular blocking agents. Succinylcholine is hydrolyzed by plasma pseudocholinesterase.[194]

Pseudocholinesterase is a human plasma enzyme that has no known action other than the degradation of succinylcholine. Patients with little or no pseudocholinesterase do not metabolize succinylcholine well, and so its action is prolonged. Idiopathic pseudocholinesterase deficiency occurs in 1 in 2800 persons and is homozygous for an autosomal recessive gene. Any patient with a prolonged recovery time from succinylcholine should be tested for pseudocholinesterase activity. This can be done easily in most hospital laboratories checking plasma pseudocholinesterase level and dibucaine number.

Prolonged block after succynylcholine may also occur in patients with liver damage, and those on drugs which inhibit plasma pseudocholinesterase: nitrogen mustard, neostigmine, pyridostigmine, trimethaphan and hexaflourenium. Local anesthetics and quinidine may potentiate the effect of depolarizing neuromuscular blocking agents.[195]

Hyperkalemia

Succinylcholine causes hyperkalemia in patients with muscle and bone injuries and may lead to cardiac arrest. This may occur three weeks post injury to the time of complete healing. Paraplegics, quadraplegics, and patients with peripheral nerve injuries or lower motor neuron disease, such as poliomyelitis, are at risk up to 12 months after injury.

Muscle Pain

Postoperative muscle pain is a frequent and annoying problem after the use of succinylcholine. A small dose of non-depolarizing neuromuscular blocking agent 3 minutes prior to the injection of succinylcholine may prevent muscle pain.

Fahmy and Malek pretreated patients with diazepam (0.05 mg/kg) and found diminished levels of serum K^+ and CPK, as well as reduction of muscle fasciculation and postoperative pain.[195a]

Causes of Prolonged Neuromuscular Block

Non-depolarizing neuromuscular blocking agents may be reversed by anticholinesterase agents (neostigmine, pyridostigmine), which act by inhibiting the destruction of acetylcholine. Prolonged neuromuscular block from non-depolarizing agents may be influenced by many factors. Inhalation of anesthetic agents potentiate the effect. Patients receiving halothane require one-third less relaxant, and patients receiving enflurane require one-half to two-thirds less.

Quinidine and local anesthetics may enhance the action of non-depolarizing agents. Since neuromuscular blocking agents are mainly excreted by the kidneys, patients with renal disease may have prolonged paralysis.

Antibiotics may potentiate the activity of the non-depolarizing drugs. Neomycin, streptomycin, kanomycin, polimixin, lincomycin and gentomycin are capable of prolonging the blockade. Penicillin, erythromycin, and the cephalosporins do not affect it.[195] This has been discussed further in Chapter I of this book.

Treatment of Prolonged Neuromuscular Blockade

Adequate respiratory function is the desired end point of reversal of neuromuscular blockade. (Measures to evaluate muscle function, such as head lift and hand grip, measures of tidal volume, or thumb twitch, may be used.) Any patient with inadequately reversed neuromuscular block requires respiratory support with endotracheal intubation and mechanical ventilation until the respiratory function is adequate.

Alkylating drugs used in the treatment of malignancy are also additive or act synergistically with non-depolarizing blocking agents. Bennett et al[195] report a case of a patient with malignant cystadenoma of the ovary and myasthenia gravis being treated with pyridostygmine. Administration of pancuronium for muscle relaxation resulted in prolonged neuromuscular blockade with a cholinergic crisis. Succinylcholine used in conjunction with anti-cancer drugs has resulted in prolonged apnea.

Residual Curarization

Residual curarization in the recovery room is more common than usually thought. Viby-Mogensen et al[196] found that 42% of their patients were not adequately reversed. The restless or depressed postoperative patient should be evaluated for evidence of inadequate reversal of neuromuscular blocking agents and should be treated before further complicating his recovery with narcotics.

Monitoring-Arterial Cannulization

New advances in monitoring capabilities provide useful information during anesthesia and surgery, and they add to post-anesthetic neurologic problems.

Cannulization of the jugular vein, subclavian vein, and radial arteries have become common practice in surgery and in critical care units. While these techniques offer the opportunity for accurate monitoring of a patient's blood pressure and cardiac output, they are not without potential hazard. Complication of internal jugular vein cannulization include pneumothorax, hematoma, Horner's syndrome, and ipsilateral mydriasis.[197] Recurrent laryngeal nerve paresis usually results from pressure from hematomas, trauma, or extravasation of fluid. There are reports of extravasation around an indwelling jugular catheter causing injury to the sympathetic chain, cervical plexus, and the cervical nerves. These neurologic defects result in pulmonary aspiration, which may be fatal if unrecognized. Cannulization of the radial artery results in an incidence of 88% transient thromboses with 0-50% hematoma formation; however, permanent ischemic injury is rare.[198] Neurologic injury is secondary to ischemia resulting from thrombosis.

Marshall et al [198a] recently reported median nerve compression following radial artery puncture. This resulted from hematoma formation during attempted puncture of the radial artery which leaked into the carpal tunnel causing compression of the medial nerve. Only sensory impairment was noted in this patient. The motor nerves, which are larger and more resistent to pressure, were not affected in this case.

Miscellaneous Neurologic Complications

Convulsions

Water Intoxication

Water intoxication during trans-urethral resection of prostate (TURP) is a well-known and serious complication when non-electrolyte irrigating solutions are used, resulting in intravascular absorption of the fluid. Classical signs of water intoxication are wide pulse pressure, bradycardia, hypertension, mental agitation, headache, confusion, dyspnea, and convulsions.

The amount of water absorbed depends upon the hydrostatic pressure of the fluid used for surgery, the number and size of venous sinuses opened during the dissection, and the length of surgery.

Measures to prevent iatrogenic hyponatremia are (1) maintaining the hydrostatic pressure of the irrigating fluid below 70 cm H_2O, and (2) keeping the total resection to one hour or less. Hurlbert and Wingard[199] recently reported a case of grand mal seizures after 15 minutes resection time secondary to iatrogenic hyponatremia.

Seizures occur if the serum Na^+ level falls rapidly 20 to 30 mEq/L or falls to below 120 mEq/L.

Most TURP surgery is done under spinal anesthesia, so that the patient may become agitated and confused as the syndrome of water intoxication begins. The anesthesiologist must be alert to subtle changes in the patient's condition to make an early diagnosis before seizures or circulatory collapse occurs. However, with very rapid changes in serum Na^+ levels, grand mal seizures may be the first indication of trouble.

Treatment

Saline solutions of 3% are given in 200 to 300 ml increments to return serum Na^+ levels to normal. Packed erythrocytes may be indicated to replace blood loss. The treatment of iatrogenic hyponatremia requires repeated serum electrolyte determinations to assure adequate replacement of Na^+.

Hypertensive Encephalopathy

Hypertensive encephalopathy is an uncommon complication of anesthesia due to an acute rise in arterial pressure in patients with malignant hypertension, eclampsia, and glomerulonephretis causing acute cerebral edema and ischemia.

Signs of headache, nausea, convulsions, hemiplegia, aphasia, papilledema, and respiratory depression may result.[200] Treatment of hypertensive cerebral edema includes diuretics, steroids, anti-hypertensive drugs, and mechanical ventilation, if needed.

Excitement

Emergence delirium or excitement is frequently seen in the post-anesthesia room. Eckenhoff et al[201] in their series of 14,436 patients admitted to the recovery room found an incidence of 5.3% emergence delirium. They found an increased relationship between the incidence of excitement and age, ranging from 13% in the 3 to 9 year age group to 2.4% in the 70-year-and-older group. Incidence was generally proportional to physical status: 6.3% of patients classified as physical status 1 (healthy, normal patients) to no excitement in patients classified as physical status 3-4 (debilitated patients with life-threatening illness). Patients who received barbiturate scopolamine premedication had the highest incidence of excitement 7.9%; those who received barbiturate-atropine premedication, 4.5%; and patients who received narcotic premedication, 1.6%. The type of surgery had an effect on postoperative excitement. There was an incidence of 14% after T and A surgery, 13.6% after thyroid surgery, and 1.6% after intracranial or spinal surgery.

Postoperative restlessness or excitement is enhanced by hypoxia and pain. Narcotics in the preoperative period, or used in balanced anesthesia, allow a slower awakening, so that patients have less agitation in the recovery room.[202]

Shivering

Postoperative shivering is a frequent complication of anesthesia. During anesthesia significant heat loss occurs through the lungs and surgically exposed organs, resulting in shivering and increased oxygen consumption in the postoperative period. Pediatric patients and those having long vascular operations lose significant heat during surgery if precautionary measures are not taken. Warming mattresses are useful to prevent major heat loss; however, shivering still occurs. Warmed, humidified gases during anesthesia will maintain the patient at normothermic levels. Low gas flows with closed system anesthesia is also effective. Warm blankets and warmed, humidified oxygen in the recovery room will minimize shivering.

Treatment of Excitement and Shivering

Physostigmine

The young healthy patient who is thrashing about in the recovery room is a difficult nursing problem and has the potential to injure himself and others. Physostigmine (1 mg IV; slowly, and 1 mg IM) will usually calm the very excited patient in a few minutes. Physostigmine has been used to reverse the central nervous system effects of neuroleptics, antihistamines, belladonna alkaloids, tricyclic antidepressants, general anesthetics, and anti-parkinsonism drugs. It acts by activating the central cholingergic pathways, but also has potential muscarinic side effects. These include nausea, vomiting, salivation, bradycardia, and bronchospasm. For this reason, the routine use of physostigmine for postoperative restlessness should be avoided, reserving it for the really difficult patient.[203,204]

Oxygen

Nearly every post-operative patient is a candidate for O_2 therapy in the recovery room. Anesthesia depresses the cardiovascular and respiratory system. Hypoxia of some degree exists in the postoperative patient. Restlessness is a sign of hypoxia so that all restless patients should receive O_2 in the recovery room until they are awake and calm.

Narcotics

Postoperative pain will contribute to excitement and is treated with narcotics. In the immediate postoperative period, we prefer to use one-half the dose the patient is to receive after his recovery from anesthesia. Large doses of narcotics in the recovery room add to respiratory depression that may already exist.

Delirium after Drugs Used in Conjunction with Anesthesia

Delirium has been reported from the use of scopolamine and other belladonna drugs, such as phenothiazines, tricyclic depressants, antihistamines, and benzodiazepines.[203,205]

Benzquinomide was first introduced as a tranquilizer and recently has been widely used in recovery rooms as an antiemetic.

Side effects have been reported as delirium and involuntary movements similar to extrapyramidal reaction. Tranquilizers, such as benzquinomide, can produce dual response and the clinical symptoms may be similar; the central anticholinergic syndrome is manifest by delirium, anxiety, hyperactivity, seizures, hallucinations, illusions, disorientation, and recent memory impairment. The extrapyramidal effects are akinesia (mask-like facies, rigidity, tremors, lethargy) and akathesia (dystonia, hypertonicity of muscle groups). With extrapyramidal reaction, consciousness is not impaired. Diazepam and atropine are useful to treat extrapyramidal symptoms.[206] This has been discussed further in Chapter VI in this book.

Physostigmine is a useful anticholinesterase for the anticholinergic syndrome reaction, since it easily crosses the blood brain barrier.

It is interesting that patients in the recovery room may be given physostigmine for somnolence or excitement, which is followed by the side effect of nausea and vomiting, at which point benzquinomide is given. Any postoperative patient deserves a careful evaluation and the conservative therapy of time and oxygen to treat minor problems first, before injecting a drug that is thought to be a panacea, but which has potentially dangerous side effects.[206]

Malignant Hyperthermia

Malignant hyperthermia is a condition that is characterized by fever, skeletal muscle rigidity and tachycardia during anesthesia. This condition occurs approximately 1 in 14,000 administrations of general anesthesia and carries with it a mortality rate of between 50-75%. It is triggered in susceptible patients by the administration of succinylcholine and halothane. Rare instances have been reported where malignant hyperthermia was triggered by other agents; however, the most common triggering agents are succinylcholine and halothane. Initial symptoms are tachycardia and tachypnea along with marked elevation in temperature. In modern surgical suites, the temperature is usually maintained at a maximum of 21°C. With temperatures of this degree, it is unusual for patients to have marked increases in body temperature, and any patient with a temperature increase during anesthesia of 0.5°C should be suspect as having an onset of malignant hyperthermia.

Rigidity occurs immediately after the administration of succinylcholine and may be the warning sign that the syndrome is beginning. In any surgical procedure where rigidity follows the administration of succinylcholine, the anesthetic should be terminated, particularly if there has been previous tachycarida, tachypnea and fever. Other symptoms associated with malignant hyperthermia are cyanosis, skin mottling, arrythmias, and profuse sweating. Signs of malignant hyperthermia include central venous desaturation, central venous hypercarbia, metabolic acidosis, respiratory acidosis, hyperkalemia, myoglobinemia, and elevated creatine phosphokinase (CPK). The exact etiology of malignant hyperthermia is unkown; however, it does appear to be primarily a disease of muscle.[207-208]

Treatment of Malignant Hyperthermia

1. Discontinue the triggering agents (i.e., halothane, succinylcholine).

2. Dantrolene, 1-2 ml/kg IV in man is given as soon as the diagnosis is made.

3. Treatment of acidosis with sodium bicarbonate intravenously. Acidosis should be followed with arterial blood gases.

4. Cooling measures necessary to lower the temperature should be aggressive. The patient may be packed in ice, given gastric or peritineal lavage, or iced intravenous fluids.

5. Maintain urinary output by using adequate volume and diuretics.

6. The value of steroids has not been established; however, they are usually given and may be of help during some of the severe stress reactions.

Complications of Malignant Hyperthermia

1. Retriggering of malignant hyperthermia. This occurs when the initial dose of dantrolene is redistributed and repeated dosages of dantrolene are required.

2. Bleeding may occur secondary to disseminated intravascular coagulation. Disseminated intravascular coagulopathy is difficult to diagnose and treat, and one must be aware of this complication.

3. Renal failure resulting from low cardiac output or from myoglobinemia.

4. Pulmonary edema may occur secondary to volume overload or cardiac failure.

5. Hyperkalemia occurs from increased release of K^+ from muscle cells. This reverses rapidly with successful treatment with dantrolene.

6. Muscle edema may require fasciotomy.

7. Neurologic sequelae (coma, paralysis) may occur secondary to hypoxia and inadequate perfusion.

References

1. Henderson Y, Haggard HW: *Noxious Gases.* New York, The Chemical Catalog, Co. 1917, p 146.
2. Health U.S.: *PHS* **80**:12-30, 1979.
3. Goldstein A Jr, Keats AS: The risk of anesthesia. *Anesthesiology* **33**: 130-143, 1970.
4. *Los Angeles Times,* Sunday, November 9, 1980, p 2.
5. Utting JE, Gray TC, Shelley FC: Human misadventure in anesthesia. *Can Anaesth Soc J* **26**:472-478, 1979.
6. Dripps RD, Lamont A, Eckenhoff JE: The role of anesthesia in surgical mortality. *JAMA* **178**:261-266, 1971.
7. Keats AS: What do we know about anesthetic mortality? *Anesthesiology* **50**:387-392, 1979.
8. Hunter CR, Dornette WHL: Neurologic injuries in the unconscious patient. *Clin Anesth* **18**:351-367, 1972.
9. Steen PA, Michenfelder JD: Neurotoxicity of anesthetics. *Anesthesiolo-*

gy **50**:437-453, 1979.

10. Ames A, Wright RL. Kowada M, et al: Cerebral ischemia: The no-reflow pehnomenon. *Am J Pathol* **52**:437-453, 1968.

11. Brodersen P, Jorgensen EO: Cerebral blood flow and oxygen uptake, and cerebrospinal fluid biochemistry in severe coma. *J Neurol Neurosurg Psych* **37**:384-391, 1974.

12. Smith AL: Barbiturate protection in cerebral hypoxia. *Anesthesiology* **47**:285-293, 1977.

13. Haugen FP: The failure to regain consciousness after general anesthesia. *Anesthesiology* **22**:657-664, 1961.

14. Hossman KA, Kleihaus P: Reversibility of ischemic brain damage. *Arch Neurol* **29**:375-384, 1973.

15. Smith AL, Wollman H: Cerebral blood flow and metabolism: Effects of anesthetic drugs and techniques. *Anesthesiology* **36**:378-400, 1972.

16. Smith AL, Hoff JT, Nielsen SL, et al: Barbiturate protection in acute focal cerebral ischemia. *Stroke* **5**:1-7, 1974.

17. Farhat SM, Schneider RC: Observations on the effect of systemic blood pressure on intracranial circulation in patients with cerebrovascular insufficiency. *J Neurosurg* **27**:441-445, 1967.

18. Eckenhoff JE, Enderby GEH, Larson A, et al: Human cerebral circulation during deliberate hypotension and headup tilt. *J Appl Physiol* **18**:1130-1138, 1963.

19. Frost EAM: Anesthesia for neurosurgical procedures in the sitting position. Princeton, *Weekly Anesth Update* 1:Lesson 4:2-8, 1977.

20. Edelman JD, Wingard DW: Air embolism arising from burr holes. *Anesthesiology* **53**:167-168, 1980.

21. Adornato DC, Gildenberg PL, Ferrario CM, et al: Pathophysiology of intravenous air embolism in dogs. *Anesthesiology* **49**:120-127, 1978.

22. White RI, Alexander JK: Body oxygen consumption and pulmonary ventilation in obese subjects. *J Appl Physiol* **20**:197-201, 1965.

23. Holley HS, Milio-Emili J, Becklake MR, et al: Regional distribution of pulmonary ventilation and perfusion in obesity. *J Clin Invest* **46**:475-481, 1967.

24. Tsueda K, Debrand M, Zeok SS, Wright BD, Griffin WO: Obesity supine death syndrome: Reports of two morbidly obese patients. *Anesth Analg* **58**:345-347, 1979.

25. Smith N Ty: Monitoring the circulation in the operating room. 1978 ASA Annual Refresher Courses, 204-B, 1978.

26. 26th Joint Commission on Accreditation of Hospitals, *Accreditation Manual for Hospitals*, Chicago, Illinois. AMH, 1981, pp 5-10.

27. Carlsson C, Hagerdal M, Siesjo B: Protective effect of hypothermia in cerebral oxygen deficiency caused by arterial hypoxia. *Anesthesiology* **44**:27-35, 1976.

28. Kramer RS, Sanders AP, Lesaga AM, et al: The effect of profound hypothermia on preservation of cerebral ATP content during circulatory arrest. *J Thorac Cardiovasc Surg* **56**:699-709, 1968.

29. White RJ: Cerebral hypothermia and circulatory arrest, reviews and commentary. *Mayo Clinic Proc* **53**:450-458, 1978.

30. Frost EAM: Update on therapeutic barbiturate coma. Miami, *Curr Rev Clin Anesth* 1:Lesson 1:3-7, 1980.

31. Stanski DR, Mihm FG, Rosenthal MH, Kalman SM: Pharmacokinetics of high-dose thiopental used in cerebral resuscitation. *Anesthesiology* **53**:169-171, 1980.

32. Havill JH: Barbiturates in cerebral resuscitation. *Europ Cong Obstet Anesth Analg* (abstract), 1979.
33. Millar RA: Neurosurgical anaesthesia in the sitting position. *Anaesthesia* **44**:495-504, 1972.
34. Whitby JD: Electrocardiography during posterior fossa operations. *Brit J Anaesth* **35**:624-630, 1963.
35. Hardy CA, Fischbach HP: Delayed postanoxic encephalopathy. *Anesthesiology* **43**:694-695, 1975.
36. Wylie WD, Churchill-Davidson HC: *A Practice of Anesthesia.* 3rd edition: Chicago, Year Book Medical Publishers, 1972, pp 1106-1111.
37. Lincoln JR, Sawyer HP Jr: Complications related to body positions. *Anesthesiology* **22**:800-809, 1961.
38. Michaels DD, Zugsmith GS: Optic neuropathy following cataract extraction. *Ann Ophth* **5**:303-306, 1973.
39. Givner I, Jaffe NS: Occlusion of central retinal artery following anesthesia. *Arch Ophth* **43**:197-201, 1950.
40. Cole WH: Partial anesthesia of scalp following general anesthesia. *Med J Aust* **2**:372, 1965.
41. James FM III: Hypesthesia of the tongue. *Anesthesiology* **42**:359-362, 1975.
42. Dripps RD, Eckenhoff JE, Vandam LD: *Introduction to Anesthesia, the Principles of Safe Practice,* 2nd edition: Philadelphia, WB Saunders Co., 1961, pp 280-281.
43. Bageant TE, Tondini D, Lysons D: Bilateral hypoglossal nerve palsy following a second carotid endarterectomy. *Anesthesiology* **43**:595-596, 1975.
44. Budinger K: Über Lahmunger nach Chloroformnarkosen. *Arch Klin Chir* **47**:121-145, 1894.
45. Horsley V: On injuries to peripheral nerves. *Practitioner* **63**:131, 1899.
46. Halstead AE: *Anesthesia Paralysis.* Wisconsin MJ, Milwaukee, 1907-1908, vi, pp 511-515.
47. Dhuner KG: Nerve injuries following operations: A survey of cases occurring during a six-year period. *Anesthesiology* **11**:289-293, 1950.
48. Jackson L, Keats AS: Mechanism of brachial plexus palsy following anesthesia. *Anesthesiology* **26**:190-194, 1965.
49. Adelman M, Pratilas V: Unexplained brachial plexus palsy. *Anesthesilogy* **51**:479-480, 1979.
50. Patel RI, Thein RMH, Epstein BS: Costoclavicular syndrome and the sitting position during anesthesia. *Anesthesiology* **53**:341-342, 1980.
52. Ellul JM, Notermans SLH: Paralysis of the circumflex nerve following general anesthesia for laparoscopy. *Anesthesiology* **41**:520-521, 1974.
52. Britt BA, Gordon RA: Peripheral nerve injuries associated with anesthesia. *Can Anaesth Soc J* **11**:537-548, 1964.
53. Wadsworth TG: The cubital tunnel and external compression syndrome. *Anesth Analg* **53**:303-308, 1974.
54. Schmidt CR: Peripheral nerve injuries with anesthesia. *Anesth Analg* **45**:748-753, 1966.
55. Ellis PDM, Pallister WK: Recurrent laryngial nerve palsy and endotracheal intubation. *J Laryn* **89**:823-826, 1976.
56. Salem M, Wong A, Baranger VC, et al: Post-operative vocal cord paralysis in pediatric patients. Reports of cases and a review of possibly idiologic factors. *Brit J Anaesth* **43**:696-700, 1971.

57. Shapiro SL: The traumatic sequelae of endotracheal anesthesia. *EENT Month* **53**:94-98, 1974.
58. Komorn RM, Smith CP, Erwin JR: Acute laryngeal injury with short-term endotracheal anesthesia. *Laryngoscope* **83**:683-690, 1973.
59. Oldham KW: An unusual complication of the reversed Trendelenburg position. *Anaesthesia* **28**:451-454, 1973.
60. Newberry JM: Paraplegia following general anaesthesia. *Anaesthesia* **32**:78-79, 1975.
61. Carron H: Successful regional anesthesia: Management of common complications. ASA Anual Refresher Course, 112E:1-2, 1978.
62. Lichtiger M, Moya F, eds.: *Introduction to the Practice of Anesthesia.* New York, Harper & Row, 1974.
63. Moore DC: Are systemic toxic reactions to all local anesthetic agents the same? *Acta Anaesth Scand,* Suppl **XXV**:48-53, 1966.
64. Moore DC: *Complications of Regional Anesthesia.* Springfield, Illinois, Charles C. Thomas, 1955, p 90.
65. Bridenbaugh PO: Complications. *Regional Anesth* **5**:6-8, 1980.
66. Usubiaga JE, Wikinski J, Ferrero R, Usubiaga LE, Wikinski R: Local anesthetic-induced convulsions in man...an electro-encephalographic study. *Anesth Analg* **45**:611-620, 1966.
67. Scott DB: Evaluation of the toxicity of local anaesthetic agents in man. *Brit J Anaesth* **47**:56-61, 1975.
68. Munson ES, Pugno PA, Wagman IH: Does oxygen protect against local anesthetic toxicity? *Anesth Analg* **51**:422-427, 1972.
69. Moore DC, Balfour RE, Fitzgibbons D: Convulsive arterial plasma levels of bupivacaine and the response to diazepam therapy. *Anesthesioloty* **50**:454-456, 1979.
70. Munson ES, Wagman IH: Diazepam treatment of local anesthetic-induced seizures. *Anesthesiology* **37**:523-527, 1972.
71. Maekawa T, Sakabe T, Takeshita H: Diazepam blocks cerebral metabolic and circulatory responses to local anesthetic-induced seizures. *Anesthesiology* **41**:389-391, 1974.
72. DeJong RH, Heavner JE: Convulsions induced by local anaesthetic: Time course of diazepam prophylaxis. *Can Anaesth Soc J* **21**:153-158, 1974.
73. DeJong RH, Heavner JE: Diazepam prevents local anesthetic seizures. *Anesthesiology* **34**:523-531, 1971.
74. Klein HO, Jutrin I, Kaplinsky E: Cerebral and cardiac toxicity of a small dose of lignocaine. *Brit Heart J* **37**:775-778, 1975.
75. Munson ES, Martucci RW, Wagman IH: Bupivacaine and lignocaine-induced seizures in rhesus monkeys. *Brit J Anaesth* **44**:1025-1029, 1972.
76. Korevaar WC, Burney RG, Moore PA: Convulsions during stellate ganglion block: A case report. *Anesth Analg* **58**:329-330, 1979.
77. Breithardt G, Seipel L, Lauternschlager J, Schulte H: Cerebral convulsions and cardiac arrest during local anesthesia in patients on antiarrhythmic treatment. *Chest* **67**:375-376, 1975.
77a. Aldrete JA, Daniel W: Evaluation of premedicants as protective agents against convulsive (LD 50) doses of local anesthetic agents in rats. *Anesth Analg* **50**:127-130, 1971.
78. Moore DC, Bridenbaugh LD: Oxygen: the antidote for systemic toxic reactions from local anesthetic drugs. *JAMA* **174**:842-847, 1960.
79. Moore DC: Administer oxygen first in treatment of local anesthetic-

induced convulsions. *Anesthesiology* 53:346-347, 1980.

80. Gjerris F: Transitory procaine-induced Parkinsonism. *J Neurol Neurosurg Psychiat* 34:20-22, 1971.

81. Shnider SM, Asling JH, Holl JW, Margolis AJ: Paracervical block in anesthesia in obstetrics, I: Fetal complications and neonatal morbidity. *Am J Obstet-Gynec* 107:619-625, 1970.

82. Craft JB, Bishop N, Shnider SM: Regional anesthesia for vaginal delivery. Princeton, *Weekly Anesth Update* 2:Lesson 28:2-11, 1979.

83. Peterson AW Jr, Jacker LM: Neonatal tetany during anesthesia. A case report. *Anesth Analg* 52:555-557, 1973.

84. Pash MP, Pickering BG, Tweed WA, Palahniuk RJ: Pressure passive cerebral blood flow in the non-asphyxiated fetus. *Anesthesiology* 51: 3S, S293 (September), 1979.

84a. Bier A: Versucheiiber Cocainsirung des Ruckenmarkes. *Dentscheztschr f Chir* 51:361-369 (ap), 1899.

85. Dripps RD, Vandam LD: Long-term follow-up of patients who received 10,098 spinal anesthetics: Syndrome of decreased intracranial pressure (headache and ocular and auditory difficulties). *JAMA* 161:586-591, 1956.

85a. Moore DC, Brindenbaugh LD: Spinal (subarachnoid) block. *JAMA* 195: 907-912, 1966.

86. Greene BA: A 26-gauge lumbar puncture needle: Its value in the prophylaxis of headache following spinal analgesia for vaginal delivery. *Anesthesiology* 11:464-469, 1950.

87. Phillips OC, Ebner H, Nelson AT, Black MH: Neurologic complications following spinal anesthesia with lidocaine: A prospective review of 10,440 cases. *Anesthesiology* 30:284-289, 1969.

88. Katz JD: Atypical responses to spinal anesthesia. Princeton, *Weekly Anesth Update* 1:Lesson 3-6:6, 1977.

89. Greene HM: Lumbar puncture and the prevention of post-puncture headache. *JAMA* 86:391-392, 1926.

90. McCarthy AC, Raney BB: Preventing post-lumbar puncture headache. *Kentucky Med J* 43:165-169, 1945.

91. Jones RJ: The role of recumbency in the prevention and treatment of postspinal headache. *Anesth Analg* 53:788-796, 1974.

92. Sikh SS, Agarwal G: Postspinal headache. *Anaesthesia* 29:297-300. 1974.

93. Nelson MO: Postpuncture headaches: A clinical and experimental study of the cause and prevention. *Arch Dermat Syph* 21:615-627, April 1930.

94. Oxdil T. Powell WF: Post lumbar puncture headache: An effective method of prevention. *Anesth Analg* 44:542-545, 1965.

95. Gormley JB: Treatment of post-spinal headache. *Anesthesiology* 21:565-566, 1960.

96. Tavakoli M, Habeeb A, Fitzpatrick WO: Postspinal headache: Use of epidural blood patch. *Southern Med J* 72:767-768, 1979.

97. Cass W. Edelist G: Postspinal headache: Successful use of epidural blood patch 11 weeks after onset. *JAMA* 227:786-787, 1974.

98. Davies JR: Epidural blood patch for post-lumbar-puncture headache. *Anesthesiology* 42:518, 1975.

99. Walpole JB: Blood patch for spinal headache. *Anesthesiology* 30:783-785, 1975.

100. Stevens JJ: Another indication for an epidural blood patch. *Anesthesiology* 51:96, 1979.

101. Loeser EA, Hill GE, Bennett GM, Sederberg JH: Time vs. success rate

for epidural blood patch. *Anesthesiology* **49**:147-148, 1978.

102. Abouleish E: Epidural blood patch for the treatment of chronic post-lumbar-puncture cephalgia. *Anesthesiology* **44**:291-292, 1978.

103. Ostheimer GW, Palahniuk RJ, Shnider SM: Post-lumbar-puncture headache. *Anesthesiology* **41**:307-308, 1974.

104. Doctor N, DeZoysa S, Shah R, Modi K, Hussaine SZ: The use of the blood patch for post-spinal headaches. *Anesthesiology* **31**:794-795, 1976.

106. Venus R: Entwicklung and ergebnisse der lumbalanashtesie sammel-referat. *Wien Klin Wchnschr* **20**:566-606, 1907.

107. Lee JJ, Roberts RB: Paresis of the fifth cranial nerve following spinal anesthesia. *Anesthesiology* **49**:217-218, 1978.

108. Robles R: Cranial nerve paralysis after spinal anesthesia. *Northwest Med* **67**:845-847, 1968.

109. Edelman JD, Wingard DW: Subdural hematomas after lumbar dural puncture. *Anesthesiology* **52**:16-167, 1980.

110. Alfery DD, Marsh ML, Shapiro HM: Post-spinal headache or intracranial tumor after obstetric anesthesia. *Anesthesiology* **51**:92-94, 1979.

111. McCutchen JJ: Olfactory groove meningioma-herniation following spinal anesthesia. *J Arkansas Med Soc* **62**:306-309, 1966.

112. Phillips OC: Aseptic meningitis following spinal anesthesia. *Anesth Analg* **49**:866-871, 1970.

113. Goldman WW, Sandford JP: An "epidemic" of chemical meningitis. *Amer J Med* **29**:94-101, 1960.

114. Winkelman NW: Neurologic symptoms following accidental intraspinal detergent injection. *Neurology* **2**:284-291, 1952.

115. DiGiovanni AM, Lathrop GD: Chemical meningitis. Scientific Exhibit, ASA Annual Meeting, 1969.

116. Seigne TD: Aseptic meningitis following spinal analgesia. *Anesthesiology* **25**:402-407, 1970.

117. Kadrie H. Driedger AA, McInnis W: Persistent dural cerebrospinal fluid leak shown by retrograde radionuclide myelography: Case report. *J Nuclear Med* **17**:797-799, 1976.

118. Mulroy MF: Spinal headache and air travel. *Anesthesiology* **51**:479, 1979.

119. Dykes MHM, Sears BR, Caplan LR: Transient global amnesia following spinal anesthesia. *Anesthesiology* **36**:615-617, 1972.

120. Massey Kawkins CJ: An Analysis of the complications of extradural and caudal block. *Anaesthesia* **24**:554-563, 1969.

121. Kim YI, Mazza NM, Marx GF: Massive spinal block with hemicranial palsy after a "test dose" for extradural analgesia. *Anesthesiology* **43**:370-372, 1975.

122. Mandlekar WM: Accidental total spinal (intradural) block. *Anaesthesia* **25**:393-396, 1970.

123. Abram SE, Cherwenka RW: Transient headache immediately following epidural steroid injection. *Anesthesiology* **50**:461-462, 1979.

124. Famewo CE: Headache following epidural anaesthesia for obstetrical delivery: A case report. *Can Anaesth Soc J* **22**:370-372, 1975.

125. Janis KM: Epidural hematoma following postoperative epidural analgesia: A case report. *Anesth Analg* **51**:689-692, 1972.

126. Helperin SW, Cohen DD: Hematoma following epidural anesthesia: Report of a case. *Anesthesiology* **35**:641-644, 1971.

127. Bonica JJ: *The Management of Pain*, Philadelphia, Lea & Febiger, 1953,

p 493.
128. Gingrich TF: Spinal epidural hematoma following continuous epidural anesthesia. *Anesthesiology* **29**:162-163, 1968.
129. Saady A: Epidural abscess complicating thoracic epidural analgesia. *Anesthesiology* **44**:244, 1976.
130. McManus F, Sheehan JM: Cauda equina compression following epidural injection for disc prolapse. *Irish J Med Sci* **144**:447-448, 1975.
131. Cotev S, Robin GC, Davidson JT: Back pain after epidural analgesia. *Anesth Analg* **46**:259-263, 1967.
132. Harrison PD: Paraplegia following epidural analgesia. *Anesthesiology* **30**:778-782, 1975.
133. Urguhart-Hay D: Paraplegia following epidural analgesia. *Anaesthesia* **24**:461-470, 1969.
134. Davies A, Solomon B, Levene A: Paraplegia following epidural anaesthesia. *Brit Med J* **2**:654, 1958.
135. Bromage PR: Paraplegia following epidural analgesia: A misnomer. *Anaesthesia* **31**:947-949, 1976.
136. Lund PC: Peridural Anesthesia. *Acta Anesth Scand* **6**:143-159, 1962.
137. Foldes FF, Colavincenzo JW, Birch JH: Epidural anesthesia; reappraisal. *Anesth Analg* **35**:89-100, 1956.
138. Bonica JJ, Backup PH, Anderson CE, et al: Peridural block: Analysis of 3637 cases and a review. *Anesthesiology* **18**:723-784, 1957.
139. Lund PC, Cwik JC, Quinn JR: Experiences with epidural anesthesia: 7730 cases. Part I, *Anesth Analg* **40**:153-163, 1961.
140. Delany TJ, Carron J, Rowlingson JC, et al: Effect of epidural steroids on nerves and meninges. *Anesthesiology* **51**:3S, S226, 1979.
141. Neumark J, Feichtinger W, Gassner A: Epidural block in obstetrics followed by aseptic meningoencephalitis. *Anesthesiology* **52**:518-519, 1980.
142. Prentiss JE: Cardiac arrest following caudal anesthesia. *Anesthesia* **50**:51-53, 1979.
143. Yamashiro H: Bupivicaine-induced seizure after accidental intravenous injection, a complication of epidural anesthesia. *Anesthesiology* **47**:472-473, 1977.
144. Collier CB: Horner's syndrome following obstetric extradural block analgesia. *Brit J Anaesth* **47**:1342, 1975.
145. Evans JM, Gauci CA, Watkins G: Horner's syndrome as a complication of lumbar epidural block. *Anaesthesia* **30**:774-777, 1975.
146. Woolley EJ, Vandam LD: Neurological sequelae of brachial plexus nerve block. *Ann Surg* **149**:53-60, 1959.
147. Selander D, Edshage S, Wolff T: Paresthesiae or no paresthesiae? Nerve lesions after axillary blocks. *Acta Anaesth Scand* **23**:27-33, 1979.
148. Selander D, Brattsand R, Lundborg G, et al: Local anesthetics: Importance of mode of application, concentration and adrenaline for the appearance of nerve lesions. *Acta Anaesth Scand* **23**:127-136, 1979.
149. Markham JW: Sudden loss of vision following alcohol block of the infraorbital nerve. *Neurosurg* **38**:655-657, 1973.
150. Kepes ER, Foldes FF: Transient abducens paralysis following therapeutic nerve blocks of head and neck. *Anesthesiology* **38**:393-394, 1973.
151. Hyams SW: Oculomotor palsy following dental anesthesia. *Arch Ophth* **94**:1281-1282, 1976.
152. Blaxter PL, Britten MJA: Transient amaurosis after mandibular nerve block. *Brit Med J* **18**:681, 1967.

153. Aass AS, Tenicela R: Inadvertent abducens nerve block during therapeutic trigeminal nerve block. *Acta Anaesth Scand* **20**:359-360, 1976.
154. Tiwari IB, Keane T: Hemifacial palsy after inferior dental block for
dental treatment. *Brit Med J* **1**:798, 1970.
155. Seltzer JL: Hoarseness and Horner's syndrome after interscalene brachial
plexus block. *Anaesth Analg* **56**:585-586, 1977.
156. Otto CW, Wall CL: Total spinal anesthesia: A rare complication of
intrathoracic intercostal nerve block. *Ann Thorac Surg* **22**:289-292, 1976.
157. Moore DC, Mather LE, Bridenbaugh PO, et al: Arterial and venous
plasma levels of bupivicaine following epidural and intercostal nerve
blocks. *Anesthesiology* **45**:39-45, 1976.
158. Peng ATC, Bufalo J, Blancato LS: Rare complication during stellate
ganglion block: A case report. *Can Anaesth Soc J* **17**:640-642, 1970.
159. Keim HA: Cord paralysis following injection into traumatic cervical
meningocele: Complication of stellate ganglion block. *NYSJ Med* **70**:
2115-2116, 1970.
160. Superville-Sovak B, Rasminsky M, Finlayson MH: Complications of
phenol neurolysis. *Arch Neurol* **32**:226-228, 1975.
161. Galizia EJ, Lahiri' SK: Paraplegia following coeliac plexus block with
phenol. *Brit J Anaesth* **46**:539-540, 1974.
161a. Winters WD, Mori K, Spooner CE, Bauer RO: The new physiology
of anesthesia. *Anesthesiology* **28**:65-80, 1967.
162. Domino EF, Chodoff P, Corssen G: Pharmacologic effects of CI-581,
a new dissociative anesthetic, in man. *Clin Pharmacol Ther* **6**:279-291,
1965.
163. Atkinson RS: Trichloroethylene anaesthesia. *Anesthesiology* **21**:67-77, 1960.
164. Feldman RG, Mayer RM, Taub A: Evidence for peripheral neurotoxic
effect of trichloroethylene. *Neurology* **20**:599-606, 1970.
165. Elder BF, Feal H, DeWald W, Cobb S: Exacerbation of subclinical
myasthenia by occupational exposure to an anesthetic. *Anesth Analg*
50:383-387, 1971.
166. Chang LW, Dudley AW Jr, Lee YK, Katz J: Ultrastructural changes
in the nervous system after chronic exposure to halothane. *Exp Neurol*
45:209-219, 1974.
167. Chang LW: Pathologic changes following chronic exposures to halothane: A review. *Environ Health Perspec* **21**:195-210, 1977.
167a. Bruce DL: Trace anesthetic effects on perceptual and cognitive skills.
Anesth Rev **1**:24-25, 1974.
168. McDowell SA, Dundee JW, Pandit SK: Para-anaesthetic headache in
female patients. *Anaesthesia* **25**:334-340, 1970.
169. Tyrrell MF, Feldman SA: Headache following halothane anaesthesia. *Brit
J Anaesth* **40**:99-102, 1968.
170. Zohairy AFM: Postoperative headache after nitrous oxide-oxygen-halo-
thane anaesthesia. *Brit J Anaesth* **41**:972-976, 1969.
171. Smith PA, MacDonald TR, Jones CS: Convulsions associated with
halothane anaesthesia. *Anaesthesia* **21**:229-233, 1966.
172. Conway CF, Hoffmann RJ: Tetany during deep halothane anaesthesia.
Anaesthesia **22**:142-146, 1967.
173. Curelaru I, Stanciu St, Nicolau V, Fuhrer H, Iliescu M: A case of recovery from coma produced by the ingestion of 250 ml of halothane. *Brit
J Anaesth* **40**:283-288, 1968.
174. Furgang FA, Sohn JJ: The effect of thiopentone on enflurane-induced

cortical seizures. *Brit J Anaesth* **49**:127-132, 1977.

175. Ohm WW, Cullen BF, Amory DW, Kennedy RD: Delayed seizure activety following enflurane anesthesia. *Anesthesiology* **42**:367-368, 1975.

176. Darimont PC, Jenkins LC: The influence of intravenous anaesthetics on enflurene-induced central nervous system seizure activity. *Can Anaesth Soc J* **24**:42-55, 1977.

177. Kruczek M, Albin MS, Wolf S, Bertoni JM: Post-operative seizure activity following enflurane anethesia. *Anesthesiology* **53**:175-176, 1980.

178. Perel A, Davidson JT: Recurrent hallucinations following ketamine. *Anaesthesia* **31**:1081, 1976.

179. Meyers FF, Charles P: Prolonged adverse reactions to ketamine in children. *Anesthesiology* **49**:39-40, 1978.

180. Corssen G, Little SC, Tavakoli M: Ketamine and epilepsy. *Anesth Analg* **53**:319-335, 1974.

181. Fine J, Weissman J, Finestone SC: Side effects after ketamine anesthesia: Transient blindness. *Anesth Analg* **53**:72-74, 1974.

182. Crumrine RS, Nulsen FE, Weiss MH: Alterations in ventricular fluid pressure during ketamine anesthesia in hydrocephalic children. *Anesthesiology* **42**:758-761, 1975.

183. Winters WD: Epilepsy or anesthesia with ketamine. *Anesthesiology* **36**:309-312, 1972.

184. Johnson BD: Psychosis and ketamine. *Brit Med J* **1**:428-429, 1971.

185. Stanley TH: Pitfalls and problems in using narcotics for anesthesia. ASA Annual Refresher Courses, 214, 1978.

186. Finck AD: Opiate receptors: Significance for anesthesiology. ASA Annual Refresher Courses, 224, 1978.

187. Weller M, Perry RH: Unusual cardiac and neurological reactions to narcotics. *Lancet* **1**:799-801, 1973.

188. Courville CB: *Untoward Effects of Nitrous Oxide Anesthesia.* Mountain View, California, Pacific Press, 1939.

189. Waun JE, Sweitzer RS, Hamilton WK: Effect of nitrous oxide on middle ear mechanics and hearing acuity. *Anesthesiology* **28**:846-850, 1967.

190. Layzer RB: Myeloneuropathy after prolonged exposure to nitrous oxide. *Lancet* **2**:1227-1230, 1978.

191. Kitahata LM, Collins WF: Meningitis as a complication of anesthesia in a patient with a basal skull fracture. *Anesthesiology* **32**:282-284, 1970.

192. Hashimoto Y, Shima T, Matsukawa S, Satou M: A possible hazard of prolonged neuromuscular blockade by amikacin. *Anesthesiology* **49**: 219-220, 1978.

193. Yao F-S, Seidman SF, Artusio JF Jr: Disturbance of consciousness and hypocalcemia after neomycin irrigation, and reversal by calcium and physostigmine. *Anesthesiology* **53**:69-71, 1980.

194. Owens WD: Anesthetic side effects and complications: Seeking, finding, and treating. *Int Anesth Clin* **18**:1-9, 1980.

195. Bennett EJ, Schmidt GB, Patel KP, Grundy EM: Muscle relaxants, myasthenia, and mustards? *Anesthesiology* **46**:220-221, 1977.

195a. Fahmy NR, Malek NS: Adverse effects of succinylcholine administration: Their modification with diazepam. *Clin Pharmacol Ther* **26**(3):395-398, 1979.

196. Viby-Mogensen J, Jorgensen BC, Ording H: Residual curarization in the recovery room. *Anesthesiology* **50**:539-541, 1979.

197. Forestner JE: Ipsilateral mydriasis following carotid-artery puncture

during attempted cannulation of the internal jugular vein. *Anesthesiology* 52:437-439, 1980.

198a. Marshall G Edelstein G, Hirshman CA: Median nerve compression following radial artery puncture. *Anesth Analg* 69:953-954, 1980.

198. Mangano DT, Hickey RF: Ischemic injury following uncomplicated radial artery catheterization. *Anesth Analg* 58:55-56, 1979.

199. Hurlbert BJ, Wingard DW: Water intoxication after 15 minutes of transurethral resection of the prostate. *Anesthesiology* 50:355-356, 1979.

200. Pollard JA: Hypertensive encephalopathy following anaesthesia. *Brit J Anaesth* 41:640, 1969.

201. Eckenhoff JE, Kneale DH, Dripps RD: The incidence etiology of postanaesthetic excitement. *Anesthesiology* 22:667-673, 1961.

202. Bastron RD, Moyers J: Emergence delirium. *JAMA* 200:883, 1967.

203. Chapin JW, Wingard DW: Physostigmine reversal of benzquinamide-induced delirium. *Anesthesiology* 46:364-365, 1977.

204. Smiler BG, Bartholomew EG, Sivak BJ, Alexander GD, Brown EM: Physostigmine reversal of scopolamine delirium in obstetric patients. *Am J Obstet Gynecol* 116:326-329, 1973.

205. Crawford RD, Baskoff JD: Fentanyl-associated delirium in man. *Anesthesiology* 53:168-169, 1980.

206. Ghoneim MM: Antagonism of diazepam by physostigmine. *Anesthesiology* 52:372, 1980.

207. Gronert G: Malignant hyperthermic management. ASA Annual Refresher Courses, 119C, 1978.

208. Ryan JF: Malignant hyperpepexia: Recognition. ASA Annual Refresher Courses, 119B, 1978.

209. Beasley H: Hyperthermia associated with ophthalmic surgery. *Amer J Opth* 77:76-79, 1974.

Chapter VIII

Neurological Complications
of General Surgery

Jack H. M. Kwaan, M.D.

Introduction

Unlike triumphs and successes, complications and failures frequently imply errors and omissions and thus resemble an unwanted stepchild. While its presence is acknowledged, its legitimacy is often questioned. It is especially distressing to encounter neurological complications where the resultant deficiency can be more profound than the original disorder, without mentioning the medicolegal implications of such therapeutic misadventures. In this chapter on the neurological complications resulting from surgical procedures, an attempt will be made to classify this problem into three general categories.

The first group includes those patients whose neurological dysfunction is the direct consequence of inadvertent transection, retraction or excessive manipulation at operation. Comprehensive knowledge of the anatomical course of the peripheral nerves in the specific area is of prime importance in preventing such occurrences. Unexpected and atypical nerve pathways should be anticipated where there is tissue distortion from tumor, scarring or irradiation.

The second group comprises those patients with nerve injury following excessive stretch or traction. This complication can be avoided by proper positioning of the patient on the operating table. Unfortunately, this much belittled task of patient positioning is often delegated to the most junior member of the operating team.

Finally, a third group consists of those patients where neurological dysfunction has primarily been caused by devascularization or ischemia. This includes patients with thrombosis or embolism to critical vessels supplying either the brain, the spinal cord or peripheral nerves during an operative procedure.

269

Neurological Complications Resulting from Direct Surgical Trauma

The cranial nerves, and in particular, the facial, vagal, accessory and hypoglossal nerves are susceptible to iatrogenic injury during oper- ations in the head and neck region.

Facial Nerve

Because of its close proximity, injuries to the facial nerve can occur with operations upon the parotid gland. Facial nerve dysfunction can be both cosmetic and functional. The frequency of permanent weakness of a major facial branch (3-6%) was noted to be more common after total than after superficial parotidectomy.[1] Where weakness and palsy of the facial nerve has occurred following parotidectomy and clear identifica- tion of the nerve throughout its course has been made at surgery, reexplo- ration is generally unfruitful and return of neurological function can be expected in three to six months. However, if inadvertent transection has occurred, microsurgical technics have been especially valuable in nerve reapproximation. Interruption of the mandibular branch of the facial nerve can result from operations over the upper neck. Indentification of this nerve tributary can avoid the consequences of an unsightly lip deformity.

Frey's Syndrome

A gustatory sweating in the parotid area may be observed following superficial parotidectomy. This complication is referred to as Frey's Syndrome and usually appears several weeks following operation, but once present is usually permanent.[2] Involvement of the greater auricular or the auricular temporal nerve is generally implicated. Sections of these nerves or division of the tympanic plexus (Jacobsen's nerve) have been used to correct this malady with varying degrees of success.

Vagus Nerve

The vagus nerve and its branches are within the operative field in surgical exposure of the thyroid gland, larynx, cervical lymph node chain or the carotid vessels. More commonly known are injuries to the superior laryngeal or the recurrent laryngeal divisions of the vagus nerve. The superior laryngeal nerve divides into internal and external branches. The internal branch provides sensory innervation to the larynx and epiglottis, and can produce disturbances in degluttition if involved. The external branch, however, controls motor function of the inferior constrictor and cricothyroid muscles and hoarseness results from injury to this branch. Although the superior laryngeal nerve is generally not within the operative field, it can be subjected to pressure, compression and retraction. The recurrent laryngeal nerve ascends in the tracheo-esophageal groove and passes in close relation to the inferior thyroid artery as it enters to supply intrinsic muscles of the larynx.[3] Attention should also be drawn to the anomalous "non-recurring" laryngeal nerve occurring in 1% of the patients and which can easily be mistakenly ligated with the inferior thyroid artery.[4] The recurrent nerve is not only vulnerable during thyroid and parathyroid surgery, but can be injured in its intrathoracic course in pulmonary or aortic procedures. Routine identification of the recurrent laryngeal nerve is a preferred approach during thyroidectomy because this would eliminate further reexploration should laryngeal function deficits occur postoperatively. Immediate reapproximation of the recurrent nerve is desirable where inadvertent transection has occurred. Such early treatment will result in return of function within 12 to 16 monts.[5] The great auricular nerve has been used as donor where interruption has involved excessive loss of nerve tissue. If dennervation is permanent, Teflon injection of the vocal cord area for improvement of dysphonia and airway difficulties has met with varying degrees of success.[6]

Accessory Nerve

Although rare, injury involving the spinal accessory nerve has been reported following minor surgical procedures.[7] The surperficial course of the nerve and its proximity to the lymph node chains where biopsies are performed renders the accessory nerve particularly susceptible to iatrogenic injury in the posterior cervical triangle. The resultant weakness of the shoulder girdle movements can be disabling, but early reexploration and nerve repair can restore muscle function.

Phrenic Nerve

It is fortunate that phrenic nerve crush procedures for treatment of pulmonary tuberculosis has become a relic of the past. Injury to the nerve in the supraclavicular region can occur in scalene node biopsy procedures. Phrenic nerve section leads to paralysis of diaphragmatic movements and the resultant paradoxical motion may be especially disabling to the patient who already has respiratory compromise.

Hypoglossal Nerve

The hypoglossal nerve in its course through the upper cervical and submandibular triangle, is exposed to surgical trauma in operations on the upper neck or the carotid vessels. Transection of this nerve results in ipsilateral loss of motor function with subsequent atrophy. Surprisingly, little disability results and the patient is rarely inconvenienced.[8] If transected, however, repair of this nerve should be attempted.

Other peripheral nerves may also be involved.

Long Thoracic Nerve

The advent of lesser procedures such as lumpectomy, or simple mastectomy for breast cancer have lessened the incidence of exposure of the long thoracic nerve at operation. The classical wing scapula deformity results from transection of the nerve during the course of a radical mastectomy. Treatment for this condition had mainly been supportive.

Intercostal Nerve

Intercostal pain over a thoracotomy incision or following tube thoracostomy can be a disquieting experience. Relief with local nerve block confirms the diagnosis. Corrective therapy such as surgical excision of a neuroma is occasionally necessary, but the condition is generally self-limiting.

Ilioinguinal Nerve

The ilioinguinal nerve enters the inguinal canal after piercing the transversus abdominis and internal oblique musculature at the level of the iliac crest. Trauma to this nerve during inguinal herniorrhaphy may lead to sensory loss or severe pain over the groin area. Schneck[9] described a 37-year-old physician who developed massive gastrointestinal bleeding following anticoagulant therapy for suspected thrombophlebitis. This apparently was a misdiagnosis and the correct diagnosis was made when the patient developed burning pain over the upper thigh with sensory loss coupled also with a previous history of inguinal herniorrhaphy. His symptoms of ilioinguinal neuralgia was relieved following neurolysis.

Genitofemoral Nerve

The genitofemoral nerve descends in its retroperitoneal course over the psoas major muscle to divide into the genital and femoral branches.

The genital branch distributes its terminal twigs to the scrotum or labia and adjacent thigh, while the femoral branch supplies the skin over the femoral triangle. Operative procedures that involve the retroperitoneum such as lumbar sympathectomy, vascular reconstruction or even appendectomy[10] can lead to severance or entrapment of this nerve with resultant neuralgia. Neurolysis may be necessary for the relief of symptoms.

Femoral and Sciatic Nerves

Direct injuries to these nerve trunks have been reported following orthopedic procedures such as hip arthoplasty[11] or manipulation associated with hip fractures.[12] Nerve damage during hip arthoplasty has been attributed to the heat of the setting cement or overflow of the methylmethacrylate used on the prosthetic acetabulum. Delayed entrapment from the acrylic material has been reported as late as 7 months following the procedure.[13] Electrophysiological testing can be a useful adjunct in the management of these patients in deciding such needs as braces, exercise programs as well as prognostic indications with respect to recovery.[14]

Saphenous Nerve

The saphenous nerve, which is a branch of the femoral nerve, descends alongside the superficial femoral artery. Below the popliteal fossa, the nerve is in the company of the long saphenous vein. Because of its intimate association with these two structures, involvement of the saphenous nerve leading to neuralgia not infrequently complicates arterial reconstructive procedures or vein stripping. This complication of saphenous neuralgia can be an extremely uncomfortable and persistent experience and is probably more common than reflected in the current literature.[15] Awareness of this troublesome and painful complication should alert the surgeon to minimize trauma or preserve this small but important nerve branch, as there is no direct curative treatment of this problem.

Neurological Injury Following Excessive Stretch or Traction

Although this condition is sometimes classified as post-anesthetic palsy, discovery of a new neurological deficit following a surgical procedure would place the immediate responsibility upon the operating surgeon. Most lamentable has been the fact that these postoperative neuropathies, which are the cause of much patient distress and legal action, can so readily be prevented.

Brachial Plexus Palsy

Brachial plexus palsy was recognized as early as 1894,[16] and since then, a number of reports have appeared in the literature (Table I). This complication is infrequent but its occurrence can be a painful and anguishing experience, not only to the patient, but perhaps to the operating surgeon as well. The author's first encounter with this complication involved a 59-year-old male who sustained total loss of motor and sensory functions of his right upper extremity following a three-and-one-half hour esophagectiomy procedure.[17] The patient was placed in the left lateral position (inclined 60°) with the right side up. The arm being attached to the ether screen was therefore abducted 90° and extended 30°. It was fortunate that this patient regained function of his hand by the third postoperative day and was fully recovered by the end of two months.

Clausen[18] credited Gerdy as the first to promote the theory of traction and this view is shared by Stephen and others.[19,20] Objective measurements on cadavers also clearly demonstrated increased tension or stretch of the nerve bundle in commonly used positions on the operating table.[17]

Maximum stretch of the brachial plexus was also observed where arm abduction was beyond 90° and especially in combination with extension, where bilateral arm abduction is involved or where there is concurrent contralateral head rotation and arm abduction. In the prevention of this complication, such positions involving increased tension to the brachial plexus should be judiciously avoided. Compression of the plexus can be an additional factor if there are other anomalous defects such as cervical ribs, scalenous anticus hypertrophy or other narrowing or constrictive factors of the thoracic outlet. Because brachial palsy has occurred with operations of short intervals, the time factor probably only plays a secondary role.

Treatment of this complication is mainly supportive. During the acute phase, the use of cortisone is beneficial, as the initial injury is very likely one of traumatic neuritis.[21] Massage, stretching or active physical therapy during this period can be harmful. Immobilization in the position of optimum function is recommended, and passive motion to maintain muscle tone during the period of recovery is advisable. Electrophysiological findings are a useful adjunct in the follow-up or as an indicator of improvement.[22]

Brachial plexus palsy following median sternotomy approach to intracardiac operations has been reported.[23] In this instance, arm positioning could not have been a contributing factor, and nerve injury was attributed to excessive spread of retractors causing stretch to the brachial plexus.

The prognosis of postoperative brachial palsy is excellent and recovery can generally be expected as permanent injury is the exception rather than the rule. Awareness of this condition with knowledge of appropriate preventive measures is the best solution to this neurological complication.

Sciatic and Peroneal Palsy

Stretch to the sciatic or peroneal nerve has been observed in pelvic procedures with the patient in the lithotomy position. These include both general, gynecological or urological operations. The resultant sensory or motor deficit can be disabling. Burkhart and Daly[24] attributed this to excessive external rotation of the hip and also to extension of the knee. Treatment, as in the brachial plexus injury, is supportive and prognosis for complete recovery is extremely good.

The neuropathies produced by improper positioning have also been discussed in Chapter VII in this book.

Neurological Complications Resulting from Ischemia or Devascularization of Brain, Spinal Cord or Peripheral Nerves

Carotid Artery

Stroke Following Carotid Artery Ligation

Erosion of the carotid artery often leads to a fatal hemorrhage. Extensive neck dissection and high dose radiation for treatment of head and neck tumors is a frequent cause of this complication. Because carotid artery rupture has resulted from necrosis and infection, arterial reconstruction is generally inadvisable and the only alternative entails proximal and distal ligation of the carotid vessel. The adequacy of cerebral collateral circulation then becomes extremely important. The lack of sufficient collateral through the circle of Willis would merely convert the castastrophe of death from exanquination in these patients to the agony of lifelong disability from stroke or hemiplegia.

The incidence of neurological deficit following unilateral carotid interruption was examined in 125 consecutive patients who underwent carotid endarterectomy.[25] Only 19.2% had apparently failed to tolerate test clamping of the carotid artery and developed temporary loss of consciousness or hemiplegia. In another study,[26] of 61 patients who underwent

Table I
Reported Cases of Postoperative Brachial Plexus Palsy

Author(s)	No. of Cases	Type of Operation	Arm Position	Operation Time	Injury	Recovery Period
Stephens[a]	3	Intracardiac procedures cardiopulmonary bypass	Abduction at shoulder	Not stated	Upper roots	Not stated
Ewing[b]	3	Abdominoperineal resection	Arm abduction, Trendelenberg	2-3½ hr	Upper roots or bilateral total paralysis	3-9 mo
	2	Cholecystectomy and sigmoid resection	Bilateral arm abduction	1½-2½ hr	Upper roots	1-5 mo
Cotton and Allen[c]	4	Appendectomy, hip operation	Bilateral arm abduction	3/4-2 hr	Total paralysis	Several months
Kiloh[d]	4	Cholecystectomy	Bilateral arm abduction 90°	1½-2 hr	Total/partial paralysis	4-7 mo
Raffan[e]	2	Hysterectomy	Arm abduction 90°, Trendelenberg	1-1½ hr	Total paralysis	2-4 mo

Woodsmith[f]	1	Cystectomy	Arm abduction 90°, Trendelenberg	3 hr	Upper roots	3 mo
Clausen[g]	8	Abdominoperineal resection	Arm abduction, Trendelenberg	2-3 hr some not stated	Mostly upper roots	6 weeks-11 mo
	1	Chest lobectomy	Arm abduction (marked)	2½ hr	Upper roots	7 mo
Dhuner[h]	11	Not stated	Mostly bilateral abduction 90°	40 min and not stated	Upper roots	Few weeks-3 mo

[a] See, Ref. 19.

[b] Ewing MR: Postoperative paralysis in the upper extremity. *Lancet* 1:99-103, 1950.

[c] Cotton FJ, Allen SW: Brachial paralysis, post narcotic. *Boston Med Surg J* 148:499-502, 1903.

[d] Kiloh LG: Brachial plexus lesions after cholecystectomy. *Lancet* 1:102-105, 1950.

[e] Raffan AW: Postoperative paralysis of the brachial plexus. *Brit Med J* 2:149, 1950.

[f] Woodsmith FG: Postoperative brachial plexus paralysis. *Brit Med J* 1:1115-1116, 1952.

[g] See Ref. 18.

[h] Dhuner KG: Nerve injuries following operations. *Anesthesiology* 11:289-293, 1950.

From Kwaan, JHM, Rappaport I: Postopertive brachial plexus palsy. *Arch Surg* 101:612-615, 1970, with permission. Copyright 1970, American Medical Association.

unilateral carotid artery ligation for hemorrhage during tumor resection, 28% developed neurological complications. However, in 27 patients who were hypotensive, cerebral complications following carotid artery interruption rose to 87%. These reports do not define any specific treatment modality for this condition, but do provide some predictable expectation of stroke complication which occurs in approximately one fifth of patients undergoing unilateral carotid interruption.

Stroke Following Carotid Endarterectomy

It is ironical that carotid endarterectomy, a frequently performed surgical procedure for the prevention of stroke, can in itself produce stroke as an operative complication. Although mortality and morbidity for carotid endarterectomy have continued to decline, the reported stroke rate following such an operation continues to vary between 2 and 14%.[27,28] The mechanism of neurological deficit developing during the immediate postoperative period is not known, but cerebral ischemia and carotid thrombosis is generally suspected. A recent report on the successful management of early stroke after carotid endarterectomy placed special emphasis on the value of instant reoperation.[29] The favorable outcome in this report was attributed to the avoidance of any delay by omitting preoperative arteriography, reexploration under local anesthesia and rapid restoration of cerebral flow by insertion of a shunt. With improved selection such as avoiding operations upon patients with progressive acute strokes, and better cerebral protection during the surgical procedure, the incidence of this complication can be reduced to a minimum.

Ischemia to Spinal Cord

Operation upon the abdominal aorta is a common vascular procedure whether it be for aneurysm or arteriosclerotic occlusion. Although aortic grafting or endarterectomy is relatively safe, the most dreaded, though infrequent complication of paraplegia following aortic revascularization, remains a menace to the operating surgeon. Seldom mentioned in the standard surgical text[30] and receiving equally brief attention in the current literature, this problem is also rarely discussed in the preoperative consent request and can thus be the source of much misunderstanding and litigation.

The etiology of this condition is often explained as interruption of an anomalous infrarenal origin of the arteria redicularis magnus with diminished collateral flow. Ischemic necrosis of the anterior and lateral horns of the spinal cord has been found on postmortem examination.[31] Recovery from this complication is rare and no beneficial treatment is known at this time. Preoperative angiography in demonstrating a large lumbar artery may indicate the predominant blood supply of the lower spinal cord to be an infrarenal arteria radicularis magna.[32] Preventive measures such as reimplantation of the lumbar vessel or even the possibility of considering conservative management should be entertained. This problem is discussed in greater detail in Chapter IX in this book.

Ischemia to Spinal Nerves

Ischemic neuropathy developing following embolectomy or revascularization procedure is uncommon, but can be a distressing postoperative problem. The cause can be attributed to arterial interruption at surgery. Symptoms vary from numbness to causalgic pain. The pathophysiology is not dissimilar to arterial occlusion and involves segmental demyelination from local ischemia and occlusion of the vasa nervorum.[33] Management is primarily supportive, but prospects of permanent relief especially with causalgic pain remain dismal.

References

1. Nichols RD, Stine PH, Bartsclic LR: Facial function in 100 consecutive parotidectomies. *Larygoscope* **89**:1930-1934, 1979.
2. Gordon AB, Foddoam RV: Frey's syndrome after parotid surgery. *Amer J Surg* **132**:54-58, 1976.
3. Anscom BJ, McVay CB: *Surgical Anatomy*, 5th Edition. Philadelphia, W.B. Saunders Co., 1971.
4. Stewart GR, Mountain JC, Colcock BP: Non recurrent laryngeal nerve. *Brit J Surg* **59**:379-381, 1972.
5. Peters LL, Gardner RJ: Repair of recurrent nerve injuries. *Surgery* **71**:865-867, 1973.
6. Dedo HH, Urrea RD, Lawson L: Intracordial injection of Teflon in the treatment of 135 patients with dysphonia. *Ann Otol* **82**:661-667, 1973.
7. Dunn AW: Trapezius paralysis after minor surgical procedures in the posterior cervical triangle. *S Med J* **67**:312-315, 1974.
8. Warpeha RL: Symposium on complications of general surgery, head and neck surgery. *Surg Clin N Amer* **57**:1357-1363, 1977.
9. Schneck SA: Peripheral and cranial nerve injuries resulting from general surgical procedures. *Surgery* **81**:855-859, 1960.
10. Magee RK: Genitofemoral causalgia (a new syndrome). *Can Med Assn J* **46**:326-328, 1942.
11. Weber ER, Danbe JR, Coventry MB: Peripheral neuropathies associated with total hip arthroplasty. *J Bone Joint Surg* **58A**:66-69, 1976.
12. Campbell RD, Mason JB, Wade PA: The use of intramedullary prosthetic replacement in fractures of femoral neck. *Amer J Surg* **99**:745-755, 1960.
13. Casagrande PA, Danahy PR: Delayed sciatic nerve entrapment following the use of self curing acrylic. *J Bone Joint Surg* **53A**:167-169, 1971.

14. Echternach JL: Peripheral nerve lesions following total hip replacement. *Phys Ther* **57**:1034-1036, 1977.
15. Adar R, Meyer E, Zweig A: Saphenous Neuralgia. *Ann Surg* **190**:609-613, 1979.
16. Budinger K: Ueber Lahmingen Nach Chloroform Narkosen. *Arch Klin Chir* **47**:121-145, 1894.
17. Kwaan JHM, Rappaport I: Postoperative brachial plexus palsy. *Arch Surg* **101**:612-615, 1970.
18. Clausen EG: Postoperative paralysis of the brachial plexus. *Surgery* **12**:933-942, 1942.
19. Stephens JW: Neurological sequelae of congenital heart surgery. *Arch Neurol* **7**:450-459, 1962.
20. Jackson L, Keats AS: Mechanism of brachial plexus palsy following anesthesia. *Anesthesiology* **26**:190-194, 1965.
21. Adler JB, et al: Erb's palsy. *J Bone Joint Surg* **49**:1052-1063, 1967.
22. Trojaborg W: Electrophysiological findings in pressure palsy of the brachial plexus. *J Neurol Neurosurg Psychiat* **40**:1160-1167, 1977.
23. Kirsh MM, Magee KR, Gago O, et al: Brachial plexus following median sternotomy incision. *Ann Thor Surg* **11**:315-319, 1971.
24. Burkhart FL, Daly JW: Sciatic and peroneal nerve injury: A complication of vaginal operations. *Obstet Gynec* **28**:99-102, 1966.
25. Kwaan JHM, Peterson GJ, Connolly JE: Stump pressure — an unreliable guide for shunting during carotid endarterectomy. *Arch Surg* **115**:1083-1085, 1980.
26. Ketcham AS, Hoye RC: Spontaneous carotid artery hemorrhage after head and neck surgery. *Amer J Surg* **110**:649-655, 1965.
27. Easton JD, Sherman DG: Stroke and mortality rate in carotid endarterectomy. *Stroke* **8**:565-568, 1977.
28. Thompson JE: Internal carotid and vertebral artery occlusive disease. In: Hardy JE, ed: *Rhoad's Textbook of Surgery*, 5th Edition. Philadelphia, JB Lippincott Co., 1977.
29. Kwaan JHM, Connolly JE, Sharefkin JB: Successful management of early stroke after carotid endarterectomy. *Ann Surg* **190**:676-678, 1979.
30. Golden GT, Wellon HA, Muller WH: Paraplegia and operations upon the abdominal aorta. *Surg Gynec Obstet* **141**:424, 1975.
31. Szilagyi DE, Hagerman JH, Smith RF, et al: Spinal cord damage in surgery of the abdominal aorta. *Surgery* **83**:38-56, 1978.
32. Kwaan JHM, Connolly JE, Vandermolen R, et al: The value of arteriography before aneurysmectomy. *Amer J Surg* **134**:108-114, 1977.
33. Eames RA, Lange LS: Clinical and pathological study of ischemic neuropathy. *J Neurol Neurosurg Psychiat* **30**:215-226, 1967.

Chapter IX

Neurologic Complications of Aortic Surgery

Gerald T. Golden, M.D., F.A.C.S., and
Sandra J.A. Golden, R.N.

Introduction

Serious neurologic complications of aortic surgery are uncommon, usually unexpected, and occur in the face of strict adherence to accepted standards of surgical judgement and technique. The neurologic defects vary from minimal to severe and may be transient or permanent; their effects, however, are invariably psychologically devastating to both the patient and surgeon. The fact is, fewer than one-half dozen scientific publications have addressed any aspect of this subject in the past five years[1-4] which reflects our stagnant and incomplete understanding of several key factors in this area. The three neurologic defects which may complicate aortic surgery are brain injury, paraplegia, and disturbances of sexual function. In this chapter, the pathophysiology, prognosis and prevention of these complications will be discussed.

Brain Injury

Brain injury may be the result of cerebral embolism by clot or atheromatous debris which attends surgical manipulation of the thoracic aorta. In some instances, air is introduced into a system of extracorporeal shunts and causes cerebral damage by air embolism. In addition, elderly patients with cerebral arteriosclerosis may experience thrombosis of one or more intracranial arteries because of hypotension with diminished blood flow and stasis. When high aortic cross-clamping is necessary, excessive pressure in the intracranial arterial system can occur causing focal or widespread hemorrhage within the brain. The effects of the foregoing may vary from a transient hemiplegia

281

to an unrelenting decerebrate or decorticate state and death. Prevention of such complications is not always possible, is strictly related to technical considerations, and its discussion is beyond the scope of this chapter. The treatment of brain injury following air or atheromatous embolism, cerebral thrombosis, or intracranial hemorrhage is largely supportive and aimed at reducing further insult and the reduction of intracranial pressure. Rarely, a large, localized cortical hemorrhage can be evacuated surgically.

Paraplegia

The pathophysiologic postulates explaining brain injury following manipulation of the aortic arch are relatively straight forward. When thrombosis or embolism occurs, the occluded artery can usually be identified once the neurologic deficit has been accurately assessed. When paraplegia complicates the surgical repair of aortic disease, the pathophysiology is, at best, abstruse. For example, paraplegia may unexpectedly follow elective operation for coarctation or an abdominal aortic aneurysm performed under the best of circumstances. Obviously, the complication is due to finite or permanent interruption of the blood supply to the spinal cord. Despite what is considered an adequate understanding of the cord's blood supply, the rare and sporadic occurrence of paraplegia following aortic surgery remains baffling.

The first accurate descriptions of the spinal arteries were provided by Adamkicwicz[5] and Kadyi[6] at the end of the nineteenth century and more recent clinical and radiographic studies have confirmed their accuracy.[7-11] The blood supply to the cord originates from the anterior and posterior spinal branches of the vertebral arteries, and the posterior inferior cerebellar arteries. Anteriorly, the confluence of vessels courses down the cord in the median longitudinal fissure from the cervical region to the filum termenale as the anterior spinal artery. The posterior spinal arteries are paired, originating principally from the posterior inferior cerebellar arteries. They are perfused above from both the vertebral and posterior inferior cerebellar arteries and course downward in the posterolateral sulci (Fig. 1).

In the early human embryo, there is extensive segmental reinforcement of the anterior spinal artery by cervical, intercostal, and lumbar arteries. During development, this segmental system undergoes extensive modification and at birth, only a few segmental vessels remain. These arteries are usually single and arise from the left intercostal or lumbar arteries. Passing posteriorly, they ultimately pass through the intervertebral foramina to the anterior spinal artery. They average eight in number and are present in a ratio of roughly one artery to each four spinal roots.

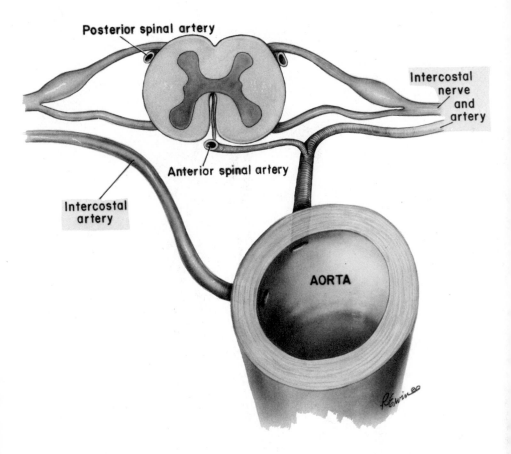

Figure 1. The relationship of the anterior and posterior spinal arteries to the spinal cord and aorta.

Of the six or eight persistent radicular branches, three to five may be in the cervical or upper thoracic region (Fig. 2). Between the levels of the eighth cervical and the ninth thoracic vertebrae, there are usually two unilateral, inconsistently located, small branches to supply this long section of cord.[12]

The principal segmental vessel in the region of the lower thoracic and lumbar portions of the spinal cord is through a large lumbar segmental branch called the *arteria radicularis magna* (ARM).[5,9-11] Radiographic studies by Doppman and DiChiro[9,10] indicate that the anastomosis between the ARM and the anterior spinal artery is usually present between the ninth thoracic and second lumbar veretebrae. During development, the vertebral column grows more rapidly than the spinal

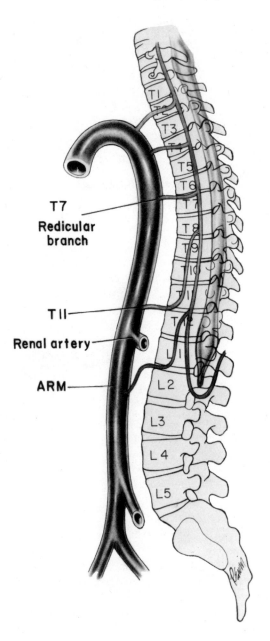

Figure 2. The variable segmental blood supply to the spinal cord and the relative cephalad position of the cord with respect to the aorta. Note the *Arteria Radicularis Magna* arising from the aorta in the lumbar region of the spinal cord.

cord and there is progressive cephalad displacement of the conus medullaris. For this reason, the ARM arises from the aorta several segments below its anastomosis with the anterior spinal artery and ascends the intervening distance at a very acute angle with the spinal cord (Fig. 2). The studies of Kadyi[6] indicate that the ARM arises with equal frequency above and below the renal arteries.

The anterior spinal artery has a variable diameter throughout its lengthy course from the foramen magnum to the filum terminale and may not be uniformly patent throughout this distance. This creates a physiologic "watershed" that renders this vessel a poor source of collateral blood flow in some patients especially if a critical segmental branch is occluded. Therefore, occlusion of a segmental branch may be harmless in one patient and disastrous in another.[13] These anatomic inconsistencies have also been demonstrated experimentally in other mammals.[14-17]

The posterior spinal arteries course down the dorsal aspect of the cord in the posterolateral sulci. They originate as branches of the vertebral and posterior inferior cerebellar arteries. These vessels have little in the way of segmental reinforcement, and the posterior portions of the spinal cord in the cervical and upper thoracic regions are almost totally dependent upon their parent arteries. For the remainder of their thoracic and lumbar course, these arteries are dependent upon their vital inferior anastomoses with the terminal branches of the anterior spinal artery.

The anterior spinal artery provides multiple nutrient branches which supply the greater part of the cross-sectional area of the cord. Nutrient branches of the posterior spinal artery are confined to the dorsal white matter and the dorsal most portions of the posterior horns of gray matter. There are few, if any, anastomoses between the two systems within the substance of the spinal cord.[12]

When there is inadequate blood flow to the anterior spinal artery for a significant period of time, the effects are somewhat variable. When the infarction is large and located in the thoracic cord, there is usually permanent paraplegia with loss of pain and temperature perception below the lesion as well as disturbances in vesical and rectal sphincter control. This paraplegia may be of the flaccid type for days or weeks but ultimately spasticity of the lower limbs supervenes with hyperreflexia with extensor plantar responses and tends to be permanent.[18]

When the anterior spinal syndrome complicates occlusion of a lumbar segmental branch, the effects are more variable. Although the paraplegia may be complete and permanent, there is a clinical spectrum which includes partial and even complete recovery in some patients.[1,12]

In our review[12] of 19 patients with paraplegia following aortic aneurysm repair, the ultimate result varied from permanent paraplegia to total recovery.[7,19-30] In two patients treated at the University of Virginia Medical Center with this complication,[12] both had persistent weakness and one was continent of feces but incontinent of urine. The second patient also had marked bladder dysfunction. In our review, however, we discovered three patients in whom the paraplegia was transient and the recovery complete.[22,23,29] In the remaining patients reviewed in this series, there was either permanent paraplegia or varying degrees of permanent dysfunction below the level of the infarction. The syndrome of transient paraplegia with complete recovery was later described in two additional patients by Ferguson and his colleagues.[1] These workers believe that the occurrence of partial paraplegia with complete recovery in one of their patients indicated sparing of the conus medularis and sacral fibers from the ischemic process. Moreover, the increased knee and ankle jerks present initially in this patient are difficult to explain. The authors postulate that there are common anomales which occur and favor the development of spinal cord ischemia in the arteriosclerotic population which are, as yet, not fully understood.

Clinical Considerations

Fortunately, paraplegia infrequently complicates aortic surgery. When significant cord ischemia occurs, it is presumably due to division of a significant segmental supporting vessel, significant reduction in flow for a critical period of time (usually considered 20 minutes or longer)[13] or the intraluminal occlusion of such a vessel by thrombosis or embolization of atheromatous material. Significant cord ischemia has occurred as a complication of virtually every operation on the thoracic and abdominal aorta including the surgical correction of coarctation of the aorta,[13] and the correction of thoracic[31-34] and abdominal[1,12,16] atherosclerotic aneurysms. Moreover, paraplegia has occurred spontaneously in patients with coarctation[13] and secondary to hypotension unrelated to aortic disease,[35] dissecting aortic aneurysm[32] and as a complication of intra-aortic balloon assistance.[3]

In 1968, Brewer and his associates[13] surveyed a large number of surgeons across the country regarding the incidence of paraplegia complicating the surgical correction of coarctation of the aorta. In this collected series of 12,532 patients, paraplegia occurred in 51, an incidence of 0.41%. In this review, the number of intercostal arteries sacrificed during the coarctation repair and the duration of aortic cross clamping did not seem to be an important factor in those patients who developed paraplegia. Summarizing this vast review, Brewer concluded that the adequacy of collateral flow in the distal aorta as assessed by clinical and manometric means before and after cross clamping provided the most certain means of predicting possible difficulty. In those patients in whom poor collateral circulation is present, he recommended additional supportive measures such as left heart bypass, femoral vein-pump oxygenator to femoral artery bypass, aorto-aorta jump grafts, surface hypothermia, or other adjunctive measures. Despite these measures, Brewer concedes that even the briefest cross clamping time may result in paraplegia in some patients, even in the presence of adequate collateral flow. Moreover, the use of adjunctive measures to perfuse the distal aorta failed to prevent paraplegia in some patients in this series.

The incidence of paraplegia in the treatment of atherosclerotic aneurysms of the descending thoracic aorta is much higher than that following operations for coarctation. As with coarctation, the use of measures to maintain intra-operative perfusion of the distal aorta have failed to eliminate neurologic complications entirely. DeBakey and associates[33] used left atrial to femoral bypass in 36 patients, but two developed partial paraplegia, an incidence of 5.5%. Bloodwell and his colleagues[31] reported a 17% incidence of paraplegia in 17 patients with thoracic aneurysms in whom femoral vein to femoral artery bypass had been used with pump oxygenation. Despite the use of an external shunt composed of Tygon tubing by Kahn[34] in 26 patients, a patient became paraplegic. These facts prompted Crawford and Rubio[32] to review the experience at Baylor University Medical Center over a 16-year period. They reviewed 84 patients with thoracic aneurysms arising distal to the left subclavian artery. During the early part of this series, some type of bypass was routinely employed, but during the final 6 years, no bypass was employed. In 38 patients in this series, some type of bypass was used and in 45 patients adjunctive distal aortic perfusion was not used. Both groups were roughly comparable with respect to age, general health and extent of aortic involvement. In the bypass group, three cases of permanent partial paraplegia occurred compared to one case in the non-bypassed group. The authors concluded that there was no value to distal aortic perfusion in their patients. They believed that temporary inadequate collateral circulation due to hypotension was a key factor in their series as well as permanent interruption of an "end artery" segmental branch.[32]

The marked difference in incidence of paraplegia between operated patients with coarctation and arteriosclerotic aneurysms is probably best explained by the absence of significant arteriosclerosis in patients with coarctation. The arteriosclerotic collateral vessels in older patients with thoracic aneurysm would seem to be at much greater risk for thrombosis during periods of relatively poor perfusion, compared to the undiseased dilated collaterals present in patients with coarctation.

The incidence of ischemic injury of the spinal cord complicating operations for atherosclerotic aneurysms of the abdominal aorta is much less common than that following operations for thoracic aneurysms. In a six-year period at the University of Virginia Medical Center in which more than 250 aortic aneurysms were repaired, paraplegia occurred in only two instances.[12] In both cases, the patients recovered from their operations but had residual neurologic sequelae. The occurrence of paraplegia in two patients in our series prompted a review of the literature. We were able to discover only 18 prior reported cases in this review.[7,19-30] Two years later, Ferguson and his co-workers[1] added five additional patients to the total reported experience. If we again reflect upon the anatomy of the blood supply of the lower spinal cord, an obvious hypothesis to explain paraplegia following abdominal aortic aneurysm repair would be division of *arteria radicularis magna* during the operation. However, if this alone could account for all cases, one would expect a much higher instance of the complication since this vessel originates with equal frequency above and below the renal arteries. Obviously, the role of collateral circulation in the blood supply to the spinal cord in this region cannot be precisely defined from either laboratory studies or clinical experience. For instance, after cross clamping the aorta, incision of the aneurysm and removal of atheromatous debris from the posterior aortic wall, there is invariably vigorous back bleeding from at least one or two lumbar arteries. The orifices of these vessels were presumably previously occluded and extensive collateral circulation must be present to account for both the back bleeding and the absence of spinal cord ischemia prior to operation. In this situation, it is almost certain that either the ARM or anterior spinal artery has been supported exclusively through collateral circulation.

In our review of the literature,[12] the age range for all patients was 46 to 82 years and the majority were men with evidence of extensive atherosclerosis. Seven patients died and the postmortem examination confirmed the presence of spinal cord infarction. Ten of the nineteen patients had ruptured aneurysms with significant peri-operative hypotension. Under these circumstances, it is probable that thrombosis or significant reduction in flow in delicate collaterals occurred as suggested by Crawford.[32] Further credence to this concept is provided by concurrent large bowel ischemia which occurred in one of our patients and two additional patients reported in the literature. This suggests reduced flow with or without thrombosis in multiple collateral channels fed by the supra-renal aorta. In individuals who did not experience significant hypotension during their illness, paraplegia is probably best explained by arteriosclerotic narrowing of necessary collaterals which are subsequently unable to maintain the necessary blood flow to prevent ischemia. The role of temporary supra-renal occlusion cannot be adequately assessed from the available clinical experience as it was reviewed, since supra-renal control is usually mandatory in instances of ruptured aneurysms.

Preoperative visualization of the arteria radicularis magnus has been recommended to prevent paraplegia by Doppman and his group.[9] However, in the face of a ruptured aneurysm, such a procedure is not plausible for obvious reasons. Moreover, this procedure is perfomed in only a few centers and in itself carries a risk of spinal cord infarction. Finally, there is also no evidence that once one has identified the vessel he would be able to significantly alter the surgical approach to an abdominal aneurysm.

The available data suggests a very vague and unclear relationship between the level of the ARM artery and the occurrence of paraplegia following abdominal aneurysm repair. Moreover, paraplegia has occurred in patients in whom surgery of the infra-renal aorta was performed for occlusive disease other than aneurysm. In essence, the multifactorial complex which comprises each patient's clinical picture clouds a precise specific cause for paraplegia in these cases. As pointed out by Ferguson and his group,[1] neither hypotension, steel phenomenon nor emboli are necessary for completion of the syndrome.

Impairment of Sexual Function

Impotence may occur as a feature of severe atherosclerotic disease of the aorta and its pelvic collateral vessels. Often, however, impotence and retrograde ejaculation complicate reconstructive aortic surgery. May and his colleagues reported a 21% incidence of impotence following aortic aneurysmectory and a 34% incidence following aorto-iliac reconstruction for occlusive disease.[36] The same authors reported retrograde ejaculation in 63% of the former group and 49% of the latter. Obviously, these distressing symptoms are a complication of the surgical procedure and not the underlying disease process. Spiro and Cotton[37] believed impotence following aorto-iliac surgery to be due to interruption of the hypogastric sympathetic plexus which is located in front of the left common iliac vein and continuous with the branches of the sympathetic plexus around the inferior mesenteric artery above. A detailed review of this subject was published by Weinstein and Machleder in 1975.[4] These investigators believe that technical features of the operation may definitely contribute to postoperative sexual dysfunction. It is well-established that bilateral ablation of the L1 and L2 sympathetic ganglia produces impotence and similarly, that ablation of the L3 and L4 ganglia causes retrograde ejaculation. Weinstein and Machleder therefore recommend careful nerve sparing technique in both aneurysmectory and aorto-iliac reconstruction. These include a nerve sparing right lateral aortotomy for endarterectomy and an aortotomy above the inferior mesenteric artery for aorto-femoral bypass. Strict avoidance of dissection in the region of the left common iliac vein is also stressed. During aortic aneurysm repair, the endo-aneurysmorrhaphy technique of Creech is recommended to protect both the hypogastric and inferior mesenteric sympathetic plexus. Although the author's clinical series of 20 patients was small, their detailed analysis and scholarly literary research strongly supported their conclusions. Until more is known about this area, the precautions they propose seem quite appropriate.

Summary and Conclusions

The neurologic complications of aortic surgery vary from the well understood to the abstruse. Embolism of air or atheromatous material may occur with manipulation of the aortic arch or during cardiopulmonary bypass. Operations on the aorta beyond the left subclavian artery may be complicated by paraplegia. The reasons for this are poorly understood and probably multifactorial. The anterior spinal artery is not always a continuous vessel and its variable segmental arterial reinforcement renders it a poor source of collateral circulation especially in the face of arteriosclerotic reinforcing vessels. Available information tenuously supports the use of measures to supplement distal aortic circulation in patients with coarctation in whom there is clinical or manometric evidence of poor collateral circulation. However, supplemental aortic perfusion has not eliminated paraplegia in either patients with coarctation or arteriosclerotic thoracic aneurysms and its value in the latter group of patients has been seriously questioned. Paraplegia following abdominal aortic surgery is rare and partial to complete recovery may be expected in some patients. Sexual dysfunction following aortic surgery is quite common and may be prevented in some patients by minor modifications in operative technique.

References

1. Ferguson LRJ, Bergan JJ, Conn J: Spinal ischemia following abdominal aortic surgery, *Ann Surg* **181**:267-272, 1975.
2. Grace RR, Mattox KL: Anterior spinal artery syndrome following abdominal aortic aneurysmectomy, *Arch Surg* **112**:813-815, 1977.
3. Tyras DH, Willman VL: Paraplegia following intra-aortic balloon assistance. *Ann Thorac Surg* **25**:164-168, 1978.
4. Weinstein MH, Machleder HI: Sexual function after aorto-iliac surgery. *Ann Surg* **181**:787-790, 1975.
5. Adamkiewicz A: Die Blutefässe des menschlichen Rukermarkesober-

fläche. *Sitz Akad Wiss Wien Math Natur Klass* 85:101-110, 1882.

6. Kadyi H: Über die Blutefässe des menschlichen Rukermarkes, nach einer im XV. Bander der Denkschriften der Math. Natur. Classe der Akademic der Wissenschaften in Krakau Ershienenin Monographie. Aus dem Polnischen übersetz von Verfasser, 152 pp. 10-46, Lemberg. Gubrinowicz and Schmidt, 1889.

7. Adams HD, van Geertruyden HH: Neurologic complications of aortic surgery. *Ann Surg* 114:574-610, 1956.

8. Bolton B: Blood supply of human spinal cord. *J Neurol Psychiat* 2:137-148. 1939.

9. Doppman JL, DiChiro G, Morton DL: Arteriographic identification of spinal cord blood supply prior to aortic surgery. *JAMA* 204:172-173, 1968.

10. Doppman J, DiChiro G: The *Arteria Radicularis Magna*: Radiographic Anatomy in the adult. *Brit J Radiol* 41:40-45, 1968.

11. Suh TH, Alexander L: Vascular system of the human spinal cord. *Arch Neurol Psychiat* 41:659-687, 1939.

12. Golden GT, Sears HF, Wellons HA, Jr, Muller WH, Jr: Paraplegia complicating resection of aneurysms of the infrarenal abdominal aorta. *Surgery* 73:91-96, 1973.

13. Brewer LA, III, Fosburg RG, Mulder GA, Verska JJ: Spinal cord complications following surgery for coarctation of the aorta. *J Thorac Cardiovasc Surg* 64:368-381, 1972.

14. Field EJ, Graysen J, Roger AF: Observations on the blood flow in the spinal cord of the rabbit. *J Physiol (Lond)* 114:56-70, 1951.

15. Fried LC, DiChiro G, Doppman JL: Ligation of major thoracolumbar spinal cord arteries in monkeys. *J Neurosurg* 31:608-614, 1969.

16. Killen DA, Edwards RH, Adkins RB, Boehm FH: Spinal cord ischemia following mobilization of canine aorta from posterior parietes. *Ann Surg* 162:1063-1068, 1965.

17. Killen DA: Paraplegia in the dog following mobilization of the abdominal and lower thoracic aorta from the posterior parietes. *Surgery* 57:542-548, 1965.

18. Moossy J: Anterior spinal artery syndrome. In: Baker AB, ed: *Clinical Neurology*. Hagerstown, Harper and Row, pp 12-13.

19. Bates T: Paraplegia following resection of abdominal aortic aneurysm. *Brit J Surg* 58:913-917, 1971.

20. Coupland GAE, Reeve TS: Paraplegia: A complication of excision of abdominal aortic aneurysm. *Surgery* 64:878-881, 1968.

21. Edmondson HT, Gindin RA: Paraplegia as a complication of abdominal aortic resection. *Amer Surg* 36:383-387, 1970.

22. Gump FE: Paraplegia after resection of aneurysm. *N Engl J Med* 281:798-800, 1969.

23. Hara M, Lipin RJ: Spinal cord injury following resection of abdominal aortic aneurysm. *Arch Surg* 80:419-424, 1960.

24. Hogan EL, Romanul FCA: Spinal cord infarction occurring during insertion of aortic graft. *Neurology* 16:67-74, 1966.

25. Lake PA: Paraplegia after resection of aneurysm. *N Engl J Med* 281:798-799, 1969.

26. Mehrez IO, Nabseth DC, Hogan EL, Deterling RA: Paraplegia following resection of abdominal aortic aneurysm. *Ann Surg* 156:890-898, 1962.

27. Pasternak BM, Boyd DP, Ellis FH, Jr: Spinal cord injury after procedures

on the aorta. *Surg Gynec Obstet* **135**:29-34, 1972.
28. Sher MH, Healy EH: Paraplegia following infrarenal aneurysmorrhaphy, *Vasc Surg* **5**:171-178, 1971.
29. Skillman JJ, Zervas NT, Weintraub RM, Mayman C: Paraplegia after resection of aneurysms of the abdominal aorta. *N Engl J Med* **281**:422-431, 1969.
30. Zuber WF, Gaspar MR, Rothschild PD: Anterior spinal syndrome — a complication of abdominal aortic surgery: report of five cases and a review of the literature. *Ann Surg* **172**:909-917, 1970.
31. Bloodwell RD, Hallman GL, Cooley DA: Partial cardiopulmonary bypass for pericardiectomy and resection of descending thoracic aortic aneurysms. *Ann Thorac Surg* **6**:46-55, 1968.
32. Crawford ES, Rubio PA: Reappraisal of adjuncts to avoid ischemia in the treatment of aneurysms of descending thoracic aorta. *J Thorac Cardiovasc Surg* **66**:693-704, 1973.
33. DeBakey ME, Cooley DA, Crawford ES, Morris GC: Aneurysms of the thoracic aorta: analysis of 170 patients treated by resection. *J Thorac Surg* **36**:393-420, 1958.
34. Kahn DR: Discussion: reappraisal of adjuncts to avoid ischemia in the treatment of thoracic aortic aneurysms. *Surgery* **67**:182-183, 1970.
35. Madow L, Alpers BJ: Involvement of the spinal cord in occlusion of the coronary vessels. *Arch Neurol* **61**:430-439, 1949.
36. May AG, DeWeese JA, Rob CG: Changes in sexual function following operation on the abdominal aorta. *Surgery* **65**:41-53, 1969.
37. Spiro M, Cotton LT: Aorto-iliac thrombo-endarterectomy. *Brit J Surg* **57**:161-165, 1970.

Chapter X

Neurological Complications of Open Heart Surgery

Kyösti A. Sotaniemi, M.D.

Introduction

The introduction of the operative treatment of the heart valves some three decades ago made it possible for the first time to significantly influence the course of cardiac disease. Thereafter, the development of cardiac surgery has improved the chances to prolong life and also, undoubtedly, the quality of life of the cardiac patient.[1] The history of major intracardiac surgery was initiated with a closed heart technique which achieved notable alleviation of cardiac symptoms. This technique was relatively inexpensive and simple to use but it had evident limitations in offering no ways for reparative procedures. The closed heart technique was commonly used until the development of a method involving extracorporeal circulation (ECC); this opened a new era in cardiac surgery, making open heart operations possible. Open heart procedures have now been performed for over twenty years. The ECC forms the essential basis for modern cardiac and major cardiovascular surgery and its applications are routine today.

Evaluated from the surgical and cardiac points of view, the development of operative methods, techniques and equipment during the past two decades has been epochal and the strides forward have been enormous. Unfortunately, however, these new, effective and often necessarily life-saving methods occasionally prove to have some less favorable side effects manifesting themselves in the form of disorders in the function of various parenchymal organs of which the nervous system is clearly the most vulnerable. These complications may sometimes mar an otherwise successful outcome. Together with more complicated procedures, the patient, in addition to having previously been liable to neurological complications related to the cardiac disease itself, now faces also the eventual risks related both to the operative treatment and to the investigatory

293

procedures necessary prior to surgery. Hence the development of cardiac surgery, as magnificent as it has been, has created new problems while solving others.

Open heart procedures and the applications of ECC, to which the neurological complications have most commonly been attributed, are becoming ever more widely used and operative treatment is initiated in more and more new units. Therefore, since the neurological problems of cardiac surgery have by no means been eliminated despite recent advances, there is a constant need to recognize the potential threat of neurological complications and to consider the factors which determine the outcome. This chapter reviews the features associated with the occurrence, detection and prediction of neurological disorders in open heart surgery.

Neurological Manifestations in Cardiac Disease

Valvular disease carries an increased risk of cerebral disorders particularly due to embolic complications,[2,3] which may even be the first manifestations in otherwise clinically asymptomatic diseases.[4] The occurrence of cerebral emboli, however, is not necessarily a function of the duration or severity of the cardiac disease.[5] Information available on the prevalence of neurological disturbances in adult cardiac disease patients in general is scarce and no systematic studies considering various cardiac conditions and central nervous system (CNS) abnormalities related to them have been published. For example only a few authors have paid attention to preoperative neurological findings in cardiac surgery patients; the reported prevalence varying between 7%[6] and 13%.[7] On the other hand, neurological manifestations are known to be frequent in congenital heart disease; prevalence values up to 25% having been reported.[8] The general aspects of neurological disorders related to heart diseases have been reviewed recently.[5,9] Briefly, a preoperative history of cerebrovascular disorders has been encountered in from 6%[10] to 11%[7] of valvular disease cases, of which transient ischemic attacks (TIA) form roughly one-half.[7]

Preoperative neurological complaints are indeed common: in one study [7] of 100 adult valvular replacement patients, various neurological symptoms were reported during the year before surgery in 55% of the cases, migraine (12%), other forms of headache (11%), vertigo and dizziness (11%), and syncope (9%) being the most common symptoms.

The high prevalence values of cerebrovascular accidents, TIAs and other circulatory disturbances in cardiac patients clearly reflect the extensiveness of their CNS risks; the values given above markedly exceed the known prevalence of cerebrovascular occurrences in the general population. Accordingly, these observations confirm the necessity of improving cardiac surgical procedures from the neurologist's point of view as well.

Neurological Complications of Cardiac Investigatory Procedures

Our knowledge concerning the complications related to the investigatory measures used to diagnose heart disease are confined to the information of only a few reports on cardiac catheterization. Prevalence values for overall complications are of the magnitude of from 3.4%[12] to 1.5%,[11] of which less than a quarter are neurological in nature. In a more recent and larger study,[13] ten cases of CNS disorders were described among over 10,000 catheterizations, and the mechanisms thought to be responsible for the neurological disturbances were: nerve trauma, toxic reaction to contrast agent, thrombosis related to pre-existing disease, dehydration or hypotension, and embolization from the vessels or catheter.

Clinical Aspects of Neurological Complications

Neurological complications following open heart surgery have been described ever since the earliest operations more than twenty years ago.[14-16] Although the nature of disturbances has become noticeably less serious due to technical improvement, the occurrence of these complications still remains one of the main problems of cardiac surgery.[5,7,17]

The reported prevalence of neurological complications involving the CNS varies widely. In prospective investigations, prevalence values of from 3% to 53% have been reported.[7,18-22] In postoperative neurological assessments, however, it is important to note that there are essential differences in the clinical criteria used :[5,7] some register only the obvious and most severe signs such as overt hemiplegia, while others take account of all detectable disturbances. Moreover, most of the studies with low complication rates (i.e., below 10%) have been retrospective, the neurological data being collected from case histories. Additionally it should be noted that patients have not always undergone a thorough and relevant neurological examination made by a neurologist, neither pre- nor postoperatively. These disparities make comparisons between the results of different centers and evaluations of the effects of altered operative conditions and presumed technical and surgical improvements extremely difficult. Considering the available studies with proper neurological evaluation, 23% seems to be the lowest prevalence value reported.[21] The influence of the varying clinical criteria is illustrated in a recent prospective study:[7] taking account of all detectable CNS disorders independent of their severity, abnormalities were found in 37%, but when the definition of CNS disorder was less stringent and embraced only those disturbances detected by the routine postoperative care unit staff (including doctors), the prevalence of complications for the same group of patients would have been only 9%. One may question the significance of minor disturbances, but it should be remembered that the main aims of such investigations are to learn to indicate and recognize the neurological disorders in order to find their determinants and eliminate them. If the disorders are inadequately detected, obviously the determinants will also be missed.

Despite the criteria of evaluation, the timing of the postoperative investigations has varied. Most commonly, the patient is examined either immediately after regaining consciousness or during the first postoperative day and additional further examinations are made only if required. The timing of the evaluation creates additional problems when the results of different authors are compared. Some mild and rapidly reversible signs may be missed if the first postoperative investigation is made some days after surgery; on the other hand, great difficulties in neurological practice are met in examining patients with several cannulae and connected to technical surveillance equipment. A complete neurological examination can only rarely be performed in the immediate postoperative phase. Particularly difficult is the recognition of mild, but not necessarily at all insignificant disorders which either may easily escape the attention of non-neurologists or may be overlooked [6] or misdiagnosed as psychiatric manifestations. Early recognition of such abnormalities would of course be valuable in the later evaluation and rehabilitation of the patient. The proportion of neurological disorders recognized in regular postoperative care unit surveillance is thought to have been from 24% [7] to 38%.[6]

From the practical point of view, it is to be highly recommended that every cardiac surgery patient should undergo neurological investigation both preoperatively and immediately postoperatively, i.e., at the time the patient has or should have regained consciousness. This would prepare one for eventual emergency procedures.[23] However, it is equally important to perform a proper neurological examination in a later phase when the patient's condition allows consideration of all the functional levels of the nervous system.[7]

The clinical picture of complications attributable to open heart surgery has been extremely variable and disorders from all the levels of the nervous system have been described. Among the most commonly reported findings are disturbances of consciousness and orientation, hemiparetic signs, visual field defects, gnostic and practic disorders, aphasia, cranial nerve signs, cerebellar and brain stem symptoms and convulsive disorders.[5,7,10,14-23] Psychiatric disturbances appearing with or without neurological signs are also relatively frequent.[18,24] Peripheral neurological complications are not uncommon but they have been given attention in only a few communications.[7,25-27] These peripheral disorders, however, should not be overlooked: first, because they seem to cause considerable annoyance;[7] second, because they are potentially avoidable;[26] and third, because they may be misdiagnosed as CNS complications.[25] Mononeuropathy or multiple peripheral nerve or nerve plexus involvement predominantly in the upper extremities are the most commonly reported [25-27] peripheral manifestations. Signs attributable to affections of the lower part of the brachial plexus seem to be relatively frequent.[7,27] This problem has already been discussed in Chapters VII and VIII in this book.

Generally, the neurological complications have been described as mild and often as relatively rapidly reversible. Most communications report a favorable recovery in the majority of cases by the time of discharge from hospital. However, persistent deficits are not uncommon; they are encountered in from 2% to 15% of the survivors[7,10,19,28] but the number of them as well as the number of severe complications seems to be continuously decreasing.[28,29] The number of patients who die from cerebral damage has fallen to the level of 0.3-2% during the last few years, [7,28,29] having been considerably greater some ten years ago. Slight clinical disturbances and psychiatric symptoms manifesting themselves as exaggerated tendon reflexes, abnormal plantar extensor reflex, disorientation and delirium are very common.[5-7,10,18-21] However, the clinical picture may be very complex and concomitant signs reflecting multiple lesions may occur. The recovery rate during the first days seems astonishingly rapid and thus might reflect a metabolic and non-structural etiology of involvement. On the other hand, the course of the more severe signs such as hemiplegia or aphasia do not, according to the present author's experience, differ from the course of similar manifestations due to spontaneous occurrences.

Beyond the occurrence of overt neurological complications one should also pay attention to subclinical disturbances; these are often forgotten but actually represent the very maximum acceptable level of iatrogenic neurological disorders. It is evident that what we find clinically is just a small fraction of the total number of CNS events and disturbances. Several electroencephalographical (EEG) studies[30-33] and neuropsychological investigations[17,21,34,35] have in fact shown that our concepts and understanding of the cerebral events related to open heart surgery procedures are still far from satisfactory. The occurrence of subclinical events also emphasizes the relativity of the significance of the complication prevalence values obtained from investigations which take account of only overt clinical findings. Therefore, greater emphasis should be put on multidimensional studies which allow consideration of several functional aspects of the nervous system simultaneously.[17,22,36]

Some evidence has accumulated regarding differences between the dominant and non-dominant hemispheres in their ability to tolerate an open heart operation. In several investigations,[7,10,19,32,37] the non-dominant hemisphere seems to have been somewhat more vulnerable than the dominant hemisphere although the differences have not been given attention in all the mentioned reports. The lack of evidence of any recognizable pre-, intra- or postoperative factor favoring non-dominant (right) hemisphere involvement with the multiplicity of right-sided predominance of dysfunction elicits the suggestion either that the hemispheres, though equally affected, are different in tolerating extraordinary strains such as are operant during ECC, or that they are different in generating clinical manifestations. This disparity might be based on differences in metabolic functions, the existence of which might be concluded from the well-known neuropsychological and neurophysiological characteristics of the hemispheres. The background of this disparity needs further research. The results might be useful not only in the recognition of the determinants of cerebral dysfunction related to ECC but also in achieving a better understanding of the hemispheral functional differences.

Determinants of Neurological Disorders Related to Open Heart Surgery

Despite extensive literature on the subject during the past two decades the determinants of neurological disorders in open heart surgery seem to be somewhat controversial. In part this may be due to the above-mentioned differences in the clinical criteria, the investigational designs, and the patient materials.[5,7,10] The possibility of several coexistent factors contributing to disturbed circulatory and metabolic conditions and the difficulty in pointing out the role of a given single determinant make the etiological considerations complicated. Additionally, the preoperative state of a patient and the obvious interindividual differences in tolerating exceptional conditions such as ECC are often neglected in the evaluation of the operative measures.[17] Among the factors most commonly claimed to be involved in determining the neurological outcome are: advanced age,[10,19] long duration of ECC,[7,10,19,22] cardiological factors,[10,17,39] hypotension during operation,[19,20,40] a history suggestive of previous neurological diseases,[7,10,20] and technical factors in the ECC equipment.[7,10,41,42] Some of the factors and conditions considered most important are dealt with in more detail below.

Operative Determinants of Cerebral Complications

Duration of ECC (i.e., perfusion time). The duration of the perfusion seems to be one of the most clearly verified factors of postoperative outcome.[7,10,19,22,40,42] A critical time threshold of two hours has been stated in several reports;[7,10,19] for instance, in one of these studies[7] a statistically highly significant (p = 0.0001) rise in the occurrence of neurological complications was encountered after perfusion times exceeding two hours. On the other hand, a definitely safe lower time limit has not been found in any study. Although the perfusion time does not in itself indicate any specific harmful factor, and although it is evident that a number of factors and occurrences tend to occur together with advancing time, these observations give indisputable evidence that at least some of the determinants of CNS disorders are attributable to ECC. Furthermore, it is widely recognized that while all potentially harmful factors may each individually be innocuous, they are nevertheless cumulative. Thus, although this information is non-specific, there is a simple practical conclusion: to pursue as short a perfusion time as possible.

Embolism from the heart or the perfusion apparatus is among the most commonly suggested determinants of cerebral injury. In manipulating the heart and in excisioning the valves, calcified debris may unknowingly be dislodged and subsequently embolize in the arterial system when the bypass is terminated. Embolization of calcium particles or fragments from the excised valve used to be common in closed heart surgery but corresponding macroemboli have been encountered only occasionally after open heart procedures.[18,40] On the other hand, microembolization originating from the body tissues or the technical equipment may occur. Moreover, fat may be released during sternotomy or during excision of the mediastinal tissues, drain into the pericardial sac and be sucked into the perfusion system, thus causing cerebral infarction.[41,42] Antifoam or silicone embolism has also been reported.[43] Gaseous emboli may be produced either from air suspended in stored cold blood, causing bubbles when the blood is rewarmed, or from the air trapped in the heart or the great vessels entering the circulation, or from foaming occurring in the oxygenator.[41] Regions of subatmospheric pressure in the perfusion devices have also been described as causing nitrogen liberation from blood and the solutions used.[44] Embolization has also been reported as occurring as a result of protein denaturation leading to the formation of red cell aggregates.[45] Other kinds of aggregates consisting of either blood elements such as platelets, leucocytes and fibrin strands[46] or cholesterol[47] have also been verified.

Oxygenators have been shown to differ from each other in the production of emboli. The number of particulate matter emboli has been reported[48] as being smaller in membrane oxygenators than in bubble oxygenators. Although membrane oxygenators seem to be more advantageous as to the patient's neuropsychological outcome,[49,50] the reverse has also been reported.[22] Besides the type of oxygenator, *the type of blood flow* during ECC has also been considered important; pulsatile flow being claimed more beneficial both in EEG changes[51] and experimentally.[52] However, the clinical neurological significance of the choice of oxygenator and blood flow[53] still seems uncertain.

Changes in *cerebral blood flow* and oxygen *metabolism* during ECC have been observed in experimental studies[54,55] but only a little information is available on these subjects in man. Cerebral blood flow has been found[56] to fall considerably at the onset of cardiopulmonary bypass; this fall was found to occur despite high flow rates but could be partially corrected by an increase in arterial carbon dioxide pressure. The conclusion was drawn that the combination of hypotension, a fall in cerebral blood flow, and a reduction in hematocrit due to hemodilution, obviously causes a serious impairment in oxygen availability at tissue level, resulting in a fall in cerebral metabolic rate. The available information concerning microcirculatory and metabolic alterations undoubtedly occurring in the CNS during ECC is scanty and the clinical implications of the observations mentioned above remain unclear. Furthermore, no investigations on the relationship between clinical and intraoperative blood flow or metabolic alterations have so far been published.

Consideration of the possible role of *anesthetics* has also so far been disregarded and no attention has been paid to the matter in reports assessing the neurological, neuropsychological, psychiatric or EEG outcome after cardiopulmonary bypass. While the intraoperative changes in EEG dependent on the type and level of anesthesia are well known and while some reports[57,58] have discussed the intraoperative EEG changes also in open heart surgery patients, the alterations have not been correlated to the postoperative course.

Hypothermia is used in cardiac surgery in order to protect the brain from ischemic and hypoxic injury, but it is generally believed[59-61] that postoperative complications cannot be attributed to hypothermia.

Information on the role of arterial blood pressure and *hypotension* during cardiopulmonary bypass seems to be controversial. Hypotension has been considered one of the major determinants of cerebral dysfunction by some authors[19,20,62] and less important by others.[7,10,17,18,22,32,33] It is self-evident that extreme hypotension is disastrous to the brain but it has not seemingly been possible to state any definitely critical mean arterial blood pressure limit, [7,10,18,56] though the value of 50 mmHg has been proposed in some communications.[19,20,63] It would seem possible to conclude that the effects of at least moderate systolic hypotension above 40-50 mmHg alone is not necessarily a major factor of brain damage and that the effects of such hypotension are dependent on the etiology and rapidity of the pressure changes. Moreover, the outcome is undoubtedly determined by an individual's abilities to tolerate hypotension and to respond to it.

Since circulatory conditions are also significantly affected by venous pressure, the use of *perfusion pressure* (mean arterial pressure - central venous pressure) would seem to be recommended. In a study[64] using clinical, EEG and neuropathological investigations it was shown that the most significant determinants of cerebral vulnerability were: the reperfusion pressure established after hypotensive episodes, postoperative blood pressure, cardiac output and brain temperature at the time of hypotension. The question of arterial hypotension does not yet seem to be settled definitely; but the necessity of maintaining an adequate blood pressure, especially in old, hypertensive or arteriosclerotic patients, needs to be emphasized.[22]

The whole procedure of ECC and surgical maneuvers is very complicated and despite all advances the hazards of technical disturbances still seem to remain. Indeed *unexpected intraoperative occurrences* are among the most detrimental factors of cerebral damage.[7,10,20,65]

In addition to the numerous factors already discussed there still remains a large group of items possibly no less important than those mentioned above but less well documented. Factors such as, to mention only a few, the nature of the solution used to prime the ECC,[10,17] mean flow rate,[10] valvular calcifications[7,10,68] and cardiac rhythm,[33] should certainly be remembered when evaluating the causes of cerebral dysfunction.

Despite the vast literature devoted to the neurological complications related to cardiac surgery our knowledge of the final harmful causes operant during ECC, excepting some definitely obvious occurrences such as, e.g., massive air embolism or obstruction of cannulae, etc., still lacks depth and certainty and in fact some of the causes may even still be unrecognized. In the future, further investigations should be focused on the nerve cell level and on the regulators of cell metabolism in order to obtain a better understanding of the actual basic events determining the outcome.

Age

Some authors[10,19,20] have emphasized the importance of age on the postoperative outcome while some others[7,18,21,66] have considered its influence to be less prominent. The effects of perfusion time and intraoperative hypotension have been reported to be independent of age in one study[7] on 100 patients aged 15-65 years. It seems to be justified to presume that age itself is not a matter of importance but rather the state of the regulatory mechanisms of circulation and metabolism modifying the ability to adapt to exceptionally strenuous conditions such as ECC.

Sex

The clinical neurological outcomes of the sexes seem equal but some studies[17,21,67] report a less favorable neuropsychological or psychiatric outcome in women when compared with men. The causes of this difference remain unexplained and may not be directly attributable to sex but, for instance, to cardiological factors[17] or to educational or psychic characteristics.[21,67]

Cardiac Factors

Relatively little attention has been paid to the possible cardiac factors affecting the neurological outcome. Multiple valve replacements are known to be followed by cerebral complications more often than single valve replacements[7,10,21,68] and this does not seem to be solely a function of the duration of perfusion.[21] Mitral valve patients have been reported[17,35,67] to experience a less advantageous postoperative outcome of the higher cerebral functions than aortic patients, but this phenomenon cannot be connected with the perfusion time because it is generally considerably shorter in mitral than in aortic operations. The observed differences may be attributed to the fact that the general postoperative benefit and cardiological outcome of the mitral patients is also usually less marked than that of the aortic patients.[69] It is well known that mitral disease is more often complicated by embolic complications than aortic valve disease,[3] and that the mitral patients usually come to operation several years later than the aortic patients. Accordingly, the duration of the symptoms of heart disease has been found to show some correlation to the postoperative outcome.[21] Congenital heart disease patients have been observed to display more severe EEG changes[32,33] and a less advantageous postoperative neuropsychological course than those with acquired heart disease. Prolonged exposure to repetitive episodes of inadequate cerebral blood flow resulting in hypoxia,[70] and particularly occurring in association with conditions of physical stress,[71] might explain the lowered tolerance towards such exceptional strains as the cardiopulmonary bypass in the mitral and congenital disease patients. On the other hand, the preoperative cardiac status has not been confirmed as having any significant influence on the postoperative neurological outcome.[34,68]

The role of the cardiac factors and their influence on operative practice needs further research. Considering the above observations, one could speculate that it might be possible to obtain information useful for evaluating the risks and advantages associated with various types of heart disease and with its operative treatment. This in turn might lead to a better understanding of the criteria indicating potential cerebral dysfunction and the ability to determine a proper time for surgical intervention.

Postoperative Aspects

Generally, the neurological disorders related to heart operations have been so closely attributed to intraoperative occurrences and factors that the influence of postoperative conditions has gained scarce discussion. This may be due to the fact that the clinical evaluation has usually been performed in the immediate postoperative phase allowing no consideration of the possible later alterations. However, it would seem quite evident that postoperative cardiological, hemodynamic, metabolic and biochemical conditions and alterations may influence cerebral function. The consideration of these aspects has been emphasized by only a few authors.[37,72] In several communications[34,73-75] discussing psychiatric complications, the significance of the postoperative environmental conditions such as sensory and sleep deprivation has been pointed out. Late postoperative complications, such as embolization from the artificial valves, dysfunction of the valvular prosthesis, and paraprosthetic leakage causing cardiac decompensation, and the risks related to life-long anticoagulant treatment[76] have also been discussed only briefly. Types of valvular prostheses may differ in their tendencies to produce emboli and in their hemodynamic characteristics,[5] but generally they increase the risk of infectious complications.[76,77] Furthermore, some complications obviously attributable to intraoperative damage may not appear until long after clinical signs have improved, epilepsy being one example.[7]

Determinants of Peripheral Neurological Disorders

The causes of peripheral neuropathic manifestations following open heart procedures perhaps deserve more attention than they have received so far. Although their clinical picture is less dramatic than that of CNS complications, they may cause long-term annoyance.[7] Prolonged malposition on the operating table resulting in a compressive nerve injury is the most commonly proposed cause[25] but ischemic damage due to inadequate perfusion cannot be excluded.[25,26] However, the peripheral disorders which are particularly common in the upper extremities may be due to a stretching injury of the brachial plexus resulting from retraction of the sternum, which, in turn, displaces the clavicle posteriorly.[27]

Neuropathological Observations

The neuropathological aspects will be discussed only briefly in this context. The first communications[16,18,41] on neuropathological findings after open heart surgery described either diffuse lesions typical of cerebral anoxia of focal damage caused by hemorrhage or embolism. The present concepts or the pathological changes are based for the most part on the observations of Aguilar, et al[40] who investigated 206 cases of patients dying after open heart surgery. They observed a variety of lesions, many of which were found to appear coexistently: intracerebral or subarachnoidal hemorrhages, focal or diffuse neuronal degeneration, focal infarcts, emboli of fibrin, platelets, fat and miscellaneous origin. The emboli consisted of fat in 78%, fibrin and platelet aggregates in 20%, crystalline material in 12% and other matter in 9%. The presence of nonfat emboli showed a significant correlation with the duration of perfusion. The authors emphasized that all of the mentioned lesions must be looked for, that there may be wide-ranging pathogenetic mechanisms underlying the ischemic, anoxic, toxic, metabolic and other processes that give rise to the observed lesions.

Neuropathological lesions are nearly always found in patients dying after open heart surgery even if the death has not been attributable to clinical cerebral damage.[78] This would suggest that surviving patients may also have cerebral damage with or without clinical manifestations and emphasizes the necessity to use methods of neurological assessment other than routine clinical examination alone.

Higher Cerebral Functions

Despite the clinical somatic outcome, the patient's postoperative course is greatly influenced by the state of the higher cerebral functions. It is evident that clinical or EEG methods are only rough indicators of the CNS functions, and therefore more refined methods are necessary for investigating intellectual and cognitive conditions. Neuropsychological investigations often show a decline in intellectual functions, the most often reported impairment being observed in visual perception, perceptual-motor coordination, attention span, visuoconstructive ability and perceptual speed.[17,35,68,72,79,80] The neuropsychological changes, just like the clinical signs, have generally been described as mainly reversible. Test scores designed to measure intellectual performance seem to rise significantly in later postoperative follow-up studies.[17,35,68] One would readily regard the increased test score as an indicator of improved cognitive functions due to a supposed enhancement of cerebral circulatory and metabolic conditions, but there does not seem to be any justification for drawing such a promising conclusion. On the contrary, these beneficial changes generally seem to be attributed to the practice effects.[34,68] On the other hand, remembering the unquestioned beneficial long-term effects[1,31,33,76] of cardiac surgery, one should perhaps not deny the possibility of some real improvement in higher cerebral functions.

Neuropsychological impairment may occur with or without clinical symptoms. The interrelationship between these two kinds of complications has been widely discussed, some authors[17,20,68,79] describing the parallelism of the findings, others[34,35,72] reporting the contrary. It is clear that the clinical and neuropsychological manifestations differ from each other as to the origin and extensiveness of the damage but they should not be regarded as separate phenomena. What we see clinically is merely a narrow reflection of the actual events. The determinants of neuropsychological complications do not differ from those of the clinical disorders.[17,29,34,68,72]

Reference has already been made to the finding that the cerebral hemispheres, at least in certain patient materials, tend to display characteristics reflecting their probable differences in ability to tolerate the strains of ECC. Interestingly, some recent neuropsychological observations have given tentative support to these findings. Certain tests presumed to measure non-dominant hemisphere dysfunction have been claimed[17,35] to display more marked impairment than the dominant hemisphere tests. The possible interhemispheric differences, however, must be re-evaluated in larger patient materials than those referred to above to allow further conclusions to be drawn.

There is a vast literature devoted to the psychiatric problems related to open heart surgery,[21,24,34,67,72-74,79-83] delirium being the most common psychiatric disturbance in the early postoperative phase. Details of these complications, however, will not be discussed here.

The above described observations show that much may be missed if only clinical neurological aspects are considered and they suggest that the extent of the subclinical occurrences may be quite large. Subclinical events may generate only slight and reversible cognitive disorders without leading to persistent defects, but even so they should not be overlooked. The eventual involvement of the intellectual and cognitive functions may cause embarrassment and lead to successive consequences affecting the patient's adaptability to postoperative conditions. Neglecting the consideration of these functions may well lead to erroneous interpretations. For instance, in the present author's experience it is not a rarity to see dyspractic or dysphasic symptoms considered as psychiatric manifestations in the postoperative care unit. The outcome of the higher cerebral functions is naturally of the greatest importance when the patient's rehabilitation needs to be evaluated and his capacity to return to work is assessed.

EEG Findings in Cardiac Surgery Patients

The EEG has been widely used in assessing the CNS functions in open heart surgery patients, particularly intraoperatively, and some kind of intraoperative EEG surveillance is routine in many operative centers. Preoperative EEG investigations in patients undergoing cardiac surgery have revealed very high prevalences of abnormal findings. Prevalences of from 60%[33] to 74%[84] have been encountered in congenital heart disease and up to 44%[33] in acquired valvular disease. Mitral and multiple valve patients have been described[32,33] as displaying EEG abnormalities more often than aortic patients, possibly reflecting the higher susceptibility of embolic complications in mitral disease[3] or the duration of the cardiac affection before coming to operation, usually longer in mitral than in aortic disease. The most common preoperative EEG abnormalities consist mainly of theta range disturbances appearing predominantly in the left temporal regions and being episodic in nature.[33] This is also the usual finding in vascular diseases.[85]

The EEG is of valuable help in intraoperative surveillance of the cerebral functions, making early detection of harmful events possible.[28,30,39,51,66] Both conventional EEGs[30,63,86,87] and computerized EEG (cerebral function monitor) have been used.[39,51] Each of the methods has its own advantages and disadvantages. The cerebral function monitor is costly and offers only a rough insight to the quantified EEG, but it is often nonetheless the first indicator of disturbances in, for instance, cerebral blood flow. On the other hand, in order to give reliable information, the continuous recording of conventional EEG requires considerable knowledge of clinical neurophysiology. New and more practical surveillance devices are being developed in several centers and marked progress can be expected in the near future.

Investigations on the postoperative EEG have revealed considerable changes, of which slowing of the dominant activity and an increase or appearance of slow wave abnormalities are among the most common.[30,33,38,78,87] Significantly, these changes do not appear only in association with clinical signs but are often encountered without any other manifestations reflecting the magnitude of subclinical disorders.[31-33] The abnormalities may be either local or diffuse. No one region has been described as having a special predilection to dysfunction. The duration of perfusion and the extensiveness of the EEG deterioration have been found to show some correlation,[32,33,78] particularly in the impairment of the dominant EEG frequency values[32,33] but also in the nature of episodic abnormalities.[33] In general, the severity of the EEG changes corresponds well with clinical symptoms, the interrelationship becoming more reliable as the EEG deterioration increases.[31,78] The postoperative EEG has been claimed to have some prognostic clinical value in some studies

[31,66,78] although this is denied in some other reports.[30,86] Differences in the timing of the investigations and in the EEG criteria, however, make comparisons difficult.

The postoperatively observed EEG disturbances are reported to display a distinct tendency towards recovery,[14,30,33,63,86] suggesting that the EEG changes reflect, at least in part, temporary and non-structural disturbances in the CNS after ECC. In one series,[33] the preoperative prevalence of abnormal EEGs was 49%; 10 days postoperatively it had risen to 80% but 5 months after surgery it was 36%, and one year postoperatively only 25% of the EEGs were classified as abnormal. Hence, the EEG did not only recover but it also improved when compared with the preoperative state. In this series, the improvement was mainly due to a decrease of episodic theta range disturbances while the dominant activity remained unchanged. Interestingly, aortic patients seemed to achieve a more beneficial EEG outcome than mitral valve patients.

The development of methods for quantitative EEG (QEEG) analysis has brought new insights into EEG evaluation: QEEG gives objective information and allows the use of statistical procedures. The QEEG has been proven to yield additional useful information in the evaluation of the cerebral functional conditions and the determinants of their changes also in cardiac surgery patients.[17,32]

EEG phenomena can be divided into the following successive stages: first, the preoperative state which reflects the consequences of prolonged exposition to inadequate circulatory conditions; second, the intraoperative phase depending on a number of surgical and anesthesiological variables; third, the early postoperative phase representing the effects of operative strains on previously existing impaired tolerance; fourth, the phase of recovery characterizing the capacity of the compensatory mechanism; and finally, fifth, the phase of stabilization in which the expected advantages of treatment are weighed. The beneficial long-term EEG outcome is encouraging. The negative consequences of prolonged circulatory inadequacy and even occasional operative cerebral damage seem to be at least partially reversible and to be eventually outweighed by the overall benefits.[31]

Prediction of the Neurological Complications

Realizing the frequent occurrence of cerebral disorders and the marked role played by the intraoperative determinants of damage, any preoperative predictive information would be of great interest. However, these aspects have been given very little attention in the otherwise extensive literature on open heart surgery. A previous history of neurological disease has been claimed[10,69,74] to impair the clinical prognosis, but according to some authors[20] this is only true when clinical abnormalities attributable to a previous disease are still present at operation. Previous major cerebrovascular accidents seem to be important but less dramatic signs such as syncope[7] have also been claimed to impair the prognosis.

Preoperative EEG investigations have been considered to have no predictive value in some reports[14,30,66] while certain predictive measures seem to have been extracted in others.[31,33] For example, preoperative occurrence of delta or sharp wave abnormalities or a low frequency (≤ 8.5 Hz) of the dominant activity in the conventional EEG[31] and low values (≤ 7 Hz) of quantitative EEG mean frequency[32] have been described as being associated with an unfavorable outcome. The last mentioned observations, however, are based on a relatively small patient material and must be considered with some reservations. However, the fact that the use of the above-mentioned EEG criteria alone could correctly predict the clinical disorders in 15 cases out of the 19 which displayed the criteria gives some indication of the probable interrelation of certain kinds of EEG manifestations and lowered tolerance of ECC.

In accordance with the EEG findings, the preoperative neuropsychological measures have also previously been evaluated[88] to be of no predictive use. More recently, however, tentative signs of predictive significance have been described.[17,81,82]

When evaluating the possible importance of the proposed predictive measures, one should remember that the conclusions made on the basis of information obtained from studies which approach the subject with purely clinical neurophysiological or neuropsychological tools reflect only very limited data. The whole matter of predictive assessment reaches entirely new levels and ranges, however, when several cerebral functional levels are considered simultaneously and when the conclusions are drawn by uniting the information from the different levels. Only by this kind of investigation can one hope to obtain something more than only a faint impression of the CNS events related to cardiac disease and its operative treatment. An attempt has in fact been made[89] to adopt this kind of multidimensional approach by re-evaluating as an entity both the predictive references in some of the studies mentioned above[7,17,31-33] and their results. It appeared that when using clinical EEG, QEEG and neuropsychological criteria the manifestation of postoperative cerebral dysfunction could be correctly predicted with an accuracy of 83% (19 cases out of 23; $p = 0.02$).

What would be the use of predictive information in practice? The information would be of especial importance when alternative methods of treatment are weighed against each other. Prognostic correlates would also be useful in detecting cases with particularly high risks, indicating those patients needing special consideration and extraordinary procedures of pre-, intra-, and postoperative surveillance. It might indeed be found advisable for high risk cases to be forwarded for operation to certain special centers only. Furthermore, the evaluation of the need for operative treatment may hopefully come to be based on wider insights than the purely cardiological terms now used almost exclusively.

Our present knowledge of the predictive measures is unfortunately inadequate and more research is needed if we are ever to reach a practically significant level of prediction for at least the most severe cases.

Prevention of the Neurological Complications

Advances in surgical techniques and improvements in equipment have been shown to decrease the risk of cerebral complications, particularly of overt disorders.[22,28,29,40,49,50,68,90,91] Development of the filters used in the cardiopulmonary bypass preventing embolization of air and particulate matter, [28,40,90,91] development of the prostheses[5] and oxygenators, [49,50] changes in the priming techniques, [22,28] procedures to prevent hypotension[28] and gaseous microemboli[51] at the onset of cardiopulmonary bypass, the use of a cerebral function monitor,[28,38] and the introduction of cardioplegia[92] have been among the most effective factors responsible for the advantageous results of recent years. In one series,[28] the introduction of prophylactic measures was followed by a reduction in the prevalence of cerebral damage from 19.2% to 7.4%, and the prevalence of neurological injury which could not be attributed to any specific feature of the operative period fell from 11.5% to 3.4%. Correspondingly, other studies[22,29] report a reduction of cerebral complications from 14.5% to 2% during the years since 1972. The importance both of investigating the condition of the precerebral vessels before heart operation if vascular lesion is suspected and of reconstructing hemodynamically significant lesions prior to cardiopulmonary bypass has been emphasized.[93,94] The postoperative use of anticoagulant treatment is now routine but the benefits of additionally used dipyridamole[95] seem to be open to discussion as is the recently reported use of prostacyclin.[96] In instances of air embolism, hyperbaric treatment might be useful.[97,98] Prompt recognition of potentially correctable complications such as intracranial surface hemorrhages should be kept in mind.[23] Finally, prevention of peripheral neurological injuries involves careful consideration of the mechanical conditions and of patient positioning on the operating table, particularly when there are also coincident factors rendering neuropathy more likely.

Summary

The extensive literature devoted to the neurological complications of open heart surgery reflects the multiplicity of the risk factors to which the patient is exposed before, during and after operation. Both the ever increasing number of procedures which use ECC and the expected and justified more exacting demands and requirements oblige us to develop effective methods to prevent iatrogenic complications. Several factors in the operative treatment with all its complicated maneuvers can be recognized as potentially harmful but a definite single cause of complications can be reliably pointed out only rarely. However, the positively advantageous results achieved by advances in surgical techniques and operative procedures have shown that at least the more severe neurological complications which threaten a valuable surgical outcome can to a certain extent be minimized. Moreover, neurological investigatory methods have also been developed concurrently, and the earlier and more accurate recognition of subclinical dysfunction has now become possible.

It is obvious that emphasis should now be put on investigations at the nerve cell level, on the metabolic changes and their determinants. Only this level will give us answers to the questions arising from the clinical observations. At the same time more attention should be given in neurological investigations to the higher cerebral functions and subclinical consequences. Quite obviously progress involves the use of multidimensional investigatory procedures which comprise clinical, neuropsychological, electroencephalographical, and psychiatric assessment. Thorough clinical examinations should particularly concentrate on the preoperative condition in order to reveal possible predictive measures and indicators of disturbed cerebral circulation and, particularly, occlusive precerebral arterial disease. Electroencephalography is of value in both pre- and postoperative evaluation but also especially in intraoperative patient surveillance because it is the only safe method to indicate the cerebral functional status during operation and the most effective method to warn of disturbances at the earliest possible stage. Neuropsychological and psychiatric investigations may reveal predictive information and together with the EEG represent the subclinical scope. It seems justified to presume that the present cardiopulmonary bypass methods are still too imperfect to replace the normal cardiorespiratory functions and that therefore the open heart procedure almost invariably results in a certain amount of cerebral dysfunction. Whether or not the consequences are detectable, detected or recognized, depends on the degree of the disorder, on the individual compensatory mechanisms and, essentially, on the investigatory methods used. It seems evident that without using several methods for the simultaneous measurement of different CNS functional levels, one can obtain only a rough impression of the cerebral events. The role of neurological surveillance in open heart surgery must not be considered as merely a reassuring one, indicating the probable nature of the surgical and cardiological outcome. On the contrary neurological surveillance will lead to a greater awareness and understanding of the neurological benefits resulting from the correction of major cardiac diseases.

References

1. Ross JK, Monro JL, Diwell AE, et al: The quality of life after cardiac surgery. *Brit Med J* 282:451-453, 1981.
2. Kannel W, Dawber T, Cohen M, McNamara P: Vascular disease of the brain. Epidemiological aspects: the Framingham study. *Amer J Publ Hlth* 55:1355-1366, 1965.
3. Karp HR: Cerebral vascular disease and neurologic manifestations of cardiovascular disease. In: Hurst JW, ed: *The Heart,* Fourth Edition, New York, McGraw-Hill, 1978, p. 1890.
4. Bannister RB: The risks of deferring valvotomy in patients with mitral stenosis. *Lancet* 2:329-332, 1960.
5. Mohr JP: Neurological complications of cardiac valvular disease and cardiac surgery including systemic hypotension. In: Vinken PJ, Bruyn GW, eds: *Handbook of Clinical Neurology, vol. 38,* New York, Elsevier North-Holland, 1979, pp 143-171.
6. Silverstein A, Krieger HP: Neurologic complications of cardiac surgery *Arch Neurol* 3:601-605, 1960.
7. Sotaniemi KA: Brain damage and neurological outcome after open-heart surgery. *J Neurol Neurosurg Psychiat* 43:127-135, 1980.
8. Tyler HR, Clark DP: Incidence of neurological complications in congenital heart disease. *Arch Neurol Psychiat* 77:17-22, 1957.
9. Tyler HR: Neurological disorders related to congenital heart disease. In: Vinken PJ, and Bruyn GW, eds: *Handbook of Clinical Neurology, vol. 38,* New York, Elsevier North-Holland, 1979, pp 119-142.
10. Branthwaite MA: Neurological damage related to open-heart surgery. *Thorax* 27:748-753, 1972.
11. Adams MJT: Multiple calcific embolism following mitral valvotomy. *Brit Heart J* 23:333-336, 1961.
12. Braunwald E, Swan JH: Cooperative study on cardiac catheterization. *Circulation* 37:1-113, 1968.
13. Dawson DM, Fisher EG: Neurologic complications of cardiac catheterization. *Neurology* 27:496-497, 1977.
14. Torres F, Frank GS, Cohen M, et al: Neurological and electroencephalographic studies in open-heart surgery. *Neurology* 9:174-183, 1959.
15. Egerton N, Kay JH: Psychological disturbances associated with open-heart surgery. *Brit J Psychiat* 110:433-439, 1964.
16. Björk VO, Hultquist G: Brain damage in children after deep hypothermia for open-heart surgery. *Thorax* 15:284-291, 1960.
17. Sotaniemi KA, Juolasmaa A, Hokkanen TE: Neuropsychologic outcome after open-heart surgery. *Arch Neurol* 38:2-8, 1981.
18. Gilman S: Cerebral disorders after open-heart operations. *N Engl J Med* 272:489-498, 1965.
19. Javid H, Tufo HM, Najafi H, et al: Neurological abnormalities following open-heart surgery. *J Thorac Cardiovasc Surg* 58:502-509, 1969.
20. Tufo HM, Ostfeld AM, Shekelle R: Central nervous system dysfunction following open-heart surgery. *JAMA* 212:1333-1340, 1970.

21. Lee WH, Brady MP, Rowe JM, Miller WC: Effects of extracorporeal circulation upon behaviour, personality and brain function. *Ann Surg* **173**:1013-1023, 1971.

22. Åberg T, Kihlgren M: Cerebral protection during open-heart surgery. *Thorax* **32**:525-533, 1977.

23. Humphreys RP, Hoffman HJ, Mustard WT, Trusler GA: Cerebral hemorrhage following heart surgery. *J Neurosurg* **43**:671-675, 1975.

24. Speidel H, Dahme B, Flemming B, et al: Psychische Störungen nach offenen Herz-operationen. *Nervenarzt* **50**:85-91, 1979.

25. Keates JRW, Innocenti DM, Ross DN: Mononeuritis multiplex. A complication of open-heart surgery. *J Thorac Cardiovasc Surg* **69**:816-819, 1975.

26. Honet JC, Raikes JA, Kantrowitz A, et al: Neuropathy in upper extremity after open-heart surgery. *Arch Phys Med Rehabil* **75**:264-267, 1976.

27. Vandersalm TJ, Cereda JM, Cutler BS: Brachial plexus injury following median sternotomy. *J Thorac Cardiovasc Surg* **80**:447-452, 1980.

28. Branthwaite MA: Prevention of neurological damage during open-heart surgery. *Thorax* **30**:258-261, 1975.

29. Åberg T, Kihlgren M, Jonsson L, et al: Improved cerebral protection during open heart surgery. Paper presented at Second International Symposium on Psychopathological and Neurological Dysfunctions following Open Heart Surgery, Milwaukee, 1980.

30. Lorenz R, Hehrlein F: Electroencephalographic findings in heart surgery. *Minn Med* **53**:1069-1076, 1970.

31. Sotaniemi KA: Clinical and prognostic correlates of EEG in open-heart surgery. *J Neurol Neurosurg Psychiat* **43**:941-947, 1980.

32. Sotaniemi KA, Sulg IA, Hokkanen TE: Quantitative EEG as a measure of cerebral dysfunction before and after open-heart surgery. *Electroenceph Clin Neurophysiol* **50**:81-95, 1980.

33. Sotaniemi KA: The benefits of open-heart surgery as reflected in the EEG. *Scand J Thorac Cardiovasc Surg*, **15**:205-212, 1981.

34. Frank KA, Heller SS, Kornfeld DS, Malm JR: Long-term effects of open-heart surgery on intellectual functioning. *J Thorac Cardiovasc Surg* **64**:811-815, 1972.

35. Juolasmaa A, Outakoski J, Hirvenoja R, et al: The effect of open-heart surgery on intellectual performance. *J Clin Neuropsychol* **3**:181-197, 1981.

36. Sotaniemi KA, Hokkanen TE: Cerebral dysfunction following open-heart surgery. *Acta Neurol Scand* **62, suppl 78**:199-200, 1980.

37. Sachdev NS, Carter CC, Swank RL, Blachly PH: Relationship between post-cardiotomy delirium, clinical neurological changes and EEG abnormalities. *J Thorac Cardiovasc Surg* **54**:557-563, 1967.

38. Salerno TA, Lince DP, White DN, et al: Monitoring of electroencephalogram during open-heart surgery. *J Thorac Cardiovasc Surg* **76**:97-101, 1978.

39. Schwartz MS, Colvin MP, Prior FP, et al: The cerebral function monitor. *Anesthesiology* **28**:611-618, 1973.

40. Aguilar MJ, Gerbode F, Hill J: Neuropathologic complications of cardiac surgery. *J Thorac Cardiovasc Surg* **61**:676-685, 1971.

41. Brierley JB: Neuropathological findings in patients dying after open-heart surgery. *Thorax* **18**:291-304, 1963.

42. Wright ES, Sarkozy E, Dobell ARC, Murphy DR: Fat globulemia in extracorporeal circulation. *Surgery* **53**:500-504, 1963.

43. Helmsworth JA, Call EA, Perrin EV, et al: Occurrence of emboli during perfusion with an oxygenator pump. *Surgery* **53**:177-185, 1963.

44. Bass RM, Longmore DB: Cerebral damage during open-heart surgery. *Nature* **222**:30-33, 1969.
45. Lee WH, Krumhaar D, Fonkalsrud EW, et al: Denaturation of plasma proteins as a cause of morbidity and death after intracardiac operations. *Surgery* **50**:29-39, 1961.
46. Connell RS, Page US, Bartley TD, et al: The effect of pulmonary ultrastructure of dacron-wool filtration during cardio-pulmonary bypass. *Ann Thorac Surg* **15**:217-229, 1973.
47. Williams IM: Intravascular changes in the retina during open-heart surgery. *Lancet* **2**:688-691, 1971.
48. Solis RT, Kennedy PS, Beall AC, et al: Cardio-pulmonary bypass. Microembolization and platelet aggregation. *Circulation* **52**:103-108, 1975.
49. Carlson RG, Landé AJ, Landis B, et al: The Landé-Edwards membrane oxygenator during heart surgery. *J Thorac Cardiovasc Surg* **66**:894-905, 1973.
50. Boccalon H, Puel P, Rous De Feneyrols A, et al: Comparison of psychometric findings following use of bubble and membrane oxygenator. Paper presented at Second International Symposium on Psychopathological and Neurological Dysfunctions following Open Heart Surgery, Milwaukee, 1980.
51. Kritikou PE, Branthwaite MA: Significance of changes in cerebral electrical activity at onset of cardiopulmonary bypass. *Thorax* **32**:534-538, 1977.
52. Wright G, Sanderson JM: Brain damage and mortality in dogs following pulsatile and non-pulsatile blood flows in extracorporeal circulation. *Thorax* **27**:738-749.
53. Singh RKK, Barratboyes BG, Harris EA: Does pulsatile flow improve perfusion during hypothermic cardiopulmonary bypass. *J Thorac Cardiovasc Surg* **79**:827-832, 1980.
54. Brennan RW, Patterson RH, Kessler J: Cerebral blood flow and metabolism during cardiopulmonary bypass: evidence of microembolic encephalopathy. *Neurology* **21**:665-672, 1971.
55. Henningsen P: Ilt- og kuldioksidtensionens betydning for haemodynamik og iltoptagelse under ekstrakorporal cirkulation med opbygning og stimulering af et automatisk kontrolsystem. F.A.D.L.'s Forlag A/S, Copenhagen, 1973.
56. Branthwaite MA: Cerebral blood flow and metabolism during openheart surgery. *Thorax* **29**:633-638, 1974.
57. Kavan EM, Brechner VL, Walter RD, Maloney JV: Electroencephalographic patterns during intracardiac surgery using cardiopulmonary bypass. A comparison of two anaesthetic drugs. *Arch Surg* **78**:151-156, 1959.
58. Branthwaite MA: Detection of neurological damage during open-heart surgery. *Thorax* **28**: 464-472, 1973.
59. Reilly EL, Brunberg JA, Doty DB: The effect of deep hypothermia and total circulatory arrest on the electroencephalogram in children. *Electroenceph Clin Neurophysiol* **36**:661-667, 1974.
60. Messmer BJ, Schallberger U, Gattiker R, Senning A: Psychomotor and intellectual development after deep hypothermia and circulatory arrest in early infancy. *J Thorac Cardiovasc Surg* **72**:495-502, 1976.
61. Cohen ME, Olszowka JS, Subramanian S: Electroencephalographic and neurological correlates of deep hypothermia and circulatory arrest in

infants. *Ann Thorac Surg* **23**:238-244, 1977.

62. Kolkka R, Hilberman M: Neurologic dysfunction following cardiac operation with low-flow, low-pressure cardiopulmonary bypass. *J Thorac Cardiovasc Surg* **79**:432-437, 1980.

63. Arfel G, Weiss J, Dubouchet N: EEG findings during open-heart surgery with extra-corporeal circulation. In: Gastaut H, Meyer JS, eds: Cerebral anoxia and the electroencephalogram. Springfield, Charles C Thomas, 1961, pp. 231-249.

64. Stockard JJ, Bickford RG, Myers RR, et al: Hypotension-induced changes in cerebral function during cardiac surgery. *Stroke* **5**:730-746, 1974.

65. Ross Russell RW, Bharucha N: The recognition and prevention of border zone cerebral ischaemia during cardiac surgery. *Quart J Med* **17**:303-323, 1978.

66. Hansotia PL, Myers WO, Ray JF, et al: Prognostic value of electroencephalography in cardiac surgery. *Ann Thorac Surg* **19**:127-134, 1975.

67. Tienari P, Outakoski J, Hirvenoja I, et al: Psychic complications following open-heart surgery. A prospective study. Paper presented at Second International Symposium on Psychopathological and Neurological Dysfunctions following Open Heart Surgery, Milwaukee, 1980.

68. Åberg T, Kihlgren M: Effect of open-heart surgery on intellectual function. *Scand J Thorac Cardiovasc Surg*, Suppl. 15, 1974.

69. Burggraf GW, Craige E: Echocardiographic studies of left ventricular wall motion and dimensions after valvular heart surgery. *Amer J Cardiol* **35**:473-478, 1975.

70. Gottstein Y, Bernsmeier A, Blömer H, Schimmler W: Die zerebrale Hämodynamik bei Kranken mit Mitralstenose und kombiniertem Mitralvitium. *Klin Wochenschr* **38**:1025-1030, 1960.

71. Kamp A, Troost J: EEG signs of cerebrovascular disorder, using physical exercise as a provocative method. *Electroenceph Clin Neurophysiol* **45**:295-298, 1978.

72. Lee WH, Miller W, Rowe J, et al: Effects of extracorporeal circulation on personality and cerebration. *Ann Thorac Surg* **7**:562-569, 1969.

73. Gilberstadt H, Sako Y: Intellectual and personality changes following open-heart surgery. *Arch Gen Psychiat* **16**:210-214, 1967.

74. Sveinsson IS: Postoperative psychosis after heart surgery. *J Thorac Cardiovasc Surg* **70**:717-726, 1975.

75. Orr WC, Stahl ML: Sleep disturbances after open heart surgery. *Amer J Cardiol* **39**:196-201, 1977.

76. Björk VO, Henze A, Gernandez J, et al: 10 years experience with the Björk-Shiley tilting disc valve. *J Thorac Cardiovasc Surg* **78**:331-342, 1979.

77. Marus H, Johnson WD: Prosthetic valve endocarditis. *J Thorac Cardiovasc Surg* **80**:31-37, 1980.

78. Witoszka MM, Tamura H, Indeglia R, et al: Electroencephalographic changes and cerebral complications in open-heart surgery. *J Thorac Cardiovasc Surg* **66**:855-864, 1973.

79. Shealy AE, Walker DR: Minnesota Multiphasic Personality Inventory prediction of intellectual changes following cardiac surgery. *J Nerv Ment Dis* **166**:263-267, 1978.

80. Kimball CP: The experience of open-heart surgery. *Arch Gen Psychiat* **27**:56-63, 1972.

81. Kilpatrick DG, Miller WC, Allain AN, et al: The use of psychological test data to predict open-heart surgery outcome: a prospective study. *Psychosom Med* **37**:62-73, 1975.

82. Willner AE, Rabiner CJ, Wisoff BG, et al: Analogy tests and psychopathology at follow-up after open-heart surgery. *Biol Psychiat* 11:678-696, 1976.
83. Lipowski ZJ: Cardiovascular disorders. In: Kaplan HI, Freedman, AM, Sadock BJ, eds: *Comprehensive Textbook of Psychiatry/III. Vol. 2, 3rd Edition*, Baltimore/London, Williams & Wilkins, 1980, pp. 1891-1907.
84. Kalyanamaran K, Niedermeyer E, Rowe R, Wolf K: The electroencephalogram in congenital heart disease. *Arch Neurol* 18:98-106, 1968.
85. Obrist WD, Bissel LF: The electroencephalogram of aged patients with cardiac and cerebral vascular disease. *J Geront* 10:315-330, 1955.
86. Storm van Leeuwen W, Mechelse K, Kok L, Zierfuss E: EEG during heart operations with artificial circulation. In: Gastaut H, Meyer JS, eds: *Cerebral Anoxia and the Electroencephalogram.* Springfield, Charles C Thomas, 1961, pp 268-278.
87. Fischer-Williams M, Cooper RA: Some aspects of electroencephalographic changes during open-heart surgery. *Neurology* 14:472-482, 1964.
88. Hazan SJ: Psychiatric complications following cardiac surgery. Part I: Review article. *J Thorac Cardiovasc Surg* 51:307-310, 1966.
89. Sotaniemi KA: Cerebral predictive indices in high-risk surgery. *Acta Neurol Scand*, in press, 1982.
90. Hill JD, Osborn JJ, Swank RL, et al: Experience using a new dacron wool filter during extracorporeal circulation. *Arch Surg* 101:649-652, 1970.
91. Guidoin R, Laperche Y, Martin L, Awad J: Disposable filters for microaggregate removal from extracorporeal circulation. *J Thorac Cardiovasc Surg* 71:502-516, 1976.
92. Björk VO, Ivert T: Early and late neurological complications after prosthetic heart valve replacement. Paper presented at Second International Symposium on Psychopathological and Neurological Dysfunctions following Open Heart Surgery, Milwaukee, 1980.
93. Mehigan JT, Buch WS, Pipkin RD, Fogarthy TJ: A planned approach to coexistent cerebrovascular disease in coronary artery bypass candidates. *Arch Surg* 112:1403-1409, 1977.
94. Reis RL, Hannah H: Management of patients with severe coexistent coronary and peripheral vascular disease. *J Thorac Cardiovasc Surg* 73:909-918, 1977.
95. Sullivan JM, Harken DE, Gorlin R: Pharmacologic control of thromoembolic complications of cardiac-valve replacement. *N Engl J Med* 284:1391-1394, 1971.
96. Longmore D: The effects of prostacyclin on reducing cerebral damage following open-heart surgery. Paper presented at Second International Symposium on Psychopathological and Neurological Dysfunctions following Open Heart Surgery, Milwaukee, 1980.
97. Winter PM, Alvis HJ, Cage AA: Hyperbaric treatment of cerebral air embolism during cardiopulmonary bypass. *JAMA* 215:1786-1788, 1971.
98. Mills NL, Ochsner JL: Massive air embolism during cardiopulmonary bypass-causes, prevention and management. *J Thorac Cardiovasc Surg* 80:708-717, 1980.

Chapter XI

Neurological Side Effects of Gastrointestinal Drug Therapy

Norman Godin, M.D., Julio Messer, M.D., and
I. Richard Rosenberg, M.D.

Introduction

The gastrointestinal tract is the site of origin of multiple clinical problems, both organic, and even more commonly, functional. Because of the frequency of gastrointestinal complaints in clinical practice, drug therapy directed toward the alleviation of these symptoms, by necessity, occupies a significant place in our therapeutic armamentarium. The following discussion will outline the neurologic manifestations of these commonly prescribed agents. A brief discussion of the gastrointestinal indications and modes of action will be presented for all classifications of drugs used in treating clinical problems of gastroenterologic origin.

Antacids

Antacids are chemical agents used in an attempt to neutralize the hydrochloric acid secreted by the parietal cells of the stomach.

Gastrointestinal Indications

Antacids are effective in accelerating the healing rate of peptic ulcer disease and are also used in treating reflux esophagitis.[1-4] Aluminum and magnesium hydroxide-containing preparations are preferred for ulcer therapy since calcium carbonate causes significant calcium absorption in addition to acid rebound. Sodium carbonate causes metabolic alkalosis.

The phosphate-binding property of aluminum hydroxide (Amphogel, Dialume, Basaljel) is also used in a number of non-gastrointestinal indications, e.g., to lower serum phosphate in chronic renal failure.

Adverse Neurological Effects

Aluminum hydroxyde Al(OH)₃ can cause hypophosphatemia resulting in muscle weakness, malaise and muscle tremors.[5] This symptom
complex is seen particularly in chronic renal failure patients hemodia-
lyzed with a phosphorus-free bath. In the same population of patients, a
so-called "dialysis encephalopathy syndrome" has been reported, presumably secondary to aluminum intoxication of the brain.[6]

Magnesium Hydroxyde Mg(OH)₂. With chronic intake in the presence of renal disease, hypermagnesemia can occur and manifest itself by
CNS depression and muscle weakness.

Magnesium Trisilicate has similar side effects as Mg(OH)₂.

H-2 Blockers

Cimetidine (Tagamet) blocks the H2-histamine receptors on
the gastric parietal cell. Its chief therapeutic effect is the inhibition of
gastric acid synthesis. Cimetidine (300 mg) inhibits nocturnal acid production by 90-95% for 5 to 7 hours and effectively inhibits acid production in response to food, pentagastrin and histamine.[4]

Gastrointestinal Indications

Thus far, the approved indications for cimetidine are: (1) treatment
of duodenal ulcer (2) Zollinger-Ellison syndrome (3) systemic mastocy-
tosis (4) multiple endocrine adenomas. Cimetidine is now being evaluated for long-term treatment of duodenal ulcers, gastric ulcers, reflux
esophagitis, erosive gastritis, and upper gastrointestinal bleeding from
various causes including reducing the risk of upper gastrointestinal
hemorrhage in high-risk patients with septic shock, major burns, or
while on mechanical ventilators.

Adverse Neurological Effects

The major neurological side-effects of cimetidine are experienced by
a small but appreciable portion of patients.[7-9] Symptoms have included
mental confusion, somnolence, lethargy, restlessness, disorientation,
agitation, hallucinations, focal twitching, seizures, unresponsiveness,
and periods of apnea. Mental confusion is more frequent in the elderly,
in the very young, and in the critically ill patients with renal and
hepatic disturbances where it has been shown to pass the blood-brain
barrier possibly as a consequence of diminished capacity to metabolize
and/or excrete the drug.[9] Mental symptoms in patients receiving cimetidine may result from effects of the drug in blocking H2-receptors in the
central nervous system and possibly interfering with endogenous
enkephalins.[10,11]

It must be concluded that development of otherwise unexplained CNS abnormalities in a patient taking cimetidine should be considered an indication to discontinue or substantially reduce the dose of the drug.[7,12]

Anticholinergics

Anticholinergics inhibit competitively the effect of acetylcholine released from postganglionic parasympathetic nerves and are termed antimuscarinic agents. The prototype is atropine, a tertiary amine, which is readily absorbed from the gastrointestinal tract and crosses the blood-brain barrier. Most of the synthetic antimuscarinic drugs are cationic quatenary ammonium drugs which are poorly absorbed and do not cross to the central nervous system.

Gastrointestinal Indications

The main indications for anticholinergic agents are in the treatment of peptic ulcer disease and in the utilization of their antispasmodic properties. The resultant vagolytic effect causes a partial "medical vagotomy" by decreasing gastric acid secretion. Their efficacy in treating peptic ulcer disease is not as yet proven. These agents are also commonly used in the irritible bowel syndrome as antispasmodic agents. Bile and pancreatic secretions are not markedly modified by anticholinergic drugs.

Adverse Neurological Side Effects

In high doses, atropine causes excitation and delirium leading to convulsions. The quaternary ammonium compounds, as stated earlier, do not cross the blood-brain barrier, but at high doses they interfere with the actions of acetylcholine at autonomic ganglia and at the neuromuscular junctions, causing pupil dilation and paralyzing accomodation. This problem is also discussed in Chapters XII and XVI in this book.

Bismuth Compounds

Gastrointestinal Indications

Bismuth subsalicylate compounds have been shown to symptomatically improve "traveler's diarrhea," possibly by inactivating *E. coli* toxin. Bismuth subgallate reduces the weight of excretion of ileostomy patients. It is not clear in the case of subsalicylate bismuth if the antidiarrheal effect is due to bismuth or to the salicylates.[13]

Adverse Neurological Effects

Bismuth subgallate, subcarbonate, and subnitrate have been reported to cause a reversible psychosis, aggravated by resulting constipation and thus increasing their own absorption. The diagnosis can easily be suspected by taking an x-ray of the abdomen showing a radiodense compound in the bowel (bismuth) in the absence of previous barium studies. Blood and urine levels of bismuth can also be measured.

Anti-emetics

Nausea and vomiting are obviously one of the most common gastrointestinal complaints faced by the clinician. We do not need to consider nausea or vomiting of central origin in this discussion. Nausea and vomiting of gastrointestinal origin can originate from many causes too numerous to catalogue here.

The most common family of drugs used to control these symptoms are the phenothiazine group. The following compounds are most commonly prescribed: Prochlorperazine (Compazine), perphenazine (Trilafon), chlorpromazine (Thorazine), and promethazine (Phenergan). Trimethobenzamide (Tigan) is a widely used antiemetic not in the phenothiazine family. These compounds act on the central nervous system, probably at the hypothalamic level primarily.

Adverse Neurological Effects

Phenothiazines have been known for a long time to produce striking extra pyramidal symptoms in susceptible individuals.[14] Symptoms may include pin-rolling motions, mask-like facies, drooling, tremors, cogwheel rigidity, and shuffling gait.

Dystonic reactions secondary to phenothiazines include torticolis, spasm of neck and jaw muscles, protrusion of tongue, and extensor rigidity of back muscles which can even lead to opisthotonos.[15]

Trimethobenzamide (Tigan) has rarely been reported to cause neurological symptoms.[16]

All of the above drugs have been considered as a possible causative factor in the central nervous system involvement in Reye's syndrome. There is no reported evidence to support this association. Since nausea and vomiting often precede Reye's syndrome and these drugs are commonly used to control these symptoms, the association has been suggested.

The treatment for extrapyramidal and dystonic reaction secondary to phenothiazines is: (1) Intravenous diphenhydramine HCL (Benadryl) 50 mg IV; (2) Antiparkinsonism agents (except levodopa); (3) Dosage reduced or discontinued depending on severity of symptoms. If therapy is reinstituted, it should be at a lower dosage.

The treatment of extrapyramidal and dystonic reaction secondary to trimethobenzamide is unkown because of the extreme rarity of this complication of trimethobenzamide therapy. For further discussion of this problem, see Chapter VI in this book.

Metoclopramide

Metoclopramide is a procainamide derivative with antidopaminergic and anticholinergic effects.[17] It has been released in the USA under the trade name Reglan. Metoclopramide causes an increase in lower esophageal pressure. It increases gastric contractions in animals and humans with acceleration of gastric emptying, but has no effect on gastric secretion. Metoclopromide also accelerates smooth muscle contractions in the small bowel but not in the colon. The effect on motility of the small bowel is not associated with secretion of water or electolytes and therefore usually does not cause diarrhea.[18]

The effects of metoclopramide on motility can be reversed by levodopa and atropine.

Gastrointestinal Indications

Metoclopramide is used in treating nausea and vomiting that occurs with delayed gastric emptying, for example in diabetic gastroparesis. It has been prescribed for dyspepsia, gastroesophageal reflux, gastric and duodenal ulcers, and hiccups. It facilitates radiographic and intubation procedures, including biopsy and endoscopy.

Adverse Neurological Effects

At usual therapeutic doses adverse effects are uncommon, but somewhat more frequent in children, young adults and women.

There is a reported incidence of 11% side effects. [17,18] The most commonly seen symptoms are drowsiness, lassitude, dizziness, and lightheadedness. Extrapyramidal reactions with metoclopramide are much less common than with phenothiazines or butyrophenones. The dyskinesias, beginning within 36 hours after starting metoclopramide include trismus, torticollis, facial spasms, opisthotonos, and oculogyric crises. They disappear within a day of stopping metoclopramide and respond to anti-parkinsonian drugs such as parenteral benztropine or diazepam. Metoclopramide has not been found to aggravate the severity of Parkinson's disease or levodopa associated dyskinesias.

Overdose poisoning with metoclopramide has resulted in somnolence, disorientation, irritability, agitation, and convulsions. In severe poisoning, in addition to gastric lavage and supportive care, anticholinergics have been used to reverse the central nervous system effects.

Laxatives

Most chronic laxative abusers run the risk of developing electrolyte abnormalities — most commonly hypokalemia, with profound muscle weakness.[19] Hyponatremia, hypomagnesemia, and hypocalcemia have been reported with laxative abuse.[20]

Irritant purgatives of the anthraquinone group (cascara, senna, aloes, rhubarb, and danthron) have been reported to damage the myenteric plexuses of the gut, predominantly in the right colon and therefore, after many years of continuous use, these agents lose their efficacy and constipation worsens.[21]

Anti-Diarrheal Agents

Morphine and Derivatives

Gastrointestinal Indications

Narcotics are used in gastrointestinal therapy for their analgesic, constipating, and emetic effects. Morphine sulfate arrests gastric emptying and causes pylorospasm after a short spurt of gastric motor activity. Morphine decreases propulsive contractions in the small bowel and significantly increases intraluminal pressures in the colon causing abnormal segmentation, spasm, and constipation because of a decrease in propulsive waves. It increases the pressure in the biliary tract and the sphincter of Oddi, this effect being reversed by nitrates. The emetic effect is caused by direct action on the chemoreceptor trigger zone (CTZ) in the medulla of the brain.

Adverse Neurological Effects

Nausea and vomiting, as described, result from CTZ stimulation. Pupil constriction is characteristic and cough is suppressed. Respiratory depression, hypotension, and coma are well described in abusers.

Diphenoxylate

Diphenoxylate is a derivative of the synthetic narcotic meperidine and acts like morphine in stopping intestinal propulsion without any effect on intestinal fluid shifts. To discourage abuse, the drug is marketed in combination with a subtherapeutic dose of atropine, thus causing abusers to have unpleasant anticholinergic effects.

Gastrointestinal Indications

Diphenoxylate is used for symptomatic treatment of diarrhea. However, delayed intestinal motility can cause dangerous complications in ulcerative colitis or infectious bowel disease such as shigellosis.[22] This drug should only be prescribed after an etiological diagnosis of the diarrhea has been made.

Adverse Neurological Effects

These are similar to morphine. Further neurological complications of narcotics are described in Chapter VII in this book.

Loperamide

Loperamide is used in the symptomatic treatment of diarrhea. Its mechanism of action has not been defined.

Adverse Neurological Effects

In contrast to morphine and diphenoxylate, the dissociation of gastrointestinal effects from opiate-like central nervous system effects is almost complete in loperamide.[23] There are no reported central nervous system effects in man and loperamide does not appear to potentiate action of barbiturates or tranquilizers. Even at doses four times higher than the constipating dose, loperamide appears to be devoid of central activity.[24]

Anti-inflammatory and Immunosuppressive Agents

Corticosteroids, ACTH

Corticosteroids are 21-C cholesterol derivatives with numerous biological effects. They are used in gastrointestinal and liver disease primarily for their anti-inflammatory effect.

Gastrointestinal Indications

Corticosteroids are mainly used for the treatment of ulcerative colitis, Crohn's disease, and some forms of chronic liver disease.

Chronic active hepatitis results from three major etiologies: (1) Viral-hepatitis B and non-A-and non-B virus, (2) Autoimmune, (3) Drugs (much less common). The indications for corticosteroid therapy in chronic active hepatitis secondary to viral etiology are currently in flux. There is a strong movement away from treating this group of patients with any definitive drug therapy.

Autoimmune chronic active hepatitis remains the only form of the disease universally treated with corticosteroid agents.

Adverse Neurological Side Effects

The neurological side effects of corticosteroids are numerous.

Mental reactions to glucocorticoids can range from mild nervousness, euphoria, and insomnia to severe depression or psychosis.[25] Pseudo tumor cerebri with papilledema has also been reported as a side effect of corticosteroids, particularly upon withdrawal.[26] Steroid induced myopathy tends to involve the hip and shoulder-girdle musculature. Although the patient is weak, the muscles are not tender and muscle enzymes are usually normal. Muscle biopsy is usually not necessary to make the diagnosis and clinical judgement must dictate whether to increase or decrease steroid doses. Steroid induced myopathy can be improved by lowering glucocorticoid dosage and instructing the patient in an aggressive exercise program. Resistance to infections is decreased by glucocorticoid therapy, therefore minor infections may become systemic with central nervous system involvement; quiescent infections may become activated and organisms usually nonpathogenic may cause disease. A detailed discussion of the neurotoxicity of steroid medication is presented in Chapters II and III in this book.

Sulfasalazine

Sulfasalazine is a chemical combination of the sulfonamide sulfapyridine and the anti-inflammatory 5-amino-salicylate (5-SASA). It has been shown that of the two compounds of sulfasalazine, 5-aminosalicylate (5-SASA) is the active compound and sulfapyridine serves primarily as a means to deliver the drug to the colon, blocking absorption in the small bowel.[27,28] In the colon, colonic bacteria cleave sulfasalazine liberating the 5-SASA. Most of the side effects of the drug are related to sulfapyridine and are more frequent in slow acetylators.[29]

Gastrointestinal Indications

A number of controlled trials[30-33] have shown that sulfasalazine has a therapeutic as well as prophylactic role in the management of ulcerative colitis.

In Crohn's disease, the National Cooperative Crohn's disease study demonstrated that Crohn's colitis was especially responsive to sulfasalazine, however no prophylaxis against flare-up or recurrence could be demonstrated.

Adverse Neurological Effects

Adverse neurological effects occur in 5 to 55% of patients taking the drug and may be dose-related or sensitivity reactions.

The dose-dependent reactions occur most often in the first 8-12 weeks of therapy at doses of sulfasalazine exceeding 4 g daily, especially in slow acetylators and include among other manifestations such as nausea, vomiting, fever, arthalgias, severe headaches that subside readily as drug therapy is stopped and may not recur if restarted at lower dosage. Headache sometimes can be prevented by the concomitant use of an antihistaminic preparation.

Among the sensitivity reactions to sulfasalazine including rash, blood dyscrasias, bronchospasm and hepatotoxicity, peripheral neuropathy in both lower limbs with numbness, paresthesias, absence of knee and ankle jerks, and impairment of proprioception and vibration have been described.[34]

Azathioprine and 6 Mercaptopurine (6 MP)

6-Mercaptopurine and its imidozolyl derivative, azathioprine, are antimetabolites with antineoplastic and immunosuppressive properites. They have been tried in the treatment of Crohn's disease,[35] ulcerative colitis,[36,37] and chronic active liver disease.

In chronic active liver disease of autoimmune etiology, azathioprine had a sparing effect on steroids given on a long-term basis and reduced side effects of steroids.

Adverse Neurological Side Effects

The main adverse effects are due to increased susceptibility to infections with increased risk of central nervous system infection. Other neurological side effects of these drugs have been presented in Chapter III of this book.

Treatment of Hepatic Encephalopathy

Neomycin is an antibiotic with poor systemic absorption when given orally.

Gastrointestinal Indications

Neomycin given orally alters intestinal flora in preparation for bowel surgery, ameliorates hepatic encephalopathy by reducing ammonia forming bacteria in the gut and increases tolerance to protein in the diet of patients at risk of developing encephalopathy.[38]

Adverse Neurological Effects

Nephrotoxicity is the most serious, life-threatening toxic effect of neomycin leading to drug accumulation. Most neurological side effects such as deafness and neuro-muscular blockage have been described only with high neomycin levels often secondary to renal toxicity.[38-40] A more detailed discussion of ototoxic complications and neuro-muscular blockage of antibiotics has been presented in Chapter I in this book.

Miscellaneous

d-Penicillamine

d-Penicillamine is an orally effective chelating agent that binds metals, including copper, mercury, zinc and lead.

Gastrointestinal Indications

d-Penicillamine is the treatment of choice for chelating copper accumulated in Wilson's disease (hepatolenticular degeneration).[41,42] d-Penicillamine can arrest the progression of the characteristic brain and liver lesions of Wilson's disease and may reverse some of the manifestations of these lesions including Kaiser-Fleischer rings if started before irreversible brain damage or nodular cirrhosis have developed.[43,44]

d-Penicillamine is also currently under investigation for a number of other indications including chronic active hepatitis,[45] primary biliary cirrhosis[46] and possibly in sclerosing cholangitis, all liver diseases where increased liver copper accumulation have been documented.

Adverse Neurological Effects

l-penicillamine, either alone or when present in the dl racemate form is an inhibitor of pyridoxine. To avoid pyridoxine deficiency and its associated neuritis, only the d form is used clinically and pyridoxine supplements 12.5 to 25 mg daily are given to patients receiving d-penicillamine for Wilson's disease.

Penicillamine-associated myasthenia gravis, antiacetylcholine receptor-antibodies and antistriational antibodies have been described,[47] developing 4 to 28 months after commencing penicillamine and not modified by thymectomy.

Optical axial neuritis has also been reported as a consequence of dl-penicillamine therapy. Prompt relief was achieved by pyridoxine therapy, suggesting that the optic nerve lesions resulted from a penicillamine-induced pyridoxine deficiency.[48] Rare cases of systemic lupus erythematosis (SLE) secondary to d-penicillamine have been reported with possible central nervous system involvement.

Metronidazole

Gastrointestinal Indications

Metronidazole (Flagyl) has been proven effective in the treatment of aerobic abcesses and some protozoa infections including amoebiasis and giardiasis.[49] Metronidazole is also effective against anaerobic bacteria. Because of the potential role of anaerobes in mucosal injury and deconjugation of bile-salts, long-term therapy with metronidazole has been used to treat Crohn's disease. Preliminary reports indicate that it may be of some benefit in treating symptomatic patients with colonic involvement and perianal disease.[50-52]

Adverse Neurological Effects

Adverse effects include peripheral sensory neuropathy with paresthesias developing in half the patients treated in one series, occurring a mean of six months after metronidazole therapy was begun and disappearing six months after it was discontinued.[53] Dizziness, vertigo and, very rarely, ataxia have been described. See Chapter I for more details.

The following drugs used in gastrointestinal therapy have not been described as causing neurological side effects: simethicone, carbenoxolone, medium-chain triglycerides, surfactant laxatives, bulk foming laxatives, mineral oil, loperamide, cholestyramine (but binds other drugs in the gut), lactulose, cheno-deoxycholic acid, and deferoxamine.

References

1. Hollander D, Harlan J: Antacids versus placebo in peptic ulcer therapy. A controlled double-blind investigation. *JAMA* **225**:1181-1185, 1973.
2. Littman A, Welch RW, Fruin RC, Aronson AR: Controlled trials of aluminum hydroxyde gels for peptic ulcer. *Gastroenterology* **73**:6-10, 1977.
3. Peterson WL, Sturdevant RAL, Frankl HD, et al: Healing of the duodenal ulcer with an antacid regimen. *N Engl J Med* **297**:341-345, 1977.
4. Greenberger NJ, Arvanitakis C, Hurwitz A: *Drug Treatment of Gastrointestinal Disorders. Monographs in Clinical Pharmacology:* Vol. 2. New York, Churchill Livingstone 1979, pp 1-78.
5. Boelens PA, Norwood W, Kjellstrand C, Brown DM: Hypophosphatemia with muscle weakness due to antacids and hemodialysis. *Amer J Dis Child* **120**:350-353, 1970.
6. Alfrey AC, LeGendre GR, Kaehny WD: The dialysis encephalopathy syndrome: Possible aluminum intoxication. *N Engl J Med* **294**:184-188, 1976.
7. McGuigan J: A consideration of the adverse effects of cimetidine. *Gastroenterology* **80**:181-192, 1981.
8. Delaney JC, Ravey M: Cimetidine and mental confusion. *Lancet* **2**:719, 1977.

9. Schentag JJ, Cerra FB, Calleri G, et al: Pharmacokinetic and clinical studies in patients with cimetidine-associated mental confusion. *Lancet* 1:177-181, 1979.

10. Vogt M: Histamine H2-receptors in the brain and sleep produced by clonidine, *Brit J Pharmacol* 61:441-443, 1977.

11. Takayanagi I, Iwayama Y, Kasuya Y: Narcotic antagonistic action of cimetidine on the guinea-pig ileum. *J Pharm Pharmacol* 30:519-520, 1978.

12. Kimmelblatt BJ, Cana FB, Calleri F, et al: Dose and serum concentration relationships in cimetidine-associated mental confusion. *Gastroenterology* 78:791-795, 1980.

13. Dupont HL, Sullivan P, Pickering LK, et al: Symptomatic treatment of diarrhea with bismuth subsalicylate among students attending a Mexican university. *Gastroenterology:* 73:715-718, 1977.

14. Ayd FJ: A survey of drug induced extrapyramidal reactions. *JAMA* 175: 1054-1060. 1961.

15. Cotton DG, Newman CGH: Dystonic reactions to phenothiazine derivatives. *Arch Dis Child* 41:551-553, 1966.

16. Holmes C, Flaherty RJ: Trimethobenzamide HCl (Tigan) induced extrapyramidal dysfunction in neonate. *J Pediat* 89:669-670, 1976.

17. Pinder RM, Brogden R.N, Sawyer PR, et al: Metoclopramide: a review of its pharmacological properties and clinical use. *Drugs* 12:81-131, 1976.

18. Robinson OMV: Metoclopramide — A new pharmacological approach? *Postgrad Med J* 49(Suppl 4):77-80, 1973.

19. Flering BJ, Genuth SM, Gould AB, Kamionkowski MD: Laxative-induced hypokalemia, sodium depletion and hyperenemia. *Amer Intern Med* 83:60-62, 1975.

20. Rawson MD: Cathartic colon: *Lancet* 1:1121-1124, 1966.

21. Smith B: Effect of irritant purgatives on the myenteric plexus in man and the mouse, *Gut* 9:139-143, 1968.

22. Engback J, Ersboll J, Faurby V, et al: The constipating effect of diphenoxylate in ulcerative colitis. *Scand J Gastroenterol* 10:695-698, 1975.

23. Galambos JT, Hersch T, Schroeder S, Wenger J: Loperamide: A new antidiarrheal agent in the treatment of chronic diarrhea. *Gastroenterology* 70:1026-1029, 1976.

24. Verhaegen H, DeCree J, Schuermons V: Loperamide, a novel type of antidiarrheal agent. *Arzneim Forsch* 24: 1657-1660, 1974.

25. Haynes RC, Murad F: Adrenocorticotropic hormone; adrenocortical steroids and their synthetic analogs. In: Gilman AG, et al, eds: *Goodman and Gilman's The Pharmacological Basis of Therapeutics.* New York, MacMillan, 1980, Chapt 63 pp 1466-1496.

26. Levine SB, Leopold IH: Advances in ocular corticosteroid therapy. *Med Clin N Amer* 59:1167-1177, 1973.

27. Das KM, Eastwood MA, McManus JPA, Sircus W: Metabolism of salicylazo sulphapyridine in ulcerative colitis. *Gut* 14:631-641, 1973.

28. Das KM, Eastwood MA, McManus JPA, Sircus W. Salicylazosulfapyridine. Adverse reactions and relation to drug metabolism. *N Engl J Med* 289:491-495, 1973.

29. Klotz U, Maier K, Fischer CH, Heinkel K. Therapeutic efficacy of sul-

fasalazine and its metabolites in patients with ulcerative colitis and Crohn's disease. *N Engl J Med* **303**:1499-1502, 1980.

30. Baron JH, Connell AM, Lennard-Jones JE, Avery-Jones F: Sulphasalazine and salicylazo-sulfadimidine in ulcerative colitis. *Lancet* **1**:1094-1096, 1962.
31. Truelove SC, Watkinson G, Draper G: Comparison of corticosteroid and sulphasalazine therapy in ulcerative colitis. *Brit Med J* **2**:1708-1711, 1962.
32. Dick AP, Grayson MJ, Carpenter RG, Petrie AA: Controlled trial of sulphasalazine in the treatment of ulcerative colitis. *Gut* **5**:437-442, 1964.
33. Misiewicz JJ, Lennard Jones JE, Connell Am, et al: Controlled trial of sulfasalazine in maintenance therapy for ulcerative colitis. *Lancet* **1**:185-188, 1965.
34. Wallace IW: Neurotoxicity associated with a reaction of sulfasalazine. *Practitioner* **204**:850-851, 1970.
35. Present DH, Korelitz BI, Wisch N, et al: Treatment of Crohn's disease with 6 mercaptopurine. A long-term, random, double-blind study. *N Engl J Med* **302**:981-987, 1980.
36. Korelitz BI, Glass JL, Wisch N: Long term therapy of ulcerative colitis with 6 mercaptopurine: a personal series. *Amer J Dig Dis* **17**:111-118, 1972.
37. Wisch N, Korelitz BI: Immunosuppressive therapy for ulcerative colitis, ileitis and granulomatous colitis. *Surg Clin N Amer* **52**:961-969, 1972.
38. Conn HO, Leevy Cm, Vlahcevic ZR, et al: Comparison of lactulose and neomycin in the treatment of chronic portal-systemic encephalopathy: a double-blind controlled trial. *Gastroenterology* **72**:573-581, 1977.
39. Kunin CM, Chalmers TC, Leevy CM, et al: Absorption of orally administered neomycin and kanamycin. *N Engl J Med* **262**:380-385, 1960.
40. Last PM, Sherlock S: Systemic absorption of orally administered neomycin in liver disease. *N Engl J Med* **262**:385-389, 1960.
41. Dreiss A, Lynch RE, Lee GR, Cartwright GE: Long term therapy of Wilson's disease. *Ann Int Med* **75**:57-65, 1971.
42. Goldstein NP, Gross JB: Treatment of Wilson's disease. In: Klawans HL. ed: *Clinical Neuropharmacology Vol. 2*. New York, Raven Press, 1977, pp 99-112.
43. Scheinberg IH, Sternlieb I: The long-term management of hepatolenticular degeneration (Wilson's disease). *Amer J Med* **29**:316-333, 1960.
44. Walshe JM: Wilson's disease, a review. In: Peisach J, Aisen P, Blumberg WE, eds: *The Biochemistry of Copper*. New York, Academic Press, 1966, pp 495-498.
45. Stern RB, Wilkinson SP, William R: Controlled trial of d-penicillamine therapy in chronic active hepatitis. *Gut* **17**:390, 1976.
46. Deering TB, Dickson ER, Fleeting CR: Effect of d-penicillamine on copper retention in patients with primary biliary cirrhosis. *Gastroenterology* **72**:1208-1212, 1977.
47. Masters CL, Dankins RL, Zilkop J: Penicillamine-associated myasthenia gravis, anti-acetylcholine receptor and antistriational antibodies. *Amer J Med* **63**:689-694, 1977.

48. Tu J-B, Blackwell RQ, Lee P-F: dl-Penicillamine as a cause of optic axial neuritis. *JAMA* **185**:2 119-122, 1963.
49. Cohen HG, Reynolds TIB: Comparison of Metronidazole and chloroquine for the treatment of amoebic liver abcess. *Gastroenterology* **69**: 35-41, 1975.
50. Ursing B, Kaname C: Metronidazole for Crohn's disease. *Lancet* 1:775-777, 1975.
51. Allan R, Cooke WT: Evaluation of metronidazole in the management of Crohn's disease. *Gut* **18**:422, 1977.
52. Bernstein LH, Frank MS, Brandt LJ, Boley SJ. Healing or perineal Crohn's disease with metronidazole. *Gastroenterology* **79**:357-365, 1980.
53. Brand LJ, Bernstein L, Boley SJ, Frank M: Long term follow-up of metronidazole therapy for perineal Crohn's disease. *Gastroenterology* **80**:1115, Part 2 1981 (Abstracts).

Chapter XII

Neurological Side Effects of Local Ocular Drugs

Amos D. Korczyn, M.D., M. Sc.

Drugs used for the diagnosis or in the treatment of eye disorders are mainly used locally, and are then usually regarded as lacking systemic effects. The recognition of the possibility of such untowards action is the single most important factor to prevent their occurrence. This review will briefly outline the possible neurologically relevant actions. Drugs which are used systemically for ophthalmological purposes, e.g., corticosteroids, are discussed elsewhere in this book (see Chapters II, III, and XI) and will not be mentioned here.

A frequent assumption is that the total dose prescribed in ocular solution is so minute that it cannot produce systemic actions. However, in reality this is not the case. Most ophthalmic drop solutions come at concentrations ranging from 0.5% to as high as 10%. One drop of 2% solution or two drops of 1% collyrium, contain 1 mg of the active solute (the actual amount depends of course on the drop size, which in turn is determined by the dropper). For drugs like atropine, the ophthalmic dose therefore exceeds that adult parenteral dose. The reason that such a high amount is given, is the only a fraction of the drug penetrates the cornea and is able to reach its target. The rest may flow out of the eye and on the cheek, but more usually is either absorbed through the conjunctiva or carried over with tears in the nasolacrimal duct. The nasal mucosa is rather vascular, and drugs can easily penetrate it. Moreover, excessive tears are frequently swallowed so that any residual active drug can be absorbed from the gastrointestinal tract. Thus it is not unusual for practically all the administered dose to be absorbed systemically over a relatively short period. Another factor that can enhance systemic absorption is local inflammation in the eye, such as conjunctivitis.

Systemic effects of mydriatic eye drops are not rare, but frequently go unrecognized. Neonates, infants, and children are commonly affected.[1,2] One reason is the small volume of distribution, once the drugs got absorbed systemically, as well as immaturity of the hepatic systems which metabolize drugs. Another important consideration is that young patients may be negativistic, resist drug application, and cry. There is therefore a tendency to ensure the desired response by giving them additional drops.

Systemic effects of atropine-like drugs include flushing due to vascular dilatation in the blush area, tachycardia, lack of sweating with a consequent "dry" hyperthermia, as well as CNS effects. These may consist of disorientation, delirium, and hallucinations. The patient may be restless, aimlessly wandering, about, and aggressive, or, conversely, quiet, withdrawn and even stuporose. Hallucinations, at times apparently frightening, may occur.[3] Other patients seem to be amused by the experience. As is common in other toxic psychotic reactions, the hallucinations caused by antimuscarinics are usually visual, and may resemble delirium tremens; but auditory hallucinations were also reported.[4] Speech may be incoherent due to the psychic state or as a manifestation of dysarthria. Gross ataxia leads to a broad-based stance and occasional patients were so ataxic as to be unable to sit unaided.[5,6] Grand mal seizures, coma, and even death were reported.[7-10] However, in most cases uneventful recovery will follow cessation of therapy. The recovery may, however, be delayed for 48 hours or more. Usually subjects will be partially or totally amnestic for the period of intoxication.

The effects are particularly common in children. They were rarely reported in infants, probably being unrecognized. Psychotic reactions occur even in adults and in the elderly.[4,11,12] They were reported with atropine, homatropine, scopolamine and cyclopentolate, and probably will occur with any antimuscarinic agent which may penetrate the blood-brain barrier. Reactions seem to be dose dependent,[13] and were thought to occur particularly frequently in blond children and in those with cerebral damage.[14] A careful review of the literature does not support this view, however, although it is known that the melanin in the eye can bind drugs easily.[15]

As mentioned in Chapter XVI in this book, autonomic manifestations of muscarinic blockade usually coexist, and it is the occurrence of flushed, dry skin and tachycardia which should alert the physician to the possibility of intoxication.

Awan[16] described several cases of adults treated with cyclopentolate who developed dizziness, loss of balance and coordination, as well as nausea, vomiting, and generalized weakness. The symptoms suggest vestibular dysfunction, but apparently none of the subjects had nystagmus, and in fact antimuscarinics are not likely to impair vestibular function. It is possible that the effects were cerebellar, but a more detailed neurological examination will be needed before the pathogenesis is resolved.

Tropicamide, another widely-used antimuscarinic agent, is apparently much less liable to cause central effects, possibly due to poor penetration across the blood-brain barrier. Wahl et al,[17] reported a 10-year-old who fell unconscious immediately after drug instillation. The rapidity of onset as well as the lack of other CNS manifestations suggest that this was not a centrally-mediated effect of the drug.

Sympathomimetics are also used for mydriasis. Drugs like phenylephrine are used in high concentrations (e.g., 10%), but systemic reactions are rare. This is so because of the safety afforded by the adrenergic terminals throughout the body, which can take up the amines and thus inactivate them. In addition, most sympathomimetic drugs do not cross the blood-brain barrier. Amphetamine and some derivatives, such as phenylpropanolamine can, however, reach the brain, and psychic disturbances, including psychotic reactions have been reported.[18] Cocaine too may be absorbed and produce its own signs of CNS stimulation including excitement and anxiety.

The interest to the neurologist with regard to these drugs lies in the susceptibility of patients in whom the adrenergic terminals cannot take up the sympathomimetics. This may occur when the terminals are physically damaged, for example in the Shy Drager syndrome or in the diabetic neuropathy, [19,20] or when other drugs (such as tricyclic antidepressants) inactivate the uptake mechanism.[21] In either case, supersensitivity may develop and cause severe hypertensive responses, leading to subarachnoid hemorrhage.[22]

Guanethidine produces a Horner syndrome, whereas cocaine and other sympathomimetics cause the reverse, i.e., mydriasis and widening of the inter-palpebral fissure. Drugs acting on beta receptors lack these effects. Ptosis and pupillary dilatation may follow corticosteroid therapy.

Pilocarpine and carbachol may be used as miotics or to reduce intraocular pressure. They also may be absorbed, but with most drugs, systemic effects are uncommon. When a more prolonged action on the eye is desired, a cholinesterase inhibitor is prescribed. Physostigmine is known to cause twitching of the eyelids, probably because of local diffusion to the orbicularis oculi. The same effects can occur with non-reversible cholinesterase inhibitors, such as isoflurophate (DFP), echothiophate (Phospholine Iodide), or demecarium. All these are absorbed quickly into the systemic circulation and inhibit plasma cholinesterase.[23] The clinical syndrome mimics that of insecticide poisoning, although its degree is usually mild. Reactions are particularly common with echothiophate.[24,25] Plasma cholinesterase activity is frequently inhibited in subjects treated with these drugs who do not demonstrate clinical symptoms. This may occur after a single application of the drug and cumulative effects should be expected. One possible result is delayed recovery from succinylcholine-induced paralysis (succinylcholine is hydrolyzed by plasma cholinesterase). It is claimed the echothiophate and isoflurophate inhibit preferentially plasma cholinesterase, whereas eserine and demecarium have a greater affinity for acetylcholinesterase.[26]

Clearly, ophthalmic drugs can have systemic actions and when confronted with a patient with a suspected drug adverse reaction, the possibility that it may arise from ocular preparations, used therapeutically or for diagnostic purposes, should not be disregarded.

References

1. Caputo AR, Schnitzer RE: Systemic responses to mydriatic eyedrops in neonates. *J. Pediat Ophthal Strab* **15**:109, 1978.
2. Gray LG: Avoiding adverse effects of cycloplegics in infants and children. *J Am Optom Assoc* **50**:465, 1979.
3. Beswick JA: Psychosis from cyclopentolate. *Amer J Ophthal* **53**:879, 1962.
4. Freund M, Merin S: Toxic effects of scopolamine eye drops. *Amer J Ophthal* **70**:637, 1970.
5. Hoefnagel D: Toxic effects of atropine and homatropine eyedrops in children. *N Engl J Med* **264**:168, 1961.
6. Simcoe CW: Cyclopentolate (cyclogyl) toxicity. *Arch Ophthal* **67**:406, 1962.
7. Heath WE: Death from atropine poisoning. *Brit Med J* **2**:608, 1950.
8. Kennerdell JS, Wucher FP: Cyclopentolate associated with two cases of grand mal seizure. *Arch Ophthal* **87**:634, 1972.
9. Morton HG: Atropine intoxication: its manifestations in infants and children. *J Pediat* **14**:755, 1939.
10. Scally CM: Poisoning after one instillation of atropine drops. *Brit Med J* **1**:311, 1936.
11. Baker JP, Farley JD: Toxic psychosis following atropine eye drops. *Brit Med J* **2**:1390, 1958.
12. German E, Siddiqui N: Atropine toxicity from eyedrops. *N Eng J Med* **282**:689, 1970.
13. Binkhorst RD, Weinstein GW, Baretz RM, Clahane AC: Psychotic reaction induced by cyclopentolate. *Amer J Ophthal* **55**:1243, 1963.
14. Walsh FB: *Clinical Neuro-Ophthalmology.* 2nd edition, Baltimore Williams and Wilkins, 1957.
15. Kloog Y, Sachs DI, Korczyn AD, et al: Muscarinic acetylcholine receptors in the cat iris. *Biochem Pharmacol* **28**:1505, 1979.
16. Awan KJ: Adverse systemic reactions of topical cyclopentolate hydrochloride. *Ann Ophthal* **8**:695, 1976.
17. Wahl JW: Systemic reaction to tropicamide. *Arch Ophthal* **82**:320, 1969.
18. Norvenius G, Widerlov E, Lonnerholm G: Phenylpropanolamine and mental disturbances. *Lancet* **2**:1367, 1979.
19. Kim JM, Stevenson CE, Mathewson HS: Hypertensive reactions to phenylephrine eyedrops in patients with sympathetic denervation. *Amer J Ophthal* **85**: 862, 1978.
20. Robertson D: Contraindication to the use of ocular phenylephrine in idiopathic orthostatic hypotension. *Amer J Opthal* **87**:819, 1979.

21. McReynolds WV, Havener WH, Henderson JW: Hazards in the use of sympathomimetic drugs in ophthalmology. *Arch Ophthal* **56**:176, 1956.
22. Boakes AJ, Laurence DR, Teoh PC, et al: Interactions between sympathomimetic amines and antidepressant agents in man. *Brit Med J* **1**:311, 1973.
23. Leopold IH, Krishna N, Lehman RA: The effects of anticholinesterase agents on the blood cholinesterases levels of normal and glaucoma subjects. *Trans Amer Ophthal Soc* **57**:63, 1959.
24. Humphreys JA, Holmes JH: Systemic effects produced by echothiophate iodine in treatment of glaucoma. *Arch Ophthal* **69**:737, 1963.
25. Klendshoj N, Olmsted E: Observation of dangerous side-effect of phospholine iodine in glaucoma therapy. *Amer J Ophthal* **56**:247, 1963.
26. Havener WH: *Ocular Pharmacology*. St. Louis, C.V. Mosby, 1966.

Chapter XIII

Neurological Complications of Antiepileptic Drug Treatment

David H. Rosenbaum, M.D.

Introduction

The history of the pharmacotherapy of epilepsy has been dominated by the search for effective compounds that are low in neurotoxicity. Potassium bromide, introduced in 1857, was the first useful anticonvulsant. Its efficacy is demonstrated by the fact that 2.5 tons per year were being dispensed at the National Hospital in London by the 1870's.[1] Unfortunately, seizure control was usually accompanied by sedation and often the eventual appearance of dementia and psychosis. The introduction of phenobarbitol (PB) early in this century provided a less toxic and more effective alternative, but sedation remained a problem.

Between 1936 and 1945, in a search for a more satisfactory drug, Merritt and Putnam used the newly described maximal electroshock model of seizures in animals to screen over 700 compounds.[2] This work was a milestone in the history of clinical pharmacology, as it now became possible to evaluate chemicals experimentally prior to their administration to patients. Phenytoin (PHT) was one of the first compounds tested and it proved to be among the most potent.[3] Toxicologic studies in animals showed it to be well tolerated, and it was subjected to clinical trials. Its efficacy was reported in 1938[4] and it was introduced in the same year. Many patients whose seizures had been unresponsive to bromides and PB improved dramatically with PHT, and its relative absence of sedative effect was striking. It rapidly gained wide acceptance. Dose-related CNS toxicity, usually in the form of a syndrome of vestibulo-cerebellar dysfunction, was soon noted, but was observed to be reversible with dose reduction and most patients were able to benefit from therapeutic effects at subtoxic doses.[5] More than 40 years after its introduction, PHT remains the most widely prescribed antiepileptic drug (AED).

337

In 1944, trimethadione was observed to protect rodents against threshold seizures induced by pentylemetetrazol,[6] though it was without effect in the maximal electroshock model.[7] In the following year, Lennox delineated the syndrome of petit mal epilepsy and reported trimethadione to be effective against absence seizures in patients who had been unresponsive to other drugs, though it did not control their grand mal attacks.[8] For the first time a correlation between different experimental models and clinical seizure types was established. Trimethadione was introduced in 1946 and remained the drug of choice for petit mal absence seizures until it was replaced by ethosuximide (ETX) in 1960, which proved to have less hematologic, hepatic and renal toxicity.

Primidone (PRI), an analogue of PB (which is one of its principal metabolites) was introduced in 1956, and is felt by some to be more effective against partial seizures with complex symptomatology[9] (CPS; previously called psychomotor or temporal lobe seizures). Its CNS depressant effects are at least as great as phenobarbital and the evidence for its increased efficacy is not compelling.

For complex legal and economic reasons (reviewed by Krall et al)[10] the pace of new drug development slowed considerably after the mid-1950's and only two important new first line drugs have since appeared. Carbamazepine (CBZ), widely used in Europe since 1960 and finally marketed as an AED in the United States in 1974, has proved to be effective in a considerable number of patients previously resistant to other drugs and is widely believed to be the drug of choice for CPS.[11,12] It has been shown to be as effective as PHT and may have even less CNS toxicity.[13] The introduction of valproic acid in this country in 1978 promises to further benefit a considerable group of patients, particularly those with refractory generalized seizures, and preliminary experience suggests very little neurological toxicity.[14]

There is accumulating evidence that the introduction of these drugs and a better understanding of their pharmacology (largely secondary to the availability of serum drug level measurements) has improved the prognosis of patients with epilepsy.[15,16] They are, however, CNS active drugs which as a group have a low toxic/therapeutic ratio. (In fact, the upper end of the "therapeutic range" (TR) of blood levels is defined as the point at which toxicity becomes common.) Furthermore, the nature of the disease is such that drugs need to be taken continuously over periods of years or decades. It would not be surprising therefore if deleterious neurological effects appeared in a considerable proportion of those treated. It is remarkable how sparse the literature on this subject has been. Only in the last 10-15 years has a sensitivity to the potential for long-term toxicity surfaced in the medical community. While the current review will deal only with neurological toxicity, the example of AED related teratogenicity is illustrative: though an etiologic relationship has not been definitely established, recent reports claim an incidence of abnormalities as high as 30% or more in children born to epileptic mothers taking AED's during pregnancy.[17] Yet the possibility of teratogenic effects was not suspected until the report of Meadow in 1968.[18]

The actual prevalence of neurological toxicity in treated patients is by no means clear, as we shall see, and the question is further confounded by the fact that some of the presumed neurotoxic effects were evident in the pre-drug era and may in fact be a consequence of epilepsy itself. Nonetheless, it is probable that the effectiveness of these compounds and the clear-cut benefit they have provided to many patients, together with the relative absence of acute toxicity — particularly when compared to older drugs — has led to an insensitivity to their potential for harm.

Most of the literature in this area is concerned with PHT. To a considerable extent this is a reflection of its impressively widespread use over more than 40 years. The extent to which it reflects a potential for neurotoxicity specific to this compound is not clear, though in some instances this does appear to be a factor.

In the following pages, we shall first consider reversible neurotoxicity, both typical and atypical, and related to elevated blood levels as well as to levels within the TR. We shall then explore the relationship between syndromes of irreversible neurological damage and the chronic ingestion of AED's.

For further discussion of bromide neurotoxicity and of some barbiturate side effects see Chapter VI in this book.

Reversible Neurotoxicity Attributed to AED's

Tolerance

The most obvious example of reversible neurological effects of AED's are those side effects which appear on initiation of therapy and remit during continued administration of the same dosage. This phenomenon of "tolerance" is widely recognized in the clinical setting, and drug treatment is often initiated in gradually increasing doses to minimize side effects while it develops. Side effects to which tolerance develops are of relatively little relevance in a situation of chronic drug therapy. While this point seems obvious, a surprising number of studies cited in the literature on neurotoxicity have been carried out with volunteers or patients under conditions which did not allow adequate time for tolerance to develop.[19-22]

Dose-Related Neurotoxicity (reversible)

Occurring at Blood Levels above the Therapeutic Range

The Typical Syndrome

The acute reversible syndrome of PHT intoxication was recognized by Merritt and Putnam, shortly after the drug's introduction.[5] It consists primarily of dose related cerebellar-vestibular dysfunction, with nystagmus, occasional oscillopsia and diplopia, and gait ataxia; at higher doses sedation and mental changes may be seen. The relatively high concentration of PHT in cerebellum and brainstem may be the anatomical correlate of this clinical pattern,[23] and electrophysiologic studies indicate that Purkinje cell function is altered at therapeutic as well as toxic levels.[24,25]

It has long been recognized, however, that there is a rather poor correlation between administered dose, even expressed as mg/kg, and toxic as well as therapeutic effects. As techniques for measuring drug concentrations at the low levels found in body fluids were refined in the 1950's and 60's, it became apparent that there was a rather weak correlation between mg/kg dose of PHT and blood levels, while toxic and therapeutic effects are clearly better correlated with the latter. Kutt et al in 1964 popularized the idea of a close relation of varying degrees and manifestations of PHT intoxication with the magnitude of blood level elevation.[26] Thus, nystagmus was said to appear at levels of approximately 20 mcg/ml, ataxia at approximately 30 mcg/ml and levels greater than 40 mcg/ml are frequently associated with somnolence. Unfortunately, subsequent experience has shown the correlation to be considerably less than perfect. Rarely, patients will develop the classical syndrome of intoxication with blood levels below those generally considered to be toxic; more commonly, individuals will tolerate (or even require for adequate therapeutic response) unusually high levels. In some cases this may relate to a variation in the fraction of drug bound to plasma proteins (routine blood PHT determinations measure total drug concentration; while PHT is generally 90% protein bound,[27] it is the unbound fraction that is pharmacologically active), but in most it is due to individual variability of unspecifiable "constitutional factors." There is also a clinical impression that polypharmacy further confounds the relationship between levels of individual drugs and toxicity; patients on multi-drug regimens are occasionally observed to be intoxicated despite blood levels within the therapeutic range for each individual drug.[155,156]

Nevertheless, for most patients there is a range of PHT blood levels in which therapeutic responses can be expected to occur, and above which toxicity becomes frequent. Blood level measurement has proved a far more reliable guide than administered dose. Similar information exists for the other widely used AEDs. Unfortunately, early studies of

AED toxicity were generally done without benefit of blood levels and are consequently difficult to interpret; similarly, studies utilizing patients on multi-drug regimens are of somewhat questionable value.

Atypical Reversible Intoxication.

Encephalopathy: With the increasing clinical utilization of blood level determinations, there have been occasional observations of patients with varying neurological syndromes associated with high AED levels. Thus, a number of reports in recent years have concerned patients with mental deterioration or other "encephalopathic" features who were not intoxicated by the usual clinical criteria but were found to have elevated blood levels. In nearly all of these studies the abnormal findings remitted when the offending drug was discontinued or decreased in dose. The rare reports of irreversible deterioration will be reviewed in a subsequent section.

Merritt and Putnam noted drowsiness and psychosis in two of their first 350 patients,[5] and several reports have described an acute brain syndrome with delirium and hallucination as a manifestation of toxic psychosis.[28-30] In 1961, Roseman[31] reviewed his large experience with dose-related PHT intoxication and pointed out that in some patients the vestibulo-cerebellar disturbance was accompanied by mental abnormalities such as exhilaration, euphoria, drowsiness and depression, as well as EEG slowing. While PHT generally has no effect on the EEG background, Roseman found in these patients a slowing of the alpha rhythm and the eventual appearance of delta activity, at times in paroxysms.

In 1965, Levy and Fenichel[32] described three patients with clinical PHT toxicity who manifested an increase in seizures accompanied by slowing and increased epileptiform activity in the EEG. In one of these patients, there was a change in the character of the seizure, with episodes of tonic stiffening, stertorous breathing, and lip smacking replacing previous tonic-clonic convulsions. This patient and one other also developed focal neurological deficits and focal EEG abnormality. All toxic manifestations reversed when PHT was eliminated or decreased in dose. The authors point out that as early as 1940, opisthotonic convulsions had been observed in rats at the LD_{50} of PHT[33] and in 1958 a 2-year-old accidentally poisoned with a large dose of PHT developed stupor and frequent episodes of opisthotonous reversed by hemodialysis.[34]

Logan and Freeman[35] in 1969, introduced the concept of PHT intoxication in children manifesting itself in the guise of a progressive CNS degeneration. All of their patients were mentally retarded. Apparent progression of their underlying neurological disease was found to be related to PHT levels above 40 mcg/ml (therapeutic range = 10-20 mcg/ml) and was reversible with decrease of blood level. Drug toxicity was not at first suspected because all patients were receiving standard doses and their clinical condition precluded evaluation of or obscured the classical signs of PHT intoxication. One patient (17 months old) showed progressive developmental and neurological deterioration with hypotonia; nystagmus was not observed. A 9-year-old also had no nystagmus but had progressive ataxia, lethargy, hypotonia, and inability to speak. A 19-year-old who had occasionally manifested mild choreoathetosis in the past developed marked choreoathetosis and dystonia; nystagmus and ataxia were present in this patient. Diffuse EEG slowing was reversible in all three, and CSF protein was mildly elevated in two. Increased seizure activity was not seen. In the same year, Perlo and Schwab[36] reported five cases in which PHT intoxication was not suspected because of the absence of nystagmus. Only three patients are fully described, but the syndrome in all apparently consisted of gait ataxia with variable mental changes. EEGs were reversibly slowed and all patients had blood PHT levels greater than 20 mcg/ml.

In 1972, Glaser[37] reviewed the neurological toxicity of PHT and brought together a number of these observations under the term "diphenylhydantoin encephalopathy." He defined this as a syndrome in which the effect of the drug appears to be on "higher" cerebral activity (as opposed to vestibulo-cerebellar effects), manifesting itself with a variable combination of features, including increased seizure activity, EEG changes, alterations in mental function, and other disturbances including focal motor and sensory deficits,[32,38] hemianopia,[32] choreoathetosis,[35] increased CSF protein,[35,39] and even CSF pleocytosis.[40] External opthalmoplegia[41] and 6th nerve palsy[42] can be added to Glaser's list. He pointed out that the reaction is unusual, often occurs in the absence of nystagmus or ataxia, and though it may be present with average PHT doses, it is usually associated with elevated blood levels. All of the clinical features were felt to disappear without residua after discontinuation of the drug.

Subsequent to Glaser's important contribution, a number of reports dealing with various aspects of the encephalopathic syndrome have appeared, with movement disorder being the feature common to most. Gerber, Lynn and Oates[43] in 1972, described a patient in whom impaired DPH metabolism resulted in a blood level of 92 mcg/ml. Clinically, the patient had a vestibulo-cerebellar intoxication accompanied by abrupt, purposeless movements of all extremities. In 1974, Kooiker and Sumi[44] described two patients with a remarkably similar syndrome associated with PHT levels of 40 and 68 mcg/ml respectively. Both exhibited facial grimacing and mouthing movements, gross flailing of the arms and dystonic posturing of the trunk, together with mental confusion and slurred speech. While both were ataxic, nystagmus was absent on admission in both and appeared only transiently in one during the course of improvement. The authors point out that blood levels in their patients were higher than those required to produce the cerebellar syndrome and suggest that nystagmus may no longer be evident in this range. Although one patient carried a diagnosis of paranoid schizophrenia and detailed description of baseline mental state is not given, both were felt to have normal neurological examinations prior to intoxication and both recovered completely.

Also in 1974, McClellan and Swash[45] reported a similar movement disorder in two patients with mental retardation and intractable seizures. One had a PHT level of 37 mcg/ml and the other of 50, both had mental changes and ataxia, but contrary to Kooiker and Sumi's patients, nystagmus was prominent. One patient had asterixis in addition to choreoathetosis, and the patient with the PHT level of 50 mcg/ml had an apparent increase in seizure frequency. The authors re-emphasize the point first made by Logan and Freeman,[35] that the syndrome, with progressive mental deterioration, ataxia, movement disorder and worsening seizure status may be mistaken for a degenerative disease if drug intoxication is not considered in the differential diagnoses. Both of these patients made complete recovery.

Also appearing in the same year was a report by Shuttleworth, et al[46] of three mentally retarded patients who developed choreoathetosis with PHT levels ranging from 29-43 mcg/ml; oro-facial dyskinesia was prominent in one. Two out of the three had nystagmus and ataxia, while the former was absent in the third, who interestingly was noted to have had pre-existing mild dystonic posturing of one limb with a suggestion of athetosis. The authors discuss the relation of pre-existing brain damage to the occurrence of this particular toxic manifestation and indeed it is striking how many of the cases of dyskinesia and other atypical dose related toxic reactions have occurred in patients with static encephalopathy.

One of the earliest descriptions of asterixis in association with PHT intoxication was by Engel et al[47] in 1971, but the presence of concurrent liver failure and the lack of blood levels obscures the significance of this case report. Murphy and Goldstein in 1974,[48] emphasized asterixis as a feature of PHT encephalopathy. They reported two patients with PHT levels of approximately 40 mcg/ml who manifested prominent asterixis as well as ataxia, nystagmus, confusion, and EEG slowing; one had myoclonic jerks of the arms at rest as well. Both recovered completely when PHT was withheld, and relapsed when it was re-introduced. Asterixis has also been reported in association with elevated blood levels of phenobarbital (PB) and carbamazephine (CBZ) by Chadwick et al;[49] all patients in this series presented with ataxia and nystagmus as well, but in three patients re-challenged with the presumed offending drug, arterixis was the only sign of toxicity in two. The authors acknowledge, however, that asterixis is a common feature of a variety of metabolic and toxic encephalopathies; there would not appear to be anything specific about its association with AED encephalopathy.

Dyskinesias other than asterixis have also been observed with AED's other than PHT, though as we shall see there may be some important differences. In 1975, Kirschberg[50] reported an idiosyncratic reaction in a 15-year-old (with presumably normal baseline neurological and mental status except for primary generalized epilepsy) to a single 250 mg dose of ethosuximide (ETX). The patient developed continuous orofacial dyskinesia and prominent choreoathetosis unaccompanied by nystagmus or ataxia after one dose. She was seen in the same condition after the second dose and was given an intravenous injection of 75 mg of diphenhydramine with prompt resolution of her symptoms. The patient had also been receiving 120 mg of PB and 300 mg of PHT, and no blood levels were obtained, so it might be argued that the dyskinesia was mediated via PHT. This is unlikely because serum levels of the latter could not have been elevated so rapidly by any metabolic effect of a single small dose of ETX, and protein binding interaction leading to elevated levels of free PHT is ruled out by the extremely low affinity of ETX for plasma protein.[51]

Carbamazepine has been implicated as a cause of movement disorder in several reports. Franks and Richter[52] described psychiatric deterioration and choreoathetoid movement in a retarded seizure patient treated with 600 mg of CBZ. The condition remitted when CBZ was discontinued, but blood levels were not reported and the association in this patient, given the low dose and absence of associated findings, is somewhat tenuous. Joyce and Gunderson[53] have recently reported a patient who developed prominent orofacial dyskinesia, nystagmus and appendicular ataxia after a massive overdose (24 g) of CBZ. Unfortunately, CBZ levels were not obtained and the patient was also receiving PHT and PB with levels of 10 mcg/ml and 70 mcg/ml (TR of PB = 15-40 mcg/ml) but all symptoms were resolved within a week without CBZ. Because of recurrent seizures, CBZ subsequently was reinstituted at 400 mg/day and was increased to 600 mg/day several months later; the patient was admitted to the hospital after a series of generalized seizures and was found to have similar but less severe oro-facial dyskinesia and limb ataxia. Levels of PHT and PB were in the therapeutic range, but again CBZ was not measured. The abnormalities disappeared and did not recur on 400 mg/day; a blood CBZ level on this last dose was measured 4 months later, and found to be 1.3 mcg/ml, well below the TR of approximately 6-12 mcg/ml. As intriguing as this report is, it can only be considered suggestive because of the lack of blood level confirmation and the low dose of CBZ at the time the syndrome reappeared (it is doubtful that the blood level was even in the therapeutic range in this patient at a dose of 600 mg/day).

While CBZ has previously been used as a treatment for childhood dystonias,[158] a recent report has implicated it in the production of severe dystonia and opisthotonous in three brain damaged children.[54] In all patients the movements remitted when the drug was stopped and they reappeared in the single patient who was rechallenged. Intravenous diphenhydramine was without benefit during the acute phase in this patient. CBZ blood level was within the TR in the one patient in whom it was measured, and the authors reason that this reaction therefore need not necessarily be considered toxic. They re-emphasize the point that unusual neurotoxic manifestations of AEDs including CBZ have most often been observed in patients with pre-existing brain damage, and suggest that the expression of movement disorder may depend on prior abnormality of the basal ganglia and their connections. This suggestion is consistent with the observation, alluded to earlier, by Logan and Freeman[35] and Shuttleworth, et al[46] of dyskinesia appearing in patients with pre-existing mild extrapyramidal cerebral palsy.

The dyskinesia that occasionally accompanies intoxication with PHT and other AEDs is phenomenologically rather similar to the syndrome of tardive dyskinesia seen in the setting of chronic antipsychotic drug administration.[55] In both, oro-facial dyskinesia is prominent and may occur alone, but is often associated with limb dystonia and chorea. The mechanism underlying neuroleptic-induced tardive dyskinesia, while not well understood, appears to be related to the capacity of these compounds to block cerebral dopamine receptors.[56] Chadwick et al[49] reviewed a number of animal models in which this effect can be demonstrated, and noted that PHT has been shown to have similar effects in some of these. The inhibitory effect of PHT and chlorpromazine (CPZ) on ADH secretion in animals and man[57] may be added to the list. On the other hand, there are considerable differences between the two classes of drugs, both in some of the models cited by Chadwick et al and more obviously in their therapeutic and side effects. Even the dyskinetic syndromes produced are fundamentally different: the neuroleptic induced syndrome is frequently irreversible, often appears when the offending drug has been discontinued or decreased in dose, and is ameliorated by resumption of dopamine blockade, suggesting a long lasting sensitization of dopamine receptors.[56] The PHT related syndrome on the other hand, appears to be dose-related and has always abated as the drug left the CNS. All the same, alteration of neurotransmission, probably dopaminergic, is likely to be a common link.

This particular effect is probably unique to PHT among the AEDs. The one report dealing with ETX[50] clearly describes an idiosyncratic reaction. Most reports relating to CBZ have been rather poorly documented. All have occurred at relatively low doses with blood levels at or below the TR when reported.[52-54] The best documented cases are those of Crossley,[54] where the syndrome consisted of acute dystonic reaction quite similar to that seen acutely with antipsychotic medications and quite distinct from the syndrome of tardive dyskinesia. Interestingly, CBZ (as well as the tricyclic antidepressants) is structurally related to the phenothiazines;[58] furthermore, like PHT and CPZ, CBZ has effects on ADH secretion, but unlike the inhibitory effect seen with the first two, it stimulates ADH secretion and has been known to be an effective treatment for diabetes insipidus since 1966.[57] The precise significance of these observations is elusive; one can speculate about anatomical and pharmacological variability of dopamine receptor subtypes, but again the evidence seems to point towards an effect of AEDs on neurotransmission at specific classes of synapse.

The role of prior brain damage in the appearance of AED encephalopathy and the particular form it assumes is not clear. Certainly the great majority of affected patients have had pre-existing pathology, though some have appeared to be normal except for their seizure diathesis.

Psychiatric Disturbances: As previously mentioned, psychosis related to bromide therapy was well known in the 19th century, and psychiatric disturbances accompanying PHT intoxication have been apparent since Merritt and Putnam's 1939 report.[5] Subsequent publications have linked PHT to a variety of psychiatric disturbances including tactile and visual hallucinatory states with somatic delusions,[28] schizophrenia-like psychosis,[52,59] and even hysterical conversion reaction[60] (interpretation of "arching of the back typical of the hysterical seizure" described in this paper should be tempered by awareness of the opisthotonic component of tonic seizures that have been associated with PHT toxicity).[32-34] The better documented of these reports deal with relatively non-specific delirious states associated with toxic psychosis. In the remainder, the nature of the relationship between drug and psychosis is obscure and often dubious. For example, case 3 of Franks and Richter[52] was psychotic with a PHT level on admission of 9 mcg/ml. The patient was apparently poorly compliant in taking his prescribed dose, and on supervised administration of the same dose in the hospital, his level came up to 43 mcg/ml; he remained psychotic. With dose reduction and haloperidol therapy his psychosis cleared at a time when his PHT level was 11 mcg/ml, not significantly different from what it had been on admission.

Of greater interest is the report by Demers-Desrosier et al[61] of two patients who developed a schizophreniform psychosis with clear sensorium on withdrawal of AEDs (PRI, PB, PHT and PHT, PB,CBZ), coincident with a marked increase of EEG epileptogenic activity. Clinical status and EEG returned to baseline within 48 hours of drug re-institution in both cases without any psychotropic therapy. These patients would seem to exemplify an opposite situation to Landolt's well-known description of psychosis occurring during "forced normalization" of the EEG by AED therapy.[62] In view of the neuropharmacologic similarities between PHT and the antipsychotic neuroleptics alluded to above, it is tempting to speculate about the occurrence of rebound receptor hypersensitivity when dopaminergic blockade is abruptly removed.

One group in France has observed psychotic reactions to ETX with some frequency;[63,64] these actually are acute confusional states by description and do not seem to have been observed by others. Dalby,[65] in his report on the psychotropic effect of CBZ, described five patients with cerebral atrophy in whom the administration of CBZ was associated with the onset of severe mental disturbance, including schizophrenia-like psychosis; but again this appears to be an isolated and unconfirmed observation.

Neuropathy: A reversible slowing of nerve conduction associated with elevated blood levels of PHT has been well-documented and will be discussed in a subsequent section together with the better known non-reversible polyneuropathy.

Occurring at Blood Levels within or below the Therapeutic Range

Idiosyncratic Reactions

As discussed above, idiosyncratic reaction to ETX in the form of dyskinesia has been observed,[50] and there is reason to think that dyskinesia associated with CBZ[52-54] may also be of this nature.

Cognitive Defects

A number of reports have explored the relationship of AEDs to changes in mental performance within the therapeutic range. Tests in normal volunteers involving acute administration of drugs have often shown impairment of a variety of tasks,[19,20] but as discussed previously, these studies are of little relevance to the clinical situation as they did not allow for tolerance. The lack of blood level measurements in early studies has also been alluded to. The study of Hutt et al in 1968[66] is one of the few exceptions. A 12-day period was allowed for the development of tolerance in four normal volunteers given PB or placebo, and a correlation between PB levels and some measures of perceptual-motor performance was demonstrated. There has long been a clinical impression that phenobarbital has detrimental cognitive and behavioral effects in patients, particularly in children, but this has rarely been adequately demonstrated in a controlled study. A recent study done in Turkey compared the performance on a battery of psychological tests of 63 children before and again three months after random assignment to PB, PHT or placebo treatment groups.[67] Serum levels were measured but are unfortunately not reported. Detrimental effects of PB but not PHT were found on behavior (hyperactivity, irritability, increased sleep, and school problems) and some measures of cognitive and/or perceptual motor function.

A retrospective study of adult patients reported by Reynolds and Travers in 1974 also found negative effects.[68] They assessed a group of 57 ambulatory epileptics taking only PHT and PB. Patients with clinical toxicity, mental retardation, and evidence of gross cerebral lesions were excluded. They classified the patients as to presence or absence of psychomotor slowing, intellectual deterioration, and psychiatric illness or personality change, and found significant differences in the average blood levels of both drugs between groups with and without each type of impairment (except for psycho-motor slowing and phenobarbital). Of particular note was the fact that mean levels of both drugs were within the therapeutic range in all impaired groups. To answer the potential objection that seizure frequency would be expected to correlate with mental changes and patients with greater seizure frequency would be treated with larger drug doses, they examined a subgroup of patients with seizure frequency of less than one per month and found a similar trend, though the correlation was significantly less than 0.05 only between PHT level and intellectual deterioration and psychiatric illness.

The authors present this study as a preliminary report and are aware of some methodologic weaknesses. A large part of their evaluation was subjective and the examiners were apparently not blinded concerning AED dosage (nor to prior blood level estimations, in all likelihood). Furthermore, there is a disturbing failure of the number of patients in all of their individual categories (those with and those without relevant changes) to add up to the defined final sample size of 57; in fact the number of patients for each parameter is never the same, either for the entire group or the sub-sample with infrequent seizures. No explanation of which patients were excluded or why is offered. Finally, although the same trends were evident in the group with infrequent seizures, the actual seizure frequency for those with and without impairment is not given and one cannot be sure that it is not significantly different. Even if they were the same, this would imply that the impaired group, with higher blood levels, in fact required larger concentrations of drugs to achieve a similar degree of control and therefore had a more intense underlying epileptogenic process which could itself be a relevant variable.

A somewhat similar study was conducted more recently by Trimble and Corbett on a group of children residing in a hospital/school an epileptics.[69] Of 204 patients who had at least two IQ assessments at the interval of greater than one year, 15% had a fall of IQ of greater than 10 points (range 10 to 48). This subgroup was found to have significantly higher levels of PHT and PRI, though the mean was within TR; differences in PB and CBZ levels were not significant. Serum, but not red cell folate, was also significantly lower in the "IQ fall group." In comparing groups with blood levels above and below 15 mcg/ml for PHT and 5 mcg/ml for PRI (TR 4-10), they again found a significantly greater incidence of IQ fall in the two higher groups. In an attempt to control for seizure frequency, they eliminated patients with greater than 10 seizures per month and still found the differences to be significant in the remaining patients.

In a subsequent publication[70] the authors admit to a number of flaws in this study which hamper interpretation of its results: many patients were on polypharmacy and seizure frequency was difficult to quantitate. In fact, examination of the reports does not clarify whether the groups with and without IQ fall were comparable for number of drugs received, initial IQ and actual seizure frequency (0 to 10 seizures per month certainly does not define a homogeneous group). With reference to the last point, the objection regarding the possibility of a more intense epilepsy in the group with higher blood levels that was raised in discussing the study of Reynolds and Travers[68] might be cited again here.

In a well-designed study, Dodrill in 1975 evaluated 70 patients stabilized on PHT monotherapy;[71] he utilized the Halstead-Reitan battery as well as a marching test specifically designed to assess motor abilities. The patients were separately examined for evidence of clinical toxicity, and blood PHT level was measured. Reflecting therapeutic practice at the study institution, all patients were on rather high doses by conventional standards and many, if not most, had levels above the usually defined TR. They dichotomized the patients by blood level and also by presence or absence of clinical intoxication. A number of psychometric parameters were significantly impaired in the high level group, all related to motor performance; although the high group was consistently worse than the low on measures of higher mental function, this never attained statistical significance. The PHT level for the "high" group was defined at greater than or equal to 31 mcg/ml (mean 43.15 ± 9.8) and equal to or less than 30 for the "low" group (mean 17.44 ± 7.78). In the clinically defined groups, toxic patients were found to have a mean PHT level of 42.08 ± 12.48 and non-toxic 24.7 ± 13.79; the same trends were seen, with toxic patients tending to perform more poorly on motor tests, but there were less differences that were statistically significant, suggesting that serum levels were a more reliable predictor of impairment (in the toxic range of blood levels) than clinical observation. The authors also examined the question of whether blood levels were related to psychometric impairment in patients without clinical toxicity and found no significant differences between non-toxic patients having levels above or below 24 mcg/ml.

The findings in this well-controlled study which are most relevant to other studies with positive findings are the absence of significant impairment of higher mental function in toxic patients, somewhat surprising given the magnitude of blood PHT levels in this group, and the lack of correlation between measures of neuropsychological impairment and blood levels in patients not clinically intoxicated. It might be argued, in view of the high blood levels in the study group as a whole, that nearly all of the patients may have had some degree of impairment, and clearer effects on higher cognitive processes might have been evident if the non-toxic patients with blood levels less than 24 had been compared to the toxic group; this comparison was not made. In any case, the failure to find a relationship between mental impairment and blood levels in non-toxic patients in this well-controlled study casts doubts on the significance of Reynolds and Travers' preliminary observations.[68]

A double-blind cross-over comparison of PHT and CBZ reported by Dodrill and Troupin in 1977, on the other hand, seems to suggest some degree of neurotoxicity for the former.[72] Comparing psychometric parameters between periods on each drug, they found significant degrees of relative impairment during PHT on tests of high level complex skills requiring mental manipulation and concentration; there was no difference on simple tasks or perceptual tasks. Comparison of MMPIs revealed no significant differences for any of the scales except F, felt to be a reliable indicator of major psychopathology, which was lower during CBZ treatment. Furthermore, they found these differences not to be apparent for all patients: it was particularly a subgroup of patients with subnormal intelligence and a greater degree of psychopathology that did better with CBZ. Since Dodrill's previous study[71] of PHT had found this drug to impair motor skills exclusively, the differences found in the present study were felt to be related not to withdrawal of PHT, but to a positive effect of CBZ (there was no difference in seizure frequency during the two periods), consonant with a frequently alluded to "positive psychotropic effect" of CBZ.

This paper does not report blood levels, but an examination of the original study by Troupin[13] reveals that the average PHT level was 31.2 ±2.3, while CBZ was 9.3 ± 0.55. Since the accepted TR for PHT is 10 to 20 or 25, and that for CBZ is 4 to 10 or 12, the two groups are not strictly comparable. As in Dodrill's previous study,[71] most of the patients on PHT had toxic blood levels; in that study there was no comparison with a group having non-toxic levels, and, therefore, the observed changes when CBZ was substituted can reasonably be explained by the abatement of subtle PHT intoxication. The fact that it was principally patients with pre-existing abnormalities that improved is consistent with the often observed heightened sensitivity of these patients to PHT intoxication and the greater likelihood that intoxication will present with atypical or unsuspected manifestations. In any case, there is no indication in this study that PHT levels in the therapeutic range produce mental impairment, though it once again emphasizes the subtle forms intoxication may assume and reemphasizes the value of blood level determinations.

In a promising approach to this question, Dekaban and Lehman studied the effect of three different dose levels of AEDs on mental performance in each of 15 chronic epileptics.[73] Unfortunately, the study was seriously flawed. All patients were on multi-drug regiments, including PB, PRI and PHT in 10, PB and PHT in 4, and PB and PRI in 1. The admission doses were changed by 30 to 50% after initial testing, the direction of change being determined by clinical and blood level assessment of whether the patient was over- (8 patients) or under-medicated (2 patients): the 5 patients felt to be receiving the correct dose were first decreased and then increased. Seven to 10 days were allowed between dose change and retest. Significant differences were found for tests of vigilance and reaction time between high and low doses, with a similar but weaker pattern for memory tasks; no difference was observed in calculation and block design. Unfortunately, though blood levels were apparently measured, they are not reported, and no details regarding presence or absence of clinical intoxication at the three levels is given, so it is not possible to determine whether these differences occurred within the therapeutic range or are correlates of toxicity (either clinical or by laboratory criteria). The fact that the differences were significant only between the high and low groups suggests the latter. Furthermore, the interval between dose change and retesting was too short to allow for achievement of steady-state levels of PB, much less to allow for the development of tolerance.

A somewhat better designed study using a similar approach was performed by Macleod et al.[74] Nineteen patients on monotherapy (17 PB, 2 PRI) were studied at two different doses. The "low" level on first test is uncertain, probably due to a misprint, as the average PB level is stated to be 15.8 ± 4.77, while at another point the range is given as 8 to 15 mcg/ml. Tests designed to assess short-term memory scanning and access to long-term memory were performed at this level and again five days after the dosage was increased. At the time of retest, the PB level averaged 26.2 ± 7.89 (range 20 to 32); thus levels at the time of test and retest were both within the therapeutic range and no patients were clinically intoxicated. No effect on long-term memory access was found, while short-term memory was markedly diminished at the higher level. However, the relevance of this observation to the clinical setting is once again doubtful because of the failure to allow for tolerance. In fact PB levels would still be rising five days after a dose alteration.

There is a curiously inconsistent pattern of reports concerning mental effects of ETX. Guey et al[63] reported alarming consequences of ETX therapy in 25 patients treated for petit mal epilepsy. In a test-retest design they found global intellectual and psychiatric impairment as well as confusional states. However, patients were receiving other drugs at the onset of the study, and 15 of their 25 patients were re-tarded (an unusual finding in petit mal epilepsy). There was no control group and no blood levels were measured. This observa-tion was confirmed in a more extensive study of 100 patients by Soulay-rol and Roger,[75] who found that intellectual perfomance deteriorated in the majority. On the other hand, two well-controlled studies[76,77] did not detect any such deleterious effects, and in fact noted improved per-formance in a number of patients, probably related to enhanced seizure control.[157] The study of Smith et al in 1968[78] might also be mentioned. This was a double-blind cross-over study using small doses of ETX to treat children with 14 and 6 positive spike phenomenon and learning disabilities; they reported significant improvement in verbal and full-scale IQ compared to placebo.

In conclusion, despite the growing literature and fairly prevalent clinical impression (particularly regarding PHT) to the contrary, there are no convincing studies that establish a relation between any of the widely prescribed non-barbiturate AEDs and mental or cognitive impair-ment in seizure patients without clinical evidence of intoxication and with blood levels in the therapeutic range. While the failure to prove a hypothesis does not disprove it, certainly if non-toxic levels of these drugs do produce mental impairment, the effect must be relatively weak.

Folic Acid: The role of folic acid deficiency in the genesis of neurologi-cal AED toxicity has received much attention recently, particularly from Reynolds and co-workers (see reference 69 for review). Folic acid defi-ciency is relatively common in patients on AEDs, and its prevalence has been estimated between 27 and 91% in various studies.[80] Most AEDs that have been evaluated have been implicated and Latham[81] found low-est folate levels to be related to pheneturide, and next lowest to PRI while PHT and PB were associated with the highest levels. The mecha-nism by which these drugs produce folate deficiency is uncertain. Some studies have implicated impaired intestinal absorption or transport while others have refuted this (reviewed by Rosenberg[82]). The bulk of evidence seems to favor increased folate metabolism secondary to liver enzyme induction by AEDs.[83,84,105]

In 1952, megaloblastic anemia was first recognized as a rare compli-cation of AED therapy.[83] In the 1960's as assays for folic acid became available, the prevalence of decreased serum levels in treated patients became apparent, and it was shown that the values correlated with decreased red blood cell folate[85] (reflecting tissue stores), as well as decreased CSF folate.[86] In contrast to the well-documented neuropsychiatric manifestations associated with B_{12} deficiency, folic acid deficiency has traditionally been assumed to lack CNS manifestations. However, in 1968, Reynolds and co-workers[87] noted a high incidence of neuropsychiatric illness in patients with drug-induced megaloblastic anemia, and subsequent reports indicated that non-anemic seizure patients with mental symptoms and demantia had a greater incidence of decreased serum and CSF folate.[86,88,89] Uncontrolled trials of B_{12} and folate supplementation in such patients by Reynolds[90] and Neubauer[91] were reported to result in marked mental improvement.

These observations led Reynolds to suggest that folate deficiency might be implicated in the genesis of neurological disease, particularly dementia.[87,90,92] It has also been suggested that at least a part of the therapeutic effect of AEDs may be mediated by an "antifolate effect" based on reports of seizure exacerbation in patients treated with folate replacement,[90,93,95] as well as the experimental observation that folic acid applied to the cortex has convulsant properties,[96] and systematically administered folate antagonizes the anti-epileptic actions of PHT[97] and PB[98] in animals.

In regard to neuropsychiatric illness, it has been shown that serum and CSF folate correlate inversely with blood levels of PHT and PB,[99] and it is therefore difficult to determine whether the association with mental changes is etiologically related to folate deficiency, elevated levels of drugs, or to a more severe epilepsy necessitating higher AED doses. A number of placebo controlled studies of the effects of folic acid replacement on behavior, mood, mental state, and performance on a variety of psychometric tests have all been negative.[100-102] Although two of these were carried out over five-to twelve-month periods,[100-101] Reynolds[103] has argued that penetration of the blood-brain barrier by folate is slow and it may take many months to reach steady state levels in the CSF. A three-year placebo controlled study might in fact be required to definitively settle the issue.[83] At any rate, it has not been possible to replicate the previously reported dramatic response to replacement therapy in a controlled setting. Nor have observations of an antagonism between therapeutic effect of AEDs and folic acid been documented in placebo controlled trials.[100-102] On the other hand, some case reports of such a relationship have been rather well documented and cannot be dismissed. For example, Chanarin et al[93] described a patient seizure-free for four years who was treated with large parenteral doses of folate for correction of megaloblastic anemia; the injections resulted in severe aggravation of the epilepsy on two separate occasions. The explanation of this effect in individual cases, if it is not coincidental, may be the well-documented decrease in AED levels resulting from folic acid replacement.[83,102] Since folate is a required cofactor in drug hydroxylation, it may become a factor limiting the rate of AED metabolism in deficiency states, which results in the acceleration of drug metabolism when it is replaced.[84,105] This would explain why its epileptogenic and AED lowering effect are most often observed in the most seriously depleted patients.[83,93] This AED lowering effect might also account for the marked mental improvement which has been seen in occasional patients given folic acid supplementation, if one assumes these particular individuals to have had borderline or clinically inapparent drug intoxication before treatment.

Convincing evidence of a direct effect of folic acid or its deficiency on mental function and seizure control in humans is lacking.

Non-reversible Neurotoxicity Attributed to AEDs

All of the neurotoxic syndromes attributed to AEDs that have been discussed to this point are felt to be reversible as the offending drug is cleared from the nervous system. In addition, three irreversible toxic syndromes have been described: polyneuropathy, cerebellar degeneration, and irreversible mental deterioration. A causal relation to drug therapy is established only for the first of these.

Neuropathy

In vitro effects of PHT on conduction in peripheral nerves have been known for over 30 years,[106-109] and a clinical syndrome of reversible neuropathy accompanying PHT intoxication has been described a number of times.[109]

The best study of this phenomenon was reported by Birkit-Smith and Krogh,[110] who took advantage of an epidemic of PHT intoxication occasioned by a bio-availability difference in PHT preparations to study 24 patients with levels above 20 mcg/ml. They measured motor conduction velocity (MCV) of deep peroneal nerve in these patients before and after blood level was normalized and found a very significant correlation of reversible slowing with levels above 30 mcg/ml; all patients with levels of 20 to 30 mcg/ml had normal CVs and all abnormal CVs returned to normal with decrease of level over a period of several weeks. There was no correlation with degree of clinical intoxication. (It is not mentioned whether any patients were symptomatic and reflex status is not reported.) A sub-acute reversible neuropathy induced by PHT levels within the TR, unaccompanied by evidence of intoxication has been reported as well.[109] This 34-year-old patient developed paresthesias of her feet after 12 months on PHT, which progressed to mid-calf level over the subsequent four months, with PHT levels ranging from 9 to 17 mcg/ml. This was accompanied by disappearance of KJs and AJs, hyperesthesia, and decreased pin sensation in the feet and mild diminution of vibratory sense and joint position sense in the toes. Autonomic function was tested and was normal, as was an extensive lab work-up including serum and CSF folate and B_{12} levels. The EMG was normal, there was no weakness, and CVs and distal latencies were abnormal only in the sural nerve. Symptoms and findings resolved over about a four-week period after PHT was tapered and discontinued, though DTRs returned only after six months.

Of greater clinical importance is the occurrence of apparently irreversible polyneuropathy in patients on long-term PHT therapy. After observing six cases of neuropathy in epileptic patients on therapy,[111] Lovelace and Horwitz undertook a clinical and electrophysiological study of 50 patients (age 12 to 50) selected at random from a seizure clinic, and found a prevalence of 18% (9 patients) with lower extremity areflexia.[112] This areflexic group was supplemented with 12 further referred cases, and compared with those subjects from their original group of 50 who had normal reflexes. None of the areflexic patients had weakness; sensory loss, (mainly distal vibratory loss) was observed in 14, though only five were symptomatic, nineteen out of 20 areflexic patients showed evidence of slow conduction and denervation. The legs were generally more severely involved than the arms, and the number of nerves affected as well as degree of slowing correlated with presence of symptoms and severity of clinical findings. The normoreflexic patients on the other hand all had no findings of neuropathy on exam, and no evidence of denervation; motor nerve conduction velocities (MNCVs) were considerably faster than in the areflexic group, but there was statistically significant slowing of conduction in the posterior tibial nerve in this group as well.

A strong correlation of age, duration of therapy, and neuropathy was observed — only one areflexic patient had been treated less than 10 years. Data concerning correlation with dose was inconclusive (blood levels were not available), but 12 out of 20 areflexic patients had had their PHT dose decreased at some time because of ataxia and dizziness. No patients were anemic, though folate levels were reduced in a large proportion of both normal and areflexic patients without correlation to neuropathy. In the one patient in whom PHT was discontinued, there was no change in conduction velocity over a six-month follow-up.

The authors suggested that a progressive neuropathic dysfunction results from long-term PHT intake, initially apparent only in slowing of CVs, but progressing to areflexia of the lower extremities and eventually, though rarely, manifesting itself in some patients with sensory loss and denervation. The possibility of a correlation with dose (again, unfortunately, blood levels were not available) and episodes of clinical intoxication was raised.

Eisen, Woods, and Sherwin[113] extended this study with the addition of more sophisticated electrodiagnostic techniques as well as blood level measurements. They studied 45 seizure patients on PHT therapy for more than 10 years with normal serum B_{12} and folate levels and compared them to a matched control group. They divided seizure patients into two rather awkwardly defined groups. Group one consisted of 19 patients; 7 had PHT blood levels greater than 20 (6 out of 7 with nystagmus) 6 had levels below 20, but a total estimated PHT intake of greater than or equal to 3 kg, and the remaining 6 had levels less than 20, and intake below 3 kg but had absent ankle jerks. Group two was comprised of 26 patients with ankle jerks, levels less than 20 mcg/ml, no nystagmus, total intake less than 3 kg, and no symptoms or signs of neuropathy.

In group one, eight patients had sensory symptoms suggestive of neuropathy (five with levels greater than 20), and 12 had absent ankle jerks (confirmed electrophysiologically) associated with absent H reflex. Groups one and two cannot be compared for these important findings, since the study design excluded such patients from group two. Mean values of all electrophysiologic parameters did not differ significantly between the two groups, although the frequency of slowed lower limb CVs correlated strongly with elevated blood levels. On the other hand, the percent of patients in each group having electrodiagnostic abnormalities was much greater in group one despite the equivalence of mean values, and evidence of denervation was present in 42% of one and only 15% of two.

When the seizure group as a whole was compared with controls, a small but statistically significant slowing of CVs in the former was apparent. This study then tends to confirm the observation that long-term PHT can induce clinical and electrophysiologic evidence of neuropathy (which would appear to be primarily axonal, based on evidence of denervation), and further strengthens the suggestions that there is a correlation with blood levels as well as total cumulative dose.

Further evidence is provided by Encinoza,[114] who studied 300 patients on PHT therapy for periods of 2½ to 9 years with no manifest neuropathy. Fifty-two percent had slowed CVs, and the presence of abnormalities correlated with age, duration of therapy, and dose.

Thus, while PHT can produce acute, sub-acute, and chronic (perhaps irreversible) polyneuropathy, the occurrence of a clinically significant syndrome is extremely rare, despite the relatively high prevalence of electrophysiologic abnormalities.*

---

* Since preparation of the manuscript, two reports casting doubt upon the specificity of the relationship between neuropathy and PHT have appeared.[159,160]

More disturbing is the suggestion that AEDs can produce irreversible cerebellar degeneration and mental deterioration. It must be kept in mind, however, that unlike neuropathy, both of these conditions can also be the result of seizures and have been observed in the absence of drug therapy.

Cerebellar Degeneration

As discussed earlier, the acute reversible cerebellar syndrome of PHT toxicity was recognized and described shortly after the drug's introduction in 1938.[5] Livingston, in reviewing drug therapy for childhood epilepsy in 1957,[115] mentioned having observed three patients in whom ataxia persisted for 6 months after drug withdrawal, but no further details were given. Beginning in 1958, occasional case reports of persistent cerebellar deficits following PHT therapy began to appear.[116-120] A number of studies in experimental animals were also published implicating PHT intoxication as a cause of cerebellar degeneration.[116,117,120-122] The interpretation of case reports is complicated by the well-known fact that epilepsy itself can produce Purkinje cell loss and cerebellar degeneration as first described by Spielmeyer over 60 years ago,[123] and similar changes in the cerebellum may result from a variety of insults including ischemia-anoxia.[124] Between 1970 and 1972, Dam[125] published a series of articles comprehensively reviewing the clinical and experimental data, as well as presenting his own controlled investigations in humans and three animal species. He found no evidence of cerebellar damage related to PHT in animals, and attributed the previously observed experimental changes (including those in his own study of 1966[121]) to coma and hypoxia produced by massive overdoses, as well as possible fixation artifact and inexact estimation. He pointed out further that the experimental pathology reported was not the same as is seen clinically, as the Purkinje cell loss was never as severe as in patients and Bergmann astrocytosis did not occur. In his human material, though there was some correlation of PHT dose to Purkinje cell loss, patients on larger doses were receiving them because of greater seizure frequency, and the latter was much better correlated with cerebellar damage. Dam's contribution, summarized in a fascicle appearing in 1972,[125] seemed to settle the issue for the moment, but in the last three or four years a number of important challenges have been mounted.

In 1976, a report by Ghatak et al[126] described a woman with major motor seizures since age 16, on therapy with PHT for at least 20 years before death at age 78; a progressive cerebellar syndrome existed during the last 10 years (a period during which she averaged approximately one seizure per year). At autopsy, marked Purkinje cell loss was noted, while no atrophy was present in Ammon's horn, a region known to be equally susceptible to hypoxia, thus arguing against seizure-related hypoxia as the cause. (A similar distribution of pathology was also noted in earlier reports by Haberland[119] and Hoffman.[118]

Iivanainen[127] reported a large series of mentally retarded epileptics in whom clinical and PEG evidence of cerebellar atrophy correlated with toxic PHT levels and their duration, but the toxic patients also had more frequent seizures making the significance of the correlation uncertain.

Rapport and Shaw[128] reported an autopsy case of a patient with tuberculous meningitis treated with three antitubercular drugs who never had a seizure but who was given prophylactic PHT. No clinical signs of toxicity were noted. At autopsy, marked Purkinje cell loss was found, together with Bergmann gliosis and edema; no anoxic changes were present in the hippocampus. The authors' argument that the cerebellar damage must have been related to PHT (the co-administration in INH precipitates PHT intoxication in up to 10% of patients[129]) due to the absence of seizures is unconvincing, since hypoxia probably occurred. The patient is described as having had an episode of "ataxic respiration" requiring tracheostomy and assisted ventilation for a week, and was comatose for several weeks before death. The sparing of the hippocampi, however, is an argument against a hypoxic etiology.

Salcman, et al[130] reported cerebellar changes found in biopsy of five patients with medically intractable epilepsy who were undergoing electrode implants for cerebellar stimulation. All of these patients had been treated with high doses of PHT as well as other AEDs, but none had clinical evidence of cerebellar dysfunction at the time of biopsy (although some had experienced acute reversible episodes of intoxication), and contrast studies as well as direct visualization at operation did not suggest cerebellar atrophy. Unfortunately, no blood levels are reported. All biopsies revealed severe Purkinje cell loss, usually accompanied by Bergmann gliosis. Interestingly, two of their patients never experienced major motor convulsions. While the authors discount the possibility of PHT as an etiology, citing the work of Dam[125] as having disproved it, this series can be used as one of the more compelling arguments in its favor, particularly since hypoxia cannot be implicated in the two patients without convulsive seizures.

McClain et al[131] reported five patients who developed a clinical cerebellar syndrome while being treated with PHT at high plasma levels. Cerebellar atrophy was documented by CT in all cases. No information regarding the status of the hippocampi is available. While seizure control was poor in most, none were having convulsive seizures at the time the ataxia appeared. Although some patients showed a decrease of symptoms on reduction of blood level, all remained impaired. In three of the five patients, ataxia developed after a number of years of therapy with constant PHT doses (and presumably blood levels) which had not previously been associated with clinical intoxication; in fact, one patient had a level of 19 mcg/ml and another 23 mcg/ml at the time of examination — values which are probably within the therapeutic range. In the other two, irreversible cerebellar dysfunction supervened after clinically apparent intoxication of five to ten years duration, associated with clearly elevated blood levels.

Preliminary data from a CT study was recently reported by Koller et al[132] in which 8 patients with cerebellar atrophy who also had epilepsy (seizure type unspecified) and were on long-term PHT therapy (average duration of therapy was 14 years, no levels reported) were identified during a one-year period. None of these patients had signs of cerebellar dysfunction, and all were said to be under "good seizure control." The authors speculate, following the lead of McClain et al[131] that the atrophic process presumably induced by PHT must in many cases progress insidiously for a number of years before a functional disturbance appears. This would be consistent with the findings in Salcman's[130] patients (as well as those described by Cooper et al[133] and Rajjoub et al[134]). Though these findings are intriguing, the data presented are not sufficient to argue convincingly against epilepsy per se as an etiology, as seizure type and frequency (remote as well as recent) and hippocampal status are unknown.

The validity of Dam's experimental studies in animals has also been questioned by McClain, et al,[131] on the grounds that duration and degree of intoxication may have been inadequate. In fact, Dam specifically chose levels which would not induce coma and death,[125] but it may well be that such studies would need to be carried out with toxic blood levels for periods of months or years to be absolutely conclusive. They remain to be done.

The cogent issues raised, therefore, in the more recent studies attributing cerebellar degeneration to PHT are the following:

1. Cerebellar degeneration has occurred in patients on PHT, with signs appearing in the absence of seizure types which could be expected to produce anoxia.

2. In several cases, extensive cerebellar cortical pathology has been observed in the absence of hippocampal involvement, contrary to what has repeatedly been observed as a sequel to experimental and clinical hypoxia. In essence then, the evidence against seizure-related hypoxia as the cause of cerebellar degeneration in these cases is compelling. This, however, does not rule out the possibility that other seizure-related mechanisms may be operating.

It is beyond the scope of this review to examine in any detail recent work concerning the pathophysiology of brain damage in paralyzed, ventilated animals subjected to experimental seizures, but it is becoming increasingly evident that pathology in the distribution seen in epileptic patients can be produced in animals in the absence of hypoxia, hypotension, or hypoglycemia, though the actual mechanisms remain unclear. (See Plum[135] for a review.) Furthermore, while the relative vulnerability of various brain regions and cell types to hypoxia is predictable (Sommer sector of hippocampus, followed by Purkinje cells, followed by the neurons of neocortex, thalamus, and amygdala),[136-138] this is true only on a statistical basis in seizure patients as well as in animals subjected to experimental seizures without hypoxia.[124] Thus, it is unusual for all of the expected sites to be involved in any particular case or for them to be involved in the relative degree of severity that might be expected. The fact that hippocampal or mesial temporal sclerosis is largely unilateral in 80% of cases[136] further emphasizes the difficulty of attributing the epileptic brain damage to purely systemic etiologies. The type of epileptic insult is also of importance, as the distribution of lesions produced by experimental status in primates is different from that seen in chronic epilepsy; the hippocampus is not more commonly or severely damaged than neocortex and cerebellar structures.[139] Furthermore, some studies have found that neocortical, thalamic, and hippocampal damage occurs, but cerebellar lesions do not, in the absence of hyperpyrexia and arterial hypotension.[140] There is even experimental documentation that sustained partial seizures restricted to the limbic system can produce hippocampal damage strikingly similar to that seen in chronic patients.[141] These lines of evidence should not be construed to suggest that systemic factors such as hypotension and hypoxia are unimportant in the clinical situation, but they do indicate that much of the observed pathology can also be produced by seizures of various types in their absence.

One may speculate, as do Salcman et al,[130] about the significance of the cerebellum in the control of seizure activity. Activation[24] or inhibition[25] of Purkinje cells has been suggested as one mechanism by which AEDs may exert their therapeutic effect, and enhanced Purkinje cell activity during a seizure may, by suppression of a cerebello-thalamo-cortical loop, be one mechanism by which the brain terminates seizure activity.[142] It might be then, that chronic hyperactivity in Purkinje cells induced as a response to seizures (or to AED stimulation) can cause these cells to exceed the available supply of a critical factor, leading to their degeneration. Arguments concerning the importance of epilepsy versus drug therapy in the genesis of cerebellar degeneration may in fact be pointless, as PHT may well exacerbate a process set in motion by epilepsy. However, at this point in time, despite the accumulation of suggestive evidence, the role of PHT in the genesis of cerebellar disease remains unproved, while it is clear that seizures themselves can produce Purkinje cell loss.

Irreversible Mental Deterioration

Mental deterioration in persons with epilepsy has been observed and commented on since antiquity. In the second century, Aretaeus described epileptics as "languid, spiritless, stupid, unsociable...slow to learn from torpidity of the understanding and of the senses...either from the nature of the disease or from the wounds during the attacks."[143] In a remarkably similar vein, 1700 years later, Gowers stated[144] "the mental state of epileptics...frequently presents deterioration... In its slighter form there is merely defective memory... In more severe degree there is greater imperfection of intellectual power, weakened capacity for attention and often defective moral control... Every grade of intellectual defect may be met with down to actual imbecility." Addressing the question of etiology raised by Aretaeus he continues, "the mental state must not be regarded in all instances as entirely the effect of the disease. It is certainly in some the expression of a cerebral imperfection of which the epilepsy is another manifestation... In other cases, however, which constitute a majority of the whole, the failure must be regarded as a consequence of the disease. It distinctly succeeds the fits in point of time, and may lessen very much when the fits are arrested by treatment" (with bromides). Other authors in the 19th century recognized the importance of social and interpersonal stresses to which the epileptic was subject as factors in the patient's personality, and there was even an awareness of the role AEDs might play — specifically the association of prolonged use of bromides with "idiocy."[145] Interestingly, an "epileptic facies" was recognized in this essentially pre-drug era, [146] which is remarkably similar to recent descriptions of facial changes attributed to chronic PHT therapy[147] (including coarsening of expression, swollen prominent lips, etc.).

In the modern era, Lennox[148] in 1942 was the first to specifically examine the problem of mental deterioration in epileptics in a systematic manner. He found a great majority to be normal, and identified five etiologically relevant factors in those showing deterioration: (1) static or progressive lesions causing both seizures and mental changes, (2) heredity, (3) psychosocial and environmental influences, (4) effects of drugs (specifically bromides, phenobarbitol, and various proprietary preparations; PHT was not generally available during this study period), (5) seizures and cerebral dysrhythmia. He felt that the last was clearly the most important; although mentation was felt to be adversely affected by drugs in 15%, it was noted to be improved by drug therapy in an even larger proportion. He examined the same question in 1960[149] after PHT was in wide use, and felt drugs to be a factor contributing to decreased mental function in only 5% of patients. In these instances, the changes were assumed to be reversible and dose-related.

The first report or irreversible neurological deterioration attributed to AEDs was published by Vallarta et al in 1974.[150] These authors des-cribed 10 patients on long-term hydantoin therapy (9 PHT and 1 mephenytoin) who developed a syndrome of progressive neurological deterioration indistinguishable from a degenerative CNS disease. While the progressive deterioration abated in all cases after discontinuation of therapy and 6 patients returned to pre-therapy status, 4 patients appeared to suffer from some degree of irreversible damage. The patients were aged 9 to 16 and were epileptics residing at an institution for the mentally retarded. Five patients were thought to be intellectually normal before treatment, while 5 had varying degrees of retardation; 9 had nor-mal neurological exams (excluding mental functioning) before treat-ment while one was noted to have hyperreflexia and Babinski signs.

The nine patients treated with PHT were all receiving 300 mg per day and the one on mephenytoin, 500 mg. Duration of treatment was one to 23 years, but of the four patients who did not improve, three had been treated for over 20 years. The six who improved were treated for one to 16 years (mean 7.6), while the two who made complete recovery had been treated for only one and two years. All developed typical cere-bellar disturbance while on treatment, although nystagmus was present in only three. All appeared to be sedated and had slurred speech, and 8 out of 10 had a deterioration of intellectual function (the other two had pre-existing severe retardation and showed no further decline). Five patients developed hyporeflexia, one with clinical sensorimotor neuro-pathy, one developed bilateral Babinski signs, and one (the same patient ?) developed spastic paraparesis. Seizure frequency was increased in five. Seven patients developed behavioral abnormality (i.e. became stubborn, aggressive, destructive, confused, lethargic, withdrawn, with refusal to take care of their own needs) and two also developed psychotic behavior manifested by hallucinations, abnormal interpersonal relations, and thought disorder.

The patients were followed for two to six years after discontinua-tion of hydantoin therapy, and progression of deterioration halted in all. Of the six patients who showed marked improvement after discon-tinuation, only two returned to their pre-hydantoin status, while three had persistent broad-based gait, and one had persistent hyporeflexia. The remaining patients had no improvement and one died unexpectedly in bed of suffocation six months after medication was discontinued. Autopsy of this last patient revealed cerebellar atrophy with marked Purkinje cell loss and Bergmann gliosis, while Ammon's horn, thala-mus and dentate were spared, a distribution similar to cases described in the previous section in which cerebellar degeneration was attributed to PHT.[118,119,126,128] Seizure frequency decreased in five, increased in two, and was unchanged in two after hydantoins were stopped.

The authors also observed that nine of their patients had serum folate levels below 3 mcg/ml (normal 5 to 10 mcg/ml), one had reversible dose-related EEG slowing, and of the 7 who had CSF exams, one showed reversible protein elevation.

The authors emphasize that PHT intoxication was not seriously entertained as a diagnosis, largely because the doses were not excessive and the presentation was atypical. They note that six of the ten were referred to their institution by "reputable neurologists" who believed the patients to be suffering from an unspecified neurological degenerative disease. It is presumably this factor that allowed the long period of intoxication, the duration of which appeared to correlate with irreversibility.

While the implications of this study, particularly the suggestion of irreversible CNS damage, are most disturbing, there are some serious problems in the interpretation of its significance. A great deal of information is presented in a manner which makes detailed analysis of individual patients difficult. At least nine of ten had severe epilepsy with mixed seizures consisting of generalized tonic clonic and generalized tonic, while eight also had akinetic seizures and six absence attacks. Information regarding seizure frequency is provided for only three patients, in whom it was "three to seven per month to five to seven per year," "many per day to one per month" and "several per day to two per month;" two out of these three had episodes of status epilepticus (duration unspecified), one patient on two occasions (this was the patient with cerebellar atrophy at post mortem). It is particularly this group of patients, experiencing as many as several hundred seizures per year over the course of many years, that would be expected to be at highest risk of mental deterioration even in the absence of drug therapy. Furthermore, AED levels are not reported, and while one can accept an impression of drug intoxication when typical findings remit on the drug's removal, even if the dose is not excessive, the significance of atypical findings that do not remit is certainly less clear in the absence of documentation of high blood levels. While the authors found a suggestive correlation between duration of therapy and irreversibility, duration of therapy is obviously related to duration of epilepsy and total number of seizures.

In this connection, a study of mental deterioration in epileptic children by Chaudry and Pond[151] may be mentioned. This was a prospective controlled study of two groups of patients who showed mental deterioration, one starting with relatively normal baseline IQ and one with more or less profound retardation at the beginning of the study. Each was compared with a control group from its respective institution matched for age, sex, and brain damage. While this study is not without design problems (particularly lack of blood level measurement), analysis reveals the subjects and controls to be rather well matched. It was found that dosage of drugs and duration of therapy were not significantly different between those who deteriorated and their controls, while seizure frequency was significantly correlated with deterioration; relative lack of response to drug treatment was even more definitely related. The patients who deteriorated much more often had a combination of focal and generalized EEG abnormalities, compared to mostly focal abnormalities in the controls, and those who deteriorated were more likely to have been severely retarded at the outset. The authors also comment on the frequency of behavioral changes accompanying deterioration, and describe these in much the same terms used by Vallarta et al[150] (withdrawal of interest, dull, unresponsive, "at times frankly autistic with mannerisms typical of the psychotic child," violent tantrums and rages, speech slow and monotonous). Interestingly, in two of their patients the deterioration was halted and significant improvement occurred, in one when seizure frequency spontaneously decreased, and in the other when seizures were controlled following a temporal lobectomy. This observation led the authors to speculate that there may be a sort of tonic "subclinical epilepsy," presumably related to sub-ictal discharges, which cause deterioration. This suggestion has received some confirmation in a study by Dodrill and Wilkus reported in 1978,[152] in which generalized EEG discharges at a rate greater than one per minute were found to have a striking correlation with impaired neuropsychological performance.

A study by Dikmen and Matthews[153] of the effect of major motor seizure frequency on cognitive–intellectual function also concluded that impairment was significantly correlated with seizure frequency, and even more strikingly with age of onset and duration as well as frequency. Unfortunately, this study did not control for drugs or blood levels.

A recent study from Denmark[154] has again described encephalopathy in institutionalized mentally retarded patients, with severe epilepsy on PHT treatment. This paper is poorly written and details are therefore somewhat vague. The study group consisted of 21 severely retarded patients who deteriorated neurologically, most on multiple drugs, serum levels of which "were regularly checked and were within normal range." Encephalopathy and toxicity are never clearly defined, though the term "toxicity" apparently included serum hypocalcemia and elevated alkaline phosphatase. A number of patients manifested choreoathethosis. All patients were gradually withdrawn from PHT and choreoathetosis disappeared in all the patients in whom it had been present. Of the 17 patients who were felt to show toxicity at the beginning of the study, 12, 16, and 13 improved at reevaluation three months after discontinuance of the PHT in "contact," "motor abilitities," and "social abilities" respectively; only nine patients were available for follow-up at one year and all were improved although it is not clear how many of these patients were in the group that had improved at three months and whether or not this represented further interval improvement. In the four patients without apparent toxicity, one, one, and two respectively improved in the above categories at three months, and there was no change at 12 months in two patients followed for that time; the same unanswered questions pertain to this group as do to the toxic group. Seizure control was worse in the majority of patients after PHT was withdrawn.

To the extent that any conclusion can be drawn from this study, it would appear that "encephalopathy" was reversible in all patients, albeit slowly. Of note is the fact that it was said to occur at blood levels within the TR.

Thus the report by Vallarta et al[150] in 1974 stands alone in its attribution of irreversible encephalopathic changes to PHT. In view of the lack of confirmation thus far and the reservations about this study cited above, one has to conclude that there is no convincing evidence of a causal association, particularly since these changes are known to be associated with epilepsy independent of drug treatment.

Summary and Conclusion

The spectrum of clinical syndromes resulting from PHT toxicity clearly needs to be expanded beyond the well-known acute cerebellar syndrome. While the latter is by far the most common manifestation, a variety of less typical conditions must be recognized, particularly in patients with brain damage. And it must be kept in mind that they can occur at normal dosage levels, even rarely with blood levels in or below the TR. These conditions are subsumed under the concept of AED encephalopathy, and include any combination of mental changes, increased seizure frequency, focal neurological abnormalities, and dyskinesia, as well as neuropathy. This syndrome is, however, reversible, and has a proportional relationship to blood levels.

There is a clinical impression that some AEDs, even in the therapeutic range of blood levels, can impair higher mental function. PB and PRI are usually singled out, less often PHT. However, there has been a failure to document this effect for non-barbiturate AEDs in well-designed controlled studies.

A number of reports have appeared suggesting that AEDs may produce permanent neurologic damage. The only irreversible neurotoxic affect which has been convincingly shown to be caused by AEDs is polyneuropathy, which is generally not of clinical significance. A clinical impression, supported by a number of case reports and CT and autopsy studies, links PHT to cerebellar degeneration, but the fact that this lesion can be a result of epilepsy itself makes definite proof of a causal relation difficult. It is doubtful that irreversible mental deterioration is caused by AEDs, and it is doubtful that folate plays any role in the anti-seizure or toxic effects of AEDs.

In conclusion, we have seen that AEDs and the increasing skill of the medical profession in their use have improved the outlook and quality of life for the great majority of seizure patients. There is an increasing awareness that long-term therapy may exact the cost for some patients of inapparent intoxication and even possibly (though at most rarely) irreversible neurological damage, though it is clear that the overall benefits of drug treatment far outweigh these risks. It is to be hoped that continuing research and progress in new drug development will further minimize the deleterious side of this ratio.

In practical terms, the clinician treating patients with AEDs needs to make himself aware of these atypical toxic syndromes and must maintain an appropriate level of suspicion regarding any patient who is not in the most general sense "doing well." The usefulness of AED blood level measurement in such a patient is evident. Equally important, the avoidance of therapeutic complications is facilitated by use of the least number of drugs (ideally one) at the lowest effective dose.

References

1. Holmes G: *The National Hospital,* Queen Square, 1860-1948. Livingston, Edinburgh, 1954.
2. Merritt HH, Putnam TJ: Experimental determination of anticonvulsive activity of chemical compounds. *Epilepsia* 3:51-75, 1945.
3. Putnam TJ, Merritt HH: Experimental determination of the anticonvulsant properties of some phenyl derivatives. *Science* 85:525-526, 1937.
4. Merritt HH, Putnam TJ: Sodium diphenyl hydantoinate in the treatment of convulsive disorders. *JAMA* 111:1068-1073, 1938.
5. Merritt HH, Putnam TJ: Sodium diphenyl hydantoinate in treatment of convulsive seizures. Toxic symptoms and their prevention. *Arch Neurol Psych* 42:1053-1058, 1939.
6. Richards RK, Everett GM: Analgesic and anticonvulsive properties of 3, 5, 5- trimethyloxazolidine -2, 4- dione (Tridione), *Fed Proc* 3:39, 1944.
7. Goodman LS, Swinyard EA, Toman J: Laboratory technics for the identification and evaluation of potentially antiepileptic drugs. *Proc Am Fed Clin Res* 2:100-101, 1945.
8. Lennox WG: The petit mal epilepsies, their treatment with Tridione. *JAMA* 129:1069-1074, 1945.
9. Forester FM: Management of the epileptic patient. *Med Clin North Am* 47:1579-1590, 1970.
10. Krall RL, Penry JK, Kupferberg HJ, Swinyard EA: Antiepileptic drug development: I. History and a program for progress. *Epilepsia* 19:393-408, 1978.
11. Parsonage M: Treatment with carbamazepine in adults. In: *Complex Partial Seizures and Their Treatment,* Penry JK, Daly DD, eds. Raven Press, NY, 1975, pp 221-234.

12. Gamstorp I: Treatment with carbamazepine: children. In: *Complex Partial Seizures and Their Treatment*, Penry JK, Daly DD, eds. Raven Press, NY, 1975, pp 237-246.
13. Troupin A, Ojeman JM, Halpern L, Dodrill C, Wilkus R, Friel P: Carbamazepine — a double-blind comparison with phenytoin. *Neurology* 27:511-519, 1977.
14. Browne TR: Valproic acid. *N Engl J Med* 302:661-666, 1980.
15. Okuma T, Kumashiro H: Natural history and prognosis of epilepsy. In: *Advances in Epileptology: The 10th Epilepsy International Symposium*, Wada JA, Penry JK, eds. Raven Press, NY, 1980, pp 135-141.
16. Annegers JF, Hauser WA, Elveback LR, Kurland LT: Remission and relapse of seizures in epilepsy. In: *Advances in Epileptology: The 10th Epilepsy International Symposium*. Wada JA, Penry JK, eds. Raven Press, NY, 1980, pp 143-147.
17. Hanson JW, Myrianthopoulos NC, Harvey MAS, et al: Risks to the offspring of women treated the hydantoin anticonvulsants, with emphasis on the fetal hydantoin syndrome. *J Pediat* 89:662-668, 1976.
18. Meadow SR: Anticonvulsant drugs and congenital abnormalities. *Lancet* 2:1296, 1968.
19. Mirsky AF, Kornetsky C: On the dissimilar effects of drugs on the digit symbol substitution and continuous performance tests. *Psychopharmacologia* 5:161-177, 1964.
20. Idestrom CM, Scholling D, Carlquist U, Sjoquist F: Behavioral and psychophysiological studies: Acute effects of diphenylhydantoin in relation to plasma levels. *Psychol Med* 2:111-120, 1972.
21. Macleod CM, Dekaban HS, Hunt E: Memory impairment in epileptic patients: Selective effects of phenobarbitol concentration. *Science* 202: 1102-1104, 1978.
22. Dekaban HS, Lehman EJB: Effects of different doses of anticonvulsant drugs on mental performance in patients with epilepsy. *Acta Neurol Scandinav* 52:319-330, 1975.
23. Kokenge R, Kutt H, McDowell F: Neurologic sequelae following Dilantin overdose in a patient and in experimental animals. *Neurology* 15:823-829, 1965.
24. Julien RM, Halpern LM: Effects of diphenylhydantoin and other antiepileptic drugs on epileptiform activity and Purkinje cell discharge rates. *Epilepsia* 13:387-400, 1972.
25. Latham A, Paul DH: Combined study of the pattern of spontaneous activity of cerebellar Purkinje cells and phenytoin serum levels in the rat. *Epilepsia* 21:597-610, 1980.
26. Kutt H, Winters W, Kokenge R, McDowell F: Diphenylhydantoin metabolism, blood levels and toxicity. *Arch Neurol* 11:642-648, 1964.
27. Lunde PKM, et al: Plasma protein binding of diphenylhydantoin in man. *Clin Pharmacol Ther* 11:846-855, 1970.
28. Hoaken PCS, Kane FJ, Jr: Unusual brain syndrome seen with diphenylhydantoin and pentobarbitol. *Am J Psych* 120:282-283, 1969.
29. Swerdlow B: Acute brain syndrome associated with diphenylhydantoin intoxication. *Am J Psych* 122:100-101, 1965.
30. Theil GB, Richter RW, Powel MR, Dooland PD: Acute Dilantin poisoning. *Neurology* 11:138-142, 1961.
31. Roseman E: Dilantin toxicity. A clinical and electroencephalographic study. *Neurology* 11:912-921, 1961.
32. Levy LL, Fenichel GM: Diphenylhydantoin activated seizures. *Neurology* 15:716-722, 1965.

33. Gruber CM, Haury VG, Droke ME: The toxic actions of diphenyl-hydantoin when injected intraperitoneally and intravenously in experimental animals. *J Pharmacol Exp Ther* **68**:433-436, 1940.
34. Schreiner GE: The role of hemodialysis in acute poisoning. *Arch Intern Med* **102**:896-913, 1958.
35. Logan WJ, Freeman JM: Pseudo-degenerative disease due to diphenyl-hydantoin intoxication. *Arch Neurol* **21**:631-637, 1969.
36. Perlo VP, Schwab RS: Unrecognized Dilantin intoxication In: *Modern Neurology*. Locke S, ed. Little Brown and Co., Boston, 1969, pp 589-597.
37. Glaser GH: Diphenylhydantoin toxicity. In: *Antiepileptic Drugs*. Woodbury DM, Penry JK, Schmidt RP. eds. Raven Press, NY, 1972, pp 219-226.
38. Morris JV, Fisher E, Bergin JT: Rare complications of phenytoin sodium treatment. *Brit Med J* **2**:1529, 1956.
39. Rawsen MD: Diphenylhydantoin intoxication and cerebrospinal fluid protein. *Neurology* **18**:1009-1011, 1968.
40. Dutton P: Phenytoin toxicity with associated meningeal reaction. *J Mental Sci* **104**:1165-1166, 1958.
41. Orth DN, Almeida H, Walsh RB, Honda M: Opthalmoplegia resulting from diphenylhydantoin and primidone intoxication. *JAMA* **201**:485-487, 1967.
42. Manlaplaz JS: Abducens nerve palsy in Dilantin intoxication. *J Pediatr* **55**:73-77, 1959.
43. Gerber N, Lynn R, Oates J: Acute intoxication with 5, 5 diphenylhydantoin associated with impairment of biotransformation. *Ann Intern Med* **77**:765-771, 1972.
44. Kooiker JC, Sumi SM: Movement disorder as a manifestation of diphenyl-hydantoin intoxication. *Neurology* **24**:68-71, 1974.
45. McLellan DL, Swash M: Choreoathetosis and encephalopathy induced by phenytoin. *Brit Med J* **2**:204-205, 1974.
46. Shuttleworth E, Wise G, Paulson G: Choreoathetosis and diphenyl-hydantoin intoxication *JAMA* **230**:1170-1174, 1974.
47. Engel J, Cruz M, Shapiro B: Phenytoin encephalopathy? (letter). *Lancet* **2**:824-825, 1971.
48. Murphy MJ, Goldstein MN: Diphenylhydantoin induced asterixis. *JAMA* **229**:538-540, 1974.
49. Chadwick D, Reynolds EH, Marsden CD: Anticonvulsant induced dyskinesias: a comparison with dyskinesias induced by neuroleptics. *J Neurol Neurosurg Psychiat* **39**:1210-1218, 1976.
50. Kirschberg G: Dyskinesia — an unusual reaction to ethosuximide. *Arch Neurol* **32**:137-138, 1975.
51. Goodman LS, Gilman A: *The Pharmacological Basis of Therapeutics*. Macmillan, NY, 1980, p 220.
52. Franks RD, Richter AJ: Schizophrenia-like psychosis associated with anticonvulsant toxicity. *Am J Psych* **136**:973-974, 1979.
53. Joyce RB, Gunderson CH: Carbamazepine-induced orofacial dyskinesia. *Neurology* **30**:1333-1334, 1980.
54. Crossley CJ, Swerder PT: Dystonia associated with carbamazepine administration: experience with brain damaged children. *Pediatrics* **63**:612-615, 1979.
55. Marsden CD, Tarsy D, Baldessarini RJ: Spontaneous and drug induced movement disorders in psychotic patients. In: *Psychiatric Aspects of*

Neurological Disease. Benson FD, Blumer D eds. Grune and Stratton, NY, 1975, pp 219-266.

56. Marsden CD: The neuropharmacology of abnormal involuntary movement disorders. In: *Modern Trends in Neurology* — 6. Williams D, ed. Butterworths, London, 1975, pp 141-166.

57. Moses AM, Miller M, Streeten DHP: Pathophysiologic and pharmacologic alterations in the release and action of ADH *Metabolism* 25:697, 1976.

58. Goodman LS, Gilman A: *The Pharmacological Basis of Therapeutics,* Macmillan, NY, 1980, p 211.

59. Peters HA: Anticonvulsant drug intolerance. *Neurology* 12:299, 1962.

60. Niedermeyer E, Blumer D, Holscher E, Walker BA: Classical hysterical seizures facilitated by anticonvulsant toxicity. *Psychiatrica Clinica* 3: 71, 1970.

61. Demers-Desrosiers LA, Nestros JN, Vaillancourt P: Acute psychosis precipitated by withdrawal of anticonvulsant medication. *Am J Psych* 135:981-982, 1978.

62. Landolt H: Serial electroencephalographic investigations during psychotic episodes in epileptic patients and during schizophrenic attacks. In: *Lectures on Epilepsy.* Lorenz de Haas AM ed. Elsevier, Amsterdam, 1958.

63. Guey J, Charles C, Roger J, Soulayrol R: Study of the psychological effects of ethosuximide on 25 children suffering from petit mal epilepsy. *Epilepsia* 8:129-141, 1967.

64. Roger J, Grangeon J, Guey J, Lob H: Incidences psychiatriques et physiologiques du traitment par l'ethosuccimide chez les epileptiques. *L'encephale* 5:407-438, 1968.

65. Dalby MA: Antiepileptic and psychotropic effects of carbamazepine in the treatment of psychomotor epilepsy. *Epilepsia* 12:325-334, 1971.

66. Hutt SJ, Jackson PM, Belsham A, Higgins G: Perceptual-motor behavior in relation to blood phenobarbitone level: a preliminary report. *Develop Med Child Neurol* 10:626-632, 1968.

67. Ozdirim E, Renda Y, Epir S: Effects of phenobarbitol and phenytoin on the behavior of epileptic children. In: *Advances in Epileptology-1977.* Meinardi H, Rowan AJ eds. Swets & Zeitlinger, Amsterdam, 1978, pp 120-123.

68. Reynolds EH, Travers RD: Serum anticonvulsant concentrations in epileptic patients with mental symptoms. *Brit J Psychiat* 124:440-445, 1974.

69. Trimble M, Corbett J: Anticonvulsant drugs and cognitive function. In: *Advances in Epileptology: the Xth Epilepsy International Symposium.* Wada JA, Penry JK eds. Raven Press, NY, 1980, pp 113-120.

70. Trimble MR, Thompson PJ, Huppert F: Anticonvulsant drugs and cognitive abilities. In: *Advances in Epileptology: XIth Epilepsy International Symposium.* Canger R, Angeleri F, Penry JK eds. Raven Press, NY, 1980, pp 199-204.

71. Dodrill CB: Diphenylhydantoin serum levels, toxicity and neuropsychological performance in patients with epilepsy. *Epilepsia* 16:593-600, 1975.

72. Dodrill CB, Troupin AS: Psychotropic effects of carbamazepine in epilepsy: A double-blind comparison with phenytoin. *Neurology* 27:1023-1028, 1977.

73. Dekaban AS, Lehman EJB: Effects of different dosages of anticonvulsant drugs on mental performance in patients with chronic epilepsy. *Acta Neurol Scandinav* 52:319-330, 1975.

74. Macleod CM, Dekaban AS, Hunt E: Memory impairment in epileptic patients: selective effects of phenobarbitol dose. *Science* 202:1102-1104, 1978.

75. Soulayrol R, Roger J: Effets psychiatriques defavorables des medications anti-epileptiques. *Revue Neuropsychiat Infant* 18:591-598, 1970.

76. Buchanan RA: Ethosuximide toxicity. In: *Antiepileptic Drugs.* Woodbury DM, Penry JK, Schmidt RP, eds. Raven Press, NY, 1972, p 449.

77. Browne TR, Dreifuss FE, Dyken PR, et al: Ethosuximide in the treatment of absence (petit mal) seizures. *Neurology* 25:515-525, 1975.

78. Smith WL, Philipus MJ, Guard HL: Psychometric study of children with learning disability and 14-6 positive spike EEG patterns treated with ethosuximide and placebo. *Arch Dis Child* 43:616, 1968.

79. Reynolds EH: Neurological aspects of folate and vitamin B_{12} metabolism. In: *Clinics in Hematology, Vol 3.* Hoffbrand AV, ed. WB Saunders, Phila, 1976, pp 661-696.

80. Reynolds EH: Diphenylhydantoin. Hematologic aspects of toxicity. In: *Antiepileptic Drugs.* Woodbury et al eds. Raven Press, NY, 1972, pp 247-262.

81. Latham AN, Milbank L, Richens A, Rowe DJE: Liver enzyme induction and its relation to disturbed calcium and folic acid metabolism. *J Clin Pharmacol* 13:337-342, 1973.

82. Rosenberg IH: Absorption and malabsorption of folates. In: *Clinics in Hematology, Vol 3.* Hoffbrand AV, ed. WB Saunders, Phila, 1976, p 589.

83. Richens A: *Drug Treatment of Epilepsy.* Henry Kimpton, London, 1976, pp 119-153.

84. Makki KA, Perucca E, Richens A: Metabolic effect of folic acid replacement therapy in folate deficient epileptic patients. In: *Advances in Epileptology: XIth Epilepsy International Symposium.* Canger R, Angeleri F, Penry JK, eds. Raven Press, NY, 1980, pp 429-430.

85. Preece J, Reynolds EH, Johnson AL: Relationship of serum to red cell folate concentrations in drug-treated epileptic patients. *Epilepsia* 12: 335-340, 1971.

86. Reynolds EH, Preece J, Chanarin I: Folic acid and anticonvulsants. *Lancet* 1:1264-1265, 1969.

87. Reynolds EH, Chanarin I, Matthews DM: Neuropsychiatric aspects of anticonvulsant megaloblastic anemia. *Lancet* 1:394-397, 1968.

88. Callaghan N, Mitchell R, Cotter P: The relationship of serum folic acid and vitamin B_{12} levels to psychosis in epilepsy. *Irish J Med Sci* 2: 497-500, 1969.

89. Smith RP, Mehta S, Raby AH: Serum folate and vitamin B_{12} in epileptics with and without mental illness. *Brit J Psych* 116:179-183, 1970.

90. Reynolds EH: Effects of folic acid on the mental state and fit frequency of drug treated epileptic patients. *Lancet* 1:1086-1088, 1967.

91. Neubauer C: Mental deterioration in epilepsy due to folate deficiency. *Brit Med J* 2:759-761, 1970.

92. Reynolds EH, Rothfeld P, Pincus JH: Neurological disease associated with folate deficiency. *Brit Med J* 2:398-400, 1973.

93. Chanarin I, Laidlaw J, Loughbridge LW, Mollin DL: Megaloblastic

anemia due to phenobarbitone. The convulsant effect of folic acid. *Brit Med J* 1:1099-1102, 1960.

94. Wells DG: Anticonvulsants and folic acid. *Lancet* 1:46, 1968.
95. Dennis J, Taylor DC: Epilepsy and folate deficiency. *Brit Med J* 4:807-808, 1969.
96. Hommes OR, Obbens EAMT: The epileptogenic action of Na folate in the rat. *J Neurol Sci* 16:271-281, 1972.
97. Woodbury DM, Kemp JW: Pharmacology and mechanism of action of diphenylhydantoin. *Psychiat Neurol Neurochir* 74:91-115, 1971.
98. Lacey JR, Smith DB: The effect of folic acid and citrovorum factor on the anticonvulsant activity of phenobarbitol. *Epilepsia* 14:96, 1973.
99. Reynolds EH, Mattson RH, Gallhager BB: Relationship between CSF anticonvulsant drug and folic acid concentration in epileptic patients. *Neurology* 22:841-844, 1972.
100. Grant RHE, Stores OPR: Folic acid in folate deficient patients with epilepsy. *Brit Med J* 4:644-648, 1970.
101. Jensen ON, Oleson OV: Subnormal serum folate due to anticonvulsive therapy. *Arch Neurol* 22:181-182, 1970.
102. Mattson RH, Gallhager BB, Reynolds EH, Glass D: Folate therapy in epilepsy. A controlled study. *Arch Neurol* 29:78-81, 1973.
103. Reynolds EH: Anticonvulsants, folic acid and epilepsy. *Lancet* 1:1376-1378,. 1973.
104. Norris JW, Pratt RF: A controlled study of folic acid in epilepsy. *Neurology* 21:659-664, 1971.
105. Maxwell JD, Hunter J, Stewart DA, Ardeman S, Williams R: Folate deficiency after anticonvulsant drugs: an effect of hepatic enzyme induction? *Brit Med J* 1:297-299, 1972.
106. Toman JEP: The neuropharmacology of antiepileptics, *EEG Clin Neurophys* 1:33-34, 1949.
107. Korey SR: Effects of Dilantin and Mesantoin in the giant axon of the squid. *Proc Soc Exp Biol* 6:297-299, 1951.
108. Morell F, Bradley W, Ptashne M: Effect of diphenylhydantoin on peripheral nerve. *Neurology* 8:140-144, 1958.
109. Dobkin B: Reversible subacute neuropathy induced by phenytoin. *Arch Neurol* 34:189-190, 1977.
110. Birkit-Smith E, Krogh E: Motor nerve conduction velocity during diphenylhydantoin intoxication. *Acta Neurol Scand* 47:265-271, 1971.
111. Lovelace R, Horwitz S: *Trans Am Acad Neurol* 92:262, 1967.
112. Lovelace R, Horwitz S: Peripheral neuropathy in long-term diphenylhydantoin therapy. *Arch Neurol* 18:69-77, 1968.
113. Eisen A, Woods J, Sherwin A: Peripheral nerve function in long-term therapy with diphenylhydantoin. *Neurology* 24:411-417, 1974.
114. Encinoza O: Nerve conduction velocity in patients on long-term diphenylhydantoin therapy. *Epilepsia* 15:147-158, 1974.
115. Livingstone S: Drug therapy for childhood epilepsy. *J Chronic Dis* 6:45-80, 1957.
116. Utterback RA: Parenchymatous cerebellar degeneration complicating diphenylhydantoin therapy. *Arch Neurol Psych* 58:312-314, 1958.
117. Utterback RA, Ojeman R, Malek J: Parenchymatous cerebellar degeneration with Dilantin intoxication. *J Neuropath Exp Neurol* 17:516-519, 1958.
118. Hoffman WW: Cerebellar lesions after parenteral Dilantin administra-

tion. *Neurology* 8:210-214, 1958.
119. Haberland C: Cerebellar degeneration with clinical manifestation in chronic epileptic patients. *Psychiat et Neurol* 143:29-44, 1962.
120. Kokenge RH, Kutt H, McDowel F: Neurological sequelae following Dilantin overdose in a patient and in experimental animals. *Neurology* 15:823-829, 1965.
121. Dam M: Organic changes in phenytoin intoxicated pigs. *Acta Neurol Scand* 42:491-494, 1966.
122. Del Cerro MP, Snider RS: Studies on Dilantin intoxication — ultrastructural analogies with the lipoidoses. *Neurology* 17:452-466, 1967.
123. Spielmeyer W: Über einige Beziehungen Zwischen Ganglien Zelveranderungen and gliosen Erscheinungen, besonders im Kleinhirn. *Z ges Neurol Psychiat* 54:1-38, 1920.
124. Meldrum BS: Neuropathology and pathophysiology. In: *A Textbook of Epilepsy.* Laidlaw J, Richens A, eds. Churchill Livingstone, Edinburgh, 1976, pp 314-354.
125. Dam M: The density and ultrastructure of Purkinje cells following diphenylhydantoin treatment in animals and man. *Acta Neurol Scandinav* (Suppl) 49:3-65, 1972.
126. Ghatak NR, Santoso RA, McKinney WM: Cerebellar degeneration following long-term phenytoin therapy. *Neurology* 26:818-820, 1976.
127. Iivanainen M, Viukari M, Helle EP: Cerebellar atrophy in phenytoin treated mentally retarded epileptics. *Epilepsia* 18:375-386, 1977.
128. Rappaport RL, Shaw CM: Phenytoin related cerebellar degeneration without seizures. *Ann Neurol* 2:437-439, 1977.
129. Kutt H, Winters W, McDowell F: Depression of hydroxylation of diphenylhydantoin by antituberculous chemotherapy. *Neurology* 16:594-602, 1966.
130. Salcman M, Defendini R, Correll J, Gilman S: Neuropathological changes in cerebellar biopsies of epileptic patients. *Ann Neurol* 3:10-19, 1978.
131. McLain LW, Martin JT, Allen JH: Cerebellar degeneration due to chronic phenytoin therapy. *Ann Neurol* 7:18-23, 1980.
132. Koller WC, Glatt SL, Fox JH: Phenytoin induced cerebellar degeneration. *Ann Neurol* 8:203-204, 1980.
133. Cooper IS, Amin I, Riklan M, et al: Chronic cerebellar stimulation in epilepsy. *Arch Neurol* 53:559-570, 1976.
134. Rajjoub RK, Wood JH, VanBuren JM: Significance of Purkinje cell density in seizure suppression by chronic cerebellar stimulation. *Neurology* 26:645-650, 1976.
135. Plum F, Howse DC, Duffy TE: Metabolic effects of seizures. *Res Pub Assoc Res Nerv Ment Dis* 53:141-157, 1974.
136. Margerison JH, Corsellis JAN: Epilepsy and the temporal lobes: A clinical and neuropathological study of the brain in epilepsy, with particular reference to the temporal lobes. *Brain* 89:499-530, 1966.
137. Norman RW: The neuropathology of status epilepticus. *Med Sci Law* 4:46-51, 1964.
138. Zimmerman HM: The histopathology of convulsive disorders in children. *J Pediatr* 13:859-880, 1938.
139. Meldrum BS, Brierly JB: Prolonged epileptic seizures in primates: ischemic cell change and its relation to ictal physiological events. *Arch Neurol* 28:10-17, 1973.

140. Meldrum BS, Vigouroux RA, Brierly JB: Systemic factors and epileptic brain damage. Prolonged seizures in paralyzed artifically ventilated baboons *Arch Neurol* **29**:82-87, 1973.

141. Baldy-Moulinier M, Arias LP, Passouant P: Hippocampal epilepsy produced by ouabain. *European Neurology* **9**:333, 1973.

142. Julien RM, Laxer KD: Cerebellar responses to penicillin induced cortical cerebral epileptiform discharge. *Electroencephalogr Clin Neurophysiol* **37**:123-132, 1974.

143. (quoted by) Temkin O: *The Falling Sickness*. Johns Hopkins, Baltimore, 1945, p 43.

144. Gowers WR: *Epilepsy*. Churchill, London, 1881, pp 121-126.

145. Guerrant J, Anderson WW, Fisher A, et al: *Personality in Epilepsy*. Thomas, Springfield, 1962.

146. Putzel L: *A Treatise on the Common Forms of Functional Nervous Diseases*. Wm Wood, NY, 1880, pp 57-60. (Cited by Guerrant et al op cit)

147. Falconer MA, Davidson S: Coarse features in epilepsy as a consequence of anticonvulsant therapy. *Lancet* **2**:1112-1114, 1973.

148. Lennox WG: Brain injury, drugs and environment as causes of mental decay in epilepsy. *Am J Psychiat* **99**:174-180, 1942.

149. Lennox WG, Lennox MA: *Epilepsy and Related Disorders*. Little Brown, Boston, 1960.

150. Vallarta JM, Bell DB, Reichert A: Progressive encephalopathy due to chronic hydantoin intoxication. *Am J Dis Child* **128**:27-34, 1974.

151. Chaudry MR, Pond DA: Mental deterioration in epileptic children. *J Neurol Neurosurg Psychiat* **24**:213-219, 1961.

152. Dodrill CB, Wilkus RJ: Neuropsychological correlates of anticonvulsants and epileptiform discharges in adult epileptics. In: *Contemporary Clinical Neurophysiology*. Cobb WA, Van Duiyn H eds. Elsevier, Amsterdam, 1978, pp 259-267.

153. Dikmen S, Matthews CG: Effect of major motor seizure frequency upon cognitive-intellectual functions in adults. *Epilepsia* **18**:21-29, 1977.

154. Meistrup-Larsen KI, Hermann S, Permin H: Chronic diphenylhydantoin encephalopathy in mentally retarded children and adolescent (sic) with severe epilepsy. *Acta Neurol Scandinav* **60**:50-55, 1979.

155. Richens A, Houghton GW: Drug combinations and interactions in severe epilepsy. *Proceedings of the 6th International Symposium on Epilepsy*. Brussels, September 15-18, 1974.

156. Sutula TP, Sackellares JC, Miller JQ, Dreifuss, FE: Intensive monitoring in refractory epilepsy. *Neurology* **31**:243-247, 1981.

157. Tizard Bard, Margerison JH: Psychological functions during wave-spike discharge. *Brit J Soc Clin Psychol* **3**:6-15, 1963.

158. Geller M, Kaplan M, Christoff N: Dystonic symptoms in children: Treatment with carbamazepine. *JAMA* **229**:1755-1757, 1974.

159. Swift TR, Gross JA, Ward LC, Crout BO: Peripheral neuropathy in epileptic patients. *Neurology* **31**:826-831, 1981.

160. Danner R, Partanen VJ, Riekkinen T: Chronic anticonvulsive therapy, peripheral nerve conduction velocity, and EMG. *Epilepsia* **22**:675-687, 1981.

Chapter XIV

Neurological Complications of Anticoagulant Therapy

Allen Silverstein, M.D.

Introduction

The excessive bleeding occasionally induced by anticoagulation therapy may at times involve the nervous system. Almost any portion of the nervous system, central or peripheral, may be compromised by such bleeding which usually compresses various portions of the nervous system externally, but on occasion also from within. Anticoagulant induced bleeding may afflict the brain in the intracranial cavity, the spinal cord in the spinal column, and the nerve roots or peripheral nerves distant from the central nervous system. The peripheral nerve involved most frequently is the femoral nerve which is compressed by bleeding into the iliacus muscle.

In Chapter II of this book, Dr. Gilbert has already described many of the neurological complications of anticoagulation, and stressed several important diagnostic and therapeutic features of this condition. His recommendation for the awareness of, and high index of suspicion for, the development of neurological symptoms and signs in patients on anticoagulants is heartily endorsed in this chapter. All too often, patients are anticoagulated for complications of arteriosclerosis. When such patients develop mental changes on anticoagulants, they are frequently thought to be suffering from "cerebral arteriosclerosis." If focal manifestations such as hemiparesis appear, they are thought to have had a "CVA." The sudden symptom of back pain is sometimes ignored for days at a time. These and other errors in judgement may prevent — or delay — the true recognition of the intracranial and intraspinal complications of anticoagulant therapy. Certainly these and most peripheral nerve complications of anticoagulation should be treated promptly by discontinuing the anticoagulants and administering specific antidotes.

375

The purpose of this chapter is to review in some detail the neurological complications of anticoagulation, as they have been published in the medical literature, and to discuss some of the controversies in treatment. Much of this review and discussion has already appeared elsewhere.[1,2]

Intracranial Hemorrhage

Neurologists and neurosurgeons fear intracranial hemorrhage among patients on anticoagulants usually much more than internists and cardiologists, because it is the neurologist or neurosurgeon who is called in to care for such patients with intracranial bleeding. The recognition of the frequency of intracranial hemorrhage in anticoagulated patients began in the late 1930's and 1940's, with the knowledge that massive cerebral hemorrhage occurred not uncommonly in patients being anticoagulated for bacterial endocarditis.[3-6] The anticoagulants did not stop the occurrence of infected emboli; when they went to the brain, the areas of cerebral ischemia and infarction produced became hemorrhagic and this extended on anticoagulants. Duff and Skull[6] reviewed 23 deaths due to Dicumarol, and found that cerebral hemorrhage occurred in eight of these. In four of these patients, S.B.E. was the indication for anticoagulation. Intracranial hemorrhage was thus the major cause of fatalities induced by anticoagulants. A similar conclusion was reached in patients being anticoagulated for causes other than endocarditis by Russek and Zohman,[7] who reported 46 deaths due to intracranial bleeding among 122 anticoagulant-induced fatalities, and by Riddick[8] who had six cerebral hemorrhages among eight fatalities, among his 125 anticoagulated patients.

The reported incidences of cerebral hemorrhage in patients on long-term anticoagulants for myocardial infarction is not great. Thus, Nichol and Berg[9] reported 3% in 78 patients and Nichol et al, [10] 0.5% in 1091 patients.

By 1959, Barron and Fergusson[11] were able to collect 58 instances of intracranial bleeding during anticoagulant administration from the literature, but felt that there were many non-reported cases. Thirty-one of the 58 patients in the literature had cerebral hemorrhage on anticoagulants, not due to endocarditis, and these were well tabulated. Six additional personally observed patients with fatal intracranial hemorrhages on anticoagulants were presented, and nine further cases from the literature cited. Their own personal cases included a subdural hematoma, and hemorrhages into the cerebellum and brain stem, as well as several intracerebral hemorrhages. The authors indicated that hypertension and recent cerebral infarction were contraindications to anticoagulant therapy.

Askey[12] reviewed some 1,626 patients on long-term anticoagulant therapy and found that only 30 had intracranial hemorrhages. Twenty-one of these patients died. The incidence of intracranial bleeding was higher among hypertensives. One of the 30 patients survived with surgery for removal of a subdural hematoma.

From France, Mazars et al[13] described 64 patients with intracranial hemorrhages on anticoagulants. These were predominately in the sub-arachnoid space in 26 patients, subdural hematomas in 13 patients, and intracerebral hemorrhages in 25 patients.

From Switzerland, Levy and Stula[14] reported 22 patients with intra-cranial bleeding associated with anticoagulants. The bleeding was sub-dural in 14, and intracerebral in seven, with one patient having both intracerebral and subdural bleeding. Six of the seven patients with intra-cerebral bleeding died, as did two with subdural hematomas. Surgical evacuation of the hematomas helped the other patients.

More recently, Iizuka[15] in Germany, collected 124 patients with intracranial bleeding on anticoagulants from the literature and added 12 more cases of his own. He was able to obtain another 62 patients with intracranial hemorrhage and anticoagulant therapy from surveying the neurosurgical units in the large hospitals in three countries in Europe. Six of Iizuka's own cases were subdural hematomas, six intracerebral, and one was intracerebellar and one primarily subarachnoid bleeding. One hundred and two of the 124 published cases were subdural hematomas, while 22 were intracerebral.

Subdural Hematoma

The diagnosis of a subdural hematoma, probably the most often reported intracranial neurological complication of anticoagulants, does not require a history of prior head trauma. Actually, a history of head trauma is obtained in a minority of patients with anticoagulant-related subdurals,[16-20] or the trauma may be so minimal as to not have been recalled by the patient or his relatives. Anticoagulant therapy may well be a cause of the so-called "spontaneous" subdural hematoma.

A large literature on subdural hematomas in anticoagulated patients has appeared. Shleven and Lederer reported an early autopsy proven case in 1949.[21] Nathanson et al[17] reported three patients with subdural hematomas associated with anticoagulants in 1958. Wells and Urrea[20] included five patients with subdural hematomas in their report of cerebrovascular accidents in patients receiving anticoagulants. Further cases of subdural hematoma and anticoagulant therapy were reported by Eisenberg,[22] Barron and Ferguson,[11] Pan et al,[18] and Dooley and Perlmutter.[19]

LePoire et al[23] added two further cases of their own and collected 22 patients with subdural bleeding with anticoagulants from the literature.

Eisenberg's case was the first fatality in an anticoagulated patient to be proven at autopsy to be due to a subdural hematoma alone.[22] The patient of Prager and Kowalyshyn[24] had a subdural hematoma due to heparin therapy. Three patients with subdural hematoma induced by heparin therapy during hemodialysis were reported by Leonard et al.[25]

Seven cases of subdural hematomas related to anticoagulants were described by Wiener and Nathanson,[16] five by Hissa et al,[26] 13 by Mazars et al,[13] 14 by Levy and Stula,[14] six by Iizuka,[15] ten by Sreerama et al,[27] and 22 by Bret et al.[28] Two other patients receiving anticoagulant therapy and with subdural hematomas confined to the posterior fossa have also been described.[29,30]

By 1976, Bret et al[28] had found over 150 cases of anticoagulant related subdural hematomas reported in the literature and indicated that these account for one-third of all central nervous system complications of anticoagulation. The reported incidences of anticoagulant-related subdural hematomas among all cases of subdural hematomas observed at several medical centers varies from 4.8% to 37% and is shown in the accompanying table.

Table I
Incidences of anticoagulant-related subdural hematomas among all cases of subdural hematomas

Author, Year, & Ref. No.	Total Number of Patients with Subdurals Seen	Number of Patients with Subdurals Related to Anticoagulants	Incidence
Wiener and Nathanson,[16] 1962	50	6	12%
Levy and Klinger, 1964, (cited by Bret, et al)[28]	9	1	11.1%
Weber, 1964 (cited by Bret, et al)[28]	7	1	14%
Hissa, et al,[26] 1966	40	5	12.5%
Huguenin, 1967 (cited by Bret, et al)[28]	250	12	4.8%
Sreerama, et al 1973,[27]	30	11	36.6%
Bret, et al, 1976[28]	270	22	8.3%
Wintzen, 1982[123]	212	46	21.7%

The relative frequency of subdural bleeding among patients on anticoagulants, and the fact that this condition can usually be treated promptly with reversal of many of the neurological signs and symptoms require repetition again. Many of these patients are elderly and have enlarged cerebral ventricles and some cerebral atrophy to begin with, and are thus quite prone to the development of subdural hematoma with or without known prior head injuries. Subdural hematoma should be excluded promptly in any patient who develops cerebral signs and symptoms while on anticoagulation therapy. Dr. Gilbert has already discussed the means of doing so in Chapter II in this book.

Other Sites of Intracranial Bleeding

Epidural hematomas have apparently not been reported very often, if ever, in anticoagulated patients.[15] Primary sub-arachnoid hemorrhage does occur,[11,13,15,31] but intracerebral bleeding is much more common. Occasional reports of recovery following surgical removal of an intra-cerebral hematoma have appeared.[15,19] There have also been several reports of parenchymal bleeding into the cerebellum or brain stem.[11,14,15,32-38]

Occasional patients with hemorrhage into pineal[39] or pituitary[40] tumors in association with anticoagulant therapy have appeared.

Recent reports have described and discussed the occurrence of intracranial hemorrhage associated with the usage of anticoagulants with prosthetic heart valves.[41-43] Aortic valve prosthesis has been particularly shown to be related to hemorrhagic complications, at least in men.[43]

Spinal Cord Hemorrhage

Bleeding involving the spinal cord has also been reported quite frequently in patients on anticoagulant therapy, although somewhat less than intracranial bleeding. By far the most common form of spinal cord bleeding in an anticoagulated patient is an epidural hematoma, which may be spontaneous. The clinical picture of severe, persistent back pain, which may radiate in a root distribution, and is then followed by the usually rapid development of para- or quadri-paresis, sensory loss, and sphincteric disturbances has been well described with most case reports. On rare occasions the epidural hematoma related to anticoagulants can be painless.[44]

DeVanney and Osher discussed the first reported patient on anticoagulants who developed epidural hematoma as part of a clinical pathological conference in 1952.[45] This epidural hematoma was in the lumbar region, and the patient improved following laminectomy.

The second patient with spinal cord involvement on anticoagulants was described in 1954, by Arieff and Pyszik, who thought their patient had a hematomyelia, as spinal fluid manometrics were normal. No myelogram was performed and no definite proof of the pathology was obtained. The lesion was in the cervical area and the patient's paresis in the arms improved, while the paraplegia in the legs and sphincteric difficulties persisted.[46]

The third patient was reported by Cloward and Yuhl in 1955. This patient had some epidural, but much subdural and some subarachnoid bleeding in the low thoracic area. There was only slight improvement following laminectomy.[47]

Alderman[48] in 1956 described the fourth reported patient who improved slightly following laminectomy for a lumbar epidural hematoma. Winer et al[49] in 1959 reported an epidural hematoma in an anticoagulated patient in the middle and low thoracic region (T6-T11), the symptoms of which did not improve following laminectomy. The symptoms due to spontaneous spinal epidural bleeding were emphasized, and the urgency for therapeutic intervention stressed.

Single patients with epidural hematomas related to anticoagulant therapy were described.[50-54] Paliard et al[55] reviewed three other cases reported in the French literature and reported one of their own. Two patients each were reported by Spurney et al,[56] Strain,[57] and Busse et al,[58] and three others by Levy and Stula[14] and Jacobson et al.[59] Other patients with epidural bleeding and anticoagulant therapy have been recorded[14,15,27,44,60-74] more recently.

Almost all of the spinal cord complications of anticoagulant therapy have been caused by epidural hemorrhage. Only occasional reports of subdural bleeding compressing the spinal cord have appeared.[14,67,71,75-79] (The patients reported by Cloward and Yuhl,[47] and Messer et al[80] had some subdural bleeding probably associated with epidural hematomas.) This is probably related to anatomical reasons, including the relatively larger, less compact, and more vascular epidural space containing Batson's vertebral plexus.[79] Only two case reports of spinal intramedullary hemorrhage (hematomyelia) related to anticoagulants have been found in the literature.[81,82]

Most of the patients with spinal cord complications were on long-term anticoagulants with coumarin products; a few, however, were being anticoagulated with heparin.[44,62,74,80]

Iizuka[15] in 1972 reported finding a total of 56 patients in the literature who had extradural spinal cord hemorrhage associated with anticoagulant therapy. The total number of reported cases is now considerably higher. It has been written that anticoagulants account for 18-20%[56,59] to 37.5%[61] of all spontaneous spinal epidural hematomas.

Spinal epidural hematoma is a potentially curable disease if diagnosed early enough. As Strain[57] has written, "any patient on anticoagulant therapy who develops localized, acute, persistent pain anywhere along the spinal axis should be suspected of having an extradural hematoma." At this time fresh frozen plasma and vitamin K_1 or heparin antagonists should be administered. If numbness, weakness, or sphincteric difficulties develop, emergency myelography and possible laminectomy would be indicated. Some have delayed investigations until the prothrombin time is brought back to normal;[48] others have indicated that laminectomy may be done without myelography.[59] It is felt here that the former approach is dangerously too slow and that the latter may be too rapid. Epidural hematoma in an anticoagulated patient is a neurological emergency which should be treated promptly by reversing the effects of anticoagulation and investigated promptly to allow precise localization for definitive surgical therapy.

Peripheral Neuropathy

Just as in hemophilia and other bleeding disorders,[2] the excessive bleeding induced by anticoagulation can compress peripheral nerves. As in hemophilia, the femoral nerve is most frequently involved in hemorrhage into the iliacus muscle, but bleeding can also involve the sciatic, median, radial, and other nerves. Unlike intracranial and intraspinal complications of anticoagulants, where almost all reported hemorrhages are related to coumarin products, heparin-induced bleeding plays a significant role in the production of peripheral neuropathy.

The diagnosis of peripheral nerve compression by bleeding is suggested by motor, sensory, and reflex changes in the distribution of the involved nerve, sometimes with a palpable mass, and may be confirmed at times by electromyographic study.

The first report of peripheral neuropathy by anticoagulant induced bleeding was by Nichol et al[10] in 1958, who described four patients with sciatic or peroneal nerve involvement and subsequent neuritic pain in some. In 1959, Groch et al mentioned a patient with a sciatic neuropathy due to anticoagulant therapy.[32] Calverly and Mulder[83] in 1960 discussed femoral neuropathy due to anticoagulants, but in none of their 19 reported cases of femoral neuropathy were anticoagulants the cause. Prill[84] described two patients with sciatic neuropathy associated with anticoagulants in 1965.

In 1966, Lange reported three patients with femoral neuropathy due to hypoprothrombinemia, which was definitely related to anticoagulant therapy in two, and possibly in the third, who also had some sciatic nerve involvement,[85] and DeBolt and Jordan[86] described two patients who developed femoral neuropathy while on heparin and attributed this to retroperitoneal hemorrhage secondary to dissection from the site of injection. The same year, Hartwell and Kurtay[87] reported a patient with a carpal tunnel syndrome and median nerve neuropathy due to a hematoma while on anticoagulants. The hematoma was evacuated surgically with good results.

In 1967 two patients, one with median nerve involvement, which responded to corticosteroid therapy, and one with a sciatic nerve palsy due to anticoagulants, were described by Mehrota,[88] who called attention to a persisting severe causalgic type of pain, presumably due to fibrosis about the nerve, and Leurax[89] reported three patients on anticoagulants; one had radial neuropathy, one femoral nerve, and one lateral popliteal nerve involvement. The latter patient improved with evacuation of a hematoma compressing the nerve. The same year, Gallois et al described a sciatic and a femoral neuropathy due to anticoagulants.[90] Levrat, in discussing this paper, reported seeing a radial nerve palsy due to anticoagulants. Bilateral brachial plexus involvement associated with anticoagulants was described by Angstrum and Frich,[63] and obdurator nerve palsy by Kunze.[91]

A patient with sciatic nerve paralysis due to anticoagulant therapy was reported by Leonard,[92] who reviewed briefly a variety of 22 neuropathies in patients on anticoagulants reported in the literature by 1972.

Patients with femoral neuropathy due to coumarin type anticoagulants were reported by Angstrum and Frich,[63] Lange,[85] Gilbert and Laughlin,[93] Fearn,[94] (this patient was first mentioned by Goodfellow et al),[95] Goulon and Bigot,[96] Patten,[97] Kunze,[91] Butterfield et al,[98] Gertzbein and Evans,[99] Dhaliwal et al,[100] Steward-Wynne,[101] Young and Norris,[102] Brantigan et al,[103] and Simeone.[104]

Femoral neuropathy due to heparin alone has been described by Gallois et al,[90] Sussens et al,[105] Kettlekamp and Powers,[106] Cianci and Piscatelli,[107] Sigler et al,[108] Parkes and Kidner,[109] Alchroth and Rowe-Jones,[110] Kubacz,[111] Willbanks and Fuller,[112] Spiegel and Meltzer,[113] Stern and Spiegel,[114] (possibly the same patient as in Reference 113), Kounis et al,[115] Michael,[116] Young and Norris,[102] Cranberg,[117] and Chiu.[118]

A few patients who were receiving both oral coumarin anticoagulants and parenteral heparin, or in whom the precise anticoagulant employed was not stated when their peripheral neuropathies appeared, have been reported.

A discussion of complications in anticoagulated patients following epidural anesthesia is presented in Chapter VII, and that of complications following arterial puncture in Chapter XVIII of this book.

Simeone et al[104] showed how computerized tomography can be used to localize hematomas causing peripheral nerve involvement in anticoagulated patients. This new technique is quite helpful in showing retroperitoneal hematomas involving the femoral nerve[104] or bleeding in the buttocks involving the sciatic nerve.[119]

Electromyographic abnormalities have been described in some of the patients with peripheral neuropathy due to anticoagulant induced bleeding.[91,100,102,103,106,118]

The clinician caring for patients with this complication of anticoagulants, in addition to being aware of the possibility of a peripheral nerve involvement, may well have to obtain both electromyograms and CTT scans to localize the pathology further. Certainly, the anticoagulation should be discontinued and specific antagonists administered. There is some controversy as to what should be done next.

Many competent physicians believe that surgical evacuation of the hematomas compressing peripheral nerves should be performed early, to relieve pressure in the muscles and other tissues adjacent to these nerves, and thus to relieve pressure and ischemic effects on the nerve. There are a few reports of prompt improvement of median nerve involvement, and many of prompt reversal of femoral neuropathy with surgery.

Yet many patients with peripheral nerve compression due to anticoagulation-induced bleeding have had significant, sometimes complete, improvement when treated conservatively. Spiegel and Meltzer,[113] in their review in 1974, reported that 12 of 15 patients with femoral neuropathy had fair to complete recovery without surgery. Furthermore, the condition for which anticoagulants were administered in the first place (e.g., recent myocardial infarction) might contradict surgery.

The definitive treatment of each patient should be individually determined. If the patient shows improvement, surgery had best be deferred, at least in my opinion.

Certainly, analgesics (excluding aspirin), rest initially, and local ice applications and subsequent physiotherapy are standard forms of treatment.

One final word concerning the possible prevention of peripheral neuropathy, at least from heparin injections. DeBolt and Jordon[86] initially suggested that injections into the buttocks, thighs, or abdominal wall may contribute to retroperitoneal hemorrhage by direct extension of heparin and bleeding from intramuscular injections. Other writers have also expressed this opinion.[101,105,107,117,118] It has been recommended that injections should be made into the subcutaneous fat, rather than muscles, to prevent this.[117] It should be noted, however, that similar bleeding occurs with intravenous heparin or with oral coumarin products.

Neurologic Complications Noted in Infants Whose Mothers Received Anticoagulation During Pregnancy

A recent case report[120] described an infant born with hydrocephalus due to large bilateral subdural hemorrhages. The mother had been maintained on anticoagulants during pregnancy. An excellent recent review[121] of fetal sequelae of anticoagulation during pregnancy discussed the teratogenic effects of these drugs and reported a 3% incidence of central nervous system abnormalities in liveborn infants. Several recommendations concerning the usage of anticoagulants in pregnant women were offered.

Prevention and Treatment of Neurological Complications of Anticoagulants

It is generally accepted good medical practice to monitor carefully the prothrombin times of patients undergoing anticoagulation with coumarin products, and the partial thromboblastin times when heparin is administered. It is usually advisable to keep the values of the prothrombin times well within therapeutic ranges (2 to 2.2 times normal).

Attention should be paid to other drugs which interact with anticoagulants, and there are several, including phenylbutazone, certain antibiotics and hypoglycemic agents, which will change a previously established anticoagulant level. Some other drugs, such as aspirin, have a tendency to promote bleeding and should be avoided, if possible. Most of the intracranial and spinal complications of anticoagulants occur in patients on chronic long-range anticoagulation. If the medical condition permits, anticoagulants should be discontinued as soon as possible.

Despite maintaining adequate therapeutic ranges of anticoagulation, which should be checked frequently, neurological complications can still occur. There are many reports of bleeding involving the brain, spinal cord, or peripheral nerves of anticoagulated patients who were well controlled.[8,15,16,19,20,27,56,73,102,107,122] Possibly, this situation may be related to blood factors VII, IX, and X which can be reduced by coumarin products and are not being monitored, or to minor trauma to the nervous system. Certainly, the incidences of bleeding compressing the nervous system is much greater with trauma or with poorly controlled anticoagulation. Patients on anticoagulants should be cautioned against the possibility of trauma (avoiding contact sports, etc).

The treatment for coumarin anticoagulant-induced bleeding is cessation of anticoagulants, intravenous administration of fresh frozen plasma, and intramuscular injection of phytonadione. The latter requires six to eight hours to be effective and may not counteract coagulation abnormalities induced by coumarin products other than hypoprothrombinemia. Heparin-induced bleeding is reversed with protamine sulfate.

It is not always easy to discontinue anticoagulant therapy and to administer specific antidotes, particularly if the indication for anticoagulation initially was life-threatening, such as recurrent pulmonary embolization or acute myocardial infarction. Yet, knowledge of hemorrhage involving the brain or spinal cord or of severe bleeding compressing peripheral nerves probably would have been considered a contraindication to the start of anticoagulant therapy.

References

1. Silverstein A: Neurological complications of anticoagulation therapy. *Arch Int Med* **139**:217-220, 1979.
2. Silverstein A: Neurological complications in patients with hemorrhagic diathesis. In: Vinken PJ, Bruyn GW, eds. *Handbook of Clinical Neurology*, Vol. 38. Amsterdam, North Holland Publishing Co., 1979, pp 53-91.
3. Friedman M, Hamburger WW, Katz LN: Use of heparin in subacute bacterial endocarditis, *JAMA* **113**:1702-1703, 1939.
4. Kelson SR, White PD: A new method of treatment of subacute bacterial endocarditis using sulfapyridine and heparin in combination. *JAMA* **113**:1700-1702, 1939.
5. Cohen SM: Massive cerebral hemorrhage following heparin therapy in subacute bacterial endocarditis. *J Mt Sinai Hosp* **16**:214-230, 1949.
6. Duff IF, Skull WH: Fatal hemorrhage in dicumarol poisoning. *JAMA* **139**:762-766, 1949.
7. Russek HL, Zohman BL: Anticoagulant therapy in acute myocardial infarction. *Am J Med Sci* **225**:8-13, 1953.
8. Riddick FA, Jr: Long-term anticoagulant therapy in an out-patient department: Techniques and complications. *J Chronic Dis* **12**:622-638, 1960.
9. Nichol ES, Berg JF: Long-term dicumarol therapy to prevent recurrent coronary artery thrombosis. *Circulation* **1**:1097-1104, 1950.
10. Nichol ES, Keyes JN, Borg JF, et al: Long-term anticoagulant therapy in coronary atherosclerosis. *Am Heart J* **55**:142-152, 1958.
11. Barron KD, Fergusson G: Intracranial hemorrhage as a complication of anticoagulant therapy. *Neurology* **9**:447-455, 1959.
12. Askey JM: Hemorrhage during long-term anticoagulant drug therapy: I. Intracranial hemorrhage. *Calif Med* **104**:6-10, 1966.
13. Mazars G, Ribadero-Dumas C, Roge R, et al: Accidents hemorraciques

cerebraux au cours des traitments anticoagulants. Marseille Med **104**: 27-30, 1967.

14. Levy A, Stula D: Neurochirurgische Aspekte bei Antikoagulantien Blutungen in Zentrainervensystem. *Dtsch Med Woch* **96**:1043-1048, 1971.

15. Iizuka J: Intracranial and intraspinal haematomas associated with anticoagulant therapy. *Neurochir* **15**:15-25, 1972.

16. Wiener LN, Nathanson M: The relationship of subdural hematoma to anticoagulant therapy. *Arch Neurol* **6**:282-286, 1962.

17. Nathanson M, Cravioto H, Cohen B: Subdural hematoma related to anticoagulation therapy. *Ann Intern Med* **49**:1368-1372, 1958.

18. Pan A, Rogers AG, Pearlman D: Subdural hematoma complicating anticoagulant therapy. *Can Med Assoc J* **82**:1162-1164, 1960.

19. Dooley DM, Perlmutter I: Spontaneous intracranial hematomas in patients receiving anticoagulation therapy. *JAMA* **187**:396-398, 1964.

20. Wells CE, Urrea D: Cerebrovascular accidents in patients receiving anticoagulant drugs. *Arch Neurol* **3**:553-558, 1960.

21. Shleven ER, Lederer M: Uncontrollable hemorrhage after dicumarol therapy with autopsy findings. *Ann Intern Med* **21**:332-342, 1949.

22. Eisenberg MD: Bishydroxycoumarin toxicity. *JAMA* **170**:2181-2184, 1959.

23. Lepoire J, Montaut J, Renard M, et al: Les Hematomes sous-duraux spontanes au cours des traitments anticoagulants prolonges. *Neurochir* **7**:184-193, 1964.

24. Prager D, Kowalyshyn T: Subdural hematoma and anticoagulant treatment. *Lancet* **2**:800, 1969.

25. Leonard CD, Weil E, Scribner BH: Subdural haematomas in patients undergoing hemodialysis. *Lancet* **2**:239-240, 1969.

26. Hissa A, Pereira G, Nouaes V: Hematomas subdurais no curso de terapeutica anticoagulante. *Hospital* **69**:293-304, 1966.

27. Sreerama V, Ivan LP, Dennery JM, et al: Neurosurgical complications of anticoagulant therapy. *Can Med Assoc J* **108**:305-307, 1973.

28. Bret P, Leguire J, Lapras C, et al: Hematome sous dural et therapeutique anticoagulante. *Neurochir* **22**:603-620, 1976.

29. Zentano-Alanis GH, Corvera J, Mateos JH: Subdural hematoma of the posterior fossa as a complication of anticoagulant therapy. *Neurology* **18**:1133-1136, 1968.

30. Capistrant T, Goldberg R, Shibasaki H, et al: Posterior fossa subdural haematoma associated with anticoagulant therapy. *J Neurol Neurosurg Psychiatry* **34**:82-85, 1971.

31. McDevitt E: Anticoagulant therapy in the treatment of cerebral thrombosis. In Wright IS, Millikan C, eds. *Cerebrovascular Diseases: Proceedings of the Second Conference.* New York, Grune & Stratton, 1958, pp 125-145.

32. Groch SN, Hurwitz LJ, McDevitt E, et al: Problems of anticoagulant therapy in cerebrovascular disease. *Neurology* **9**:786-793, 1959.

33. De Angelis J: Hazards of subdural and epidural anesthesia during anticoagulant therapy: A case report and review. *Anesth Analg* **51**:676-679, 1972.

34. Brennan RW, Bergland RM: Acute cerebellar hemorrhage. *Neurology* **27**:527-532, 1977.

35. Dinsdale HB: Spontaneous hemorrhage in the posterior fossa. *Arch Neurol* **10**:200-217, 1964.

36. Ott KH, Kase CS, Ojemann RC, et al: Cerebellar hemorrhage: Diagnosis and treatment. *Arch Neurol* **31**:160-167, 1974.

37. Norris JW, Eisen AA, Branch CL: Problems in cerebellar hemorrhage and infarction. *Neurology* 19:1043-1050, 1969.
38. Mastaglia FL, Edis B, Kakulas BA: Medullary haemorrhage: A report of two cases. *J Neurol Neurosurg Psychiatry* 32:221-225, 1969.
39. Apuzzo MCJ, Davey LM, Manueliois CE: Pineal apoplexy associated with anticoagulant therapy. *J Neurosurg* 45:223-226, 1976.
40. Nourizadeh AR, Pitts FW: Hemorrhage into pituitary adenoma during anticoagulant therapy. *JAMA* 193:623-625, 1965.
41. Lieberman A, Hass WK, Pinto R, et al: Intracranial hemorrhage and infarction in anticoagulated patients with prosthetic heart valves. *Stroke* 9:18-24, 1978.
42. Wilson WR, Geraci JE, Danielson GK, et al: Anticoagulant therapy and central nervous system complications in patients with prosthetic valve endocarditis. *Circulation* 57:1004-1007, 1978.
43. Forfar JC: A 7-year analysis of haemorrhage in patients on long-term anticoagulant therapy. *Brit Heart J* 42:128-132, 1979.
44. Senelick RC, Norwood CW, Cohen CH: Painless spinal epidural hematoma during anticoagulant therapy. *Neurology* 26:213-215, 1976.
45. De Vanney JR, Osher D, in discussion, Airing CD: Neurological clinical pathological conference of Cincinnati General Hospital. *Dis Nerv Syst* 13:53-60, 1952.
46. Arieff AJ, Pyzik SW: Paraplegia following or associated with excessive dicumarol therapy. *Q Bull Northwestern U Med School* 28:221-222, 1954.
47. Cloward RB, Yuhl ET: Spontaneous intraspinal hemorrhage and paraplegia complicating dicumarol therapy. *Neurology* 5:600-602, 1955.
48. Alderman DB: Extradural spinal cord hematoma: Report of a case due to dicumarol and review of the literature. *N Engl J Med* 255:839-842, 1956.
49. Winer BM, Horenstein S, Starr AM: Spinal epidural hematoma and anticoagulant therapy. *Circulation* 19:735-740, 1959.
50. Lin TH: Paraplegia caused by epidural hemorrhage of spine. *J Int Coll Surg* 36:742-749, 1961.
51. Weigert M: Akutes spinales, epidurales hamatom als folge von Behandlung mit antikoagulantien. *Nervenarzt* 32:85-89, 1961.
52. Whaley RL, Lindner DW: Spontaneous spinal epidural hemorrhage associated with anticoagulant therapy. *Grace Hosp Bull* 40:27-32, 1962.
53. Kuznetsow ND, cited by Spurney et al: (Ref. 56).
54. Gold EM: Spontaneous spinal epidural hematoma. *Radiology* 80:823-828, 1963.
55. Paliard P, Mottin J, Goutelle A, et al: Hematome extradural medullaire au cours d'un traitement anticoagulant. *Lyon Med* 218:395-399, 1967.
56. Spurney OM, Rubin S, Wolf JW, et al: Spinal epidural hematoma during anticoagulant therapy. *Arch Int Med* 114: 103-107, 1964.
57. Strain RE: Spinal epidural hematoma in patients on anticoagulant therapy. *Ann Surg* 159:507-509, 1964.
58. Busse O, Hamer J, Paal G, et al: Spontane epidurale spinal hamotome wahrend und nach antikoagulation-medikation. *Nervenarzt* 6:318-322, 1972.
59. Jacobson I, MacCabe JJ, Harris P, et al: Spontaneous spinal epidural haemorrhage during anticoagulant therapy. *Lancet* 1:522-523, 1960.
60. Lazorthes G, Boulard C, Epagno J, cited by Iizuka J: (Ref. 15).
61. Harik SI, Raichle ME, Reis DJ: Spontaneously remitting spinal epidural

hematoma in a patient on anticoagulants. *N Engl J Med* **284**:1355-1357, 1971.

62. Simmons EH, Grobler LJ: Acute spinal epidural hematoma: A case report. *J Bone Jt Surg* **60A**:395-396, 1978.

63. Angstrum H, Frich E, Nil Nocere: Neurologische Komplikationen bei Antikoagulantientherapie. *Munch Med Wschr* **20**:1103-1109, 1967.

64. Oldenkott P, Driesen W: Spontanes epidurales hamaton in brustwirbelkanal wahrend antikoagulantien — Langzeit behandlung. *Med Welt* **17**:305-307, 1966.

65. Posner S, Ritter G: Der Antikoagulantien-Zwischenfall in der Neurologie *Fortschr Med* **92**:1146-1168, 1974.

66. Schicue R, Seitz D: Spinales epidurales hamatom unter antikoagulantientherapie. *Dtsch Med Wschr* **94**:275-277, 1970.

67. Fischbach R, Kollar WA: Spontane spinale epidurale blutung unter antikoagulatien *Wien Med Wochenchr* **122**:275-276, 1972.

68. Pear BL: Spinal epidural hematoma. *Amer J Roengt* **115**:155-164, 1972.

69. Pendl VG, Horcajada J: cited by Petrov V, et al, (Ref. 71).

70. Telerman-Toppet N, Moreman C, Noterman JL: cited by Petrov, et al (Ref. 71).

71. Petrov V, Collignon J, Stevenaert A: Hematomes spinaux extra-duraux et sous-duraux au cours d'un traitment par anticoagulants. *Acta Neurol Belg* **79**:398-408, 1979.

72. McQuarrie IG: Recovery from paraplegia caused by spontaneous spinal epidural hematoma. *Neurology* **28**:224-228, 1978.

73. Zuccarello M, Scanarini M, D'Avella D, et al. Spontaneous spinal extradural hematoma during anticoagulant therapy. *Surg Neurol* **14**: 411-413, 1980.

74. Kohli CM, Palmer AH, Gray GH: Spontaneous intraspinal hemorrhage causing paraplegia: A complication of heparin therapy. *Ann Surg* **179**: 197-199, 1974.

75. Tricot R, cited by Edelson RN, Chernik NC, Posner JB: Spinal subdural hematomas complicating lumbar puncture. *Arch Neurol* **31**:134-137, 1974.

76. Dabbert O, Freeman DG, Weis AJ: Spinal meningeal hematoma, warfarin therapy and chiropractic adjustment. *JAMA* **214**:2058, 1970.

77. Diaz-Aramendi A, Paniacua JL, Hernandez J, et al: Meningococcic infection submitted to treatment. Spinal subdural hematoma. *Neurochir* **19**:641-648, 1973.

78. Schwartz PT, Sartani MA, Fox JL: Unusual hematomas outside the spinal cord. *J Neurosurg* **39**:249-251, 1973.

79. Vinters HV, Barnett HJM, Kaufmann JCE: Subdural hematoma of the spinal cord and widespread subarachnoid hemorrhage complicating anticoagulant therapy. *Stroke* **11**:459-464, 1980.

80. Messer HD, Forshan VR, Brust JCM, et al: Transient paraplegia from hematoma after lumbar puncture: A consequence of anticoagulant therapy. *JAMA* **235**:529-530, 1976.

81. Papo I, Luongo A: Massive intramedullary hemorrhage in a patient on anticoagulants. *J Neurosurg Sci* **18**:268-270, 1974.

82. Brandt M: Spontaneous intramedullary hematoma as a complication of anticoagulant therapy. *Acta Neurochir* **52**:73-77, 1980.

83. Calverly JR, Mulder DW: Femoral neuropathy. *Neurology* **10**:963-967, 1960.

84. Prill, cited by Parkes and Kidner: (Ref. 109).
85. Lange LS: Lower limb palsies with hypoprothrombinemia. *Brit Med J* 2:93-94, 1966.
86. DeBolt WC, Jordan JC: Femoral neuropathy from heparin hematoma: Report of two cases. *Bull Los Angeles Neurol Soc* 31:45-50, 1966.
87. Hartwell SW, Kurtay M: Carpal tunnel compression caused by hematoma associated with anticoagulant therapy. *Clev Clin Q* 33:127-129, 1966.
88. Mehrotra TN: Phenindione-induced neuropathy. *Brit Med J* 3:218, 1967.
89. Leurax, cited by Parkes and Kidner PH: (Ref. 109).
90. Gallois P, Dhers A, Badarou G: Deux las de paralysie nerveuse peripherique par hematome spontane au cours de traitment anticoagulant. *Lyon Med* 218:401-406, 1967.
91. Kunce K: Neuropathy in association with haemophilia. In: Vinken PJ, Bruyn GW (eds.) *Handbook of Clinical Neurology*, Vol. 7 Amsterdam, North Holland Publ. Co., 1970, pp 664-670.
92. Leonard MD: Sciatic nerve paralysis following anticoagulant therapy. *J Bone Jt Surg* 54B:152-153, 1972.
93. Gilbert GJ, Laughlin R: Hemorrhagic femoral neuropathy: Report of a case due to anticoagulant. *South Med J* 60:170-176, 1967.
94. Fearn CBD'A: Iliacus haematoma syndrome as a complication of anticoagulant therapy. *Brit Med J* 4:97-98, 1968.
95. Goodfellow J. Fearn CBD'A, Matthews JM: Iliacus hematoma. A common manifestation of hemophilia. *J Bone Jt Surg* 49B:748-756, 1967.
96. Goulon M, Bigot B, cited by Iizuka J: (Ref. 15).
97. Patten BM: Neuropathy induced by hemorrhage. *Arch Neurol* 21:381-386, 1969.
98. Butterfield WC, Neviaser RJ, Roberts MD: Femoral neuropathy and anticoagulants. *Ann Surg* 176:58-61, 1972.
99. Gertzbein SD, Evans DC: Femoral nerve neuropathy complicating iliopsoas haemorrhage in patients without hemophilia. *J Bone Jt Surg* 54B:149-151, 1972.
100. Dhaliwal GS, Schlagenhauff RE, Megahed SM: Acute femoral neuropathy induced by oral anticoagulation. *Dis Nerv Syst* 37:539-541, 1976.
101. Stewart-Wynne EG: Iatrogenic femoral neuropathy. *Brit Med J* 1:263, 1976.
102. Young MR, Norris JW: Femoral neuropathy during anticoagulant therapy. *Neurology* 26:1173-1175, 1976.
103. Brantigan JW, Owens ML, Moody FC: Femoral neuropathy complicating anticoagulant therapy. *Am J Surg* 132:108-109, 1976.
104. Simeone JF, Robinson F, Rothman SLG, et al: Computerized tomographic demonstration of a retroperitoneal hematoma causing femoral neuropathy. *J Neurosurg* 47:946-948, 1977.
105. Sussens GP, Hendrickson CG, Mulder MJ, et al: Femoral nerve entrapment secondary to a heparin hematoma. *Ann Intern Med* 69:575-579, 1968.
106. Kettlekamp DB, Powers SR: Femoral compression neuropathy in hemorrhagic disorders. *Arch Surg* 98:367-368, 1969.
107. Cianci PE, Piscatelli RL: Femoral neuropathy secondary to retroperitoneal hemorrhage. *JAMA* 210:1100-1101, 1969.
108. Sigler L, Raut PS, Vollman RW: Iliacus muscle haematoma: A complication of heparin administration. *Angiology* 21:114-115, 1970.
109. Parkes JD, Kidner PH: Peripheral nerve and root lesions developing

as a result of haematoma formation during anticoagulant therapy. *Postgrad Med J* **46**:146-148, 1970.

110. Alchroth P, Rowe-Jones DC: Iliacus compartment compression syndrome. *Brit J Surg* **58**:833-834, 1971.

111. Kubacz GJ: Femoral and sciatic compression neuropathy. *Brit J Surg* **58**:580-582, 1971.

112. Willbanks DC, Fuller GH: Femoral neuropathy secondary to retroperitoneal hematoma. *Arch Int Med* **132**:83-86, 1973.

113. Spiegel PC, Meltzer JL: Femoral nerve neuropathy secondary to anticoagulation. *J Bone Jt Surg* **56A**:425-427, 1974.

114. Stern MB, Spiegel PC: Femoral neuropathy as a complication of heparin anticoagulation therapy. *Clin Orthop* **106**:141-142, 1975.

115. Kounis NG, Macauley MB, Ghorbal MS: Iliacus hematoma syndrome. *Can Med Assoc J* **112**:872-873, 1975.

116. Michael RH: Femoral neuropathy: A complication of anticoagulation. *Md State Med J* **24**:57-58, 1975.

117. Cranberg L: Femoral neuropathy from iliac hematoma: Report of a case. *Neurology* **29**:1071-1072, 1979.

118. Chiu WS: The syndrome of retroperitoneal hemorrhage and lumbar plexus neuropathy during anticoagulant therapy. *South Med J* **69**:595-599, 1976.

119. Wallach HW, Oren ME: Sciatic nerve compression during anticoagulation therapy. *Arch Neurol* **36**:448, 1979.

120. Robinson MJ, Cameron MD, Smith MF, Bayers A: Fetal subdural haemorrhages presenting as hydrocephalus. *Brit Med J* **281**:35, 1980.

121. Hall JG, Pauli RM, Wilson KM: Maternal and fetal sequelae of anticoagulation during pregnancy. *Amer J Med* **63**:122-140, 1980.

122. Pollard JW, Hamilton MJ, Christenson WA, et al: Problems associated with long-term anticoagulant therapy. *Circulation* **25**:311-317, 1962.

123. Wintzen AR: Subdural hematoma and oral anticoagulant therapy. *Arch Neurol* **32**:69-72, 1982.

Chapter XV

Neurological Complications of Anti-Parkinson Drug Therapy

Roger C. Duvoisin, M.D.

Introduction

The undesired effects of the drugs commonly employed in the treatment of parkinsonism are best understood within the context of the clinical disorder and its manifestations in the individual patient. They represent not only the known pharmacological properties of these drugs but also the altered susceptibility to certain drug effects attending the various clinical forms of parkinsonism. The most common form of parkinsonism encountered in practice today, Parkinson's disease, is a chronic progressive neuronal degeneration extending over a period of many years. There is, moreover, an extraordinary plethora of symptoms and great variability among patients. It is thus often difficult to determine whether a new symptom represents progression of the disease or a side effect. New symptoms following a change in medication or merely a change of dosage may represent a side effect or a re-emergence of parkinsonian symptomtology if the new regimen is less effective. In placebo controlled drug trials in parkinsonism, one often finds that patients interpret their increased symptoms while on placebo treatment as a "side-effect." For these several reasons, recognition and proper management of drug side effects in parkinsonism requires familiarity with the clinical syndrome under treatment as well as knowledge of the pharmacology of the drugs in question.

Optimum treatment can usually be obtained only at the price of a certain level of side effects. The object of therapy is to find the best possible balance between desired and undesired effects. Indeed, certain side effects such as the choreiform dyskinesia may serve as a guide to therapy. Many of the side effects are dose-dependent "normal" effects of the anti-Parkinson drugs, although dose-limiting and sometimes alarming, they are rarely dangerous and rapidly subside on withdrawal of the offending agent or on reducing the dosage. Other effects, however, are not "normal" responses to be anticipated at certain dosages and are not related to the therapeutic action but represent adverse effects which usually necessitate withdrawal of the drug. Fortunately, serious adverse effects have been quite rare.

The drug of choice in treating parkinsonism, with the exception of iatrogenic parkinsonism induced by the major neuroleptic agent, remains Levodopa. A number of centrally active anticholinergic agents are employed primarily as anti-Parkinson agents although many other anticholinergics may be equally effective. These all share a common pharmacology and can be considered collectively. Amantadine appears to be in a class by itself. Its mechanism of action has not been fully defined but its side effects are similar to those of the anticholinergics and an indirect cholinolytic effect has been demonstrated in certain preparations.[1] Finally, recently, Bromocriptine and related ergoline derivatives have been employed experimentally and appear to have a role in the treatment of parkinsonism. Although these dopamine-receptor agonists other than Bromocriptine are not yet formally approved for use in treating parkinsonism in the United States, they will probably soon be available and thus require consideration here.

Levodopa

After over a decade of widespread use, L-dopa remains the most effective and least toxic agent available for the treatment of Parkinson's disease and related disorders. It is generally given with a peripheral decarboxylase inhibitor in a combination which greatly diminishes the severity and frequency of certain side effects. Thus far, the decarboxylase inhibitors have not demonstrated any obvious effects of their own other than to potentiate the central action of L-dopa. Consequently, it is convenient to review the side effect of L-dopa itself, used alone.

All the biological effects of L-dopa are due to its metabolites, dopamine, and to a lesser extent, noradrenaline formed *in vivo*. A broad range of effects have been noted, chief among them being adventitious involuntary movements, anorexia, nausea, vomiting, and orthostatic hypotension. The major side effect encountered on first initiating L-dopa therapy is nausea. Anorexia, nausea, and vomiting comprise a spectrum reflecting the action of dopamine in the medullary vomiting center. The mildest symptom is anorexia. The patient may not complain of it, but in hospital, it is readily apparent on inspecting the patient's food tray. The patients may complain of a metallic taste or simply a foul taste. A more severe response consists of frank malaise and nausea. Often this is accompanied by "dizziness" or faintness. The response may culminate in frank vomiting. Usually this occurs about 45 to 60 minutes after dosing. The vomiting may occur abruptly, in a projectile manner with little warning. It is transient and the patient feels better soon after.

Although the review literature often lists nausea and vomiting among the gastrointestinal side effects, it is, in fact, a central effect similar to that of apomorphine[2] and many other sympathomimetic agents. It occurs following intravenous injection as well as after oral ingestion.[2,3] It is more likely to occur when the patient takes L-dopa on an empty stomach because the amino acid is absorbed more readily and the blood level rises more rapidly. Presumably, the vomiting center, like other sensory receptors, responds to the rate of change in stimulation and consequently is then more likely to trigger vomiting. Thus, this series of side effects may be prevented if the patient is careful to take L-dopa only post-prandially and also, by starting treatment with small doses, increasing gradually in small increments at intervals of days to weeks to allow tolerance to the emetic action of L-dopa to develop. When L-dopa is used alone, it usually requires one to three months to reach full therapeutic doses.[4,5] Should nausea and vomiting nevertheless continue to be a problem, concurrent administration of an anti-emetic agent will usually be effective. The preferred agents for this purpose are Trimethobenzamide (Tigan [R$_x$]) or diphenidol (Vontrol [R$_x$]).[6] The most effective anti-emetics are the dopamine-receptor blockers, such as the phenothiazine neuroleptics, but these agents, unfortunately, also block the therapeutic actions of L-dopa in the treatment of parkinsonism.

Nausea and vomiting are much less frequent when L-dopa is combined with a decarboxylase inhibitor such as carbidopa or bensarizide. These agents depend on the fact that they do not cross the blood-brain barrier and thus do not block the conversion of dopa to dopamine within the brain parenchyma.[7] However, the vomiting center is a special exception and lies outside the blood-brain barrier. Thus carbidopa and bensarizide can prevent the function of dopamine in this specialized brain area, thereby preventing the emetic response to L-dopa. This protection is only partial and some patients will still experience nausea and even vomiting, though rarely, on this combination therapy. In practice, this occurs mainly with the smaller doses of the combination tablets, e.g., the 10/100 mg Sinemet [R$_x$] tablet. The reason is that 10 mg of carbidopa is too small a dose to sufficiently inhibit the synthesis of dopamine in the vomiting center. Adding additional amounts of the decarboxylase inhibitor often suffices to prevent the emetic response in these patients. This may conveniently be done with the new 25/100 mg formulation of Sinemet containing 25 mg of carbidopa. Even with this preparation a few patients may still experience anorexia and nausea and rarely, vomiting. The anti-emetics discussed above may then be tried. Usually, they can be discontinued after a month or two as tolerance develops.

Adventitious involuntary movements represent the most frequent and most important dose-limiting side effect of L-dopa. A broad range of movement may be observed. The most common are choreiform in nature, and the entire spectrum of choreic-movements may occur.[8] The patients may not be aware of minimal movements. They are often first reported by the patient's spouse or other relatives. Automatic movements such as the associated movements of walking, movements of postural adjustment, expressive gestures, and expressive movements of the face may become more pronounced, then frankly exaggerated. When more severe these become flinging movements of the arms on walking, constant squirming and restlessness in the sitting position, facial grimacing, mouthing, and protrusion of the tongue. Head nodding and bobbing movements are particularly frequent. Swaying of the trunk and pelvis on standing, increased respiratory movements, and exaggerated stepping movements are also common.

The chorea occurs characteristically in episodes beginning an hour or so after dosing and subsiding an hour or so later as the effect of the dose subsides. It is more pronounced in patients exhibiting marked variations in clinical state (the "on-off" effect), swinging abruptly from a parkinsonian state to a choreic state. In such patients tremor may suddenly be replaced by chorea, sometimes there is a brief period when both are present together.

In a small proportion of patients slow twisting movements, i.e., "torsion spasms" may occur, usually during the "end-of-dose" or "wearing-off" period.[9] Slow sustained intense muscle contractions occur producing hyperpronation of a hand, internal rotation of the arm, an equinovarus posturing of the foot with clawing of the toes, torticollis or tortipelvis. A forceful involuntary opening of the mouth with deviation of the jaw, that is an oromandibular dystonia, has rarely been observed. The "end-of-dose" dystonic cramp of the foot is probably the most common of these phenomena. Often it occurs mainly during the night or on arising in the morning. Sometimes the cramps occur at the onset as well as at the end of the effect of a particular dose. Thus, several temporal patterns may result: a dystonia–improvement–dystonia (or D-I-D) sequence, or an improvement–dystonia–improvement (I-D-I) sequence.[10]

A rare phenomenon is the induction of involuntary eye closure on L-dopa treatment. It is dose-dependent and has on occasion precluded effective relief of other symptoms. Stammering and stuttering occur occasionally, also in a dose-dependent manner. Although they are uncommon, tic-like movements consisting of sudden shrugs of the shoulder, a facial twitch, throat-clearing noises, moans, grunts, sighs, and constant humming noises must be added to the list of dopa-induced dyskinesias.

Unfortunately, the dopa-induced dyskinesias can be eliminated only by reducing the dosage of L-dopa. No pharmacological agent has yet been found capable of diminishing these adventitious movements which does not also at the same time diminish the therapeutic benefits. Neuroleptics and cholinergic agents have been extensively tried for this purpose but have not proved effective. Consequently, the treating physician must seek the best compromise between the control of parkinsonian symptoms and the induction of dyskinesia. Both are dose-dependent phenomena inversely related in a see-saw manner. Patients, in general, prefer choreiform dyskinesia to parkinsonism, whereas their families are embarrassed by the chorea and often object to it. Explaining the nature of these phenomena to the patient and the family helps preclude undue alarm and provide reassurance regarding the meaning of the movements.

Orthostatic hypotension and other manifestations of autonomic dysfunction in combination with parkinsonian features — chiefly bradykinesia — occur in the Shy-Drager syndrome. Orthostatic hypotension is also an uncommon manifestation of classical Parkinson's disease. However, L-dopa therapy commonly produces a reduction of blood pressure[11] and in 8-10% of Parkinson's disease patients significant symptomatic orthostatic hypotension results.[5] The patient complains of dizziness, light-headedness, or faintness on standing up. Rarely, syncope may occur. Simple measures, such as the use of elastic stockings, usually prove sufficient to control this side effect. Sodium chloride tablets in a dose of 2 to 4 grams per day is effective in most cases. Alternatively, one may administer 0.1-0.3 mg fluorhydrocortisone daily with similar effects.[12] Tolerance to the hypotensive effect of L-dopa therapy may develop in time.

The mechanism of the hypotensive effect is not entirely clear. It has been suggested that as a result of flooding the peripheral autonomic nervous system with L-dopa, dopamine may displace noradrenaline so that on chronic Levodopa therapy a partial depletion of noradrenaline may result.[13,14] In addition, dopamine may function as a surrogate transmitter. It is a relatively weak alpha-adrenergic agonist and has beta-adrenergic effects, which would cause vasodilation in skeletal muscles and in the splanchnic circulation.[15] Baroreceptor function may also be impaired.[16] However, the fact that orthostatic hypotension is not diminished by the combined use of L-dopa and a peripheral decarboxylase inhibitor indicates that central mechanisms are probably of major importance to the hypotensive effect.[17]

The cardiac effects of L-dopa are not so generally appreciated as they should be. Interestingly, it has a weak inotropic effect and slows atrioventricular conduction.[14,18] These actions, however, subside after several weeks of treatment. They might be expected to increase the frequency of ventricular escape arrhythmias. Premature ventricular contractions may increase, but the most frequent effect on cardiac rhythm observed is mild sinus tachycardia. There are few data on its incidence in patients on chronic L-dopa therapy, but in the author's observation, tachycardia of

90 to 110 is relatively common. Episodes of supraventricular tachycardia are uncommon but they have occurred and must be regarded as one of the side effects of Levodopa therapy.[5,19]

Because of these cardiac effects, as well as the orthostatic hypotension described above, caution is advised in initiating Levodopa therapy in patients who have recently suffered a myocardial infarction or have evidence of progressive ischemic heart disease. However, the clinician must consider the fact that untreated Parkinson's disease with severe tremor and rigidity may impose a significant burden on the heart. Each case requires individual evaluation of the various factors involved. For example, if the parkinsonism is mild in severity, Levodopa may be withheld until the patient's cardiac status stabilizes. On the other hand, if the patient has had the disease several years or more or has severe parkinsonism, it may be better to continue Levodopa therapy. In most cases, it is probably better not to change the therapy. Possibly, the dosage of ongoing Levodopa treatment might be reduced 20-30% to diminish the occurrences of choreiform dyskinesia which might stress the heart during the acute phase of myocardial infarction.

Transient blurring of vision is an occasional complaint which may be ascribed to pupillary dilation an hour or two after a given dose.[20] The mydriasis is less marked than that produced by anticholinergic agents and much less sustained. There is little risk of aggravating or precipitating glaucoma except the narrow angle type. In either case, the glaucoma should be properly managed and treatment with Levodopa may then proceed as indicated. Visual dysfunction in Parkinson patients is often ascribed to drug therapy when, in fact, it represents disturbances in oculomotor function which are expressions of the disease process itself. For example, the complaint of difficulty reading despite normal corrected visual acuity may reflect faulty scanning of a line of print due to impaired saccadic movements of the eyes, ocular lateropulsion, diplopia, and perhaps also perceptual disorders and disturbances of spatial orientation which are not yet well understood.

The mental side effects of Levodopa therapy are complex and, as other side effects, reflect the interaction of pharmacologic manipulation and the pathophysiology of the disease.[21] Some patients complain on initiation of treatment of a sense of nervousness or jitteriness. Usually this subsides within a matter of days. Occasional patients complain, on the other hand, of drowziness and somnolence for an hour or two following each dose. An early sign of psychotoxicity is vivid dreaming and nightmares. Merely reducing or eliminating the bedtime dose may suffice to control this side effect. Agitation has been an uncommon side effect. Periods of euphoria and hypomanic behavior have been noted particularly in patients suffering from the "on-off" effect, accompanying the choreiform dyskinesia of the "on" phase. As they swing from the "on" to the "off" phase, profound depression may rapidly replace the previous euphoria.

Depression has been cited by some authors as a side effect of Levodopa therapy.[22,23] In the present author's experience this has been very infrequent, depression usually reflecting the disease itself or a reaction to its chronic disability. This should not be an indication for discontinuing Levodopa therapy but rather for instituting appropriate antidepressant therapy.

Acute delirium with hallucinations, confusion, often colored with paranoid ideation and agitation is rare. Severe psychotoxicity of this type and degree of severity are more common with anticholinergic drugs.[21] Levodopa is the least psychotoxic of the agents presently available for the treatment of parkinsonism. Thus in a patient on multiple drugs developing such psychotoxicity, the anticholinergic drugs should be reduced in dosage or withdrawn first, Levodopa last. Delirium, however, may occur with Levodopa alone. Rarely, it may occur in the absence of *any* drug therapy.

The visual hallucinations of Parkinson's disease are surprisingly consistent from patient to patient.[24] Commonly, the hallucinations consist of people, often spectral or diminutive in size, wandering about the patient's home. The same hallucinations recur in a regular pattern. They are not necessarily unpleasant and may resemble dreams. Their unreality is usually recognized. With the development of confusion, however, the patient may react to the hallucinations, *often with paranoid ideation.* Gilbert has recently called attention to their similarity to the "peduncular hallucinosis" described by l'Hermitte over a half-century ago.[25]

Latent or subclinical schizophrenia may be activated by Levodopa therapy and an acute psychotic episode may occur. In patients with post-encephalitic parkinsonism, their characteristic behavioral aberrations, including compulsive rituals and asocial behavior, may be reactivated.[21,22] Even behavior that had not been seen in several decades may suddenly re-emerge just as a good therapeutic response to Levodopa therapy is achieved.

A transient neutropenia on initiating therapy with the racemic D, L-dopa had been reported by Cotzias et al.[26] This was also observed by Yahr et al in their early observations on L-dopa.[5] However, no further notice of this phenomenon has been recorded and no instances of significant leukopenia have been reported. The frequent occurrence of a mildly positive Coomb's test on L-dopa therapy has also been noted.[27,28] However, only three instances of an acute hemolytic anemia probably induced by Levodopa have been published.[29,30,31] The second case was continued on treatment with Levodopa combined with the peripheral decarboxylase inhibitor bensarizide without recurrence. Autoimmune mechanisms were invoked in all three cases. A resemblance to the rare hemolytic anemias induced by methyldopa was suggested. A case of thrombocytopenia has apparently been associated with L-dopa therapy.[32] Steroid treatment permitted resumption of L-dopa treatment without a recurrence.

Anticholinergic Drugs

Anticholinergic agents were the principal drugs available for the symptomatic treatment of parkinsonism prior to the introduction of Levodopa. They are still widely employed as adjuncts to Levodopa and for the treatment or prevention of drug-induced parkinsonism. These include principally, trihexyphenidyl, cycrimine, biperiden, procyclidine, and benztoprine. The natural alkaloid atropines, hyoscine and hyoscyamus are now rarely employed although their effects are eventually identical. All these agents produce a pattern of side effects reflecting the antagonism of acetylcholine at many sites throughout the peripheral autonomic and central nervous system.

The side effects due to the central actions of these drugs comprise collectively the central anticholinergic syndrome. These include ataxia, dysarthria, tremor, nausea, "dizziness," drowziness, and in severe intoxication — stupor, delirium, and coma.

Disturbance of mental function is a prominent element of the "central anticholinergic syndrome" and comprises one of the most frequent side effects of the centrally active anticholinergic drugs which are commonly employed in the treatment of parkinsonism. A series of psychic changes is seen ranging in severity from a subtle impairment of attention and recent memory to a frank toxic psychosis with confusion, agitation, and hallucinations, and in extreme cases, delirium and even coma. The milder changes often pass unrecognized or are erroneously ascribed to arteriosclerosis, senility, Parkinson's disease, or other causes. Frequently, overt mental symptoms necessitate cessation of drug therapy, or at least reduction in dosage or a change to a milder agent. The more severe psychic changes including frank psychotic episodes are alarming and often unanticipated occurrences which can cause considerable distress and may necessitate hospitalization, or at least constant supervision for several days or more.

Mental disturbances are encountered in up to 20% of patients treated with routine dosages of the standard anticholinergic agents.[21,33] They occur more frequently in elderly patients and in those with more severe disease. Patients with mental impairment are especially prone to develop confusion and hallucinations.

The earliest mental change noted during anticholinergic treatment is impairment of recent memory and decreased power of concentration.

"Forgetfulness" is a frequent complaint. Restlessness and agitation are also frequent as is drowsiness. A more marked change reflecting higher dosages or increased sensitivity is the occurrence of confusion. Usually episodic, it may be accompanied by agitation, ataxia, and dysarthria. Amnesia for these episodes is usual. Illusions and hallucinations, usually visual are also quite common. Complex experiential hallucinations of people wandering about are typical. Patients may experience these hallucinations intermittently for months or years remaining aware that they are hallucinations. However, with the advent of confusion, the patient may react to these in a paranoid manner. Systematized paranoid delusions may subsequently develop and they may persist for many months following withdrawal of the offending drug and the subsidence of the hallucinations. Severe hallucinations may on occasion progress to frank delirium. Usually, this is precipitated by an abrupt change of dose or the addition of a new drug with anticholinergic properties. The patients may become acutely confused and disoriented. If handled tactfully and left to rest quietly, they lapse into somnolence or stupor. Rarely, "atropine" coma may supervene with fever and anhidrosis.

Mental disturbances can be reduced to a tolerable level by a reduction of dosage. The psychotoxicity is dose-dependent and can often be "titrated" with fair precision. Acute severe intoxication can be promptly reversed by the intravenous administration of 1-2 mg physostigmine salicylate (antilirium R_x).[34] In most cases, it is sufficient to withdraw the offending agent or reduce the dosage.

Patients sensitive to the psychotoxic effects of the anticholinergic agents will be sensitive not only to anti-Parkinson drugs, but also to other drugs such as antihistamines which also possess central anticholinergic properties. The anticholinergic actions of different drugs given together are additive. Thus a patient who is doing well on a regimen of Sinemet and trihexyphenidyl may develop an acute confusional episode on taking additionally an antihistamine prescribed for a different indication.

Large doses of the anticholinergic drugs may complicate the parkinsonian symptomatology by adding thereto some ataxia, dysarthria, and tremor. Choreiform involuntary movements are a rare but recognized manifestation of acute anticholinergic intoxication. Choreiform dyskinesia was not observed in Parkinson's disease patients prior to the advent of Levodopa therapy. However, anticholinergics may provoke adventitious movements, notably orofacial movements, in patients on a Levodopa regimen and enhance Levodopa-induced dyskinesia.[35]

The peripheral anticholinergic side effects are the familiar "atropinic" manifestations of blurred near-vision due to cycloplegia, dryness of the mouth, and constipation. The cycloplegic action carries the risk of exacerbating glaucoma. However, if the glaucoma is under proper treatment, anticholinergics may then be used if indicated. Constipation is itself a manifestation of Parkinson's disease which may be increased by anticholinergic treatment. The neurogenic bladder of parkinsonism may be adversely affected by anticholinergics. In elderly men with prostatic hypertrophy, there is a risk of precipitating acute urinary retention. Further discussion of the autonomic nervous system complications of antiparkinson medication appears in Chapter XVI of this book.

Amantadine

Amantadine, (Symmetrel), a drug whose mechanism of action in the central nervous system is not yet established, also produces a clinical picture of intoxication similar to that of the anticholinergic agents.[36] Since physostigmine can reverse delirium due to overdosage, it seems plausible to assume that its central actions are also due to cholinergic blockade.[37]

Two common side effects of amantadine are the development of livido reticularis and edema of the lower extremities, both usually occurring together.[38] Livido reticularis first appears as a faint cyanotic mottling of the skin of the legs (Fig. 1). Usually it may first be noted in the distal portion of the leg about the ankle and in the thigh near the knee. Less commonly, it may also be noted in the skin of the volar aspect of the forearm. The genesis of this phenomenon is unknown. It has been thought to be related to a peripheral vasoconstrictor effect.[39] It is more common in female patients. Following withdrawal of the drug, the pattern of cutaneous venous congestion gradually disappears. It may persist for several weeks. Edema of the lower extremities usually accompanies the livido reticularis but sometimes edema can be quite prominent in the presence of little or no livido. The edema also subsides gradually after withdrawal of amantadine.

Dopamine Receptor Agonists

The search for more effective treatment of Parkinson's disease has focused in recent years on a series of dopamine receptor agonists. These agents offer some therapeutic benefit and are likely to become important in the treatment of parkinsonism in the near future. The most promising have been the ergoline compounds Bromocriptine, Lisuride, and Pergolide. Bromocriptine has recently been approved in the United States for the treatment of parkinsonism. Although substantially less potent than Levodopa as an anti-Parkinson agent, it has the advantage of a much

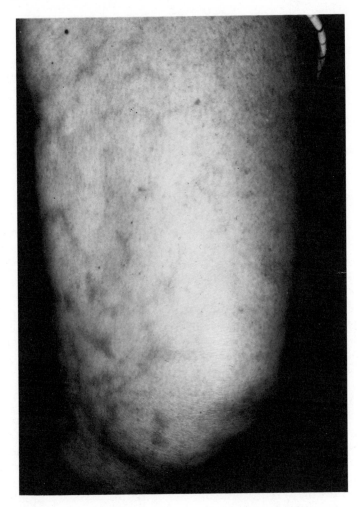

Figure 1. Livido reticularis due to amantadine treatment.

longer duration of action. Employed as an adjuvant to Levodopa, it has proved moderately useful in dealing with the "on-off" effect seen in patients enjoying only a brief relief of symptoms after each dose of Levodopa,[40,41] It has been especially helpful in minimizing the painful "end-of-dose" dystonic cramps occurring in patients with the "on-off" effect. The doses required for optimal effect range from 40 to 80 mg daily, although some benefit may occasionally be encountered with smaller doses of 15 to 20 mg daily.

The major side effects include anorexia, nausea, vomiting, orthostatic hypotension, and mental disturbances. Anorexia, nausea, and orthostatic hypotension usually occur only during the first few days or weeks of treatment. Tolerance develops very rapidly and their occurrence may be minimized by initiating therapy with small doses and gradually increasing dosage until a clinical response is obtained. Rarely the ortho-static hypotension may be quite severe, resulting in syncope and necessi-tating withdrawal of therapy.[40,42] Anorexia usually subsides within a week or two. Later, patients may develop increased appetite and gain weight.[41] A rare "initiation side-effect" has been activation of quiescent duodenal ulcer with hemorrhage and hematemesis.[41,42] Death from hemorrhagic peptic ulcer has been described in patients receiving Bromo-criptine for the treatment of acromegaly.[43] Special care should be exer-cised in patients who have a history of peptic ulceration.

Bromocriptine will enhance the choreiform dyskinesias induced by Levodopa and thus, as its dosage is gradually increased, it is usually necessary to reduce the dosage of Levodopa. A dosage of 40 to 60 mg of Bromocriptine requires approximately a 50% reduction of the dosage of Levodopa.

The most frequent and distressing side effect has been the induction of mental disturbances. Confusion, agitation, visual hallucinations, and frank delirium may occur. In some clinical trials, such mental distur-bance developed in as many as 50% of patients. Withdrawal of the drug and supportive care usually suffice to manage the psychotoxic reactions. Severe agitation may require emergency use of a narcoleptic such as Haldol.

Several side effects appear to reflect a peripheral vasoconstrictor action similar to that of ergotamine. Digital vasospasm has been observed in several female patients.[43,44] The patient may note acroparesthesiae and blanching or cyanosis of the fingers. Exposure to cold is apt to provoke the phenomenon. Rarely, an acute erythema and edema of the lower extremities may occur.[40,41] Reduction of the dose results in rapid clearing of these symptoms.

The newer drugs Lisuride and Pergolide have similar side effects but appear to be less psychotoxic.

References

1. Albuquerque EX: Amantadine: neuromuscular blockade by suppression of tonic conductance of the acetylcholine receptor. *Science* **199**:708-9, 1978.
2. Peng MT: Locus of emetic actions of epinepherine and dopa in dogs. *J Pharmacol Exptl Ther* **139**:345-349, 1963.

3. McGeer PL, Zeldowicz LR: Administration of dihydroxyphenylalamine to parkinsonian patients. *Can M Assoc J* 90:463, 1964.
4. Yahr MD, Duvoisin RC, Schear MJ, et al: Treatment of parkinsonism with Levodopa. *Arch Neurol* 21:343-354, 1969.
5. Lee JE, Sweet RD, McDowell FH: Treatment of parkinsonism with Levodopa. *Ann Int Med* 75:703-708, 1971.
6. Duvoisin RC: Diphenidol for Levodopa induced nausea and vomiting. *JAMA* 221:1408, 1972.
7. Lotti VJ, Porter CC: Potentiation and inhibition of some central actions of L-Dopa by decarboxylase inhibitors. *J Pharmacol Exptl Ther* 172: 406-415, 1970.
8. Barbeau A: Long-term appraisal of Levodopa therapy. *Neurology* 22: Part 2- 22-24, 1972.
9. Barbeau A: Diphasic dyskinesia during Levodopa therapy. *Lancet* 1: 756, 1975.
10. Muenter M, Sharpless NS, Tyce GM, et al: Patterns of Dystonia (I-D-I) and (D-I-D) in Response to L-dopa therapy for Parkinson's disease. *Mayo Clin Proc* 52:163-174, 1977.
11. Calne DB, Brennan J, Spiers ASD, et al: Hypotension caused by L-dopa. *Brit Med J* 1:474-475, 1970.
12. Hoehn MM: Levodopa-induced postural hypotension. Treatment with fluorocortisone. *Arch Neurol* 32:50-51, 1975.
13. Whitsett TL, Halushka PV, Goldberg LI: Attenuation of post ganglionic sympathetic nerve activity of L-dopa. *Circulation Res* 27:561-570, 1970.
14. Reid JL, Calne DB, George LF, et al: Levodopa and amine sensitivity in parkinsonism. *Clin Pharmacol Ther* 13:400-406, 1972.
15. McNay JL, Goldberg LI: Comparison of the effects of dopamine, isoproterenol, norepinephrine and bradykinesia on canine renal and femoral blood flow. *J Pharmacol Exptl Ther* 151:23-31, 1966.
16. Reid JL, Calne DB, George CF, et al: The action of L-dopa on baroreflexes in parkinsonism. *Clin Science* 43:851-859, 1972.
17. Calne DB, Rao S, Reid JL, et al: The action of L-alpha methyldopahydrazine on the blood pressure of patients receiving Levodopa. *Brit J Pharmacol* 44:162-164, 1972.
18. Goldberg, LI, Whitsett TL: Cardiovascular actions of Levodopa and dopamine. *JAMA* 218:1921-1923, 1971.
19. Mars H, Krall J: L-dopa and cardiac arrhythmias. *N Engl J Med* 285:1437, 1971.
20. Spiers ASD, Calne DB: Action of dopamine on the human iris. *Brit Med J* 2:333-335, 1969.
21. Duvoisin RC, Yahr MD: Behavioral abnormalities occurring in parkinsonism during treatment with L-dopa. In *L-dopa and Behavior*. Malitz S, ed. New York, Raven Press, 1972.
22. Goodwin FK: Psychiatric side effects of Levodopa in man. *JAMA* 218: 1915-1928, 1971.
23. Jenkins RB, Groh RH: Mental symptoms in parkinsonian patients treated with L-dopa. *Lancet* 2:177-180, 1970.

24. Celesia GG, Barr AN: Psychosis and other psychiatric manifestations of Levodopa therapy. *Arch Neurol* **23**:193-200, 1970.
25. Gilbert GJ: Hallucinations from Levodopa. *JAMA* **235**:597, 1976.
26. Cotzias GC, Van Woert MH, Schiffer LM: Aromatic amino acids and modification of parkinsonism. *N Engl J Med* **276**:374-379, 1967.
27. Henry RE, Goldberg LI, Sturgen P, et al: Serologic abnormalities associated with L-dopa therapy. *Vox Sang* **20**:306-316, 1971.
28. Joseph C: Occurrence of positive Coombs test in patients treated with Levodopa. *N Engl J Med* **286**:1401-1402, 1972.
29. Territo MC, Peters RW, Tanaka KR: Autoimmune hemolytic anemia due to Levodopa therapy. *JAMA* **226**:1347-1348, 1973.
30. Lindstrom FD, Lieden G, Engstrom MS: Dose-related Levodopa-induced haemolytic anemia. *Ann Int Med* **86**:298-300, 1977.
31. Gabor EP, Goldberg LI: Levodopa induced Coombs positive haemolytic anemia. *Scand J Haematol* **11**:201-203, 1973.
32. Wanamaker WM, Wanamaker SJ, Celesia GG, et al: Thrombocytopenia associated with long term Levodopa therapy. *JAMA* **226**:2217-2219, 1976.
33. Porteus HB: Mental symptoms in parkinsonism following Benhexol HCl therapy. *Brit Med J* **2**:138, 1956.
34. Duvoisin RC, Katz R: Reversal of central anticholinergic syndrome in man by physostigmine. *JAMA* **206**:1963-1965, 1968.
35. Duvoisin RC: Hyperkinetic reactions with L-dopa. In *Current Concepts in the Treatment of Parkinsonism*. Yahr MD ed. New York, Raven Press, 1974, pp 203-210.
36. Postma JV, Van Tilburg W: Visual hallucinations and delirium during treatment with amantadine (Symmetrel). *J Am Geriat Soc* **23**:212-215, 1975.
37. Casey DE: Amantadine intoxication reversed by physostigmine. *N Engl J Med* **298**:516, 1978.
38. Shealy CN, Weeth JB, Mercier D: Livido reticularis in patients with parkinsonism receiving amantadine. *JAMA* **212**:1522-1523, 1970.
39. Peerce LA, Waterbury LD, Green HD: Amantadine hydrochloride alteration in peripheral circulation. *Neurology* **24**:46-48, 1974.
40. Teychenne PE, Calne DB, Leigh PO, et al: Idiopathic parkinsonism treated with Bromocriptine. *Lancet* **2**:473-476, 1975.
41. Duvoisin RC, Mendoza MR, Yahr MD, et al: Bromocriptine as an adjuvant to Levodopa. In *Dopaminergic Ergot Derivatives and Motor Function*. Fuxe E, Calne DB, eds. New York, Pergamon Press, 1979.
42. Kissner DG, Jarrett JC: Side effects of Bromocriptine. *N Engl J Med* **302**:749, 1980.
43. Wass JAH, Thorner MO, Morris DV, et al: Long-term treatment of acromegaly with Bromocriptine. *Brit Med J* **1**:874, 1977.
44. Duvoisin RC: Digital vasospasm with Bromocriptine. *Lancet* **2**:204, 1976.

Chapter XVI

Autonomic Nervous System Complications of Therapy

Amos D. Korczyn, M.D., M.Sc.,
and Allan E. Rubenstein, M.D.

The autonomic complications of drugs used in therapeutic doses include pupillary changes, lack of salivation, orthostatic hypotension, impotence, urinary incontinence and retention, intestinal pseudo-obstruction and thermo-regulatory problems. The mechanisms which are involved in the production of these problems will be discussed, though our understanding of the physiological processes involved in normal autonomic function is incomplete.

The classical distinction between the sympathetic and parasympathetic systems, working in antagonistic manners, is of limited validity. For example, the performance of the sexual act by males necessitates simultaneous activation of both. There are also many more neurotransmitters involved in peripheral autonomic system action than the two classical agents, acetylcholine and norepinephrine.[1-3] In addition, the concept of modulation of neuro-effector transmission by pre- and post-synaptic receptors is only beginning to be explored. [4,5] Finally, our understanding of central autonomic regulation is rudimentary.

Orthostatic Hypotension

On assumption of an upright posture by man, blood tends to pool in capacitance vessels in the lower limbs and mesentric circulation, resulting in decreased cardiac filling and reduced output. The gravitational effect is immediately sensed by the carotid and aortic baroreceptors which increase sympathetic tone by reflex action. The resultant vasoconstriction counteracts the tendency of blood to pool in the lower part of the body. If this is insufficient, sympathetic tone will be increased further and cause positive chronotropic and inotropic effects on the heart, which can be experienced as palpitations. These relatively simple reflex actions are susceptible to interference by drugs at various levels.

Orthostatic dizziness is a common complaint, experienced by almost every person from time to time. Orthostatic dizziness is not necessarily associated with orthostatic hypotension (OH). Dizziness will be felt when blood supply to the brain is insufficient, and this may occur even when blood pressure is normal. Baroreceptor reflexes increase peripheral resistance so that blood pressure remains maintained, but tissue perfusion may still fall. Conversely, OH may be unaccompanied by subjective phenomena if cerebral blood flow is not excessively reduced; thus, autoregulation may maintain proper cerebral perfusion in spite of systemic hypotension.

Although OH is not always recognized subjectively, periods of suboptimal blood pressure are not necessarily innocuous. It has been speculated that OH may predispose to cerebral and cardiac ischemia and infarction,[6] and could aggravate angina pectoris. Failure of cerebral autoregulation, which occurs relatively frequently in the elderly, may make these patients more susceptible to cerebral damage from OH.[7] The view that the elderly are particularly prone to develop OH either spontaneously or in response to drugs,[8,9] was challenged recently by Myers et al.[10] Other conditions which favor the development of OH are exercise or a post-exercise period,[11] ambient heat, and debilitated state. Prolonged bed rest is also a well-recognized predisposing factor.

Three groups of drugs frequently lead to the development of OH. These are the antihypertensive, antiparkinsonian, and psychiatric drugs.

Since the advent of antihypertensive therapy, OH has been a troublesome side effect. Elderly patients appear to be more susceptible.[12] The severity of OH in antihypertensives acting directly on autonomic ganglia was a major reason for the withdrawal from the market of the drugs pentolinium, hexamethonium, and mecamylamine.[13] The adrenergic neuron blockers guanethidine, bethanidine, and debrisoquine — are not widely used for the same reason. Monoamine oxidase inhibitors (nialamide, pargyline, phenelzine, and tranylcypromine), reduce blood-pressure and may lead to OH, possibly secondarily to accumulation of octopamine as a false neurotransmitter in sympathetic terminals. Newer agents, acting mainly centrally, produce OH much less commonly, and the use of combined therapy (diuretics and beta-blockers) has further decreased its incidence.

Direct smooth-muscle relaxants which are used in the treatment of hypertension are unlikely to produce OH. This is probably because their main action is on resistance rather than capacitance vessels. An exception to this rule is prazocin.[14] OH caused by this drug is particularly common after the first exposure. This effect is dose-dependent.[15] On the other hand, drugs used as vasodilators (such as xanthines) commonly induce OH.

Beta blockers alleviate hypertension through unknown mechanisms, which are probably related to abolition of cardiovascular reflexes.[16] Although this might be expected to lead to OH, it is a rare complication of these drugs.

There is some division of opinion as to whether chronic use of diuretics may lead to OH.[10,17] Further discussion of the complications of antihypertensive medication may be found in Chapter II of this book.

Antiparkinsonian drugs may cause OH. This is true for amantadine,[18] which is also known to produce livedo reticularis and dependent edema.[19] OH, and more rarely cardiac arrhythmias, may occur during levodopa therapy; addition of benserazide does not abolish this side effect.[20] The addition of carbidopa usually helps prevent OH. Occasionally OH can occur with small doses of bromocriptine[21] which may also induce other cardiovascular disturbances such as Raynaud-like symptoms, blanching of the extremities, an erythromelalgia-like syndrome, bradycardia, left ventricular failure, and aggravation of angina pectoris.[22] The mechanism of OH in this case is thought to involve inhibition of norepinephrine release from nerve terminals.[23] Antimuscarinics are much less troublesome in that respect. See Chapter XV for more details.

OH commonly occurs in patients treated with tricyclic antidepressants[24,25] as well as with monoamine oxidase inhibitors. OH usually develops during chronic use; in a controlled trial single doses of imipramine of up to 175 mg i.v. failed to induce significant effects.[26] This is not surprising because the acute effects of tricyclic drugs would tend to increase sympathetic tone by inhibition of catecholamine reuptake, and would result in potentiation of the effect of extrinsically applied sympathomimetics.[27] Minor and major tranquilizers are also associated with OH in the elderly.[12] See Chapter VI in this book for further discussion of neurological complications of tranquilizers.

The anticancer drug cyclocytine produces OH[28] probably consequent to its absorption by sympathetic terminals.[29] OH has also been reported after the use of vincristine,[30,31] usually accompanied by manifestations of generalized neuropathy and occasionally with other autonomic problems. See Chapter III in this book for further details.

OH is one of the features of diabetic neuropathy. At times, the manifestations are exacerbated by insulin treatment. This may be due to the fact that insulin administration results in a decrease of plasma volume.[32]

Finally, hypertension accompanied by severe OH developed in patients treated with the sympathomimetic agent phenylpropanolamine used as an anorexic,[33] and OH developed subsequent to pseudoephedrine therapy.[34] The mechanism of this paradoxical effect is unknown.

Urinary Difficulties

Urination is primarily a parasympathetic action, and the drugs which commonly affect it are likely to possess antimuscarinic action. However, in normal subjects, very high doses of atropine will not necessarily result in urinary retention.

Urinary complications induced by drugs usually consist of difficulty in initiating urination, hesitancy, and frank retention. These effects are more likely to appear in elderly males, in whom mechanical factors contribute to interference with urine flow.

The major group of drugs which cause urination difficulties are the antimuscarinic agents. Several drugs used for other purposes have antimuscarinic effects such as the antihistamines (for example, cyclizine, diethazine, diphenhydramine and orphenadrine). Disopyramide, a cardiac anti-arrhythmic agent with an antimuscarinic action, can produce urinary retention.[35] Ganglion blockers may have a similar action. These effects are probably due to competitive inhibition with cholinergic transmission at the detrusor muscle, interfering with contraction of that muscle.

Some degree of urinary retention is common in patients on tricyclic antidepressants or neuroleptics, although clinical problems do not always ensue.[36,37,38] Urinary hesitancy, retention, or overflow incontinence are well-established side effects of major tranquillizers with marked antimuscarinic actions. These effects are particularly prone to develop with combined use of several drugs. Stress incontinence has also been reported with phenothiazines.[39,40]

Tricyclic antidepressants used by an expectant mother can induce urinary retention in the neonate.[41]

The action of tricyclic antidepressants on micturition is helpful in the treatment of nocturnal enuresis, though studies of the underlying mechanism of drug action in this situation cast doubt on the assumption that the effect is purely due to the antimuscarinic action of the drugs.[42]

Alpha-adrenergic stimulants, such as ephedrine, can cause urinary retention;[43] this drug has also been reported to be useful in nocturnal enuresis. Alpha-adrenergic blockers, such as phenoxybenzamine, are sometimes used to facilitate micturition in patients with neurogenic retention. Iproniazide and isoniazide are also thought to cause hesitancy. Hydralazine can induce urinary retention, as do ganglioplegic drugs used to treat hypertension.[13]

Morphine causes spasm of the smooth muscles of the urinary tract, including the sphincter. Retention of urine occurs partly because of that and partly because the patient may not realize that the bladder is full. Hypotonicity of the bladder was reported after benzodiazapines.[44]

Urinary incontinence and frequency were reported after prazocin treatment,[45] and urinary frequency was reported after the administration of dantrolene sodium.[46]

Vincristine-induced autonomic neuropathy may also lead to urinary incontinence, and a similar condition may be caused by disulfiram.[47]

Impotence

In males, erection is primarily controlled by the parasympathetic system, which also causes the propulsion of semen to the urethra. Sympathetic influences cause tonic-clonic contractions of the bulbo-cavernous muscles. Additional sympathetic effects are required to close the internal urinary sphincter in order to avoid retrograde flow of semen into the bladder. This complicated process can be interfered with by drugs which act on either part of the autonomic nervous system.

The most widely known, and probably the most common, drug effects on sexual function occur with antihypertensive drugs.[48] Ganglion blockers such as hexamethonium and pentolinium, and adrenergic neuron blockers, such as guanethidine and bethanidine, when used in amounts needed to control blood pressure, interfere with erection in more than two-thirds of patients;[49] failure of ejaculation is also common. Similar effects occur with reserpine. Other antihypertensives which may cause erectile failure are clonidine, which can also result in retrograde ejaculation in men and inability to achieve orgasm in women,[50] and alpha-methyldopa.[51] Decreased libido, impotence, and failure of ejaculation are infrequent side effects of propranolol;[52] a change to atenolol has been suggested in this situation.[53] In the case of propranolol, it has been suggested that vasoconstriction is induced in penile arteries, thus preventing successful erection.[54] The mechanism is therefore similar to that of Raynaud syndrome attributed to that drug.

Patients on antipsychotic drugs frequently develop sexual dysfunction. The pathogenesis of impotence induced by phenothiazines and related drugs is unclear. Possible mechanisms include the antimuscarinic and adrenolytic effects of the major tranquilizers and possibly elevation of serum prolactin. Hyperprolactinemic states are known to be associated with impotence and infertility.

Erectile problems and delayed orgasm are reported to occur during treatment with tricyclic antidepressants; in males these are accompanied by delayed ejaculation.[55,56] Lithium can also inhibit erection.[57]

Impotence and delayed ejaculation in males and difficulty to achieve orgasm by women were reported to occur during phenelzine treatment.[58]

Fenfluramine can induce male impotence and inhibit libido in women, particularly with high doses.[59] These effects are apparently not seen with amphetamine therapy.

Methanteline, a propantheline analogue used in the treatment of duodenal ulcer, has been reported to produce impotence relatively frequently. This may be related to its relatively strong ganglioplegic action.[60]

Disopyramide, a cardiac anti-arrhythmic agent with antimuscarinic action, was suspected to prevent erection.[61] Impotence has also been reported with clofibrate and with spironolactone and estrogens; the actions of the latter two drugs are probably secondary to endocrinologic effects.[62,63]

Male sexual dysfunction has been reported with cimetidine treatment, specifically loss of libido and later difficulties in obtaining erection.[64,65] It was speculated that hormonal factors are responsible[64] but this is an unlikely explanation.[66] Although it is usually stated that the neurotransmitter involved in erection is acetylcholine, direct evidence for this is meager and recently it was suggested that histamine may be an inhibitory transmitter leading to vasodilation and erection.[67] If this were so, then the impotence induced by cimetidine could be due to blockade receptors in the body of the penis.[68]

Morphine and other opiates (including methadone) depress sexual activity markedly. This is presumably related to lack of desire rather than to lack of ability. Erection is usually maintained while ejaculation is often delayed or absent.

Other drugs which are implicated as inducers of male sexual dysfunction include anticholinergic agents, vincristine, and abuse of opiates, barbiturates, and alcohol.[69,70]

Intestinal Pseudo-obstruction

Intestinal pseudo-obstruction is a syndrome in which the signs and symptoms of mechanical bowel obstruction are present, specifically paralytic ileus, but no mechanical cause can be found. Synonyms for this condition include idiopathic large bowel obstruction, Ogilvie syndrome, mucous colitis, megacolon, and megasigmoid.[71] Among the recognized causes of the condition, drugs play a major role. When paralytic ileus occurs, absorption of an offending oral drug may be slowed, and consequently the effect may be prolonged. Paralytic ileus may be induced by drugs with antimuscarinic activity, including phenothiazine antipsychotics, tricyclic antidepressants, and anticholinergic antiparkinsonian agents[71,72] as well as antihistamines. The syndrome is particularly likely to occur when several agents with antimuscarinic action are used simultaneously, as with Lomotil which contains both diphenoxylate and atropine. Though this condition should ostensibly be responsive to treatment with cholinesterase inhibitors or direct muscarinic agonists, treatment with physostigmine or bentanechol has been disappointing and fatalities have been reported.[76] Opiates may also be responsible for this condition, presumably by inhibiting acetylcholine release. This effect may be severe, and particularly with the use of long acting drugs (e.g. methadone) may be fatal.[73] Tricyclic antidepressants and clonidine can also cause the syndrome.[74]

Paralytic ileus was attributed to cimetidine treatment in patients suffering from severe burns.[75]

The chronic use of ganglion blockers can cause pharmacologic parasympathectomy as well as sympathectomy, and several cases of paralytic ileus were recorded when pentolinium, hexamethonium, and mecamylamine were used for the treatment of hypertension.[13,76] Constipation has been reported with monoamine oxidase inhibitors.

Vincristine may induce an autonomic neuropathy, with constipation or paralytic ileus as a manifestation.[31] The constipation is probably due to a toxic effect on the myenteric plexus;[77] it was reported to respond to lactulose.[78]

Temperature

Normal temperature depends on a delicate balance between the rate of heat production, absorption, and dissipation. Each of these factors is complex. Heat loss itself may be caused by behavioral effects (e.g. moving into a cool area), peripheral vasodilation, sweating, and hyperventilation. Heat loss is diminished by reversal of these processes and also by piloerection.

Drugs may interfere with normal temperature by changing metabolic rate, impairing peripheral mechanisms of heat loss, or by altering the function of the central "thermostat." Clinical disturbances are relatively uncommon. When a reaction does occur, however, it can be catastrophic, terminating in cardiovascular collapse and death. Rhabdomyolysis from hyperpyrexia induced by drugs has been reported.[79]

Interference with temperature regulation can induce hyper- or hypothermia, depending on factors such as generalized activity and ambient heat and humidity. Phenothiazines and other major tranquilizers which may be used clinically in the production of surgical hypothermia may lead to accidental hypothermia or severe pyrexia, either of which may cause death. It is assumed that subjects with inefficient thermoregulatory mechanisms are more sensitive to these drug effects; such reactions are more common in infants, the elderly, and in debilitated subjects. Hyperthermic effects are facilitated by concurrent administration of antimuscarinic drugs (frequently used to counteract extrapyramidal side effect of phenothiazines), because they interfere with heat dissipation through sweating.

Maternal use of clomipramine was associated with hypothermia in a neonate.[80]

The malignant syndrome following administration of major tranquilizers consists of severe hypokinetic rigidity of muscles, hyperpyrexia, hypertension, and tachycardia occasionally leading to coma and cardiovascular collapse.[81] It is thought to be due to a combination of the extrapyramidal and autonomic effects of the neuroleptics. Treatment includes withdrawal of all psychoactive drugs and administration of amantadine as well as appropriate supportive therapy.[38]

Combined treatment with lithium carbonate and diazepam was associated with profound hypothermia in a mentally retarded patient,[82] as was treatment with nitrazepam and diazepam alone in patients in their ninth decade.[9,83] The mechanism of hypothermia is probably nonspecific CNS depression, but an additional antithyroid effect has been suggested.[44] Barbiturates are also hazardous in these subjects, as is alcohol, which produces CNS depression and peripheral vasodilation. Lithium administration to an expectant mother resulted in CNS depression and hypothermia in the newborn.[84]

Febrile reactions to drugs are common, and are usually the manifestation of allergic or toxic phenomena. They may even occur with antipyretic drugs.[85] Other manifestations of hypersensitivity (rash, eosinophilia etc.) may or may not be present.[86]

Some drugs occasionally cause pyrexia through unidentified mechanisms. These include cimetidine,[87] which may act by blockade of H_2 receptors involved with thermoregulation.[88]

Other drugs which may cause fever are barbiturates, phenytoin, cocaine, antibiotics and isoniazid.[89,90]

Malignant hyperpyrexia is a rare manifestation of general anesthesia, and has previously been described in Chapter VII in this book. It occurs primarily after inhalation of halogenated hydrocarbon anesthetics (such as halothane and enflurane) and neuromuscular depolarizing blockers (e.g., suxamethonium). The syndrome consists of increased skeletal muscle activity leading to rigidity, fever, hyperpotassemia and metabolic acidosis, accompanied by hypoxia, respiratory acidosis, and cardiac abnormalities. The elevated temperature results from the hypermetabolic state. Malignant hyperthermia may be due to an insufficiency of the intracellular mechanisms of calcium inactivation. The condition is often familial, frequently affecting young patients undergoing minor surgery. Patients and affected relatives may have elevated creatine phosphokinase levels. Treatment with dantrolene sodium is probably the best available, but is still unsatisfactory.[91,92]

Patients treated with beta blockers may complain of cold extremities, and occasionally severe Raynaud phenomena may occur, including the disappearance of peripheral pulses.[93] The pathogenesis is unknown but may be due to unopposed alpha adrenergic stimulation leading to vasoconstriction.

Pupil

Mydriasis can occur after the use of antimuscarinic agents, but excessive doses have to be administered systemically to produce pupillary dilation. Antiparkinsonian drugs used in therapeutic doses do not affect pupillary size.[94] Inadvertent conjunctival application may produce mydriasis, as has been reported following the use of propantheline bromide as an antiperspirant.[95] The effect on the pupil is prolonged, being maintained for several days, and accommodation is affected to a lesser degree. The mydriasis from atropine cannot be explained solely by muscarinic blockade.[96] A simple way to distinguish this condition from other causes of mydriasis is the use of 2% pilocarpine eye drops, to which no response should occur if the mydriasis is produced by antimuscarinic drugs.[97]

Most neuroleptics, even those with marked antimuscarinic actions such as chlorpromazine do not dilate the pupil but rather cause dose-dependent miosis which has been used to analyze the bioavailability of the drug.[98] Also, significant reduction of the pupillary light reflex was observed in schizophrenic patients under long-term administration of psychotropic drugs. As this effect was observed in patients who were on phenothiazines as well as butyrophenones, it cannot be attributed purely to antimuscarinic action of the drugs. In addition, a light-near dissociation was observed in these patients, as well as more rapid redilation.[99] It is therefore likely that a central effect of the drugs contributes to these phenomena.

Corticosteroids applied locally to the eye produce mydriasis. The light reflex is preserved, and therefore the effect is unlikely to be due to interruption of parasympathetic action. The mydriasis may be accompanied by ptosis.[100,101]

A state of fatigue is accompanied by miosis and hippus, or fluctuation of pupillary size.[102] Any CNS depressant may induce miosis of a mild degree. A marked miosis, where the pupil reaches pinpoint diameter, is usually caused by opiates and is reversed by naloxone. Pupillary size and reactions have an important place in differentiating the etiology of coma, as pontine hemorrhage can also cause extreme miosis. It is interesting that in most non-human species the pupillary effects of opiates consist of dilation rather than constriction.[103] Although it was believed for a long time that tolerance does not develop to the pupillary effect of opiates, recent investigations refute this.[104]

A slight degree of miosis occurs during treatment with alpha-methyldopa,[105] as well as during treatment with cholinesterase inhibitors, such as prostigmine and pyridostigmine.

References

1. Burnstock G: Non-adrenergic, non-cholinergic nerves in the intestine and their possible involvement in secretion. In: *Mechanisms of Intestinal Secretion.* Alan R Liss, New York 1979a, pp 147-174.
2. Burnstock G: Interactions of cholinergic, adrenergic, purinergic and peptidergic neurons in the gut. In: Brooks C McC, et al, eds, *Integrative Functions of the Autonomic Nervous System,* University of Tokyo Press, Tokyo, 1979b, pp 145-158.
3. Burnstock G: Purinergic nerves. In: Bevan JA, et al, eds, *Vascular Neuro-effector Mechanisms.* Raven Press, New York, 1980a, pp 181-182.
4. Langer SZ: Presynaptic receptors and their role in the regulation of trans-mitter release. *Brit J Pharmacol* **60**:481, 1977.
5. Burnstock G: Purinergic modulation of cholinergic transmission. *Gen Pharmacol* **11**:15, 1980b.
6. Goldberg AD, Raferty EB: Patterns of blood-pressure during chronic administration of postganglionic sympathetic blocking drugs for hy-pertension. *Lancet* **1**:1052, 1976.
7. Wollner L, McCarthy ST, Soper NDW, et al: Failure of cerebral auto-regulation as a cause of brain dysfunction in the elderly. *Brit Med J* **1**: 1117, 1979.
8. Johnson RH, Smith AC, Spalding MJK: Effect of posture on blood-pressure in elderly patients. *Lancet* **1**:731, 1965.
9. Irvine RE: Hypothermia due to diazepam. *Brit Med J* **2**:1007, 1966.
10. Myers MG, Kearns PM, Kennedy DS, et al: Postural hypotension and diuretic therapy in the elderly. *Can Med Assoc J* **119**:581, 1978.
11. Talbot S, Gill GW: Exertional hypotension due to postganglionic sym-pathetic blocking drugs. *Postgrad Med J* **52**:487, 1976.
12. Jackson G, Pierscianowski TA, Mahon W, et al: *Geriat* **99**:94, 1973.
13. Grimson KS, Orgain ES, Rowe CR, et al: Caution with regard to use of hexamethonium and "Apresoline." *JAMA* **149**:215, 1952.
14. Thien Th, Koene RAP, Wijdeveld PGAB: Orthostatic hypotension due to prazocin. *Lancet* **1**:366, 1977.
15. Rosendorff C: Prazocin: severe side effects are dose-dependent. *Brit Med J* **2**:508, 1976.
16. Korczyn AD Goldberg G: Inhibition of hypertensive reflexes by pro-pranolol. *Res Commun Chem Pathol Pharmacol* **7**:145, 1974.
17. Irvine RE: When postural hypotension signals disease. *Geriat* **99**:94, 1973.
18. Sigwald J, Raymondeaud C, Gregoire J: Le traitement de la maladie de Parkinson par l'amantadine. *Therapeutique* **48**:555, 1972.

19. Silver DE, Sahs AL: Livedo reticularis in Parkinson's disease patients treated with amantadine hydrochloride. *Neurology* 22:665, 1972.
20. Gauthier G, Juge O, Birchler A: Parkinsonian syndromes. Treatment by association of l-dopa plus decarboxylase inhibitors. *Eur Neurol* 11: 133, 1974.
21. Linch DC, Saw KM, Muhlemann MF, et al: Bromocriptine-induced postural hypotension in acromegaly. *Lancet* 2:320, 1978.
22. Calne DB, Plotkin C, Williams AC, et al: Long-term treatment of parkinsonism with bromocriptine. *Lancet* 1:735, 1978.
23. Ziegler MG, Laker CR, Williams AC, et al: Bromocriptine inhibits norepinephrine release. *Clin Pharmacol TGher* 25:137, 1979.
24. Hayes JR, Born GF, Rosenbaum AH: Incidence of orthostatic hypotension in patients with primary affective disorders treated with tricyclic antidepressants. *Mayo Clin Proc* 52:509, 1977.
25. Glassman AH, Bigger JT, Giardina EV, et al: Clinical characteristics of imipramine-induced orthostatic hypotension. *Lancet* 1:468, 1979.
26. Dencker SJ, Bake BS: Investigation of the orthostatic reaction after intravenous administration of imipramine, chlorimipramine and imipramine-N-Oxide. *Acta Psych Scand* 54:74, 1976.
27. Boakes AJ, Laurence DR, Teoh PC, et al: Interactions between sympathomimetic and antidepressant agents in man. *Brit Med J* 1:311, 1973.
28. Window RA, Gottlieb JA, O'Bryan RM, et al: Myelotoxicity and orthostatic hypotension of cyclocytidine. *Cancer Treat Rep* 60:215, 1976.
29. Burks TF, Loo TT, Grubb MN: Mechanism of the cardiovascular actions of cyclocytidine. *Proc Soc Exp Biol Med* 159:374, 1978.
30. Aisner J, Weiss HD, Chang P, et al: Orthostatic hypotension during combination chemotherapy with vincristine. *Cancer Chemother Rep* 58: 927, 1974.
31. Hancock BW, Naysmith A: Vincristine-induced autonomic neuropathy. *Brit Med J* 3:207, 1975.
32. Gundersen HJG, Christensen NJ: Intravenous insulin causing loss of intravascular water and albumin and increased adrenergic nervous activity in diabetics. *Diabetes* 6:551, 1977.
33. Horowitz JD, McNeil JJ, Sweet B, et al: Hypertension induced by phenylpropanolamine (Trimolets). *Med J Aust* 1:175, 1976.
34. Beary JF: Pseudoephedrine producing postural hypotension in a pilot. *Aviat Space Environ Med* 48:369, 1977.
35. Large SH, Todd CH: Disopyramide-associated urinary retention. *Lancet* 2:1362, 1977.
36. Appel P, Eckel K, Harrer G: Veranderungen des Blasen- und Blasensphinkertonus durch thymoleptika. *Int Pharmacopsychiat* 6:15, 1971.
37. Merril DC, Markland C: Vesical dysfunction induced by the major tranquilizers. *J Urol* 107:769, 1972.
38. Korczyn AD: The major tranquilizers. In: MNG Dukes, ed *Meyler's Side Effects of Drugs.* 9th ed, Excerpta Medica, Amsterdam, 1980, p 84.
39. Shaikh A: Urinary incontinence during treatment with depot phenothiazines. *Brit Med J* 1:1698, 1978.
40. Van Putten T, Malkin MD, Weiss MS: Phenothiazine-induced stress incontinence. *J Urol* 109:625, 1973.
41. Shearer WT, Schreiner RL, Marshall RE: Urinary retention in a neonate secondary to maternal ingestion of nortriptyline. *J Pediatr* 81:570, 1972.
42. Korczyn AD, Kish I: The mechanism of imipramine in eneuresis noc-

turna. *Clin Exp Pharmacol Physiol* **6**:31, 1979.
43. Glidden RS, Dibona FJ: Urinary retention association with ephedrine. *J Pediatr* **90**:1013, 1977.
44. Korczyn AD: Hypnotics and sedatives. In: MNG Dukes, ed *Meyler's Side Effects of Drugs.* 9th ed, Excerpta Medica, Amsterdam, 1980 p 59.
45. Thien TH Delaere KPJ, Debruyne FMJ, et al: Urinary incontinence caused by prazosin, *Brit Med J* **1**:623, 1978.
46. Ostergard DR: The effect of drugs on the lower urinary tract. *Obstet Gynecol Surg* **34**:242, 1979.
47. Vincent E, Chopinet P: Trouble mictionnels sous traitment au disulfirame. *J Urol Nephrol* **79**:491, 1973.
48. Editorial: Drugs affecting autonomic functions or the extrapyramidal system. In: MNG Dukes, ed *Meyler's Side Effects of Drugs.* 9th ed, Excerpta Medica, Amsterdam, 1980, p 230.
49. Bulpitt CJ, Dollery CT: Side effects of hypotensive agents evaluated by a self-administered questionnaire. *Brit Med J* **3**:485, 1973.
50. Anonymous: Clonidine (Catapres) and other drugs causing sexual dysfunction. *Med Lett Drugs Ther* **19**:81, 1977.
51. Newman RJ, Salerno HR: Sexual dysfunction due to methyldopa. *Brit Med J* **4**:106, 1974.
52. Knarr JW: Impotence from propranolol? *Ann Intern Med* **75**:259, 1976.
53. Bathen JH: Propranolol erectile dysfunction relieved. *Ann Intern Med* **88**:716, 1978.
54. Forsberg L, Gustavil B, Hojerback T, et al: Impotence, smoking and beta-blocking drugs. *Fertil Steril* **31**:589, 1979.
55. Couper-Smartt JD, Rodham R: A technique for surveying side-effects of tricyclic drugs with reference to reported sexual effects. *J Int Med Res* **1**:473, 1973.
56. Beaumont G: Sexual side-effects of clomipramine (Anafranil). *J Int Med Res* **1**:480, 1973.
57. Vinarova E, Uhlir O, Stika L, et al: Side effects of lithium administration. *Act Nerv Super* (Praha), **14**:104, 1972.
58. Wyatt RJ, Fram DH, Buchbinder R, et al: Treatment of intractable narcolepsy with a monoamine oxidase inhibitor. *N Engl J Med* **285**:987, 1971.
59. Pinder RM, Brogden RN, Sawyer PR, et al: Fenfluramine: A review of its pharmacological properties and therapeutic efficacy in obesity. *Drugs* **10**:241, 1975.
60. Dukes MNG: Drugs affecting autonomic functions or the extrapyramidal system. In: MNG Dukes, ed, *Meyler's Side Effects of Drugs.* 9th ed, Excerpta Medica, Amsterdam, 1980, p 230.
61. McHaffie DJ, Guz A, Johnston A: Impotence in patient on disopyramide. *Lancet* **1**:859, 1977.
62. Zarren HS, Black P McL: Unilateral gynecomastia and impotence during low-dose spironolactone administration in men. *Milit Med* **140**:417, 1975.
63. Loriaux DL: Spironolactone and endocrine dysfunction. *Ann Intern Med* **85**:630, 1976.
64. Paden NR, Cargill JM, Browning MCK, et al: Male sexual dysfunction during treatment with cimetidine. *Brit Med J* **1**:659, 1979.
65. Wolfe MM: Impotence on cimetidine treatment. *N Engl J Med* **300**:94, 1979.
66. Barber SG: Male sexual dysfunction and cimetidine. *Brit Med J* **1**:1147, 1979.

67. Adaijkan PG, Karim SMN: Effects of histamine on the human penis muscle in vitro. *Eur J Pharmacol* 45:261, 1977.
68. Adaijkin PG, Karim SMN: Male sexual dysfunction during treatment with cimetidine. *Brit Med J* 1:1282, 1979.
69. Levine SB: Marital sexual dysfunction: erectile dysfunction. *Ann Intern Med* 88:716, 1976.
70. Hollister LE: Drugs and sexual behavior in man. *Life Sci* 17:661, 1977.
71. Striam K, Schumer W, Ehrenpreis S, et al: Phenothiazine effect on gastrointestinal tract function. *Am J Surg* 137:87, 1979.
72. Daggett P, Ibrahim SZ: Intestinal obstruction complicating orphenadrine treatment. *Brit Med J* 1:21, 1976.
73. Rubenstein RB, Wolff WI: Methadone ileus syndrome. *Dis Colon Rectum* 19:357, 1976.
74. Zenther-Munro PL, Northfield TC: Drug-induced gastrointestinal disease. *Brit Med J* 1:1263, 1979.
75. Watson WC, Kutty PK, Colcleugh RG: Does cimetidine cause ileus in the burned patient? *Lancet* 2:720, 1977.
76. Becker KL, Sutnick AI: Paralytic ileus simulating acute intestinal obstruction due to pentolinium tartrate (Ansolysen). *Ann Intern Med* 54:313, 1961.
77. Smith B: The myenteric plexus in drug-induced neuropathy. *J Neurol Neurosurg Psychiatry* 30:506, 1967.
78. Smolen VF, Murdock HR, Williams EJ: Bioavailability analysis of chlorpromazine in humans from pupillometric data. *J Pharmacol Exp Therap* 195:404, 1975.
79. Mason J, Thomas E: Rhabdomyolysis from heat hyperpyrexia. *JAMA* 235:633, 1976.
80. Ben Musa A, Smith CS: Neonatal effects of maternal clomipramine therapy. *Arch Dis Child* 54:405, 1979.
81. Greenblatt DJ, Gross PL, Harris J, et al: Fatal hyperthermia following haloperidol therapy of sedative-hypnotic withdrawal. *J Clin Psychiatry* 39:673, 1978.
82. Naylor GL, McHarg A: Profound hypothermia on combined lithium carbonate and diazepam treatment. *Brit Med J* 2:22, 1977.
83. Impallomeni M, Ezzat R: Hypothermia associated with nitrazepam administration. *Brit Med J* 1:223, 1976.
84. Tunnessen WW, Hertz CG: Toxic effects of lithium in newborn infants. *J Pediatr* 81:804, 1972.
85. Mandell B, Shen HS, Hepburn B: Fever from ibuprofen in a patient with lupus erythematosus. *Ann Intern Med* 85:209, 1976.
86. Tierney L: Drug fever. *West J Med* 129:321, 1978.
87. Ramboer C: Drug fever with cimetidine. *Lancet* 1:330, 1978.
88. Nistico G, Rotiroti D, Sarro A, et al: Mechanism of cimetidine-induced fever. *Lancet* 2:265, 1978.
89. Bystryn JC: Drug fever. *Am J Med Sci* 264:47, 1972.
90. Davis RS, Stoler BS: Febrile reactions to I.N.H. *N Engl J Med* 297:337, 1977.
91. Kanpe H: General anaesthetics and therapeutic gases. In: Dukes MNG, ed. *Meyler's Side Effects of Drugs*. 9th ed, Excerpta Medica, Amsterdam, 1980, p 165.
92. Korczyn AD, Shavit S, Schlosberg I: The chick as a model for malignant hyperpyrexia. *Eur J Pharmacol* 61:187, 1980.

93. Marshall AJ, Roberts CJC, Barritt DW: Raynaud's phenomenon as side effect of beta-blockers in hypertension. *Brit Med J* 1:1498, 1976.
94. Korczyn AD, Rubenstein AE, Yahr MD: Pupillary responses in Parkinsonism. In preparation, 1982.
95. Nissen SH, Nielsen PG: Unilateral mydriasis after use of propantheline bromide in an antiperspirant. *Lancet* 2:1134, 1977.
96. Korczyn AD, Laor N: A second component of atropine mydriasis. *Invest Ophthalmol Vis Sci* 16:231, 1977.
97. Thompson HS: Pupil in clinical diagnosis. *Trans Am Acad Ophthalmol Otolaryngol* 83:840, 1977.
98. Smolen VF, Murdock HR, Williams EJ: Bioavailability analysis of chlorpromazine in humans from pupillometric data. *J Pharmacol Exp Therap* 195:404, 1975.
99. Okada F, Kase M, Shintomi Y: Pupillary abnormalities in schizophrenic patients during long-term administration of psychoactive drugs: Dissociation between light and near vision reactions. *Psychopharmacol* 58:235, 1978.
100. Miller D, Peczon D, Whitworth CG: Corticosteroids and functions in the anterior segment of the eye. *Am J Ophthalmol* 59:31, 1965.
101. Newsome DA, Wong VG, Cameron TP, et al: Steroid-induced mydriasis and ptosis. *Invest Ophthalmol Vis Sci* 10:424, 1971.
102. Lowenstein O, Feinberg R, Lowenfeld IE: Pupillary movements during acute and chronic fatigue. A new test for the objective evaluation of tiredness. *Invest Ophthal* 2:138, 1963.
103. Korczyn AD, Boyman R, Shifter L: Morphine mydriasis in mice. *Life Sci* 24:1667, 1979.
104. Adler C, Keren O, Korczyn AD: Tolerance to the pupillary effect of opiates in mice. *J Neural Transmission* 48:43, 1980.
105. Traub Y, Korczyn AD, Sharit G: Effect of treatment with alpha-methyldopa on pupillary sympathetic activity. *Isr J Med Sci* 13:542, 1977.

Chapter XVII

Peripheral Nerve Injury from Venipuncture and Arterial Puncture

William E. Wallis, M.D., F.R.A.C.P.

Introduction

Although peripheral nerve injuries from venipuncture and arterial puncture are only reported rarely, such complications have long been recognized. Weir Mitchell commented upon these accidents and quoted Ambroise Pare's description of Charles IX, who suffered a nerve injury from blood letting.[1] The royal victim made a slow, painful recovery, resembling the course of some of the patients described in this account. The apparent rarity of these injuries is puzzling, considering the widespread use of the procedures and the proximity of peripheral nerves to the commonly chosen veins and arteries. A partial explanation may be found in a review of the pathophysiology of injection injuries to peripheral nerves.

The Mechanism of Nerve Injuries from Venipuncture and Arterial Puncture

Needle puncture of blood vessels can damage peripheral nerves *directly* by the mechanical trauma from the needle, or by neurotoxic effects of injected materials. *Indirect* injuries to the nerve may also occur presumably from tissue swelling, extravasation of blood into a confined fascial space, as well as by subsequent fibrosis. Such indirect effects are more likely to occur from arterial puncture than from venipuncture. The direct and toxic forms of nerve trauma have been well studied experimentally and clinically, but the indirect forms are poorly understood.

Animal experiments show that nerves are difficult to transfix, as they tend to roll away from the approaching needle.[2] In addition, through and through needle punctures and even injections of saline into the nerve may not necessarily produce any visible, histological changes. These factors may partially explain the relative rarity of peripheral nerve injuries from needle puncture.[2,3] The histological changes from direct needle injuries include discrete separation of nerve fibers, open canals through nerve bundles with several nerve fibers cut, herniation of nerve fibers through perineural gaps, and also endoneural hemorrhage. These changes are more likely to occur with large bore needles, particularly those with a long bevel.[2] With direct injection of drugs into nerves, the changes are understandably more impressive.[3,4,5] Here, large myelinated fibers are more susceptible to injury than smaller, thinly myelinated fibers. At the site of the injection, the changes involve the axon as well as the myelin sheath. Nevertheless, the nerve fibers distal to the injury show primarily Wallerian degeneration, rather than segmental demyelination. Histological changes may appear as early as 30 minutes after injection. The severity of the nerve injury depends upon the site of the injection, as well as the type and amount of drug injected. Intrafascicular injections invariably produce severe nerve injuries and extrafascicular injections do so rarely. There is considerable variability in the neurotoxic effects of different drugs. For example, penicillin, diazepam (or its solvent 40% propylene glycol), and chlorpromazine are more likely to produce severe nerve injury than iron, dextran, meperidine, and cephalothin. There is some evidence that the mechanism of these drug-induced injuries may be related to a break-down in the blood-nerve barrier.

In the animal experiments mentioned above, peripheral nerve regeneration subsequently occurs, even with total axonal degeneration. This is clearly not so in all human cases who have suffered peripheral nerve injuries from drug injections or needle punctures. Histological studies of irreversible nerve injuries in humans are sparse.[6] It may be that factors that prevent complete recovery include fibrosis around the nerve from an admixture of blood and drugs, damage to the microvascular supply of the nerve, traumatic neuroma formation, and ischemic nerve injury from bleeding into a confined fascial space.[6,7,8]

The Clinical Syndromes of Venipuncture and Arterial Puncture Nerve Injuries

Brachial Puncture

The median nerve as well as the medial and lateral cutaneous nerves of the forearm lie closely adjacent to the vessels commonly selected for arterial and venous puncture in the antecubital fossa. Diagnostic venipuncture may produce direct needle injuries to these nerves.[9] The injuries are rare, being estimated at only one in 25,000 diagnostic venipunctures. The resulting syndrome presents in a fairly stereotyped fashion. The patient complains of painful swelling in the antecubital fossa with painful radiation down the arm roughly in the sensory distribution of the injured nerve. Decreased sensation or dysesthesia is found in the distribution of the appropriate nerve. Total loss of sensation and motor findings are rare. Tinel's sign in the antecubital fossa is a prominent feature. Patients may also complain of cold fingers, and minor trophic changes can occur, suggesting a causalgia-like syndrome; however, a classical causalgia does not occur. Electrophysiological tests, such as motor conduction velocities and sensory evoked potentials, are usually normal. Recovery occurs spontaneously in most patients in a matter of a few weeks, but some may complain of symptoms for up to three or four months. The pain is usually relieved by anticonvulsant drugs given in dosages suitable for epilepsy.

Rarely, more severe nerve injuries may occur from venipuncture in the antecubital fossa with subsequent swelling as well as extravasation of blood into the arm. These complications are more likely to occur with infiltration of intravenous infusions, and with venipuncture in anticoagulated patients, or in those with blood dyscrasias.[10] In such cases, the author has observed alteration of sensation, not only in the median nerve distribution, but also in the radial and ulnar nerve distribution. Blood may occasionally track down from the venipuncture site in the antecubital fossa and produce compression of the median nerve in the carpal tunnel.[11]

Arterial puncture in the antecubital fossa may produce extremely severe neurological complications. This is particularly true in new-born infants, anticoagulated patients, and those with blood dyscrasias.[6-8,10,12] Massive hemorrhage may occur from the brachial arteries into confined fascial spaces in the forearm and produce potentially irreversible ischemic changes to nerve and muscle. The management of impending muscle and nerve damage from this type of injury is dealt with subsequently under the section of Management.

The radial artery and the superficial tributaries of the cephalic veins along the radial aspect of the wrist are sometimes chosen for needle puncture. The author has observed two types of injury from venipuncture at this site. The first is a nerve injury confined to the sensory branch of the radial nerve with symptoms of numbness and painful paresthesias in the appropriate distribution. The syndrome is usually trivial and resolves spontaneously in a few weeks. The second is a more wide-spread syndrome which is associated with massive infiltration of an intravenous infusion. Here the patient develops a tight, painful swelling of the wrist and hand and may complain of symptoms similar to a carpal tunnel syndrome and show decreased sensation in the median nerve distribution in the hand. Again, recovery is usually complete and apart from reassurance, no further measures are necessary. With *arterial puncture* of the radial artery, particularly in an anticoagulated patient, a compartment syndrome may ensue with serious damage to the median nerve and forearm muscles.[13]

Femoral Puncture

This procedure is almost exclusively done for diagnostic purposes. As the femoral vein and artery are closely associated to the femoral nerve, injury to the femoral nerve may occur with puncture of either of these vessels.[12] Injury to the nerve from *venous puncture* is unusual, and most complications occur from *arterial puncture*. Again, this is particularly true in anticoagulated patients and those with blood dyscrasias. In such patients, massive hemorrhage occurs into the femoral area, with compression of the femoral nerve. Rarely, the blood may track down into the pelvic cavity and damage the lumbosacral plexus.[12] The prognosis of such cases should be guarded.

Supraclavicular Fossa Puncture

Venipuncture of the subclavian vein in the supraclavicular fossa is usually performed for long-term intravenous therapy or for insertion of pressure measuring devices. Damage to the phrenic nerve, which lies just behind the junction of the subclavian and jugular veins, may occur from the needle. In one series, this complication occurred in two of 500 procedures.[14] Recognition of this cause of phrenic nerve palsy may avoid unnecessary investigations. In this type of phrenic nerve injury, recovery is usually spontaneous, although serious respiratory failure could develop if the other phrenic nerve has been previously disrupted.

Management of Injuries to Peripheral Nerves from Venipuncture and Arterial Puncture

Before discussing treatment of these conditions, some comment about their prevention is in order. Knowledge of regional anatomy may prevent damage to the nerve. For example, in venipuncture of the antecubital fossa, superficial placement of the needle laterally to the brachial artery and advancement of the needle avoiding the medial aspect of the antecubital fossa may spare damage to the median nerve. With femoral venipuncture, the needle should be introduced vertically, medially to the pulsation of the femoral artery. This will avoid damage to the femoral nerve which lies laterally to the femoral artery. Needles with short bevels may be less damaging to nerves than those with long bevels, and possibly advancement of the needle into deeper structures with the bevel in a vertical position may avoid horizontal transection of longitudinal nerve fibers.[2] Special caution should be exercised in venipuncture and arterial puncture in new-born infants, premature infants, patients receiving anticoagulants, and those with blood dyscrasias. If paresthesias occur with needle punctures, particularly if injection is contemplated, the needle should be immediately withdrawn, as these symptoms may herald impending nerve damage.[15]

Most patients with peripheral nerve damage from venipuncture will recover spontaneously and early recognition of this complication as well as reassurance will usually lead to a satisfactory clinical outcome and the subsequent avoidance of litigation. If painful neurological symptoms persist for more than a few days, treatment with anticonvulsant drugs should commence in doses such as those used for epilepsy. Carbamazepine, 400 mg b.i.d. or diphenylhydantoin, 300-400 mg nocte will usually suppress not only the painful paresthesias, but also the causalgia-like syndrome as well.[9] Blood levels of the drugs can be measured in two weeks after commencing treatment and adjustments made as necessary. It is rarely necessary to use these drugs for more than two or three months.

Nerve injury resulting from arterial puncture may produce much more serious consequences than those commonly encountered with venipuncture. More aggressive management is necessary in order to avoid irreversible, ischemic compression of the peripheral nerves and ischemic necrosis of muscle.[7,8,10,13] If the patient is anticoagulated, these drugs should be stopped. Reversible hematological abnormalities should be corrected in those patients with blood dyscrasias. If there are signs of impending muscle and nerve damage, surgical decompression by fasciotomy may be necessary to avoid irreversible damage to these tissues.

References

1. Mitchell SW: *Injuries of Nerves and Their Consequences.* American Academy of Neurology Reprint Series, Dover Publications, Inc., New York, 1965, pp 88-89.
2. Selander D, Dhuner KG, and Lundborg G: Peripheral nerve injury due to injection needles used for regional anesthesia. *Acta Anesth Scand* 21: 182-188, 1977.
3. Gentili F, Hudson A, Kline D, Hunter D: Peripheral nerve injection injury: An experimental study. *Neurosurgery* 4:244-253, 1979.
4. Gentili F, Hudson AR, Kline D, Hunter D: Early changes following injection injury of peripheral nerves. *Can J Surg* 23:177-182, 1980.
5. Gentili F, Hudson A, Hunter D, Kline D: Nerve injection injury with local anesthetic agents: A light and electron microscopic, fluorescent microscopic, and horseradish peroxidase study. *Neurosurgery* 6:263-272, 1980.

6. Pape KE, Armstrong DL, Fitzhardinge DL: Peripheral median nerve damage secondary to brachial arterial gas sampling. *J Pediatr* **93**:855-856, 1978.

7. Litter WA: Median nerve palsy — a complication of brachial artery cannulation. *Postgrad Med J* **52** (Suppl.7):110-111, 1976.

8. Neviaser RJ, Adams JP, May GI: Complications of arterial puncture in anticoagulated patients. *J Bone J Surg* **58A**:218-222, 1976.

9. Berry PR, Wallis WE: Venipuncture nerve injuries. *Lancet* **1**:1236-1237, 1977.

10. Macon WL, Futrell JW: Median nerve neuropathy after percutaneous puncture of the brachial artery in patients receiving anticoagulants. *NEJM* **228**(26):1396, 1973.

11. Kohn D, Bush A, Kessler L: Risk of Venipuncture. *Brit Med J* **2**:1133, (Letter) 1976.

12. Patten B: Neuropathy induced by hemorrhage. *Arch Neurol* **21**:381-386, 1969.

13. Halpern AA, Mochizuki R, Long CE: Compartment syndrome of the forearm following radial-artery puncture in a patient treated with anticoagulants. *J Bone J Surg* **60**:1136-1137, 1978.

14. Epstein EJ, Quereshi MS, Wright JS: Diaphragmatic paralysis after supraclavicular puncture of subclavian vein. *Brit Med J* **1**:693-694, 1976.

15. Selander D, Edshage S, Wolff T: Paresthesiae or no paresthesiae? *Acta Anesth Scand* **23**:27-33, 1979.

Chapter XVIII

Neurological Complications of Hyperbaric Oxygen Therapy*

Sidney A. Hollin, M.D., Mitchell E. Levine, M.D.,
Michael H. Sukoff, M.D., Julius H. Jacobson, II, M.D.

Introduction

Hyperbaric oxygen therapy (HBO) has been utilized in the management of a large variety of disorders. It is generally accepted to be the primary treatment for decompression sickness and air embolism, and of value in carbon monoxide poisoning and gas gangrene. More controversial indications are adjuncts to therapy of anaerobic infections, cyanide poisoning, myocardial and cerebral ischemic disorders, organ transplantation, cerebral and spinal cord trauma, cutaneous ulcerations, respiratory distress of the newborn, burns, shock, osteomyelitis, and osteoradionecrosis. The value of HBO in cardiac and carotid surgery is still under study. Clinical evaluation of therapeutic effects of HBO is impeded by a paucity of controlled trials. Benefits of breathing one hundred percent oxygen at elevated rather than atmospheric ambient pressures may be too marginal to justify the added expense, risks, and difficulties in administering hyperbaric therapy for many of the preceding conditions.[1,2] The literature concerning possible applications of HBO is voluminous, but much pertinent material is in the *Proceedings of the International Hyperbaric Conference*[3-8] and standard texts.[9-14]

Two main types of hyperbaric facilities in general use are in the individual patient (monoplace) chamber and the walk-in (multiplace) chamber. Individual patient chambers[15] resemble either an iron lung or a bed with a Plexiglas bubble around it. The patient is placed within

* Acknowledgements: The authors wish to thank Ms. Babe Stevens for her invaluable assistance in the preparation of this manuscript. We are also grateful to Dr. Melvin E. Prostkoff, scuba diver and neurosurgeon, for his contribution to the section on inner ear barotrauma.

the chamber and ambient pressure is raised by adding one hundred percent oxygen. Monoplace chambers have the advantage of relatively low initial and maintenance costs, simplicity of operation, and avoidance of personnel exposure to hyperbaria.[16] However, should a respiratory or other emergency arise, the physician faces a choice of rapidly decreasing ambient pressure, with the risk of decompression sickness, or decompressing slowly, with a resultant delay in treatment.

The walk-in type of chamber[17] consists of a large tank accomodating both patient and personnel. This chamber is pressurized with air which medical attendants breathe. The patient receives oxygen by mask, oxygen head tent or endotracheal tube. Despite high initial and operating costs and the necessity for personnel exposure, walk-in chambers have the advantage of permitting better nursing and medical care for the patient during treatment. Frequent monitoring and neurological examinations can be performed. Mixed gas treatments may be administered. The multiplace chamber is used as a combination operating room, recovery room, and intensive care unit. Pressurization of a multiplace chamber with one hundred percent oxygen, as in the case with individual patient chambers, is hazardous. While oxygen is not explosive, a spark of static electricity may be responsible for catastrophic fires which spread too rapidly for effective fire control techniques.[18,19]

In addition to fire hazards, possible complications of HBO therapy are accidental explosive decompression, accumulation of toxic vapors if there is inadequate chamber ventilation, middle ear or paranasal sinus barotrauma, decompression sickness, oxygen toxicity, "burst lung" with air embolism, nitrogen narcosis, late bone marrow necrosis, aggravation of viral infections,[20-22] anemia, and "rebound" phenomenon with deterioration of neurological status. Despite this imposing list of potential problems, the present authors conclude that HBO therapy is relatively safe if proper precautions are taken. In The Mount Sinai Medical Center over 24,000 individual compressions and decompressions in the multiplace chamber, including 1,300 operations, were performed without serious permanent sequelae directly attributable to HBO.[23] Ledingham and Davidson,[24] Hart et al,[20,21] and others[25-28] confirm the reasonable safety of hyperbaric oxygenation with proper procedural techniques.

Treatments may be administered several times a day with pure oxygen breathing lasting for several hours. Levels up to six atmospheres absolute (ATA) are required for certain cases, such as severe decompression sickness or air embolism. Because HBO profoundly influences the nervous system, an understanding of the physiology and complications of this form of therapy is of value to neurologists and neurosurgeons.

Pressure Terminology

The degree of pressurization is referred to in terms of "atmospheres absolute" (ATA). In space, a vacuum exists and pressure is zero atmospheres absolute. At sea level, the weight of air pressing on the earth's surface is 14.7 lbs per square inch (760 mmHg or torr) or one atmosphere absolute, and pressure gauges register as zero pounds per square inch gauge (psig). A gauge pressure of 14.7 psig equals one atmosphere gauge pressure but 2 ATA. Absolute atmospheres and gauge pressures are also expressed as depths of a dive in sea water. A dive of 10.5 meters or 33 feet in sea water (fsw) is equivalent to a gauge pressure of one atmosphere, or 2 ATA. A dive of 66 feet is equal to a gauge pressure of 29.4 psig or 3 ATA.

The Physiological Basis of Hyperbaric Oxygenation

The physical phenomena inherent to HBO are explained by an understanding of the gas laws of Boyle, Dalton, and Henry. A compressed air environment modifies inspired gas volume, exerts physical pressure, and alters gas density and viscosity.

Boyle's law states that for a given gas sample at constant temperature, the product of gas pressure and volume always has the same value, i.e., gas volume is inversely proportional to its pressure. Compression of an ideal gas decreases its volume in direct proportion to increases of pressure. Conversely, with gas decompression there is a proportional volume increase.

$$P_1 V_1 = P_2 V_2$$

In a breath holding subject, ambient pressure elevation proportionately reduces pulmonary volume. When residual pulmonary volume decreases below normal, there is tissue distortion and eventual hemorrhage ("pulmonary squeeze"). With normal breathing or ventilation, lung volume remains constant. However, the number of gas molecules per unit volume (gas density and viscosity) rises. The work of moving air through the respiratory tract at 4 ATA is approximately double that of 1 ATA.[29] Thus, patients with decreased respiratory reserve, endotracheal tubes, or tracheotomy may have significant problems at elevated ambient pressures.

At times, air is trapped in the paranasal sinuses or middle ear during compression because of respiratory passage anatomical deformities or eustachian tube blockage by inflammatory congestion (as with a common cold). With mild barotrauma, there is ear and paranasal sinus discomfort, capillary congestion, and edema. In more severe forms, mucosal hemorrhage or ear drum rupture with permanent hearing damage sometimes follows. Conscious hyperbaric chamber occupants accelerate equilibration by air swallowing or the Valsalva maneuver. Unconscious patients are unable to equilibrate in this manner. Our previous policy was to perform myringotomies on uncooperative patients or those about to be compressed under anesthesia. More recently, myringotomy was uneventfully omitted in a large number of such patients.

During decompression, the outside environment is at lower pressure and trapped gas expands. The presence of pulmonary emphysema, or lung cysts increase the incidence of pneumothorax, subcutaneous emphysema, or air embolism. Therefore, chest X-rays are performed on potential hyperbaric chamber occupants. In actual practice, these complications are rare even though many patients with severe emphysema have been treated.

Dalton's law states that each gas in a mixture behaves independently and exerts pressure as if it were alone in the same volume. The pressure exerted by a gas is termed its partial pressure. Total pressure of a gas mixture equals the sum of partial pressures.

$$pTotal = p1 + p2 + p3 + pN$$

where p1, p2, p3 and pN represent partial pressures of various gases in the mixture.

Under normal conditions, alveolar air, upon which the gas content of blood depends, consists of approximately 5.6% CO_2, 14% O_2 (reduced from the original 20.94% due to respiratory dead space), 80.4% nitrogen and water vapor.

$$pTotal\ (760\ mmHg) = \quad pO_2\ (100\ mmHg)* + pN_2\ (573\ mmHg)$$
$$+ pH_2O\ (47\ mmHg) + pCO_2\ (40\ mmHg)$$

Inhalation of one hundred percent oxygen eliminates nitrogen from both alveolar air and respiratory dead space. At 1 ATA, alveolar pO_2 becomes 673 mmHg.

$$pTotal = pO_2 + pCO_2 + pH_2O$$
$$pO_2 = pTotal\ (760\ mmHg) - pCO_2\ (40\ mmHg) - pH_2O\ (47\ mmHg) =$$
$$673\ mmHg$$

When 100% O_2 is inhaled at 3 ATA, alveolar pO_2 rises to 2193 mmHg.

$$pO_2 = pTotal\ (3 \times 760\ mmHg) - pCO_2\ (40\ mmHg) - pH_2O\ (47\ mmHg)$$
$$= 2193\ mmHg$$

At elevated atmospheric pressures, pCO_2 and pH_2O remain essentially unchanged, since pCO_2 is a function of alveolar ventilation

---

* pTotal (760 mmHg) − pH$_2$O (47 mmHg) × 0.14 = pO$_2$ (100 mmHg)

and the respiratory control system and pH_2O is regulated by body temperature.

In a healthy subject, arterial oxygen tension is slighty lower than that of alveolar gas because of pulmonary venous admixture secondary to impaired diffusion, ventilation perfusion inequalities, anatomic shunts, and alveolar collapse. Normally, 3 to 5% of cardiac output is not oxygenated. Discrepancies in expected and actual arterial oxygen tensions at times are considerable in pathologic states which increase admixture. At hyperbaric pressures, there is also a limitation of pulmonary capillary oxygen uptake.[30] Therefore, arterial pO_2 must be directly measured, since knowledge of ambient pressure and percent of inspired oxygen is frequently inadequate.

Henry's law states that the concentration of gas in a liquid is directly proportional to its partial pressure above solution. Gases enter physical solution independently of each other. The amount of gas physically dissolved in solutions, such as blood or plasma, increases directly with ambient pressure and is a function of inspired gaseous tension. In addition, it is related to the solubility coefficient, which is the amount of gas that dissolves in one milliliter of fluid per atmosphere (760 mmHg) of gas pressure. The solubility coefficient affects molecular activity of dissolved gases and thus varies with body temperature. More oxygen dissolves in whole blood (0.0236 ml O_2/ml blood/atm) than plasma (0.0214 ml O_2/ml plasma/atm) because of the higher physical solubility of oxygen in red blood cells compared to plasma.[31]

Healthy individuals breathing air at sea level have an arterial oxygen content of approximately 20 vol %. Virtually all oxygen is carried in chemical combination with hemoglobin with 0.3 vol % dissolved in plasma. Hemoglobin is almost completely saturated with oxygen during air breathing at sea level. Further elevations in oxygen tension of inhaled air do not significantly alter the quantity of oxyhemoglobin. However, oxygen in physical solution increases in proportion to its partial pressure. Breathing one hundred percent oxygen at normal atmospheric pressure theoretically adds in solution an additional 2 vol % of oxygen in blood. Breathing one hundred percent oxygen at 3 ATA increases dissolved oxygen content in blood to approximately 6 vol %, equivalent to about 30% of the amount carried by hemoglobin in normal blood at 1 ATA.[32] Since the average arterial-venous difference in oxygen content is approximately 4.5 to 6 vol %, it is theoretically possible to abolish the need for hemoglobin as a factor in oxygen transport.[33,34]

HBO and The Nervous System

Delivery of highly oxygenated arterial blood to the brain changes cerebral blood flow (CBF), metabolism, and intracranial pressure. Breathing one hundred percent oxygen at 3 ATA has the potential to elevate arterial pO_2 levels to about 2,000 mmHg. Because of oxygen utilization during cell metabolism, capillary pO_2 decreases as blood progresses toward the venous end of the capillary system.[30] Oxygen diffuses from capillaries to cells in the tissues where it is reduced. Most oxygen reduction probably takes place in the mitochondria of cytochromes,[35] although a considerable part is by flavoproteins elsewhere in the cell. Enhanced oxidation of cytochrome aa_3, the terminal component of the electron transport system, has been reported in animals exposed to HBO.[36] Polarographic electrodes inserted into or on the surface of cerebral or spinal cord tissue record a marked rise of pO_2 with HBO.[37-41] Technical difficulties related to direct measurements of oxygen tension by needle electrodes limit its usefulness.[39,42,43]

Cerebral tissue pO_2 is less than that of jugular venous blood and cerebrospinal fluid (CSF), which represents an overestimation but important indication of cellular oxygenation.[44-46] Lambertsen,[47,48] who studied normal volunteers breathing one hundred percent oxygen at 3.5 ATA, found a rise in jugular venous pO_2 of 75 mmHg compared to 38 mmHg with air at 1 ATA. Similar alterations during HBO were reported by Jennett et al,[49] Saltzman et al,[50] and others.[51,52] The addition of CO_2 to inspired gas during HBO increases venous pO_2 elevation.

Hyperventilation in man[53] or animals[52] profoundly decreases jugular venous pO_2 due to vasoconstriction and decreased CBF. However, with HBO, venous pO_2 is elevated despite marked hyperventilation. During normobaric hyperventilation and secondary hypocapnia, CSF and brain lactates increase, indicating augmentation of anaerobic metabolism. EEG slowing is also present. Both the EEG and metabolic responses to hypocapnia may be reversed by HBO.[54]

An increase in ventricular, cisternal, and to a lesser degree, lumbar CSF oxygen tensions, accompanies the rise in arterial CSF pO_2.[39,52,55,56] Under hyperbaric conditions, cisternal pO_2 is approximately 30% of arterial levels.[57] Some investigators[58,59] believe that cisternal CSF pO_2 is a reasonable reflection of average cerebral oxygen tension or "available oxygen to the brain."

Whether HBO causes cerebral vasoconstriction by direct action of oxygen, or secondarily by hypocapnia,[47] brain oxygenation is usually enhanced despite reduced CBF.[60-64] This conclusion is based upon pO_2 elevations of jugular venous or sagittal sinus blood, CSF and cerebral tissue, mitochondrial enzyme oxidation, depressed cerebral and CSF lactate, and EEG improvement during HBO.

HBO decreases CBF by cerebral vasoconstriction,[47,65-67] and thus reduces intracranial pressure (ICP).[28,51,57,68-71] The response of ICP to HBO is variable, but seems most effective with moderate elevations. With narcosis, right-to-left cardiac shunts, inadequate ventilation or pulmonary dysfunction, CO_2 accumulation may produce cerebral vasodilation and negate the expected ICP decrease. HBO is unable to control ICP when there is vasomotor paralysis from major brain damage, prolonged high ICP, or major ischemia-hypoxia. Failure of ICP to react to hypocapnia or osmotic agents correlates well with the response to HBO. When severe intracranial hypertension is present (ICP greater than 50 mmHg), decreased cerebral perfusion pressure below the limits of autoregulation is associated with ventricular and cisternal CSF pO_2 tensions which do not respond normally to arterial pO_2 elevation. Under these conditions, during CO_2 administration, there is a less than the anticipated rise in jugular venous and CSF pO_2.[51]

The same HBO effects which help control elevated ICP are important in the management of cerebral edema.[28,57,71-74] Vasodilation in the presence of cerebral edema further increases intracranial pressure, ischemiahypoxia, and edema formation. HBO breaks this cycle by vasoconstriction in the presence of adequate or increased brain oxygenation.

The usefulness of HBO in the treatment of cerebrovascular conditions has been investigated. When neurons lose function but are not irreversibly destroyed, it might be assumed that an increase in cerebral tissue oxygenation could help facilitate recovery of impaired neurological function. At 3 ATA breathing 100 percent oxygen, Brown et al[1] estimated theoretical extension of total circulatory occlusion time as less than two minutes. Jacobson and Lawson[75] did not find protection against experimental infarction by HBO at 2 ATA. Clinical reports of sustained benefits are inconclusive.[50,76-78] Holbach et al[79] observed a more favorable outcome in stroke patients treated at 1.5 ATA compared to 2 ATA, where anaerobic metabolism increased. HBO has also been proposed as a method for selecting suitable patients for microsurgical superficial temporal-middle cerebral artery anastomosis. Neurological and EEG responses were correlated with the efficacy of surgery.[80-82] In a recent review of the current treatment of acute stroke, Millikan and McDowall[83] were of the opinion that "The problems of the mechanics of hyperbaric oxygenation, as well as possible complications, taken with the lack of enthusiasm for the treatment, even by those reporting some benefit from it, has resulted in a situation where hyperbaric oxygenation is not used in treatment."

In addition to physical injury to neural elements and blood vessels, there is considerable evidence of spinal cord ischemia, hyperemia, edema, and altered metabolism after trauma. HBO increases the partial pressure of oxygen in the spinal cord[84-87] and therefore is of potential value in facilitating recovery of marginally injured structures. Reduction of cavitation and necrosis, an increase in the number of regenerating nerve fibers,[88-90] and an improved return of spinal cord evoked potentials rostral to the site of the lesion[91] were demonstrated after HBO administration in experimental cord trauma. These protective effects may be related to a reversal of hypoxia or a reduction in tissue edema. While the therapeutic potential of HBO is encouraging[79,92] clinical trials are still in the preliminary stage.[93-96]

Oxygen Toxicity

A serious obstacle to oxygen breathing at high partial pressures is oxygen toxicity, which is influenced by ambient pressure and duration of exposure. A narrow margin exists between therapeutic benefits and toxicity of oxygen. As atmospheric pressure is increased, exposure time to oxygen must be decreased to avoid toxicity. There is a marked variation in individual susceptibility, but tolerance to oxygen below a partial pressure of 425 mmHg (0.56 ATA) appears to be unlimited.[97,98] Breathing pure oxygen under normobaric conditions may cause substernal distress and mild impairment of neuromuscular coordination after six hours and bronchopneumonia after 24 hours.[97] Following inhalation of one hundred percent oxygen at 2 ATA there are essentially no significant CNS abnormalities, but approximately 20% of subjects have pulmonary dysfunction within five hours of exposure.[99] At or above 3 ATA, neurological effects limit exposure time, while at lower pressures, pulmonary changes predominate.[100-102] Lower extremity muscle spasms were observed after 50 minutes of oxygen breathing at 3 ATA[103] and facial twitching within 15 minutes at 4 ATA. Seizures are not common before three hours at 3 ATA, but have been reported after 45 minutes at 4.5 ATA.[105]

The exact mechanisms of oxygen toxicity are unknown but seem to be related to disturbances in oxidative reactions of cellular metabolism and activity of essential enzymes. Several investigations suggest an initial excessive production of superoxide, H_2O_2 and other oxidizing free radicals.[106-109] Antioxidant activity of protective enzymes and cytoplasmic antioxidants eventually becomes inadequate. Oxidation of sulfhydryl-containing proteins and pyridine nucleotides,[109,110] a decrease in ATP and phosphocreatine levels secondary to disturbances of phosphorylation reactions of the respiratory chain,[110,111] free radical damage to structural and enzymatic properties of membranes,[112,113] and exhaustion of gamma-amino-butyric acid (an inhibitory neurotransmitter)[114] have been postulated as mediators of toxic oxygen effects.

Oxygen toxicity is modified by a number of agents. In animals, hypophysectomy,[115-118] adrenalectomy,[119-124] and adrenergic-blocking agents protect against toxicity.[119,112-127] Oxidative cyclization of epinephrine to highly reactive indoles (aminochromes) apparently contributes to toxic effects of oxygen on the brain.[128-132] It appears that formation of complexes between serotonin and catecholamines decreases oxidation of catecholamine to aminochromes. Reduction in plasma serotonin, and thus a potential increase in aminochrome formation, has been observed during prolonged HBO.[133]

Reserpine and chlorpromazine suppress hypothalamic adrenocortical and sympathetic nervous system activity thereby diminishing toxic effects of oxygen.[134-139] In addition, reserpine acts by catecholamine depletion and chlorpromazine by its adrenalytic activity.[138]

The onset of oxygen toxicity is delayed by ganglionic blocking agents,[125,140] reducing agents[141,142] (such as cysteine and reduced glutathione), chelating agents that bind metal ions,[143,144] intracellular buffering agents (tris-buffer) presumably by combating electrolyte derangement secondary to loss of hemoglobin buffering,[145-149] antioxidants such as vitamin E,[150-153] depleted metabolites (gamma-amino-butyric acid)[154-156] and substances (ATP) entering into the Krebs cycle. Although most drugs are not of clinical value, some success was reported with vitamin E and disulfiram, a free radical scavanger.[157]

Since inhalation of CO_2 increases oxygen toxicity by cerebral vasodilation and delivery of more oxygen to the brain,[158-163] it is not routinely recommended during HBO therapy. The effect of increased brain pCO_2 and lowered pH, per se, is minor.[164,165]

Oxygen itself is a CNS depressant.[166] Thus, elimination of this oxygen suppressing factor sometimes predisposes to seizures during decompression or following removal of an oxygen mask ("mask off" effect).[167] Breathing one hundred percent oxygen at 2 ATA was reported to depress auditory evoked responses without adversely affecting mental performance. Bennett and Ackles[166] considered this finding an indication of CNS depression at pressures insufficient to produce convulsions but capable of causing minimal narcosis.

Periodic reduction of inspired oxygen during HBO therapy increases oxygen tolerance.[168-174] During the latency period before symptoms of oxygen toxicity appear, cellular metabolic changes are initially easily reversed. Apparently, interludes of air breathing allow reconstitution of biochemical factors that protect against oxygen toxicity.

Holbach and Careli[175] studied the effects of HBO on the oxygen tolerance and oxygenation state of injured human brain. Oxidative glucose metabolism furnishes approximately twenty times more energy than glycolysis (anaerobic glucose metabolism). Only 5-10% of glucose delivered to brain normally undergoes anaerobic glycolysis.[176] With injury-induced interference in energy formation by oxidative glucose metabolism, there is a compensatory increase in glycolysis. This hypoxia in the presence of increased inspired oxygen ("hyperoxia hypoxidosis") is reflected by an abnormal glucose oxidation quotient, a rise in CSF and cerebral venous blood lactate, an elevated lactate/pyruvate ratio, a low bicarbonate level (a product of oxidative matabolism), and a decrease in pH secondary to lactacidosis. Holbach and Careli[175] found oxidative metabolism was enhanced at 1.5 ATA but inhibited at 2 ATA. More of their patients had clinical improvement after HBO treatments at 1.5 ATA than 2 ATA.

The latent period and clinical signs and symptoms of CNS oxygen toxicity are extremely variable. Initially, there may be dizziness, nausea, malaise, apprehension, euphoria, anxiety, confusion, myoclonus, paresthesias, and twitching of facial muscles. The major manifestation of CNS oxygen toxicity is a seizure.[177,178] After multiple HBO treatments at 2 or 3 ATA, approximately 2-3% of patients convulse.[21,25,179] Sometimes there are no preceding premonitory symptoms. EEG changes are inconsistent and not of major value in predicting seizures.[180] Hyperventilation, barbiturates, anticonvulsant medication, neuromuscular blocking agents, and general anesthesia reduce overt seizure activity but do not necessarily prevent direct cellular oxygen toxicity.

In addition to immediate reduction of inspired oxygen by switching to air breathing, usual measures for seizure therapy are instituted. It is important not to decompress the patient during the actual seizure. Decompression while breath-holding, especially with associated laryngospasm or bronchial secretions, expands pulmonary air and predisposes to cerebral embolism. After ventilation returns, the patient may be safely decompressed.

Progressive contraction of visual fields,[181] pupillary inequality, photophobia, and distortion of objects may be caused by HBO. Miller[182] detected no visual acuity or field disturbances after four hours of oxygen breathing at 1 ATA. During one hundred percent oxygen breathing at 3 ATA there is marked attenuation of retinal arterioles and venules with disappearance of small vessels.[183] The color of retinal veins becomes closer to that of arteries, suggesting increased retinal oxygen content despite vasoconstriction. At 3 ATA, there is prolongation of dark adaptation after twenty minutes,[184] visual field constriction after two and one-half to three hours,[185,186] and visual cell destruction in experimental animals after four hours.[187]

With oxygen toxicity, light and electron microscopy demonstrate hyperchromatosis and cytoplasmic pyknosis of brain cells, mainly bilaterally, in the globus pallidus, substantia nigra, superior olivary complex, ventral chochlear nuclei, and nucleus of the spinal tract of V.[188,189] The neocortex and striatum are spared in contrast to their susceptibility in anoxic ischemia.

A fairly high (17/76) percentage of rats exposed for one hour a day on consecutive days to 60 psig (5 ATA) of oxygen develop spinal cord necrosis involving part or nearly all of the gray matter. Similar changes take place with a single exposure at 30 psig (3 ATA) oxygen for five continuous hours.[190]

A reduction in peripheral nerve action potentials with eventual conduction block was produced by oxygen administration for two hours at 13 ATA.[191] This finding is not clinically significant in view of the required ambient pressure and length of exposure time.

Decompression Sickness

Decompression sickness (DCS) is a syndrome in which undesirable effects are created by release of dissolved gases from physical solution during reduction of ambient pressure. Dysbarism is a general term referring to disorders related to altered pressures. Clinical features of DCS were initially described in caisson workers by Pol and Watelle[192] in the mid-nineteenth century (thus the term "caisson disease"). These authors noted that depth and time of compression and rate of decompression influenced the severity of the illness. They recommended as treatment recompression followed by slower decompression.

With elevation of ambient pressure, there is a corresponding rise in alveolar gas partial pressures. Equilibration takes place between the dissolved and undissolved phases of nitrogen. Nitrogen becomes supersaturated in blood, tissues, and body cavities. The amount of dissolved nitrogen depends on ambient pressure and nitrogen solubility. Nitrogen capacity of various body tissues is also influenced by local blood flow.[193,194]

During decompression, there is a disequilibrium between the environment and dissolved gas, which now has a higher partial pressure than ambient pressure. Nitrogen leaves the dissolved phase in blood and tissues and is eliminated via the lungs. Lipid rich bone marrow, white matter of brain and spinal cord and other fatty tissues have a high nitrogen solubility and capacity, and take longer to release contained nitrogen. It would not be possible to reduce ambient pressure exposure unless blood and tissues were capable of holding some gas in supersaturated solution without bubble formation.[195-197] With slow decompression, there is gradual diffusion of gas, which is asymptomatically eliminated through the respiratory system. If decompression is too rapid, excessive bubbles form and symptoms of DCS take place.

Bubble formation initially occurs mainly in interstitial spaces, lymphatics, capillaries, and venules. Thereafter, bubbles tend to accumulate in larger veins.[198-200] Doppler ultrasonic techniques demonstrate more bubbles in the inferior vena cava than in the aorta.[201] Gas in venous blood becomes trapped in pulmonary capillaries and the patient

may experience respiratory distress ("chokes"). Some bubbles pass beyond the lungs to enter the systemic arterial system, obstructing capillaries of the brain and other organs. Pulmonary capillaries are an effective gas trap, except for the smallest bubbles. Bubbles bypass the pulmonary capillary bed by direct flow from the venous to arterial system
via Thebesian veins (which drain from the myocardium into the left side
of the heart), from the bronchial circulation by way of pulmonary veins,
and other shunting mechanisms.[198,202] In addition to venous shunting, it
has been proposed that bubbles in the pulmonary circulation reduce vasomotor tone, thereby decreasing the effectiveness of the pulmonary filter.[12] Passage of gas through the pulmonary circulation may be enhanced when hypoxia, hypercapnia, or hyperoxia exist. Bubbles also
enter the systemic arterial circulation in the presence of certain pathological states, such as patent foramen ovale. After standard decompression
procedures, bubbles are infrequently found in the arterial system but are
observed following explosive decompression.[203,204] Glass beads and other
objects injected into the venous system of animals were recovered in the
arterial circulation.[12,205] Some investigators[206,207] were unable to confirm
this finding.

Bubbles initially create problems by their presence in cells and tissues or by vascular obstruction. Separation of gas from solution is the
primary event, but additional factors seem to be important in the pathogenesis of DCS. These include the release of humoral agents, such as
bradykinin and other vasoactive substances,[208-211] vascular spasm with
secondary ischemic changes, the formation of tissue breakdown products, thrombotic adhesions with decreased thrombocytes and increased
intravascular clotting,[212] abnormal gas-induced tissue osmotic changes,[213] red blood cell agglutination with tendency to agglomerate and
adhere to vessel walls,[211,214-216] alterations of the blood/brain barrier,[217,218] fat emboli from bone marrow, adipose tissue or blood lipoprotein disruption,[198,200,211,219] increased capillary permeability with
hypovolemia, hemoconcentration and edema,[219-222] and the possible importance of prostaglandins in later stages of plasma extravasation.[223]

Decompression sickness is less likely to affect the patient in the
chamber breathing one hundred percent oxygen than air breathing medical personnel. While DCS is almost invariably produced by nitrogen
bubbles, on rare occasions it occurs while breathing pure oxygen.[224,225]
The tendency to bubble formation with oxygen is less than with compressed air, helium-oxygen, or argon-oxygen mixtures. This is consistent with the theory that oxygen diffusion to hypoxic areas leads to a reduction in size of gas emboli. However, oxygen bubbles can occlude
blood vessels, decrease blood flow, and cause local hypoxia.[226]

Subclinical bubble formation can be found by ultrasonic Doppler
systems.[201,203,227] For earliest detection, precordial rather than peripheral

monitoring is preferred.[204] Asymptomatic venous gas emboli may be cleared by oxygen breathing.

Over half the cases of DCS have clinical symptoms within one hour following decompression, 85% by the end of six hours, and only approximately 0.3% after 24 hours.[228] Signs and symptoms vary considerably and manifestations of this disorder are protean. Behnke[200] referred to the bubble as "the great imitator." Skin itching and rashes are probably related to bubble formation in subcutaneous nerves or lymphatics. Joint pains ("bends"), are the most common symptom. As bubbles increase in size and number, fatigue, fever, sweating, cough, dyspnea, substernal distress, and shock may occur. Late bone necrosis may take place.[229-231]

The central nervous system is affected in about 30% of cases of DCS.[228,232-234] The most common site is the thoracic region of the spinal cord.[228,235] Cord disturbances in DCS usually follow depth but not altitude exposure.[236] In the past, cord damage was attributed to systematic arterial bubble embolization. In other clinical conditions, such as fat embolism, subacute bacterial endocarditis, or left atrial mural thrombus, the cord is rarely the site of arterial embolization. Considering the large brain bulk and proportion of blood flow it receives compared to the cord, a much higher incidence of cerebral involvement would be anticipated. Haymaker and Johnston[237] suggested that bubbles forming in epidural and retroperitoneal fat enter the vertebral venous system and increase the probability of embolization via cord precapillaries and arterioles because of venous congestion and flow retardation. Hallenbach et al[238] favored blockage of the epidural venous system as the cause of cord infarction. This was supported by cinemographic studies and pathological changes predominantly in white matter with gray matter sparing. These authors considered their findings compatible with acute venous rather than arterial cord infarction from nutrient artery occlusion. However, Frankel[239] was of the opinion that pathologic observations in his cases were not typical of venous cord infarction.

Signs and symptoms of cord dysfunction comprise motor, sensory, and reflex disturbances in a variety of combinations. In a review of 935 cases of DCS, Rivera[228] found numbness or paresthesias ("pins and needles") in 21.2%, muscle weakness in 20.6% and paralysis in 6.1%. Bowel and bladder incontinence or any other manifestation of myelopathy are possible.

The brain is less commonly affected than the spinal cord in decompression sickness. EEG slowing without overt signs of cerebral dysfunction (reported in submarine escape training[240] and patients treated for joint bends[198]) suggests that brain involvement is more frequent than previously appreciated. Headaches, incoherent speech, restlessness, agitation, convulsions, hemiplegia, aphasia, impaired mentation with confusion and personality changes, and deterioration of level of consiousness to coma have been described.[228,241-244] Consiousness is lost in 1 or 2% of cases of DCS.[228,236,245] The relative lack of focal seizures may be related to bubble scavenging by increased blood perfusion of cortical areas and the generation of more gas bubbles in white matter, which is higher in lipid content and nitrogen storage capability.[246] Most cerebral symptoms are probably caused by arterial gas embolization to the brain.[12] However, some follow hypotension secondary to vasodepressor mechanisms, hemoconcentration, or hypovolemia.[247]

Visual symptoms, present in about 7% of DCS cases,[228,248] include visual field changes, blurred vision, reduced acuity, and scotomas. These findings are often preceded by skin lesions, "chokes," or "bends." Scotomas sometimes have scintillating characteristics resembling migraine attacks, perhaps from gaseous obstruction and segmental vasospasm of posterior cerebral artery branches or secondarily from tissue breakdown products.[249] Like migraine, scotomas of DCS are sometimes relieved by CO_2 inhalation. Anderson et al[250] reported three chamber personnel (0.2% incidence of decompressions) with temporary homonymous hemianopsia. The average exposure was 29 psig (3 ATA) for about one hour. In one instance, visual field changes lasted three weeks.

Vestibulocochlear disorders were previously considered a relatively unimportant part of DCS, primarily associated with other CNS manifestations.[251,252] Recently, it has become apparent that isolated inner ear DCS may occur, especially after exposure to deep depths.[231,253-256] Cochlear and vestibular involvement tend to take place separately rather than simultaneously.

The vestibular system ("staggers") is affected in about 5 or 10% of DCS cases.[228,257,258] Lesions are essentially of peripheral origin unless CNS dysfunction is extensive and obvious. Bubbles commonly form in the labyrinth, and rarely in vestibular pathways, vestibulo-spinal tract, or cerebellar cortex. After deep dives, a Meniere-type syndrome is not uncommon[254,259] and may appear before limb bends. This pattern is infrequent with other types of CNS DCS. Nausea, vomiting, nystagmus, dizziness, vertigo, and incoordination are observed. Auditory disturbances with tinnitus and hearing loss comprise less than 1% of cases.[228]

Tearing or compression of vessels and other local structural deformities by intralabyrinthine bubble formation, intravascular gaseous obstruction, hydrostatic pressure differentials by gas diffusion from the middle ear into perilymphatic fluid, and gas-induced osmosis between perilymphatic and endolymphatic fluids have been implicated in inner ear DCS.[12,260-262] Blockage of inner ear microcirculation by bubbles leads to vasospasm, vascular stasis, thrombosis, ischemia, infarction, and hemorrhages.[262,263] Capillary and venule obstruction increases vascular permeability and exudate formation. In the opinion of Landolt et al,[261] pathological findings are more compatible with interference of venous drainage than arterial gaseous obstruction.

Switching inert gases at stable depths creates labyrinthine disturbances similar to DCS. After substituting nitrogen for helium without altering inspired oxygen concentration, there may be sudden nausea, vertigo, and nystagmus,[264,265] possibly from intralabyrinthine osmotic pressure differentials or counter-diffusion of inert gases with inner ear bubble formation.[269]

Numbness, paresthesias, muscle weakness, and other manifestations of peripheral nervous system dysfunction are sometimes difficult to differentiate from those of CNS origin. This may partially account for discrepancies in the reported percentage of peripheral nerve involvement in various series.[228,232,233,257,267,268] In the peripheral nervous system, bubbles are confined to the myelin sheath.[269]

The incidence of DCS is minimized by careful gradual reduction of chamber pressure according to standard USN decompression tables.[270] Even with strict adherence to these tables, a small number of cases will occur.[271] The rate of safe decompression depends on the length of time and depth to which the patient or personnel are exposed. After air breathing at 2 ATA, direct ascent to normobaric levels is permitted for bottom times of 310 minutes or less. Deeper depths require less bottom time in order not to exceed the "no decompression" limit.

Rapid uncontrolled or blowout decompression can produce cord or brain lesions after only a few minutes of exposure to ambient pressures over 6 ATA.[272] Such an episode of explosive reduction of high pressure (4 ATA) occurred in 1976 when a patient in a multiplace chamber developed a CNS air embolism.[273,274] During the ensuing confusion, the chamber was suddenly opened. Five patients also in the chamber at that time died from DCS.

Following compression, residual amounts of partially saturated nitrogen remain in the body for 24 hours or more. Therefore, special decompression schedules are necessary for repetitive dives.[275]

Intermittent oxygen inhalation, interspersed with periods of air breathing to avoid oxygen toxicity, shortens decompression time.[276,277] Oxygen breathing increases the efficiency of inert gas elimination and tends to maintain adequate tissue oxygenation during incipient bubble formation.[278-281]

In addition to oxygen breathing and prior exposure to dysbaric conditions, age, sex, general physical condition, obesity, and degree of physical exertion during pressurization influence the susceptibility to DCS.

Recompression treatment schedules and their manner of application vary considerably. Standard tables are found in the USN Diving Operations Manual.[270] Recompression is instituted to at least 1 ATA over the pressure which relieves symptoms, but not over 6 ATA. Higher pressures prolong decompression, do not materially improve circulation, and unduly delay the administration of oxygen to reduce decompression time.[282] Oxygen therapy is not used above 3 ATA because of the relatively short interval before toxicity. Substitution of helium for nitrogen with proper control of oxygen partial pressures allows extension of time limits at higher pressures during treatment of serious DCS.[282]

Heparin,[283,284] low molecular weight dextran and other plasma volume expanders,[219,285,286] anticonvulsants, and steroids have been recommended as adjuncts to therapy. Heparin, in addition to its anticoagulation effect, may be useful as a lipid clearing agent. Low molecular weight dextran decreases blood viscosity, improves tissue perfusion, and reduces platelet clumping. When DCS affects the spinal cord, venous obstruction may be accompanied by an elevation of CSF pressure.[238] In the past, multiple spinal taps and CSF drainage were advised.[287] However, with more modern techniques of controlling increased ICP, spinal drainage is now rarely required.

CNS DCS is a medical emergency. To be effective, therapy must be rapidly instituted. The purpose of recompression is to reduce bubble size, decrease tissue distortion, and restore blood flow by relieving vessel occlusion. Therapy is less successful as tissue damage increases. Rivera[228] reported a 13% residual CNS deficit when treatment was started after six hours in contrast to 1% within 30 minutes. In the series of Polland et al,[235] there was complete recovery in 74% of divers treated for CNS DCS.

Vestibulocochlear DCS requires treatment within approximately 45 minutes or damage may be permanent.[266]

Cerebral Air Embolism ("Burst Lung")

Although bubbles reach the brain during DCS, an even more dramatic source of cerebral air embolism is "burst lung." With decompression, pulmonary air expands and alveoli hyperdistend when there is a voluntary breath-holding, involuntary glottal spasm, inadequate ventilation, plugging of segmental bronchioles by secretions, stenotic bronchioles, lung cysts, or emphysematous blebs. During reduction of ambient pressure, it is important that freely breathing patients avoid breath-holding or an attempt to equalize ear pressure by Valsalva maneuver. As previously mentioned, patients should not be decompressed during a seizure because of possible glottal spasm, accumulation of pulmonary secretions, and involuntary breath-holding. Air embolism is a potential danger during accidental rapid decompression, such as with a broken chamber window or failed valve.

If the transpulmonic pressure (the differential between the extra-thoracic space and intra-alveolar gas) exceeds approximately 100 mmHg,[288] air passes across the alveolar membrane to the pulmonary capillaries and veins, the left side of the heart, and systemic arteries. Bubbles reach the brain by way of the carotid and/or vertebral arteries and initially tend to occlude smaller arterioles. Blood flow interruption may be temporary as gas emboli pass into the venous system.[289] Intravascular air leads to vessel dilation and venous engorgement. Air bubbles have been observed in arterioles and pial vessels up to 48 hours after embolization. There may be associated cerebral arterial spasm, with secondary local vasodilation, stasis and perivascular hemorrhage, primarily in relation to small capillaries and veins. Occasionally there is diffuse subarachnoid hemorrhage.[290]

Postmortem examination usually demonstrates marked distention rather than actual disruption of alveoli.[288] Gas may be found in the pulmonary veins, mediastinum, subcutaneous spaces, and pleural cavity. In the brain, pale and red infarcts are most prevalent in border zones between the distribution of major cerebral arteries. These are areas of relatively low cerebral perfusion pressure.[291] Microscopic findings are similar to those in patients with cerebral air embolism from other causes, such as following open heart surgery, head and neck operations, diagnostic thoracentesis, or hemodialysis. Changes are compatible with neuronal ischemia and include microvacuolization, cell shrinkage, hyperchromasia, and triangular nuclear configuration.[292]

During free ascent training of submarine personnel, a situation analogous to decompression after HBO therapy at low atmospheric pressures, incidences of lung rupture from 1 to 3.5% were reported by Lindemark[293] and Ingvar et al.[294] It is important to realize that "burst lung" has followed decompression from depths of only 11 feet in scuba diving trainees.[288]

With cerebral air embolism, the patient may initially experience chest pain, headache, nausea, dizziness, and visual complaints. There is often an abrupt loss of consciousness during or shortly after the decrease in barometric pressure. Ten of the 14 patients studied by Ingvar et al[294] had focal neurological signs. Asymmetric unilateral or bilateral limb weakness or paralysis, spotty discrete brain stem signs, and other indications of generalized diffuse brain involvement are present in many cases.[295]

A common and frequently presenting manifestation of cerebral air embolism is a seizure.[296] Convulsions are generalized or focal. Oxygen toxicity is a more likely etiological factor when seizures begin during compression or at a fixed ambient pressure. Problems in differential diagnosis arise especially during or after decompression when either cerebral embolism or oxygen toxicity can cause seizures. A case described by Bond[288] illustrates this diagnostic difficulty. A patient undergoing HBO therapy was rapidly decompressed following onset of an oxygen toxicity seizure. He continued to have focal convulsions after removal from the monoplace chamber. At autopsy, the diagnosis of cerebral air embolism was made.

With massive, acute cerebral air embolism, the EEG may be electrically silent over the entire affected hemisphere. More commonly, there is asymmetrical slowing.[297] Even in the absence of overt neurological disturbances, emboli sometimes produce EEG changes and therapy should be initiated.[294] Delayed EEG changes, hours after embolization, are frequently irritative in nature.[297] EEG abnormalities may persist for months in asymptomatic patients.[294]

Farmer[266] was of the opinion that previous to 1977 there was no documented case of inner ear injury secondary to embolization of the labyrinthine arterial system. However, Caruso et al[255] found evidence of peripheral vestibular and CNS dysfunction in a patient who suffered a cerebral air embolism during sport diving.

Therapy consists of lowering the head to a dependent position followed by immediate recompression to 6 ATA.[288] Intermittent oxygen is administered at lower pressures.

With prompt adequate treatment, complete resolution of neurological findings and restitution of function without significant sequelae is possible in the majority of patients.[294-296] Results are less satisfying when there are delays in therapy or inadequate recompression, but even after several hours, full recovery can be obtained. There were no mortalities in the 14 cases reported by Ingvar et al.[294] However, nine of the 79 patients in Gillen's series[295] died, four prior to the institution of therapy. With aggressive management, and in the absence of major multiple organ system involvement, cerebral air embolism has a potentially good prognosis.

Nitrogen Narcosis

The effects of increased amounts of physically dissolved nitrogen in blood are of importance to the patient undergoing HBO therapy and personnel in the pressurized chamber.

The phenomenon of nitrogen narcosis was first described in 1835 by Junod[298] who noted disturbances in mental function after breathing compressed air. It was not until 1935 that Behnke et al[299] attributed this narcosis to nitrogen. It is now known that "narcotic" effects are not specific for nitrogen. Other metabolically inert gases such as helium, neon, argon, krypton, and xenon at high enough pressures affect the nervous system in a similar manner.[300] Helium is the least narcotic of the noble gases. Even oxygen at elevated ambient pressures has narcotic properties.[301]

In an attempt to elucidate mechanisms of action in narcosis, some of the physiochemical characteristics that have been investigated are molecular weight,[302] partial molar free energy,[303] boiling point,[304] polarizability,[305] van der Waals forces,[304] hydrate disassociation pressure,[306] and lipoid solubility.[307] The Meyer-Overton hypothesis states that all gaseous substances induce narcosis if a definite molar concentration is reached in cell lipids.[308] The excellent correlation between lipoid solubility and narcotic potency for a given gas is a compelling line of evidence in support of this hypothesis.

The site of action of nitrogen and other inert gases is thought to be at the synaptic membranes,[309,310] where there are configurational changes and transmission is blocked.[311-313]

Signs and symptoms of nitrogen narcosis progressively increase as ambient pressure rises. It is generally accepted that clinically significant nitrogen effects are not present until 4 ATA is reached, although minor changes begin at 2 ATA.[47,299,314] An attempt has been made to quantitate the early impairments seen in nitrogen narcosis. Errors in a card-sorting test during air breathing at 2 ATA by Poulton et al[315] were not verified in a similar but double-blind experiment.[316] Abnormal (near field) auditory evoked potentials observed in the compressed air environment at 2 ATA may be related to diminished intensity input signals[317-319] secondary to increased gas density rather than auditory pathway dysfunction.

Since there are usually no major problems below 3 ATA, productive work is not compromised. Most HBO treatments and surgical procedures are at 3 ATA or less. At pressures in the range of 3 to 5 ATA, air breathing subjects report a feeling resembling the pleasant effects of alcohol. Every atmosphere over 4 ATA is said to be equivalent to two to three martinis.[1] Laughing spells occur, but the mood is controlled and, with effort, normal conduct is maintained. Feelings of overconfidence, exhilaration, idea fixations, and difficulty with recollection and concentration are described.[299] Abnormal reactions to auditory, visual, olfactory, and tactile stimuli initially recorded by Behnke et al[299] at 3 ATA, were seen in all subjects tested at 4 ATA. At this level, Adolfson[320] demonstrated decreased hand/foot and manual dexterity and diminished associative strength.

AT 6 to 8 ATA, garrulousness, joviality, uncontrolled laughter, hysteria, mistakes in simple tasks, and numbness and tingling sensations may occur. Certain disorders such as DCS or cerebral air embolism are treated at 6 ATA where both patients and staff may be affected by nitrogen narcosis. Most experienced medical attendants are not incapacitated at 6 ATA, but there may be interference with decision-making.

By the time 10 ATA is reached, there is marked impairment of judgement, manic/depressive behavior, disorientation, ataxia, and decreased levels of consciousness.[321] The average depth where consciousness is lost is approximately 12 ATA.

There is a wide variation in individual susceptibility. Emotionally stable subjects who have undergone frequent exposures have a greater tolerance for the compressed air environment. Narcotic effects of nitrogen are potentiated by increased CO_2 and/or oxygen inhalation,[322] alcohol, fatigue, apprehension, and fast compression time.[323,324] Replacing nitrogen with helium aids in reducing nitrogen narcosis.[302,325]

"Rebound" Phenomenon

The neurological condition of some patients deteriorates after HBO therapy in the absence of obvious causes, such as DCS or cerebral air embolism. In a study by Hart et al[21] of 600 patients who underwent 12,000 compressions between 2 and 3 ATA, 2% were more lethargic after decompression. Several cases reported by Morgami et al[70] became significantly worse after HBO therapy. Ingvar and Lassen[76] described a patient with a focal cerebral ischemic lesion, admittedly in poor pretreatment condition, who responded during HBO administration but died 30 minutes after therapy was completed. Although deterioration may have been inevitable because of the intracranial pathology, the possible role of increased ICP was suggested.

Reduction of ICP elevation and brain edema by HBO is primarily by cerebral vasoconstriction, which decreases CBF and intracranial blood volume. Even with moderate increases of ICP the effectiveness of HBO diminishes with time. Furthermore, upon cessation of HBO therapy, ICP sometimes rises above pretreatment levels.[68,76] However, Sukoff and Ragatz[28] found such an ICP elevation in only one of ten monitored patients treated for traumatic encephalopathy.

"Rebound" has been attributed either to the underlying cerebral disorder or to direct toxic effects of oxygen with exacerbation of metabolic disturbances in an injured brain. Prolonged HBO alters brain water content and its sodium distribution thereby increasing cerebral edema and elevating ICP.[76] Lactacidosis during oxygen breathing at 2 or more ATA[79] and redistribution of cellular CO_2 and O_2 with a resulting osmotic gradient[12] are possibly associated with disturbed brain energy metabolism and changes in ionic permeability of neural cells.

Inner Ear Barotrauma

Trauma to the middle ear secondary to changes in ambient pressure is well known. There is a failure to equalize middle ear pressure through the eustachian tube, most often during compression when gas space contracts (Boyle's law). With decompression, middle ear barotrauma is not a frequent occurrence, since the eustachian tube tends to allow free exit of gas. Barotitis media is a source of conductive hearing loss in approximately 2 or 3% of cases undergoing HBO therapy.[21,25] Permanent loss of hearing is rare.

Inner ear barotrauma is less common than, and often concomitant with, middle ear disturbances.[326-331] At times, it is not evident that the inner ear is injured until days after signs of barotitis media subside.[266] Sensorineural cochlear disorders and vestibular dysfunction with partial or total hearing loss, dizziness, and vertigo are sequelae of inner ear barotrauma.[266] Damage to intralabyrinthine structures, such as Reissner's membrane, vascular stasis, exudates, and hemorrhages have been described.[328,332]

During compression, the middle ear membranes bulge inward if there is inadequate pressure equalization through the eustachian tubes. The "implosive" theory suggests that the inner ear is injured by sudden outward movement of the tympanic membrane and stapes during a rigorous Valsalva maneuver, which has rapidly cleared the middle ear.[330] The "explosive" theory[333,334] postulates that the ICP rises following a Valsalva maneuver, distorts, and at times, ruptures the thin round window membrane.[335,336] The oval window is much less implicated.[255] With deeper dives, a Valsalva maneuver is not necessary to rupture the round window, if the pressure differential between the middle and inner ear is sufficiently large.

Intracranial pressure is probably transmitted to the inner ear perilymph and thus to the membranous labyrinth by way of the cochlear aqueduct. Experimentally, following intracranial and secondary endolymphatic pressure elevation, there is loss of auditory nerve electrical activity.[337] In addition to impaired cochlear and vestibular function, possible complications of inner ear barotrauma and perilymphatic fistulae are CSF otorrhea and meningitis.[338] A potential communication exists between the subarachnoid and perilymphatic spaces via the cochlear, and to a lesser extent, vestibular aqueducts.[339-343] The cochlear aqueduct originates at the scala tympani and terminates in the petrous portion of the temporal bone between the jugular bulb and internal auditory canal. It is not a free pathway unless there is a breakdown or paucity of arachnoidal connective tissue which normally fills this structure.

Treatment of round window fistula begins with head elevation and avoidance of straining at stool, nose blowing, exercise, and other maneuvers which increase intralabyrinthine and CSF pressure. Exploratory tympanotomy and repair of round window fistula may be necessary if symptoms do not subside after 24 hours of conservative therapy.[344]

It is important to differentiate between inner ear barotrauma and isolated vestibulocochlear DCS, since the management of these conditions differs significantly. DCS occurs during or after ambient pressure reduction following relatively deep dives. Recompression up to 165 feet is required to adequately reduce bubble size and restore hearing loss or vestibular function. Inner ear barotrauma often takes place during compression at relatively shallow depths where DCS would not be expected.[266,327,336] Most HBO therapy is carried out at 2 or 3 ATA. At these levels, sensorineural vestibulocochlear disturbances are more likely to be associated with inner ear barotrauma for which recompression is contraindicated.

In addition to inner ear barotrauma and DCS, sensorineural hearing loss in divers may be related to background noise trauma.[345,346] These patients do not have evidence of middle ear barotrauma, are exposed to sound intensities above acceptable limits, and tend to exhibit bilateral high frequency hearing loss.[327]

Summary

Both therapeutic effects and complications of HBO depend upon the gas laws of Boyle, Dalton, and Henry. A marked elevation of the partial pressure of alveolar oxygen is accompanied by a similar but somewhat smaller increase in arterial pO_2. Thus, there is potential enhancement of tissue oxygenation which could be beneficial in a number of clinical conditions. The actual degree of improved cellular oxygenation is not clear. Oxygen is not actively transported but diffuses from capillary blood into surrounding tissues. Even under hyperbaric conditions, theoretical calculations show distinct limitations of oxygen reserve and diffusion distances. Animal experiments demonstrate only a few minutes of additional protection after total cerebral circulatory occlusion. The secondary vasoconstriction seen in HBO is of some value in decreasing cerebral edema and reducing ICP. Conclusions regarding the role of HBO in the treatment of a variety of disorders are limited by lack of controlled clinical trials.

A rather fine line exists between therapeutic and toxic levels of oxygen administration. At 2 ATA, there are indications of increased anaerobic brain metabolism (glycolysis) which suggest subclinical incipient oxygen toxicity. Because of these findings, some investigators recommend HBO at 1.5 ATA rather than the more routine 2 to 3 ATA.

The incidence of neurological complications in HBO therapy is difficult to determine. Few publications attempt to tabulate and analyze this problem. Some complications are not reported in the literature, and others, such as visual field defects, may not be readily apparent without a systematic search for them. Therefore, much information regarding potential dangers of HBO requires extrapolation from naval experience, and that of scuba divers and tunnel workers.

It appears that severe neurological disturbances are infrequent with HBO therapy as currently practiced. Oxygen toxicity seizures seem to be the most common and are usually easily controlled. More routine use of prophylactic anticonvulsants, especially when treating patients with cerebral dysfunction, would probably reduce the number of seizures encountered.[28]

DCS is largely avoided by proper adherence to standard decompression tables, although a small number of cases will still not be prevented. Most reported DCS following HBO does not involve the nervous system but consists of skin rashes or joint bends. Visual field defects have been observed in medical attendants. Accidental explosive decompression is a serious hazard but, fortunately, is rare.

Cerebral air embolism is a dangerous complication which can be caused by reduction of ambient pressure during a convulsion or breathholding. It is a more likely event when there are underlying pulmonary disorders, such as plugged segmental bronchioles or emphysematous blebs. "Burst Lung" may take place after decompression from rather shallow depths.

Nitrogen narcosis is generally not clinically significant below 3 ATA. Above this level, the judgement of medical attendants is at times impaired, and important decisions may have to be made by someone outside the chamber. Since most HBO therapy and surgery is carried out at 2 to 3 ATA, nitrogen narcosis is not often a difficult problem.

Occasionally, patients have increased neurological deficits after HBO therapy. In some instances, this deterioration is related to an ICP elevation to a higher level than was present prior to initiation of treatment. This "rebound" may be secondary to electrolytic, osmotic, and cell membrane disturbances. It is possible, but as yet unproven, that the likelihood of "rebound" phenomenon will decrease if HBO is administered at lower ambient pressures.

Middle ear disturbances not infrequently follow HBO treatment. Tympanic membrane rupture and middle ear infection may occur. Inner ear injury has been observed with barotitis media and after vigorous

Valsalva maneuvers. Such inner ear disturbances in divers are sometimes associated with round window membrane rupture, perilymphatic fistulas, potential CSF leaks, and meningitis. At present, we are unaware of reports in the literature describing this sequence of events after HBO therapy.

References

1. Brown IW, Fuson RL, Mauney FM, et al: Hyperbaric oxygenation (hybaroxia), current status, possibilities and limitations. In: Welsch CL, ed. Adv in Surg. Vol I. Chicago: Yearbook Publishers, 1965, pp 285-349.
2. Maloney JV: Cardiovascular surgery. *Surg Gynecol Obstet* **120**:268-272, 1965.
3. Boerema I, Brummelkamp WH, Meijne NG, eds: Clinical application of hyperbaric oxygen. *Proceedings of the First International Congress, Amsterdam, September 1963.* Amsterdam/London/New York, Elsevier Publishing Co., 1964.
4. Ledingham IMcA, ed: Hyperbaric oxygenation. *Proceedings of the Second Congress, Glasgow, September 1964.* Edinburgh/London, E & S Livingstone, Ltd., 1965.
5. Brown IW, Cox BG, eds: *Proceedings of the Third International Conference on Hyperbaric Medicine.* Washington, D.C., National Academy of Sciences, National Research Council, Publication #1404, 1966.
6. Wada J, Iwa T, eds: *Proceedings of the Fourth International Congress on Hyperbaric Medicine.* Baltimore, The Williams and Wilkins Co., 1970.
7. Trapp WG, Banister EW, Davison AJ, Trapp PA, eds: *Fifth International Hyperbaric Congress Proceedings, Vol. I & II, 1973.* Burnaby 2, B.C., Canada, Simon Fraser University, 1974.
8. Smith G, ed: *Proceedings of the Sixth International Congress on Hyperbaric Medicine.* Aberdeen University Press, 1978.
9. Bennett PB, Elliott DH, eds: *The Physiology and Medicine of Diving and Compressed Air Work.* Baltimore, The William & Wilkins Company, 1969.
10. Davis JC, Hunt TK, eds: *Hyperbaric Oxygen Therapy.* Bethesda, Maryland, Undersea Medical Society, 1977.
11. *Fundamentals of Hyperbaric Medicine.* Washington, D.C., National Academy of Sciences, National Research Council, Publication #1298, 1966.
12. Hills BA: Decompression sickness. Vol. I. In: *The Biophysical Basis of Prevention and Treatment.* New York, John Wiley and Sons, 1977.
13. Innes, GS: *The Production and Hazards of a Hyperbaric Environment.* Oxford, Pergamon Press, 1970.
14. Meijne NG: *Hyperbaric Oxygen and its Clinical Value.* Springfield, Illinois, Charles C. Thomas, 1970.
15. Hart GB, Kindwall EP: Hyperbaric chamber clinical support: monoplace. In: Davis JC, Hunt TK, eds. *Hyperbaric Oxygen Therapy.* Bethesda, Maryland, Undersea Medical Society, 1977.

16. Hart GB: Treatment of decompression illness and air embolism with hyperbaric oxygenation. *Aerospace Med* 45:1190-1193, 1974.
17. Sheffield PJ, Davis JC, Bell GC, Gallagher TJ: Hyperbaric chamber clinical support: multiplace. In: Davis JC, Hunt TK, eds. *Hyperbaric Oxygen Therapy*. Bethesda, Maryland, Undersea Medical Society, 1977.
18. Clamann HG: Fire hazards. *Ann NY Acad Sci* 117:814-123, 1965.
19. Bond GF: Safety factors in chamber operation. In: *Fundamentals of Hyperbaric Medicine*. National Academy of Sciences, National Research Council, Publication #1298, Washington D.C., 1966.
20. Hart GB, Broussard ND, Goodman DB, Yanda RL: Treatment of burns with hyperbaric oxygen. *Surg Gynecol Obstet* 139:693-696, 1974.
21. Hart GB, Lee WS, Rasmussen BD, O'Reilly RR: Complications of repetitive hyperbaric therapy. In: Trapp WG, Banister EW, Davison AJ, Trapp PA, eds. *Fifth International Hyperbaric Cong Proceedings, 1973, Vol. II*. Burnaby 2, B.C. Canada, Simon Fraser University, 1974, pp 867-873.
22. Schmidt JP, Ball RJ: Atmospheric oxygen: effect on resistance of mice to pneumococcal pneumonia. *Aerospace Med* 41:1238-1239, 1970.
23. Jacobson II, JH: Unpublished data.
24. Ledingham IMcA, Davidson JK: Hazards in hyperbaric medicine. In: Wada J, Iwa T, eds. *Proceedings of the Fourth International Congress on Hyperbaric Medicine*. Baltimore, The Williams and Wilkins Co., 1970.
25. Slack WK, Hanson GC, Chew HER, et al: Analysis of complications of hyperbaric oxygen therapy in 455 patients treated in single-person hyperbaric oxygen chambers. In: Wada J, Iwa T, eds. *Proceedings of the Fourth International Congress on Hyperbaric Medicine*. Baltimore, The Williams and Wilkins Co., 1970, pp 505-509.
26. Kuyama T: Clinical studies on the hyperbaric oxygenations at Kyoto University. In: Wada J, Iwa T, eds. *Proceedings of the Fourth International Congress on Hyperbaric Medicine*. Baltimore, The Williams and Wilkins Co., 1970, pp 481-486.
27. Lamy ML, Hanquet M: Application opportunity for OHP in a general hospital. A 2-year experience with a monoplace hyperbaric oxygen chamber. In: Wada J, Iwa T, eds. *Proceedings of the Fourth International Congress on Hyperbaric Medicine*. Baltimore, The Williams and Wilkins Co., 1970, pp 517-522.
28. Sukoff MH, Ragatz RE: Hyperbaric oxygenation for the treatment of acute cerebral edema. *Neurosurgery* 10:29-38, 1982.
29. Marshall R, Lanphier EH, DuBois AB: The resistance to breathing in normal subjects during simulated dives. *J Appl Physiol* 9:5-10, 1956.
30. Nairn JR, Power GG, Hyde RE, et al: The measurement of the apparent pulmonary diffusing capacity for carbon monoxide (DL_{CO}) at hyperbaric pressures. *Physiologist* 7:211, 1964.
31. Fasciola JC, Chiodi H: Arterial Oxygen pressure during pure O_2 breathing. *Amer J Physiol* 147:54-65, 1946.
32. Lanphier EH, Brown IW: The physiological basis of hyperbaric therapy. In: *Fundamentals of Hyperbaric Medicine*. Chapter IV. Washington, D.C., NAS, NRC, 1966, pp 33-55.
33. Boerema I, Meyne NG, Brummelkamp WH, et al: Life without blood. *J Cardiovasc Surg* 1:133-146. 1960.
34. Dittmer DS, Grebe RM, eds: *Handbook of Respiration*. WADC Tech-

nical Report. (58-352) 1958, pp 56-58.

35. Green DE, Hatefi Y: The mitochondrion and biochemical machines. *Science* **133**:13-19, 1961.

36. Hempel FG, Jobsis FF, LaManna JL, et al: Oxidation of cerebral cytochrome aa₃ by oxygen plus carbon dioxide at hyperbaric pressures. *J Appl Physiol* **43**:873-879, 1977.

37. Bean JW: Cerebral O_2 in exposures to O_2 at atmospheric and higher pressure, and influence of CO_2. *Am J Physiol* **201**:1192-1198, 1961.

38. Bennett PB: Cortical CO_2 and O_2 at high pressures of argon, nitrogen, helium, and oxygen. *J Appl Physiol* **20**:1249-1252, 1965.

39. Jamieson D, Van Den Brenk HAS: Measurement of oxygen tensions in cerebral tissues of rats exposed to high pressures of oxygen. *J Appl Physiol* **18**:869-876, 1963.

40. Maeda N: Experimental studies on the effect of decompression procedures in hyperbaric oxygenation for the treatment of spinal cord injury. *J NARA Med Assoc* **16**:429-447, 1965.

41. Sonnenschein RR, Stein SN, Perot PL: Oxygen tension of the brain during hyperoxic convulsions. *Am J Physiol* **173**:161-163, 1953.

42. Davies PW, Bronk DW: Oxygen tension in mammalian brain. *Federation Proc* **16**:689-692, 1957.

43. Adams JE, Severinghaus JW: Oxygen tension of human cerebral grey and white matter. The effect of forced hyperventilation. *J Neurosurg* **19**: 959-963, 1962.

44. Forster RE: Oxygenation of the tissue cell. *Ann NY Acad Sci* **117**:730-735, 1965.

45. Bergofsky EH, Jacobson JH, Fishmen AP: The use of lymph for the measurement of gas tensions in interstitial fluid and tissues. *J Clin Invest* **41**:1971-1979, 1962.

46. Van Liew HD: Tissue gas tensions by microtonometry: results in liver and fat. *J Appl Physiol* **17**:359-363, 1962.

47. Lambertsen CJ: Oxygen toxicity. Effects in man of oxygen at 1 and 3.5 atmospheres upon blood gas transport, cerebral circulation and cerebral metabolism. *J Appl Physiol* **5**:471-486, 1953.

48. Lambertsen CJ, Ewing JH, Kough RH, et al: Oxygen toxicity. Arterial and internal jugular blood gas composition in man during inhalation of air, 100% O_2 and 2% CO_2 in O_2 at 3.5 atmospheres ambient pressure. *J Appl Physiol* **8**:255-263, 1955.

49. Jennett WB, Ledingham IMcA, Harper AM, et al: The effects of hyperbaric oxygen on cerebral blood flow during carotid artery surgery. In: Wada J, Iwa T, eds: *Proceedings of the Fourth International Congress on Hyperbaric Medicine*. Baltimore, The Williams and Wilkins Co., 1970.

50. Saltzman HA, Anderson BJ, Whalen RE, et al: Hyperbaric oxygen therapy of acute cerebral vascular insufficiency. In: Brown IW, Cox BG, eds. *Proceedings of the Third International Conference on Hyperbaric Medicine*. Washington, D.C., National Academy of Sciences, National Research Council, 1966, pp 440-445.

51. Katsurada K, Minami T, Onji Y: Effect of hyperbaric oxygenation on CSF pO_2 in patients with head injury. In: Trapp WG, Banister EW, Davison AJ, et al, eds. *Fifth International Hyperbaric Congress Proceedings, Vol. I & II, 1973*. Burnaby 2, B.C., Canada, Simon Fraser University, 1974.

52. Plum F, Posner JB, Smith WW: The effect of hyperbaric-hyperoxic hy-

perventilation on blood, brain, and CSF lactate. *Am J Physiol* **215**: 1240-1244, 1968.
53. Gotok F, Meyrs JS, Takagi Y: Cerebral effects of hyperventilation in man. *Arch Neurol* **12**:410-423, 1965.
54. Reivich M, Cohen PJ, Greenbaum L: Alterations in the electroencephalogram of awake man produced by hyperventilation: effects of 100% oxygen at 3 atmospheres (absolute) pressure. *Neurology* **16**:304, 1966.
55. Yarnell P, Merril CR, Charlton G, et al: Cerebral fluid cavity oxygen tension. Preliminary report of observations in man. *Neurology, Minneap* **17**:659-669, 1967.
56. Yarnell P, Charlton G, Merril CR, et al: Dynamics of oxygen tension in the cisternal cerebrospinal fluid of the Rhesus monkey. *J Neurosurg* **27**:515-524, 1967.
57. Hollin S, Espinosa OE, Sukoff MH, et al: The effect of hyperbaric oxygenation on cerebrospinal fluid oxygen. *J Neurosurg* **29**:229-235, 1968.
58. Bloor BM, Fricker J, Hellinger F, et al: A study of cerebrospinal fluid oxygen tension. Preliminary experimental and clinical observation. *Arch Neurol, Chicago* **4**:37-46, 1961.
59. Jarnum S, Lorenzen I, Skinhoj E: Cisternal fluid oxygen tension in man. *Neurology, Minneap* **14**:703-707, 1964.
60. Fuson RL, Moor GF, Smith WW, et al: Hyperbaric oxygenation in experimental cerebral ischemia. *Surg Forum* **16**:416-418, 1965.
61. Heyman A, Saltzman HA, Whalen RE: The use of hyperbaric oxygenation in treatment of cerebral ischemia and infarction. *Circulation* **33**:20-27, 1966.
62. Koch A, Vermeulen-Cranch DM: The use of hyperbaric oxygenation following cardiac arrest. *Brit J Anesthes* **34**:739-740, 1962.
63. Smith G, Lawson DD, Renfrew S, et al: Preservation of cerebral cortical activity by breathing oxygen at two atmospheres of pressure during cerebral ischemia. *Surg Gynecol Obstet* **113**:13-16, 1961.
64. Whalen RE, Heyman A, Saltzman H: The protective effect of hyperbaric oxygenation in cerebral anoxia. *Arch Neurol* **14**:15-20, 1966.
65. Jacobson I, Harper AM, McDowell DG: The effects of oxygen under pressure on cerebral blood-flow and cerebral venous oxygen tension. *Lancet* **2**:549, 1963.
66. Tindall GT, Wilkins RH, Odam GL: Effect of hyperbaric oxygenation on cerebral blood flow. *Surg Forum* **16**:414-416, 1965.
67. Harper AM, Jacobson I, McDowell DG: The effect of hyperbaric oxygen on the blood flow through the cerebral cortex. In: Ledingham IMcA, ed. *Proceedings of the Second Congress, Glasgow, September 1964.* Edinburg/London, E & S Livingstone, Ltd, 1965, pp 184-192.
68. Hayakawa T, Kanai N, Kuroda E, et al: Reponse of cerebrospinal fluid pressure to hyperbaric oxygenation. *J Neurol Neurosurg Psychiat* **34**: 580-586, 1971.
69. Miller JD, Fitch W, Ledingham IMcA: Reduction of increased intracranial pressure. Comparison between hyperbaric oxygen and hyperventilation. *Arch Neurol* **24**:210-216, 1971.
70. Mogami H, Hayakawa T, Kanai N, et al: Clinical application of hyperbaric oxygenation in the treatment of acute cerebral damage. *J Neurosurg* **31**:636-642, 1969.
71. Sukoff MH, Hollin SA, Espinosa OE, et al: The protective effect of hyperbaric oxygenation in experimental cerebral edema. *J Neurosurg* **29**:263-241, 1968.

72. Dunn JE, II, Connolly, JM: Effects of hypobaric and hyperbaric oxygen on experimental brain injury. In: Brown IW, Jr, Cox BG, eds. *Hyperbaric Medicine*. Washington, D.C., *Natl Acad Sci* 1966, pp 447-454.

73. Coe JE, Hayes TM: Treatment of experimental brain injury by hyperbaric oxygenation. A preliminary report. *Am Surg* 32:493-495, 1966.

74. Fasano VA, Broggi G, Urciuoli R, et al: Clinical applications of hyperbaric oxygen in traumatic coma. In: de Vet, AC, ed. *Proceedings of the Third International Congress of Neurological Surgery*. New York, Excerpta Medica Foundation, 1966, pp 502-505.

75. Jacobson I, Lawson DD: The effect of hyperbaric oxygen on experimental cerebral infarction in the dog. *J Neurosurg* 20:849-859, 1963.

76. Ingvar DH, Lassen NA: Treatment of focal cerebral ischemia with hyperbaric oxygen. Report of four cases. *Acta Neurol Scand* 41:92-95, 1965.

77. Heyman A, Saltzman HA, Whalen RE: The use of hyperbaric oxygenation in the use of cerebral ischemia and infarction. *Circulation* 33:20-27, 1966.

78. Neubauer RA, End E: Hyperbaric oxygenation as an adjunct therapy in strokes due to thrombosis. A review of 122 patients. *Stroke* 11:297-300, 1980.

79. Holbach KH, Careli A, Wassmann H: Cerebral energy metabolism in patients with brain lesions at normo- and hyperbaric oxygen pressures. *J Neurol* 217:17-30, 1977.

80. Holbach DH, Wassmann H, Hoheluchter KL, et al: Differentiation between reversible and irreversible post-stroke changes in brain tissue: its relevance for cerebrovascular surgery. *Surg Neurol* 7:325-331, 1977.

81. Holbach KH, Wassmann H, Sanchez F: EEG analysis for evaluating chronic cerebral ischemia treated by hyperbaric oxygen and microneurosurgery. *J Neurol* 219:227-240, 1978.

82. Kapp JP: Neurological response to hyperbaric oxygen. A criterion for cerebral revascularization. *Surg Neurol* 15:43-46, 1981.

83. Millikan CH, McDowell FH: Treatment of progressing stroke. *Stroke* 12:397-409, 1981.

84. Kelly DL Jr, Lassiter KRL, Vongsvivut A, et al: Effects of hyperbaric oxygenation in tissue oxygen studies in experimental paraplegia. *J Neurosurg* 36:425-429, 1972.

85. Maeda N: Experimental studies on the effect of decompression procedures and hyperbaric oxygenation for the treatment of spinal cord injury. *J NARA Med Assoc* 16:429-447, 1965.

86. Ogilvie RW, Ballentine JD: Oxygen tensions in the deep gray matter of rats exposed to hyperbaric oxygen. *Adv Exp Med Biol* 37:299-304, 1973.

87. Ogilvie RW, Ballentine JD: Oxygen tension in spinal cord gray matter during exposure to hyperbaric oxygen. *J Neurosurg* 48:156-161, 1975.

88. Gelderd, JB, Welch DW, Fief WP, et al: Therapeutic effects of hyperbaric oxygen and dimethysulfoxide following spinal cord transections in rats. *Undersea Biomed Res* 7:305-320, 1980.

89. Yeo JD, McKenzie B, Hindwood B, et al: Treatment of paraplegic sheep with hyperbaric oxygen. *Med J Aust* 1:538-540, 1976.

90. Yeo JD, Stabback S. McKinsey B: Study of the effects of hyperbaric oxygen on experimental spinal cord injury. *Med J Aust* 2:145-147, 1977.

91. Higgins AC, Pearlstein RD, Mullen JB, Nashold BS, Jr: Effects of hyperbaric oxygen therapy on long-tract neuronal conduction in the acute phase of spinal cord injury. *J Neurosurg* 55:501-510, 1981.

92. Hartzog JT, Risher RG, Snow C: Spinal cord trauma: effects of hyperbaric oxygen therapy. In: *Proceedings of the 17th Veterans Administra-*

tion Spinal Cord Injury Conference. Washington, DC, US Government Printing Office, 1971, pp 70-71.

93. Gamache FW, Jr., Myers RAM, Ducker TB, et al: The clinical application of hyperbaric oxygen therapy in spinal cord injury: preliminary report. *Surg Neurol* **15**:85-87, 1981.
94. Holbach KH, Wassman H, Hoheluchter KL, et al: Clinical course of spinal lesions treated with hyperbaric oxygenation. *ACTA Neurochir* **31**:297-298, 1975.
95. Jones RF, Unsworth IP: Hyperbaric oxygen in acute spinal cord injury in humans. *Med J Aust* **2**:573-575, 1978.
96. Linked D, Holbach KH, Wassman H, et al: Electromyographic findings in spinal cord lesions treated with hyperbaric oxygenation. *ACTA Neurochir* **31**:298-299, 1975.
97. Welch BE, Morgan TE, Clamann HG: Time-concentration effects in relation to oxygen toxicity in man. *Fed Proc* **22**:1053-1056, 1963.
98. Comroe JH, Dripps RD, Dumke PR, et al: Oxygen toxicity. The effect of inhalation of high concentrations of oxygen for twenty-four hours on normal men at sea level and at a simulated altitude of 18,000 feet. *JAMA* **128**:710-717, 1945.
99. Clark JM, Lambertsen LJ: Pulmonary oxygen toxicity: A review. *Pharmacol Rev* **23**:37-133, 1971.
100. Clark JM, Lambertsen CJ: Rate of development of pulmonary oxygen toxicity in man during oxygen breathing at 2.0 ATA. *J Appl Physiol* **30**:739-752, 1971.
101. Donald KW: Oxygen poisoning in man. I and II. *Brit Med J* **1**:667-672, 712-717, 1947.
102. Yarbrough ID, Welham W, Brinton ES, et al: Symptoms of oxygen poisoning and limits of tolerance at rest and at work. *U.S. Navy Experimental Diving Unit Rep* No. I, 1947.
103. Bornstein A, Stroink M: Über Sauerstoffvergiftung. *Dt Med Wschr* **38**: 1495-1497, 1912.
104. Thompson WAR: The physiology of deep-sea diving. *Brit Med J* **2**:208-210, 1935.
105. Behnke AR: Effects of high pressures, prevention and treatment of compressed air illness. *Med Clin North Am* **26**:1213-1237, 1942.
106. Gerschman R: Biological effect of oxygen. In: Dickens F, Neil E, eds. *Oxygen in the Animal Organism.* New York, Macmillan, 1964, pp 475-494.
107. Gilbert DL: The role of pro-oxidants and anti-oxidants in oxygen toxicity. *Radiat Res* **3**:44-53, 1963.
108. Crapo JD, Tierney DF: Superoxide dismutase and pulmonary oxygen toxicity. *Am J Physiol* **226**:1401-1407, 1974.
109. Menzel DB: Toxicity of ozone, oxygen and radiation. *Ann Rev Pharmacol* **10**:379-394, 1970.
110. Haugaard N: Cellular mechanisms of oxygen toxicity. *Physiol Rev* **48**: 311-373, 1968.
111. Baeyens DA, Hoffert JR, Fromm PO: A comparative study of the influence of oxygen on lactate dehydrogenase. *Comp Biochem Physiol* **47**: 1-7, 1974.
112. Allen JE, Goodman BP, Besarab A, et al: Studies on the biochemical basis of oxygen toxicity. *Biochem Biophys Acta* **320**:708-728, 1973.
113. Falsetti H: Effect of oxygen tension on sodium transport across isolated frog skin. *Proc Soc Exp Biol Med* **101**:721-722, 1959.
114. Wood JD, Radomski MW, Watson WJ: A study of possible mechanisms

involved in hyperbaric oxygen induced changes in cerebral gamma-aminobutyric acid levels and accompanying seizures. *Can J Biochem* **49**: 543-547, 1971.

115. Campbell JA: Effects of oxygen pressure as influenced by external temperature, hormones and drugs. *J Physiol* **92**:29-31P, 1938.

116. Bean JW: Hormonal aspects of oxygen toxicity. In: *Proc Underwater Physiol Symp* Washington DC, Natl Acad Sci, Natl Research Council Publication, No. 377, 1955, pp 13-24.

117. Bean JW, Smith CW: Hypophyseal and adrenocortical factors in pulmonary damage induced by oxygen at atmospheric pressure. *Am J Physiol* **172**:169-179, 1953.

118. Bean JW, Johnson PC: Influence of hypophysis on pulmonary injury induced by exposure to oxygen at high pressure and by pneumococcus. *Am J Physiol* **171**:451-458, 1952.

119. Bean JW: General effects of oxygen at high tension. In: Dickens F, Neil E, eds. *Oxygen in the Animal Organism*. New York, Macmillan, 1964, pp 455-472.

120. Gerschman R, Gilbert DL, Nye SW, et al: Role of adrenalectomy and adrenal cortical hormones in oxygen poisoning. *Am J Physiol* **178**:346-350, 1954.

121. Gerschman R, Gilbert DL, Nye SW, et al: Role of anti-oxidants and of glutathione in oxygen poisoning. *Fed Proc* **14**:66, 1955.

122. Smith CS, Bean JW: Adrenal factors in toxic action of O_2 at atmospheric pressure. *Fed Proc* **14**:140, 1955.

123. Taylor DW: Effects of high oxygen pressures on adrenalectomized, treated rats. *J Physiol* **125**:46-47P, 1954.

124. Taylor DW: Effects of tocopherols, methylene blue, and glutathione on the manifestations of oxygen poisoning in vitamin E-deficient rats. *J Physiol* **140**:37-47, 1958.

125. Johnson PC, Bean JW: Effects of sympathetic blocking agents on the toxic action of O_2 at high pressure. *Am J Physiol* **188**:593-598, 1957.

126. Pagni E, Zampolini M, Frullani F: Blocking of *alpha*-adrenergic receptors as a method of prevention of lesions from hyperbaric oxygen. *Minerva Anesthesiol* **33**:49-54, 1967a.

127. Matsuda T: Experimental studies on hyperbaric oxygenation. I. The oxygen poisoning by hyperbaric oxygenation. *Jap J Anesthesiol* **18**: 620-629, 1969.

128. Houlihan RT: Adaptation to chronic hyperbaric oxygen pressures. *Final Scientific Report*. Contr Nonr. 656-36. USAF School of Aerospace Medicine, September 1969.

129. Houlihan RT: Rheomelanin accumulation in the blood and lungs and hemolysis in rats poisoned by hyperbaric oxygen. *J Amer Osteopath Assoc* **69**:1040, 1970.

130. Houlihan RT, Altschule MD, Hegedus ZL: Indole metabolism of catecholamines during exposure to hyperbaric oxygen. *Preprints of Annual Scientific Meeting of Aerospace Medical Association*. 1969, pp 192-193.

131. Houlihan RT, Altschule MD, Hegedus ZL, et al: Oxidative cyclization of catecholamines following exposure to hyperbaric oxygen. *Fourth International Congress on Hyperbaric Medicine (Program)*, Sapporo, Japan, 1969, pp 14-15.

132. Houlihan RT, Zavodni J, Cross M: Effects of increased oxygen pressure on adrenal steroid and catecholamine release. In: Hannisdahl B, Sem-

Jacobsen CW, eds. *Aviation and Space Medicine*. Oslo, Universitets-forlaget, 1969.

133. van den Brenk HAS, Jamieson D: Studies of mechanism of chemical radiation protection *in vivo*. II. Effect of high pressure oxygen on radio-protection *in vivo* and its relationship to "oxygen poisoning." *Int J Radiat Biol* 4:379-402, 1962.

134. Pagni E, Novelli GP, Patumi F: Catecholamine depletion induced by reserpine as a means of preventing hyperbaric oxygen injuries. *Osp Ital Chir* 17:233-246, 1967.

135. Garwacki J: Effect of neuroplegic drugs on changes in the respiratory organs in rats breathing pure oxygen under pressure (1 atm). *Acta Physiol Pol* 11:73-85, 1960.

136. Marcozzi G, Messinetti A, Colombati M, et al: Oximetric variations and pulmonary lesions induced by inhalation of oxygen concentrations higher than that of the atmosphere. *Arch de Vecchi Anat Patol Med Clin* 32:609-636, 1960.

137. Bean JW: Reserpine and reaction to O_2 at high pressure. *Fed Proc* 15:11-12, 1956.

138. Bean JW: Reserpine, chlorpromazine and the hypothalamus in reactions to oxygen at high pressure. *Am J Physiol* 187:389-394, 1956.

139. Paton WDM: Experiments on the convulsant and anesthetic effects of oxygen. *Brit J Pharmacol Chemother* 29:350-366, 1967.

140. Grognot P, Chome J: Action de la chlorpromazine et du tetrylammonium sur les reactions pulmonaires provoquees par inhalation d'oxygene pur. *CR Seances Soc Biol* 148:1474-1475, 1954.

141. Gerschman R, Gilbert DL, Nye SW, Dwyer P, Fenn WO: Oxygen poisoning and x-irradiation: a mechanism in common. *Science* 119:623-626, 1954.

142. Gerschman R, Gilbert DL, Nye SW, et al: Role of anti-oxidants and of glutathione in oxygen poisoning. *Fed Proc* 14:66, 1955.

143. Haugaard N: The toxic action of oxygen on metabolism and the role of trace metals. In: Dickens F, Neil E, eds. *Oxygen in the Animal Organism*. New York. Macmillan, 1964, pp 495-505.

144. Gerschman R, Gilbert DL, Caccamise D: Effects of various substances on survival times of mice exposed to different high oxygen tensions. *Am J Physiol* 192:563-571, 1958.

145. Bean JW: Tris buffer, CO_2, and sympatho-adrenal system in reactions to O_2 at high pressure. *Am J Physiol* 201:737-739, 1961.

146. McSherry CK, Veith FJ: The relationship between the central nervous system and pulmonary forms of oxygen toxicity: effect of THAM administration. *Surg Forum* 19:33-35, 1968.

147. Maritano M, Cabrai M, Marchiaro G, et al: The activity of THAM during OHP. *Acta Anesthesiol Scand Suppl* 24:353-362, 1966.

148. Nahas GG: Control of acidosis in hyperbaric oxygenation. *Ann NY Acad Sci* 117:774-786, 1965.

149. Sanger C, Nahas GG, Goldberg AR, D'Allesio GM: Effects of 2-amino-hydroxymethyl-l, 3-propanediol on oxygen toxicity in mice. *Ann NY Acad Sci* 92:710-723, 1961.

150. Kann Jr. HE, Mengel CE, Smith W, Horton B: Oxygen toxicity and vitamin E. *Aerosp Med* 35:840-844, 1964.

151. Taylor DW: Effects of vitamin E deficiency on oxygen toxicity in the rat. *J Physiol* 121:47P-48P, 1953.

152. Taylor DW: The effects of vitamin E and methylene blue on the mani-

festations of oxygen poisoning in the rat. *J Physiol* **131**:200-206, 1956.
153. Taylor DW: Effects adrenalectomy on oxygen poisoning in the rat. *J Physiol* **140**:23-36, 1958.
154. Wood JD, Watson WJ: Protective action of γ-aminobutyric acid against oxygen toxicity. *Nature* **195**:296, 1962.
155. Wood JD, Watson WJ, Clydesdale FM: γ-aminobutyric acid and oxygen poisoning. *J Neurochem* **10**:625-633, 1963.
156. Wood JD, Stacey NE, Watson WJ: Pulmonary and central nervous system damage in rats exposed to hyperbaric oxygen and protection therefrom by γ-aminobutyric acid. *Can J Physiol Pharmacol* **405**-410, 1965.
157. Faiman MD, Nolan RJ: The role of cerebral energy metabolism in oxygen convulsions. In: Trapp WG, Banister EW, Davison AJ, et al, eds. *Fifth International Hyperbaric Congress Proceedings, Vol. I & II, 1973.* Burnaby 2, B.C., Canada, Simon Fraser University, 1974.
158. Gesell R: On the chemical regulation of respiration. I. The regulation of respiration with special reference to the metabolism of the respiratory center and the coordination of the dual function of hemoglobin. *Am J Physiol* **66**:5-49, 1923.
159. Hill L: Influence of CO_2 in production of oxygen poisoning. *Q J Exp Physiol* **23**:49-50, 1933.
160. Bean JW, Zee D: Influence of anesthesia and CO_2 on CNS and pulmonary effects of O_2 at high pressure. *J Appl Physiol* **20**:525-530, 1965.
161. Marshall JR, Lambertsen CJ: Interactions of increased P_{O_2} and P_{CO_2} effects in producing convulsions and death in mice. *J Appl Physiol* **16**:1-7, 1961.
162. Szam I: Pathogenesis of hyperbaric oxygen intoxication. Experimental studies on the significance of CO_2 and NH_3 accumulation in the central nervous system for the pathogenesis of hyperbaric pulmonary edema. *Anesthetist* **18**:39-43, 1969.
163. Wood CD, Perkins GF: Factors influencing hypertension and pulmonary edema produced by hyperbaric O_2. *Aerospace Med* **41**:869-872, 1970.
164. Behnke AR, Shaw LA, Shilling CS, Thomson RM, Messer AC: Studies on the effects of high oxygen pressure. I. Effect of high oxygen pressure upon the carbon-dioxide combining power of the blood. *Am J Physiol* **107**:13-28, 1934.
165. Shaw LA, Behnke AR, Messer AC: Role of CO_2 in producing symptoms of oxygen poisoning. *Am J Physiol* **108**:652-661, 1934.
166. Bennett PB, Ackles KN: The narcotic effects of hyperbaric oxygen. In: Wada J, Iwa T, eds. *Proceedings of the Fourth International Hyperbaric Congress on Hyperbaric Medicine.* Baltimore, The Williams and Wilkins Co., 1970.
167. Paton WDM: Experiments on the convulsant and anaesthetic effects of oxygen. *Brit J Pharmacol* **29**:350-366, 1967.
168. Ackerman NB, Brinkley FB: Cyclical intermittent hyperbaric oxygenation: a method for prolonging survival in hyperbaric oxygen. In: Brown, Jr. IW, Cox BG, eds. *Proceedings of the Third International Conference on Hyperbaric Medicine.* Washington, D.C., NAS, NRC Publ. No. 1404, 1966, pp 410-420.
169. Hall DA: The influence of the systematic fluctuation of P_{O_2} upon the nature and rate of the development of oxygen toxicity in guinea pigs (MS thesis). Graduate School of Arts and Sciences, University of Pennsylvania, 1967.
170. Paine JR, Lynn D, Keys A: Observations on the effects of prolonged

administration of high oxygen concentration to dogs. *J Thorac Cardiovasc Surg* 11:151-168, 1941.

171. Penrod KE: Effect of intermittent nitrogen exposures on tolerance to oxygen at high pressure. *Am J Physiol* 186:149-151, 1956.

172. Roth EM: Selection of space cabin atmospheres. I. Oxygen toxicity. Washington, D.C., NASA Technical Note D-2008, 1963.

173. Wright RA, Weiss HS, Hiatt EP, et al: Risk of mortality in interrupted exposure to 100 percent O_2: role of air vs lowered PO_2. *Am J Physiol* 210:1015-1020, 1966.

174. Lambertsen CJ: Respiratory and circulatory actions of high oxygen pressure. In: *Proc Underwater Physiol Symp.* Washington, D.C., Natl Acad Sci-Natl Res Council. Publ. No. 377, 1955.

175. Holbach KH, Careli A: Oxygen tolerance and the oxygenation state of the injured human brain. In: Trapp WG, Banister EW, Davison AJ, et al, eds. *Fifth International Hyperbaric Congress Proceedings, Vol. I & II, 1973.* Burnaby 2, B.C., Canada, Simon Fraser University, 1974.

176. Kety SS: The general metabolism of the brain *in vivo*. In: Richter D. ed. *The Metabolism of the Nervous System.* London, Pergamon Press, 1957, pp 221-237.

177. Donald KW: Oxygen poisoning in man. *Brit Med J* 1:667-672, 1947.

178. Lambertsen CJ: Oxygen toxicity. In: *Fundamentals of Hyperbaric Medicine.* Washington, D.C., National Academy of Sciences, National Research Council, Publication #1298, 1966.

179. Foster CA: Hyperbaric oxygen and radiotherapy. In: Ledingham IM, ed. *Hyperbaric Oxygenation.* Edinburgh, Livingstone, 1965, pp 380-388.

180. Cohn R, Gersch I: Changes in brain potentials during convulsions induced by oxygen under pressure. *J Neurophysiol* 8:155-160, 1945.

181. Nichols CS, Lambertsen CJ: Effects of high oxygen pressures on the eye. *N Engl J Med* 281:25-30, 1969.

182. Miller EF: Effect of breathing 100 percent oxygen on visual field and acuity. *J Aviation Med* 29:598-602, 1958.

183. Salzman HA, Hart L, Anderson, et al: The response of the retinal circulation to hyperbaric oxygenation. *J Clin Invest* 43:1283, 1964.

184. Kent PR: Oxygen breathing effects upon night vision thresholds. *US Naval Submar M Center Rep* 469:1-13, 1966.

185. Behnke AR, Forbes HS, Motley EP: Circulatory and visual effects of oxygen at 3 atmospheres pressure. *Am J Physiol* 114:436-442, 1936.

186. Rosenberg E, Shibata HR, McLean LD: Blood gas and neurological responses to inhalation of oxygen at 3 atmospheres. *Proc Soc Exper Biol Med* 122:313-317, 1966.

187. Noell WK: Studies on visual cell viability and differentiation. *Ann NY Acad Sci* 74:337-361, 1958.

188. Nolte H, Schnakenburg KV: New histological and electron microscopic results on CNS oxygen toxicity. In: Trapp WG, Banister EW, Davison AJ, et al. *Fifth International Hyperbaric Congress Proceedings, Vol. I & II, 1973.* Burnaby 2, B.C., Canada, Simon Fraser University, 1974, pp 116-125.

189. Ballentine JD: Pathogenesis of central nervous system lesions induced by exposure to hyperbaric oxygen. *Am J Path* 53:1097-1109, 1968.

190. Ballentine JD: Central necrosis of the spinal cord induced by hyperbaric oxygen exposure. *J Neurosurg* 43:150-155, 1975.

191. Perot PL, Stein SN: Conduction block in peripheral nerve produced by oxygen at high pressures. *Fed Proc* 15:144, 1956.

192. Pol B, Watelle TJJ: Memoire sur les effects de la compression de l'air, appliquees au creusement des puits a houille. *Ann Hyg Publ.* 2^e Ser. 1:241-279, 1854.

193. Behnke AR, Thomson RM, Shaw LA: Rate of elimination of nitrogen in man in relation to fat and water content of body. *Am J Physiol* **114**: 137-146, 1935.

194. Jones HB: Gas exchange and blood-tissue perfusion factors in various body tissues. In: Fulton JF, ed. *Decompression Sickness: Caisson Sickness, Diver's and Flier's Bends and Related Syndromes.* Philadelphia, Pa., 1951, pp 290-295.

195. Boycott AW, Damant GCC, Haldane JS: Prevention of compressed air illness. *J Hyg* **8**:342-443, 1908.

196. Piccard J: Aero-emphysema and the birth of gas bubbles. *Proc Staff Meeting Mayo Clinic* **16**:700-704, 1941.

197. Epstein PS, Plesset MS: On the stability of gas bubbles in liquid gas solutions. *J Chem Phys* **18**:1505-1509, 1950.

198. Cockett ATK: Effects of emboli on the neurocirculatory system in decompression sickness. In: Trapp WG, Banister EW, Davison AJ, et al, eds. *Fifth International Hyperbaric Congress Proceedings, Vol I & II, 1973.* Burnaby 2, B.C., Canada, Simon Fraser University, 1974, pp 883-889.

199. Cockett ATK, Nakamura RM, Franks JJ: Recent findings in the pathogenesis of decompression sickness (dysbarism). *Surgery* **58**:384-389, 1965.

200. Behnke AR: Decompression sickness: advances and interpretations. *Aerospace Med* **42**:255-267, 1971.

201. Spencer MP, Postles WT, Campbell SD: Clinical use of blood bubble detection in diagnosis, treatment and prevention of decompression sickness. In: Trapp WG, Banister EW, Davison AJ, et al, eds. *Fifth International Hyperbaric Congress Proceedings Vol I & II, 1973.* Burnaby 2, B.C., Canada, Simon Fraser University, 1974.

202. Cohen R, Overfield EM, Kylstra JA: Diffusion component of alveolar-arterial oxygen pressure difference in man. *J Appl Physiol* **31**:223-226, 1971.

203. Gillis MF, Karagianes MT, Peterson PL: Bends: Detection of circulating gas emboli with external sensor. *Science* **161**:579-580, 1968.

204. Spencer MP, Clark HF: Precordial monitoring of pulmonary gas embolism and recompression bubbles. *Aerospace Med* **43**:762-767, 1972.

205. Villaret M, Cachera R: *Les embolies cerebrales: etude de pathologie experimental dur les embolies solides et gaseuse due cerveau.* Paris, Masson, 1939.

206. Marchand P, van Hasse HH, Luntz CH: Massive venous air embolism. *S Afr Med J* **38**:202-208, 1964.

207. Grulke DC, Marsh NA, Hills BA: Experimental air embolism: measurement of microbubbles using the Coulter counter. *Brit J Exp Path* **54**: 684-691, 1973.

208. Chryssanthou C, Fotino S, Gottlieb S, et al: Smooth muscle-acting factor (SMAF) and its increase in compressed-decompressed (CD) animals. *Fed Proc* **25**:287, 1966.

209. Chryssanthou C, Teichner F, Goldstein G, et al: Studies on dysbarism III: a smooth muscle-acting factor (SMAF) in mouse lungs and its increase in decompression sickness. *Aerospace Med* **41**:43-48, 1970.

210. Chryssanthou C, Teichner F, Goldstein G, et al: Newer concepts on the mechanism and prevention of decompression sickness. *Abstract XXth*

International Congress of Aviation and Space Medicine. Nice, France, p 66, 1972.

211. Philp RB, Inwood MJ, Warren BA: Interactions between gas bubbles and components of the blood. Implications in decompression sickness. *Aerospace Med* **43**:946-953, 1972.

212. Philp RB, Schacham P, Gowdey CW: Involvement of platelets and microthrombi in experimental decompression sickness: similarities with disseminated intravascular coagulation. *Aerospace Med* **42**:494-502, 1971.

213. Hills BA: Clinical implications of gas-induced osmosis. *Arch Intern Med* **129**:356-362, 1972.

214. Guest MM, Wells CH, Bond TP: Changes in rheology of animals following various pressure exposures. In: Beckman EL, Elliott DH, eds. *Proc Symp Dysbaric Ostenecrosis* Washington, NIOSH, 1974.

215. End E: The use of new equipment and helium gas in a world record dive. *J Indus Hyg* **20**:511-520, 1938.

216. End E: Blood agglutination in decompression sickness. In: Lambertsen CJ. ed. *Proc 4th Symp Underwater Physiology.* New York, Academic Press, 1971.

217. Chryssanthou CM, Springer M, Lipschitz S: Blood-brain and blood-lung barrier alteration by dysbaric exposure. *Undersea Biomed Res* **4**:117-129, 1977.

218. Chryssanthou C, Graber B, Mendelson S, et al: Increased blood-brain barrier permeability to tetracycline in rabbits under dysbaric conditions. *Undersea Biomed Res* **6**:319-328, 1979.

219. Cockett ATK, Nakamura RM: Newer concepts in the pathophysiology of experimental dysbarism-decompression sickness. *Amer Surgeon* **30**:447-451, 1964.

220. Jacobs MH: Some aspects of all permeability to weak electrolytes. *Cold Spring Harbor Symp Quant Biol* **8**:30-39, 1940.

221. Hills BA: Osmosis induced by nitrogen. *Aerospace Med* **42**:664-666, 1971.

222. Malette WG, Fitzgerald JB, Cockett ATK: Dysbarism: a review with suggestions for therapy. *Aerospace Med* **33**:1132-1139, 1962.

223. Hilton JG, Wells CH: Effect of nicotinic acid on plasma volume loss of experimental dysbarism. In: *Undersea Biomedical Research.* Washington D.C., Undersea Medical Society 1976, pp 157-161.

224. Welham W, Blanch JJ, Behnke AR: A procedure for selection of diving and aviation personnel resistant to decompression sickness based on tests in a low pressure chamber. Report 282, US NRC, Comm Aviat Med. Washington, D.C., 1944.

225. Gersh I, Hawkinson GE, Rathbun EM: Tissue and vascular bubbles after decompression from high pressure atmospheres, correlation of specific gravity with morphological changes. *J Cell Comp Physiol* **24**:35-70, 1944.

226. Donald KW: Oxygen bends. *J Appl Physiol* **7**:639-644, 1955.

227. Spencer MP, Lawrence GA, Thomas GI, et al: The use of ultrasonics in the determination of arterial air embolism during open heart surgery. *Ann Thorac Surg* **8**:489-497, 1969.

228. Rivera JC: Decompression sickness among divers: an analysis of 935 cases. *Milit Med* **129**:314-334, 1964.

229. Golding FC, Griffiths P, Paton WDM, et al: Decompression sickness during the construction of the Hartford Tunnel. *Brit J Ind Med* **17**:167-180, 1960.

230. Harrison JAB: A septic bone necrosis in Naval clearance divers: radio-

graphic findings. *Proc Roy Soc Med* **64**:1276-1278, 1971.

231. Kahlstrom SC, Burton CC, Phenister DB: Aseptic necrosis of bone: infarction of bones of undetermined etiology resulting in encapsulated and calcified areas in diaphyses and in arthritis deformans. *Surg Gynecol Obstet* **68**:631-641, 1939.

232. Berry CA: Severe dysbarism in Air Force operations and training. *US Armed Forces Med J* **9**:937-948, 1958.

233. Duffner GJ, van der Aue OE, Behnke AR: The treatment of decompression sickness: an analysis of 113 cases. Research Project X-443, Report No. 3, Naval Medical Research and Experimental Diving Unit, 1946.

234. Thorne IJ: Caissons disease: a study based on the three hundred cases observed at the Queens-Midtown Tunnel, Project 1938. *JAMA* **8**:585-589, 1941.

235. Polland CL, Adams DE, Erde A: A survey of immediate and ensuing results of hyperbaric therapy for diving accidents. In: Trapp WG, Banister EW, Davison AJ, et al. eds. *Fifth International Hyperbaric Congress Proceedings, Vol. I & II, 1973*. Burnaby 2, B.C., Canada, Simon Fraser University, 1974, pp 383-388.

236. Williams LF, Jr: Dysbarism as a source of unconsciousness. *Surg Clin N Am* **48**:453-459, 1968.

237. Haymaker W, Johnston AD: Pathology of decompression sickness. *Mil Med* **117**:285-306, 1955.

238. Hallenbeck JM, Bove AA, Elliott DH: Mechanisms underlying spinal cord damage in decompression sickness. *Neurology* **25**:308-316, 1975.

239. Frankel HL: Paraplegia due to decompression sickness. *Paraplegia* **14**: 306-311, 1977.

240. Ingvar DH, Adolfson J, Lindemark C: Cerebral air embolism during training of submarine personnel in free escape: an encephalographic study. *Aerospace Med* **44**:628-635, 1973.

241. Elliott DH, Hallenbeck JM, Bove AA: Acute decompression sickness. *Lancet* Occasional Survey, p 1193, 1974.

242. Fryer DI: *Subatmospheric Decompression Sickness in Man*. U.K., Technivision Services, Slough, 1969.

243. Griffiths PD: Clinical manifestations and treatment of decompression sickness in compressed-air workers. In: Bennett PB, Elliott DH, eds. *The Physiology and Medicine of Diving and Compressed-air Work*. London, Bailliere, Tindall & Cassell, 1969, pp 451-463.

244. Kidd DJ, Elliott DH: Clinical manifestations and treatment of decompression sickness in divers. In: Bennett PB, Elliott DH. *The Physiology and Medicine of Diving and Compressed-air Work*. London, Bailliere, Tindall & Cassell, 1969, pp 464-490.

245. Dewey AW: Decompression sickness, an emerging recreational hazard. *N Engl J Med* **267**:759-765, 812-820, 1962.

246. Liske E, Crowley WJ, Lewis JA: Altitude decompression sickness with focal neurological manifestations. *Aerospace Med* **38**:304-306, 1967.

247. Flynn DE, Womack GJ: Neurological manifestations of dysbarism: a review and report of a case with multiple episodes. *Aerospace Med* **34**: 956-962, 1963.

248. Kidd DJ, Elliott DH: Clinical manifestations and treatment of decompression sickness in divers. In: Bennett PB, Elliott DH, eds. *The Physiology and Medicine of Diving and Compressed Air Work*. Baltimore, The Williams & Wilkins Company, 1969, pp 464-490.

249. Engel GL, Hamburger WW, Reiser M, et al: Electroencephalographic

and psychological studies of a case of migraine with severe headache. *Psychosomatic Med* 15:337-348, 1953.

250. Anderson, Jr. B, Whalen RE, Saltzman HA: Dysbarism among hyperbaric personnel. *JAMA* 190:87-89, 1964.

251. Farmer JC, Thomas WG, Youngblood DG, et al: Inner ear decompression sickness. *Laryngoscope* 86:1315-1327, 1976.

252. Kennedy RS: General history of vestibular disorders in diving. *Undersea Biomed Res* 1:73-81, 1974.

253. Buhlmann AA, Gehring H: Inner ear disorders resulting from inadequate decompression — "vertigo bends." In: Lambertsen CJ, ed. *Underwater Physiology V*. Bethesda, MD, FASEB, 1976, pp 341-347.

254. Buhlmann A, Waldvogel W: The treatment of decompression sickness. *Helvet Med Acta* 33:487-491, 1967.

255. Caruso MD, Winkelmann PE, Correia MJ, et al: Otologic and otoneurologic injuries in divers: clinical studies on nine commercial and two sport divers. *Laryngoscope* 87:508-521, 1977.

256. Rubenstein CJ, Summitt JK: Vestibular derangement in decompression. In: Lambertsen CJ, ed. *Underwater Physiology*. New York, Academic, 1971, pp 287-292.

257. Keays FL: Compressed air illness, with a report of 3,692 cases, researches from the Department of Medicine, Cornell University Medical College, Ithaca, New York, 1909.

258. Slark AG: Treatment of 137 cases of decompression sickness. *RNPRC Report* 63/1030, MRC, London, 1962.

259. Edmonds C, Freeman P, Thomas R, et al: *Otological Aspects of Diving*. Sidney, Australian Medical Publishing Co., 1973, pp 55-96.

260. Chiappe E: Lesioni dell'orecchio interno da decompressione. *Oto Rino Laringol Ital* 9:149-178, 1939.

261. Landolt JP, Money KE, Topliff EDL, et al: Pathophysiology of inner ear dysfunction in the squirrel monkey in rapid decompression. *J Appl Physiol: Respirat Environ Exercise Physiol* 49:1070-1082, 1980.

262. McCormick JG, Holland WB, Braver RW, et al: Sudden hearing loss due to diving and its prevention with heparin. *Otolaryngol Clin N Am* 8: 417-430, 1975.

263. Stucker FJ and Echols WB: Otolaryngic problems of underwater exploration. *Mil Med* 136:896-899, 1971.

264. Lambertsen C: Collaborative investigation of limits of human tolerance to pressurization with helium, neon and nitrogen. Simulation of density equivalent to helium-oxygen respiration at depths of 2,000, 3,000, 4,000 and 5,000 feet of sea water. In: Lambertsen C, ed. *Proceedings of the Fifth Symposium on Underwater Physiology*. Fed Amer Soc Exp Biol. Washington, 1975, pp 35-48.

265. Sundmaker W: Vestibular function. Lambertsen C, ed. Special Summary Program, Predictive Studies III, University of Pennsylvania, 1973.

266. Farmer JC: Diving injuries to the inner ear . *Ann Otol Rhinol Laryngol* Suppl 36. 86:1-20, 1977.

267. Levy E: Compressed-air illness and its engineering importance, with a report of cases at the East River Tunnels. *Tech Pap Bur Mines*, 285, Washington, p 47, 1922.

268. Behnke AR: A review of physiological and clinical data pertaining to decompression sickness. *US Naval Med Res Inst Rept No 4*, 1947.

269. Gersh I, Hawkinson GE, Jenney EH: Comparison of vascular and extravascular bubbles following decompression from high-pressure atmospheres

of oxygen, helium-oxygen, argon-oxygen and air. *J Cell Comp Physiol* **26**:63-74, 1945.

270. *US Navy Diving Manual,* NAVSHIPS, 0994-001-9010, 1979 edition, US Government Printing Office.

271. Workman RD: Standard decompression procedures and their modification in preventing the bends. *Ann NY Acad Sci* **117**:834-842, 1965.

272. Kindwall EP: Decompression sickness. In: Davis JC, Hunt TK, eds. *Hyperbaric Oxygen Therapy.* Bethesda, Maryland, Undersea Medical Society, 1977, pp 125-140.

273. Hyperbaric homicide in Hanover? *Med World News,* March 22, 1976, p 37.

274. Richter K, Loblich HJ: Letale dekompressionskrankheit nach therapeutisher überdrückbehandlung. *Z Rechtsmedizin* **81**:45-61, 1978.

275. Des Granges M: Repetitive diving decompression tables. *US Navy Experimental Diving Unit Res Rept* 1957, pp 6-57.

276. van der Aue OE, Keller RJ, Brinton ES, et al: Calculation and testing of decompression and the use of oxygen. US Navy Experimental Diving Unit. *Rept No 1,* 1951.

277. Workman RD: Oxygen decompression following air dives for use in hyperbaric oxygen therapy. US Navy Experimental Diving Unit. *Res Rept. No 2-64,* 1964.

278. Behnke AR, Shaw LA, Messer RM, et al: The circulatory and respiratory disturbances of acute compressed-air illness and the administration of oxygen as a therapeutic measure. *Am J Physiol* **114**:526-533, 1936.

279. Behnke AR, Shaw LA: The use of oxygen in the treatment of compressed-air illness. *US Naval Med Bull* **35**:61-73, 1937.

280. Goodman MW, Workman RD: Minimal recompression, oxygen breathing approach to the treatment of decompression sickness in divers and aviators. *Research Report, 5-65.* US Navy Experimental Diving Unit, Washington, 1965.

281. Yarbrough OD, Behnke AR: The treatment of compressed-air illness utilizing oxygen. *J Ind Hyg Toxicol* **21**:213-218, 1939.

282. Behnke AR: Problems in the treatment of decompression sickness (and traumatic air embolism). *Ann NY Acad Sci* **117**:843-859, 1965.

283. Cockett ATR, Saunders JC, Pouley SM: Treatment of experimental decompression sickness by heparin alone. Aerospace Medical Association, annual meeting, San Francisco, California, 1968.

284. Philp RB: The ameliorative effects of heparin and depolymerized hyaluronate on decompression sickness in rats. *Can J Physiol Pharmacol* **42**:819-829, 1964.

285. Barnard EEP, Hanson JM, Rawton-Lee AG, et al: Post decompression shock due to extravasation of plasma. *Brit Med J* **2**:154-155, 1966.

286. Cockett ATK, Nakamura RM: Treatment of decompression sickness employing low molecular weight dextran. *Rev Physiol Subaquat* **1**: 133, 1968.

287. Halbouty MR, Long DR: Neurocirculatory collapse in aircraft flight. Report of a case. *J Aviat Med* **24**:301-307, 1953.

288. Bond GF: Arterial gas embolism. In: Davis JC, Hunt TK, eds. *Hyperbaric Oxygen Therapy.* Bethesda, Undersea Medical Society, 1977, pp 141-152.

289. Meldrum BS, Papy JJ, Vigouroux RA: Intracarotid air embolism in the baboon: effects on cerebral blood flow and the electroencephalogram. *Brain Res* **25**:301-315, 1971.

290. Fries CD: Experimental cerebral gas embolism. *Ann Surg* **145**:461-470, 1957.

291. Brierly JB: Neuropathological findings in patients dying after open heart surgery. *Thorax* 18:291-304, 1963.

292. Brierley JB, Brown AW, Meldrum BS, Riche D: The time course of ischaemic neuronal changes in the primate brain following profound arterial hypotension, air embolism, and hypoglycaemia. *J Physiol* 207: 59P-60P, 1970.

293. Lindemark C: Slutrapport over intraffade medicinska komplikationer i ovningstanken vid Karlskrona Orlogsskolor 1972.02.29-03.08 (9 bil.). Kompletterar CMUC skr 1972.03.10, bil. till CKOS skr nr 724, 1972.

294. Ingvar DH, Adolfson J, Lindemark C: Cerebral air embolism during training of submarine personnel in free Europe: an electroencephalographic study. *Aerospace Med* 44:628-635, 1973.

295. Gillen HW: Symptomatology of cerebral gas embolism. *Neurology* 18: 507-512, 1968.

296. Menkin M, Schwartzman RJ: Cerebral air embolism: report of five cases and review of the literature. *Arch Neurol* 34:168-170, 1977.

297. Naquet R: Epileptic activity evoked by air embolism in cat, monkey, and man. In: Servit, ed. *Proc Int Symp Comp Cell Pathophysiol.* Amsterdam, Excerpta Medica, 1966: 27:89-102.

298. Junod T: Recherches sur les effets physiologiques et therapeutiques de la compression et de rarefaction de l'air, taut sur le corps que les membres isoles. *Ann Gen Med* 9:157, 1835.

299. Behnke AR, Thomson RM, Motley EP: The psychological effects from breathing air at 4 atmospheres pressure. *Am J Physiol* 112:554-558, 1935.

300. Bennett PB, Simon S, Katz Y: High pressures of inert gases and anesthetic mechanisms. In: Fink R, ed. *Molecular Mechanisms of Anesthesia.* Baltimore, Williams and Wilkins, 1974, pp 367-402.

301. Bennett PB, Ackles KN: The narcotic effects of hyperbaric oxygen. In: Wada J, Iwa T, eds. *Proceedings of the Fourth International Congress on Hyperbaric Medicine.* Baltimore, The Williams and Wilkins Co., 1970, pp 74-79.

302. Behnke AR, Yarbrough OD: Respiratory resistance, oil-water solubility and mental effects of argon compared with helium and nitrogen. *Am J Physiol* 126:409-415, 1939.

303. Brink F, Posternak JM: Thermodynamic analysis of relative effectiveness of narcotics. *J Cell Comp Physiol* 32:211-233, 1948.

304. Wulf RJ, Featherstone RM: A correlation of Van der Waals constants with anesthetic potency. *Anesthesiology* 18:97-105, 1957.

305. Rinfret AP, Doebbler GF: Physiological and biochemical effects and applications. In: Cook GA, ed. *Argon, Helium and the Rare Gases.* New York, John Wiley, 1961, pp 727-764.

306. Miller SL: A theory of gaseous anesthetics. *Proc Natl Acad Sci (USA)* 47:1515-1524, 1967.

307. Bennett PB: The physiology of nitrogen narcosis and the high pressure nervous syndrome. In: Straus RH, ed. *Diving Medicine.* New York, Grune and Stratton, 1976, pp 157-180.

308. Meyer HH: Theoris der alkojolnarkose. *Arch Exp Pathol Pharmacol* 42:109-118, 1899.

309. Carpenter FG: Depressant action of inert gases on the central nervous system in mice. *Am J Physiol* 172:471-474, 1953.

310. Bennett PB: Neurophysiologic and neuropharmacologic investigations in inert gas narcosis. In: Lambertsen CJ, Greenbaum LJ, eds. *Proceedings Second Symposium on Underwater Physiology.* Washington, D.C.,

National Research Council Pub 1181, 1963.

311. Miller KW, Paton WDM, Smith RA, Smith EB: The pressure reversal of general anesthesia and the critical volume hypothesis. *Mol Pharmacol* **9**:131-143, 1973.

312. French JD, Verzeano M, Magoun HW: A neural basis of the anesthetic state. *Arch Neurol Psychiat* **69**:519-529, 1953.

313. Larrabee MG, Posternak JM: Selective action of anesthetics on synapses and axons in mammalian sympathetic ganglia. *J Neurophysiol* **15**:91-114, 1952.

314. Workman RD: Other medical problems associated with exposure to pressure. In: Lambertsen LJ, ed. *Fundamentals of Hyperbaric Medicine.* Washington, D.C., National Academy of Sciences, 1966, pp 110-114.

315. Poulton EC, Catton MJ, Carpenter A: Efficiency at sorting cards in compressed air. *Brit J Industr Med* **21**:242-245, 1964.

316. Bennett PB, Poulton EC, Carpenter A, et al: Efficiency at sorting cards in air and a 20 percent oxygen-helium mixture at depths down to 100 feet and in enriched air. *Ergonomics* **10**:53-62, 1967.

317. Farmer JC, Thomas WG, Preslar MJ: Human auditory responses during hyperbaric helium-oxygen exposures. *Surg Forum* **22**:456-458, 1971.

318. Fluur E, Adolfson J: Hearing in hyperbaric air. *Aerospace Med* **57**:783-785, 1966.

319. Thomas WG, Summitt JK, Farmer JC: Human auditory thresholds during deep saturation helium-oxygen dives. *J Acoust Soc Am* **55**:810-813, 1974.

320. Adolfson J: Human performance and behavior in hyperbaric environments. *Acta Psychologica Gothoburgensia* **6**:1-74, 1967.

321. Adolfson J: Air breathing at 13 atmospheres. Psychological and physiological observations. *Sartryck ur Forsvars Med* **1**:31-37, 1965.

322. Buhlmann AA: Respiratory resistance with hyperbaric gas mixtures. In: Lambertsen CJ, Greenbaum LJ, eds. *Proceedings Second Symposium on Underwater Physiology.* Washington, D.C., National Research Council Pub. 1181. 1963, pp 98-107.

323. Hesser CM: Measurement of inert gas narcosis in man. In: Lambertsen CJ, Greenbaum LJ, eds. *Proceedings Second Symposium on Underwater Physiology.* Washington, D.C., National Research Council Pub. 1181, 1963, pp 202-208.

324. Lanphier EH: Influence of increased ambient pressure upon alveolar ventilation. In: Lambertsen CJ, Greenbaum LJ, eds. *Proceedings Second Symposium on Underwater Physiology.* Washington, D.C., National Research Council Pub. 1181. 1963, pp 124-133.

325. Bennett PB, Ackles KN, Cripps VJ: Effects of hyperbaric nitrogen and oxygen on auditory evoked responses in man. *Aerospace Med* **40**:521-525, 1969.

326. Beasley JW: Inner ear damage due to barotrauma. *Wis Med J* **73**:143-145, 1974.

327. Edmonds C: Inner ear barotrauma. In: Trapp WG, Banister EW, Davison AJ, et al, eds. *Fifth International Hyperbaric Congress Proceedings, Vol. I & II, 1973.* Burnaby 2, B.C., Canada, Simon Fraser University, 1974, pp 874-882.

328. Eichel BS, Landes BS: Sensorineural hearing loss caused by skin diving. *Arch Otolaryng* **92**:128-131, 1970.

329. Freeman P: Inner ear barotrauma. *Arch Otolaryngol* **97**:429, 1973.

330. Freeman P, Edmonds C: Inner ear barotrauma. *Arch Otolaryngol* **95**: 556-563, 1972.
331. MacFie DD: E.N.T. problems of diving. *Med Serv J Canada* **20**:845-861, 1964.
332. Vail HH: Traumatic conditions of the ear in workers in an atmosphere of compressed air. *Arch Otolaryng* **10**:113-126, 1929.
333. Goodhill V: Sudden deafness and round window rupture. *The Laryngoscope* **81**:1462-1474, 1971.
334. Goodhill V, et al: Sudden deafness and labyrinthine window ruptures: audio-vestibular observations. *Ann Otol Rhinol Laryngol* **82**:2-12, 1973.
335. Freeman P, Tonkin J, Edmonds C: Rupture of the round window membrane in inner ear barotrauma. *Arch Otolaryngol* **99**:437-442, 1974.
336. Pullen FW: Round window membrane rupture: a cause of sudden deafness. *Trans Amer Acad Ophthalmol Otolaryngol* **76**:1444-1450, 1972.
337. Simmons FB, Mongeon CJ: Endolymphatic duct pressure produces cochlear damage. *Arch Otolaryngol* **85**:43-150, 1967.
338. Althaus SR: Perilymph fistulas. *The Laryngoscope* **91**:538-562, 1981.
339. Allen GW: Endolymphatic sac and cochlear aqueduct. *Arch Otolaryngol* **79**:322-327, 1964.
340. Arnvig J: Relation of the ear to the subarachnoid space and absorption of labyrinthine fluid. *Acta Otolaryngol* (Suppl.) **96**:1-73, 1951.
341. Harker L, Norante J, Rzu J: Experimental rupture of the round window membrane. *Trans Am Acad Ophthalmol Otolaryngol* **78**:448-452, 1974.
342. Jako G, et al: An experimental study on the dynamic circulation of the labyrinthine fluids. *Ann Otol Rhinol Laryngol* **68**:733-739, 1959.
343. Jampolsky LN: In: Perlman HB, Lindsay JR. Relation of the internal ear spaces to the meninges. *Arch Otolaryngol* **29**:12-23, 1939.
344. Goodhill V: Inner ear barotrauma. *Arch Otolaryngol* **95**:588, 1972.
345. Murray T: Noise level inside navy diving chambers. *US Navy Submarine Med Center Report* 2/70, 1970.
346. Summitt JK, Reimers SD: Noise; a hazard to divers and hyperbaric chamber personnel. *Aerospace Med* **42**:1173-1177, 1971.

Index

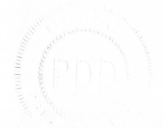